GLIOMA – EXPLORING ITS BIOLOGY AND PRACTICAL RELEVANCE

Edited by **Anirban Ghosh**

Glioma – Exploring Its Biology and Practical Relevance
Edited by Anirban Ghosh

Published by InTech
Janeza Trdine 9, 51000 Rijeka, Croatia

Publishing Process Manager Petra Nenadic

Technical Editor Teodora Smiljanic

Cover Designer InTech Design Team

Additional hard copies can be obtained from orders@intechopen.com

Glioma – Exploring Its Biology and Practical Relevance, Edited by Anirban Ghosh
p. cm.
ISBN 978-953-307-379-8

For EU product safety concerns:
IN TECH d.o.o., Prolaz Marije Krucifikse Kozulić 3, 51000 Rijeka, Croatia,
info@intechopen.com or visit our website at intechopen.com.

Meet the editor

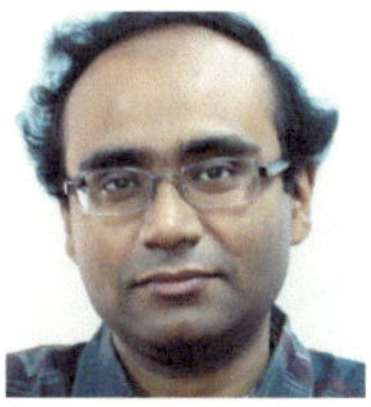

Dr. Anirban Ghosh completed his M.Sc in Zoology from University of Calcutta in 2000 and started his research in the Institute of Post Graduate Medical Education and Research (IPGMER) on brain tumor and glioma immunology. He achieved Junior Research Fellowship from Council of Scientific and Industrial Research (CSIR), Government of India after qualifying the National Eligibility Test (NET) and completed his Ph.D as Senior Research Fellow in 2007 under the guidance of Prof. Swapna Chaudhuri now at School of Tropical Medicine, Kolkata, India. From 2006 onwards, he is engaged in teaching in Zoology at Panihati Mahavidyalaya and acts as invited faculty in M.Sc and M.Phil courses on Immunology in Calcutta University and West Bengal State University. He is presently involved in research on developmental immunology in brain and acts as reviewer of different journal articles.

Contents

Preface

'Glioma' is the term that hits the human psyche with absolute despair. All our efforts to cease glioma limits it to an average of maximum 18 – 21 months of life after diagnosis and notably, this life expectancy altered marginally despite constant research of last two decades. When I was working for my Ph.D thesis and allied projects, I had to encounter a number of glioma patients and patient parties. Many of them I found first diagnosed, started treatment with surgery, radiation and chemotherapy in various combinations and after few months they disappeared. Some of them reappeared within a year with recurrence and others never turned. Rarely, a trivial number of patients were traced after 3 or 5 years. Many of those gloomy faces, their eager questions, earnest appeals, anxiety are pertinent globally and the fate varies negligibly with economic or developmental status of the society. Such an issue always provoked me to know and contribute something which is larger than my focused thesis work. As a considerable section of my work was at the interface of medical practitioners and basic scientists, I was lucky enough to observe the pattern of proceedings and attitude of both the fields at least partially. Strangely, I also sensed a fissure between these two interdependent fields. Along with, the common question of common mass that "What is medical science exactly doing against it?" is always pertinent as the problem is still unmanageable.

To face these questions and find their suitable answers, at least on the basis of current knowledge, a multitude of information from different facets of glioma research is needed to be analyzed. The fundamental biological nature of the problem, extent of its graveness as a disease, diagnostic efforts and shortcomings, level of efficiency and inefficiency of present medical interventions and therapeutics, current trends of medical research to combat glioma etc has to be scrutinized with extreme sincerity. This mammoth gathering of facts is possible if only the experts of different areas can share their expertise at the same platform. I also feel that, sometimes the gaps among medical scientists and doctors are due to the inability to build up an overview of this vast expanse as well as shortfall of awareness about this rapidly developing arena by either side. Therefore, a podium to cater the diverse problems and achievements in glioma is a much needed obligation.

In this situation, I got the offer to be involved in the effort of the book project "Glioma" by the present publisher. That was a simple but superb coincidence of my thoughts and their offer. As the subject editor of the project I had to evaluate near about 90 chapter proposals submitted from nearly every corners of the world. These worldwide contributions were then categorized and distributed into three volumes. The approach was initially to understand glioma and its biology with experimental approaches to explore the basics of the disease (vol. 1); next to share the knowledge about present diagnostic and prognostic approaches as well as current developments in modern therapeutics (vol. 2); and finally, to accustom the readers about the cutting edge basic to experimental developments and trends of biomedical research to restrict glioma (vol. 3). As the book editor I have chosen to edit the first volume, partially because of my personal background as a biomedical researcher from basic life-sciences and mostly the chapters arranged in this volume are aimed to find out the basic nature of the disease. Next two volumes are much oriented with facts that are directly relevant to medical practice to deal glioma.

The name of the first volume "Glioma – Exploring Its Biology and Practical Relevance" is indicative of its content. This introducing first volume contains 21 chapters basically intended to explore glioma biology and discussing the experimental model systems for the purpose. Under the section "Introduction" first two chapters discuss general glioma epidemiology and etiology and the next two shows the relevance of biomarkers in glioma. Following six chapters under section "Gliomagenesis" deals with different genetic, molecular and cell biological aspects of origin and development of glioma. The next section "Glioma progression" contains three chapters which discusses about glioma invasiveness which is followed by the section "Glioma Immunology" that contains two chapters. A stretch of four chapters have been clustered next in the section "Glioma Model and Culture Systems" which are devoted to present different facets of experimental models and cell culture methods that are now utilized in glioma research. In the final section "Miscellaneous" the penultimate chapter deals with oxidative stress in glioma and the final chapter of this volume talks about a special experimental approach of glioma therapeutics. It is hoped that the present volume will provide supportive and relevant awareness and understanding on the fundamental advances of the subject to the professionals from any sphere interested about glioma and deliver the momentum to the audience for the following volumes of 'Glioma'.

In this enormous task I got support from many of which only few names can be mentioned here. First and foremost, I extend my thanks to the 'InTech Open Access Publisher' for offering me the exciting opportunity to act as the subject editor of the 'Glioma' project, book editor of the present volume as well as chapter author. I enjoyed my involvement in a forum where participants are the biomedical researchers sharing their experiences and knowledge from every continents except Antarctica. To shape this gigantic effort Ms. Ana Panter and Ms. Petra Ninadic extended their continuous cooperation by building the liaison between editors, authors and the publisher. I express my heartiest thanks to them in spite of failing many 'deadline's set by them, and still getting their nonstop support to make this teamwork a success. I also express my gratitude to Prof. Swapna Chaudhuri, School of Tropical Medicine,

Kolkata, India; Prof. Ingo Bechmann, Institut für Anatomie der Universität Leipzig, Germany; Prof. Helmut Kettenmann, Max-Delbrück-Center for Molecular Medicine, Germany; Prof. Serge Rivest, Laval University, Québec, Canada and many others who helped or inspired me anyways in my recent research and activities. I am appreciative to my graduate students Nabanita Mukherjee and Payel Ghosh with other colleagues and students of my institute who cooperate me in this journey. The continuous support of the Principle of my institute Dr. Sanjoy K Ghosh and the authority made this process easier for me. Finally and most importantly, without the unparallel motivation and bearing of my wife Malabika and little son Upamanyu this effort would have never been achieved. I am dedicating this endeavor to them and all who are fighting to control glioma.

Dr. Anirban Ghosh

Assistant Professor and Head Department of Zoology
Panihati Mahavidyalaya (West Bengal State University), Kolkata,
India

Part 1

Introduction

1

Epidemiology of Glioma

Jimmy T. Efird
Center for Health Disparities Research
Department of Public Health
Brody School of Medicine Greenville, North Carolina
USA

1. Introduction

Giomas constitute a broad class of neuroectodermal tumours believed to originate from sustentacular neuroglial cells (Kleihues and Cavenee 2000). Astrocytomas form the largest group of gliomas (>75%) and glioblastoma multiforme (GBM) is the most common type of astrocytoma (CBTRUS 2011). Gliomas that share histologic characteristics with ependymal or oligodendrocyte cells are named ependymomas and oligodendrogliomas, but may not necessarily originate from the aforementioned cell types (Kleihues and Cavenee 2000). Mixed gliomas include those which consist of more than one glia cell type. For example, oligodendroglial glioblastoma multiforme (as defined by some neuropathologists) are GBM tumours with an oligodendroglioma component and generally have a significantly worse clinical outcome than GBM tumours overall (Louis et al 2007). Another mixed glioma is oligoastrocytoma, which contains both oligodendrocyte and astrocyte cells.

The Third Edition of the International Classification of Diseases for oncology (ICD-O-3) is widely used to categorize gliomas by histology (e.g., malignant glioma=9380, ependymoma NOS=9391, astrocytoma=9430, glioblastoma NOS=9440, oligodendroglioma NOS=9450) (Fritz et al 2000). Furthermore, tumours are grouped by site in the ICD-O-3 system using C-codes (e.g., cerebrum=C71.0, frontal lobal=C71.1, temporal lobe=C71.2, parietal lobe=C71.3, occipital lobe=C71.4, ventricle=C71.5, cerebellum=C71.6, spinal cord=C72.0). The World Health Organization (WHO) also has developed a classification index which grades gliomas by disease prognosis (I=best to IV=worst) (Kliehues et al 1993). Recent additions to the "WHO Classification of Tumours" include Grade I - angiocentric gliomas (predominantly occurring in children and young adults in the fronto-parietal cortex, temporal lobe, and hippocampal region), and Grade II – pilomyxoid astrocytoma (typically occurring in infants and children in the hypothalamic/chiasmatic region) (Louis et al 2007). Additionally, WHO has recognized a divergent pattern of gliomas named small cell glioblastoma characterized by EGFR amplification, p16INK4a homozygous deletion, PTEN mutations, and LOH 10q (Louis et al 2007).

2. Incidence and death rates

Gliomas comprise more than 80% of brain tumours (CBTRUS 2011), therefore, descriptive epidemiology about gliomas often is framed in the broader context of brain tumours as a whole.

2.1 Incidence

Overall, brain tumors are relatively rare events. Only 1 in 165 men and women will be diagnosed with cancer of the brain and other nervous system tumours in their lifetime (Altekruse et al 2010). The incidence rate (IR) per 100,000 person-years (100KP-Y) for malignant adult brain tumours ranges from 5.4 (95%CI =4.7-6.1) for the state of Hawaii to 12 (95%CI=12-13) for Wisconsin. IRs by state among children 0-19 years are less variable, ranging from 2 to 4. While geographic differences in IRs might suggest an environmental etiology for brain tumours, ecologic comparisons often do not account for variations in quality of reporting, diagnostic practices, and access/utilization to health care. States falling into the highest quantile for both age-adjusted incidence and death rates (DR) per 100KP-Y include Kentucky (IR=7.9, 95%CI=7.0-8.7; DR=4.9, 95%CI=4.3-5.6), Iowa (IR=7.6, 95%CI=6.7-8.6; DR=5.4, 95%CI=4.6-6.2), and Oregon (IR=7.5, 95%CI=6.7-8.4; DR=5.2, 95%CI=4.5-5.9) (Figures 1 and 2) (NCI State Cancer Profiles 2011). A noticeable cluster of states (depicted in red) with the highest death rates is located along the northern portion of the U.S. from Oregon to Iowa (Figure 2).

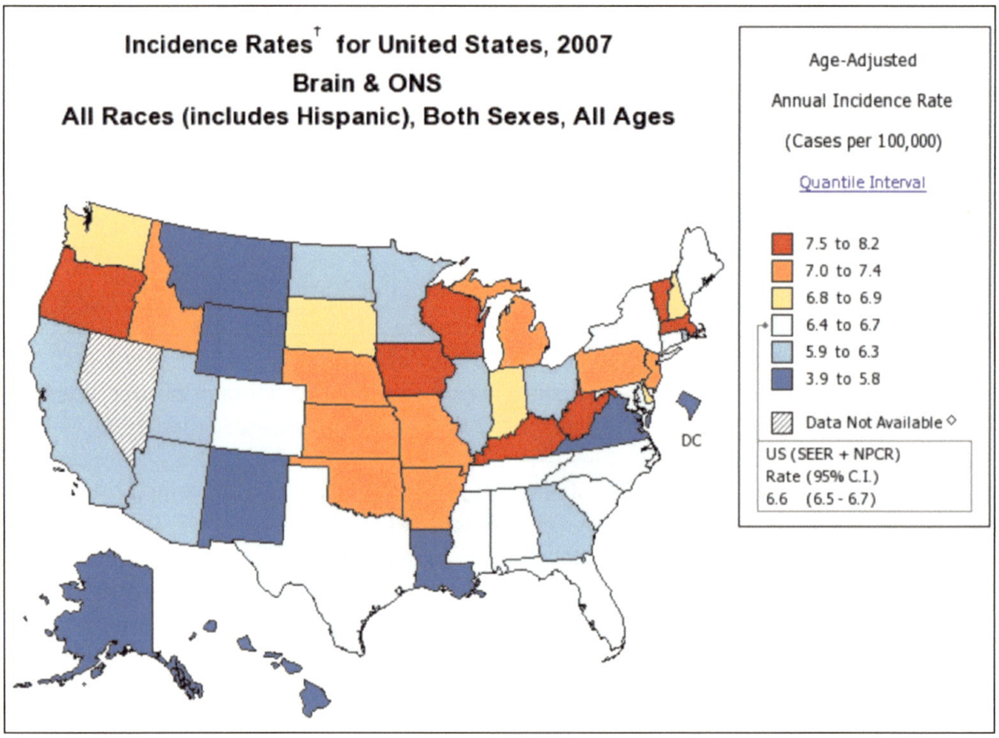

†Age-adjusted (2000 U.S. standard population) cases per 100,000 population per year. ◊Data not available for Nevada.

Fig. 1. Incidence rates (NCI State Cancer Profiles 2011).

Gliomas IRs vary by histology, race, and sex. **Histology**. For example, the age-adjusted rate per 100KP-Y for glioblastoma is 3.19 (95% CI=3.16-3.23) compared with less than 0.2 for anaplastic oligodendroglioma (IR=0.12, 95%CI=0.11-0.13) and protoplasmic/fibrillary astrocytoma (IR=0.11, 95%CI=0.10-0.11) (CBTRUS 2011). **Race**. Whites consistently have higher IR rates than blacks by histologic group (e.g., IR=3.55, 95%CI=3.52-3.59 vs. 1.64, 95%CI=1.57-1.72 for glioblastoma; IR=0.47, 95%CI=0.45-0.48 vs. 0.19, 95%CI=0.17-0.22 for anaplastic astrocytoma; IR=0.29, 95%CI=0.27-0.30 vs. 0.17, 95%CI=0.15-0.19 for ependymoma/anaplastic ependymoma) (CBTRUS 2011). **Sex**. Similarly, men consistently have higher age-adjusted IRs than women by histology (e.g., IR=3.99, 95%CI=3.94-4.04 vs. IR=2.53, 95%CI=2.49-2.57 for glioblastoma; IR=0.48, 95%CI=0.46-0.50 vs. 0.35, 95%CI=0.33-0.36 for anaplastic astrocytoma; and IR=0.27, 95%CI=0.26-0.29 vs. IR=0.25, 95%CI=0.24-0.27 for ependymoma/anaplastic ependymoma), although the latter difference is not statistically significant (CBTRUS 2011). Interestingly, the female prevalence rate (PR) for primary brain tumours per 100KP-Y (PR=264.8) is higher than males (PR=158.7), perhaps attributable to survival bias among women (Porter et al 2010).

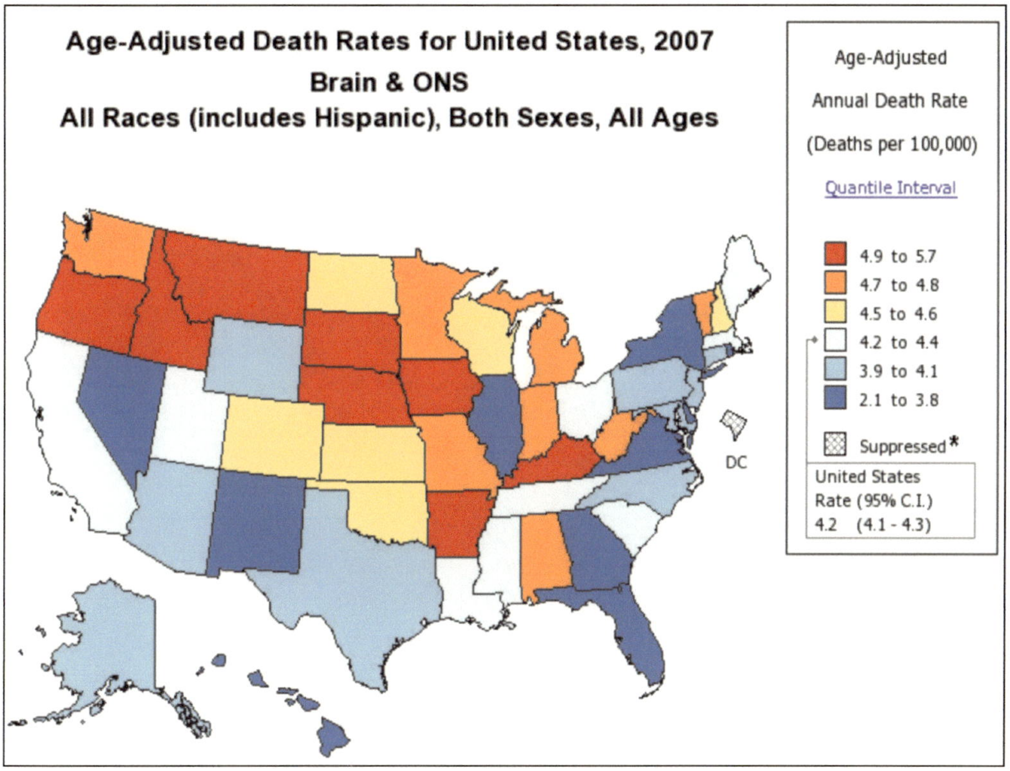

*Counts suppressed since fewer than 16 cases reported in specific area-sex-race category.

Fig. 2. Death rates (NCI State Cancer Profiles 2011).

A higher male (IR=37) to female (IR=2.6) pattern also is observed internationally (Parkin et al 2005), although U.S. rates are higher in both men (IR=7.7, 95%CI=7.5-7.8) and women (IR=5.6., 95%CI=5.5-5.7) compared with international rates (NCI State Cancer Profiles 2011). Less developed countries tend to report lower rates (e.g., Africa, Pacific Islands; IR=3.0 per 100KP-Y for males and 2.1 for females) than more developed countries (e.g., Australia, New Zealand, Europe, North America; IR=5.8 per 100KP-Y for men and 4.1 for females), possibly reflecting less access to modern medical facilities (Parkin et al 2005, CBTRUS 2011). In contrast, the standardized (age, sex, site, year at diagnosis) IR for brain tumours in Japan, a country well known for accessible MR-imaging, is relatively low (2.5 per 100KP-Y person-years) (Matsuda et al 2011). Similarly low rates have been observed in Korea (Lee et al 2010).

2.2 Death rates and survival

The annual number of brain tumour deaths at last count (2007) in the U.S. was n=7,315 for men and 5,919 for women. Age-adjusted rates steadily increased from 1975 to 1991, likely due to advances in neuroimaging, but have decreased linearly thereafter, with recent values on par with 1975 rates (Figure 3) (NCI State Cancer Profiles 2011). Overall DRs are higher among men (DR=5.1, 95%CI=5.0-5.2) than women (DR=3.5, 95%CI=3.4-3.6), however the difference is not statistically significant as was seen for IRs. The lowest DR for men and women combined was observed for the State of Hawaii (DR=2.1, 95%CI=1.4-3.0), which implemented almost complete universal health care coverage in 1994 under the Med-QUEST programme (Hawaii Department of Human Services 2011). However, Hawaii also has the largest non Caucasian population of any state (i.e., 72.8% Asian/Pacific Islander), a factor associated with lower brain tumour incidence and death rates (NCI State Cancer Profiles 2011).

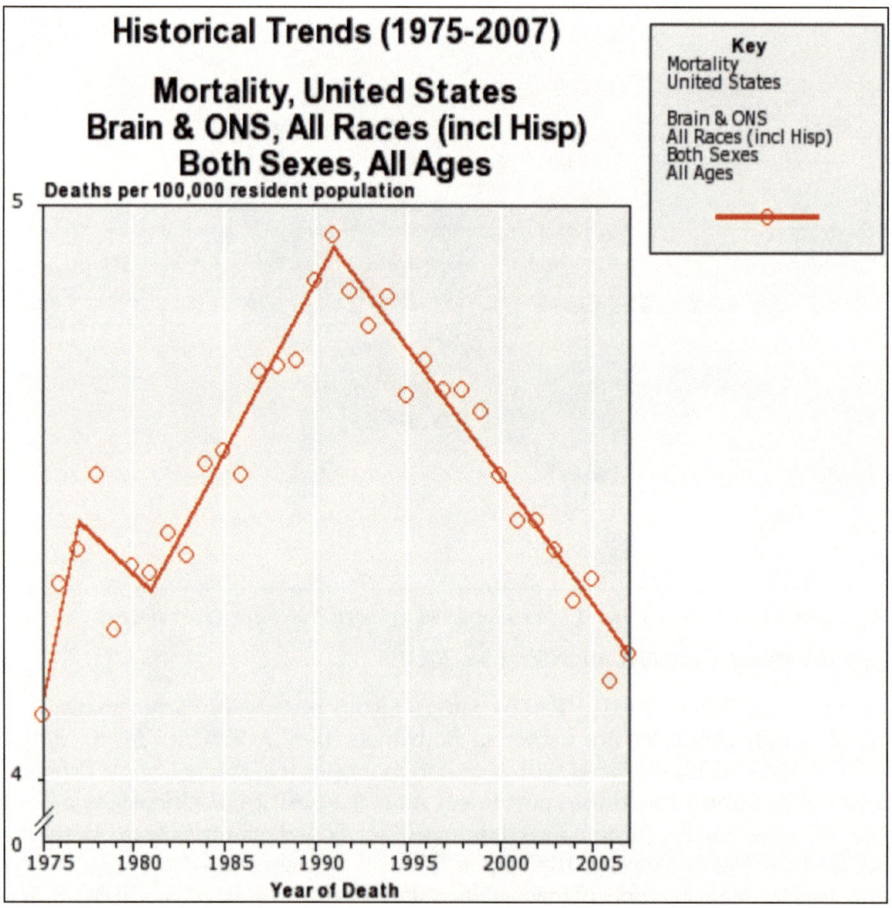

Fig. 3. Mortality trends (NCI State Cancer Profiles 2011).

Survival rates for the majority of malignant gliomas remain disappointingly low, despite decades of advances in surgical, radiation, and chemical therapies, in contrast to improvements in many other cancers. GBMs, for example, typically present as highly aggressive, difficult to treat tumours without clinical, radiologic, or morphologic forewarning of a less virulent precursor tumour (Kanu et al 2009; Ostrom and Barnholtz-Sloan 2011). Secondary GBMs account for only about 10% of all GBMs, based on the presence of IDH1/2 mutations (Ohgaki and Kleihues 2011). The infiltrating nature of these tumours makes treatment difficult. Other obstacles to effective treatment and improved survival include multi-drug resistance, radioresistance, an impermeable blood-brain barrier, a lack of preclinical models, and a rudimentary understanding of neurooncogenetics (Kanu et al 2009).

The relative survival percentages (RSP) for gliomas compared with the general U.S. population vary tremendously by histology and age at diagnosis. For example, the majority of patients diagnosed between age 0-14 years with pilocytic astrocytoma (RSP=97.3%), oligodendroglioma (RSP=95.3), protoplasmic & fibrillary astrocytoma (RSP=84.3%), and mixed glioma (RSP=75.6%) will live beyond 5 years, compared with anaplastic astrocytoma (RSP=32.0%) and glioblastoma (RSP=20.9%) (CBTRUS 2011). In contrast, 5-year relative RSPs are considerably lower across histologic types for those diagnosed between age 45-54 (e.g., RSP=82.4% for pilocytic astrocytoma; RSP=76.8% for oligodendroglioma; RSP=51.1% for mixed glioma; RSP=39.5% for protoplasmic & fibrillary astrocytoma; RSP=28.6% for anaplastic astrocytoma; and RSP=5.6% for glioblastoma). Only 0.8% of patients diagnosed between age 55-64 will be alive after 10 years.

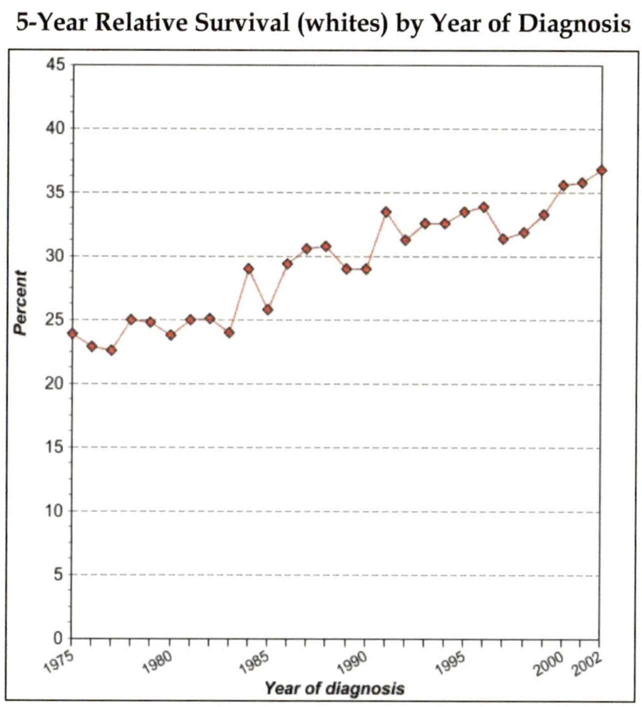

Fig. 4. Survival percent (whites) for cancers of the brain and other nervous system tumours (NCI-SEER 2011).

RSPs also vary by race and sex. Black women (44%) have the highest 5-year RSPs for cancers of the brain and other nervous system tumours, when compared with white women (36.5%), black men (34.8%), and white men (32.6%) (Altekruse et al 2010). When examined by year of diagnosis from 1975 to 2002, whites (Figure 4) consistently have lower 5-year RSPs than blacks independent of sex (Figure 5) (NCI-SEER 2011).

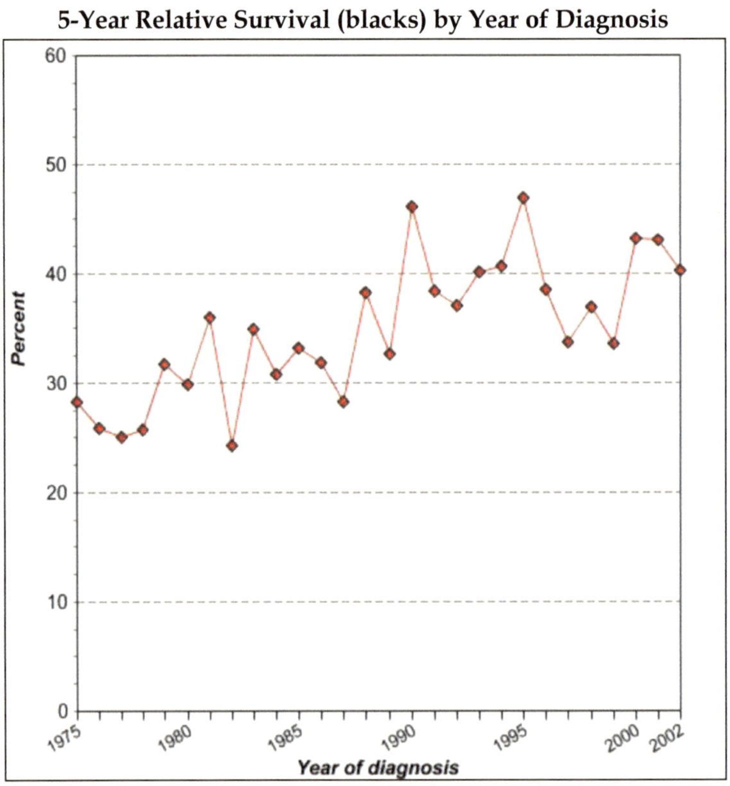

Fig. 5. Survival percent (blacks) for cancers of the brain and other nervous system tumours (NCI-SEER 2011).

Among adults, other factors associated with poorer survival include tumour site (frontal, cerebellum, multilobular), and socioeconomic status (less affluent individuals have lower survival rates) (Tseng et al 2006). The latter suggests that socioeconomic inequalities play an important role in glioma outcome, perhaps due to chronic comorbidities, inadequate access and utilization of health care, and longer wait times after surgery for adjuvant therapies (Tseng et al 2006).

While population-based relative survival statistics paint a dismal prognostic picture for certain glioma types, conditional survival rates suggest a more favorable long term outcome for patients who have already survived for a specified amount of time after diagnosis (Table 1) (Porter et al 2011). For Example, a GBM patient has a 70.4% (95%CI=55.6-81.2) relative probability of living 10 years beyond their diagnosis date if they have already survived 5 years. In comparison, the 10-year unconditional probability for GBM is less than 3% (not shown in Table).

Histologic Category	Survival upon 2 years (95%CI)	Survival upon 5 years (95%CI)
Anaplastic astrocytoma	45.4 (38.2-52.3)	73.6 (62.7-81.8)
Anaplastic oligodendroglioma	53.7 (37.8-67.2)	75.6 (51.2-89.0)
Diffuse astrocytoma	53.6 (42.9-63.2)	73.7 (59.6-83.6)
Glioblastoma multiforme	26.2 (20.6-32.1)	70.4 (55.6-81.2)
Hemangioblastoma/hemangioma	93.9 (80.5-98.2)	97.6 (69.3-99.8)
Oligodendroglioma	68.6 (63.1-73.5)	78.5 (72.5-83.3)
Pilocytic astrocytoma	95.9 (92.6-97.8)	99.2 (91.6-99.9)

Table 1. Relative probability of a patient living 10 years beyond their diagnosis date if they have already survived 2 and 5 years.

3. Risk factors

The key epidemiologic determinants of glioma risk include advancing age, male sex, and Caucasian race (Bondy and Wrensch 1996). Few environmental or lifestyle exposures, except for ionising radiation, have been found to be consistently associated with glioma risk. Suspected risk factors include lifestyle behaviors (e.g., smoking, alcohol consumption, coffee drinking), infectious agents (e.g., polyomaviruses, cytomegaloviruses, influenza, varicella zoster, *Toxoplasma gondii*), diet/vitamins (e.g., nitrosamine compounds, vitamin C, vitamin D_3), beauty products (e.g., hair dyes and lighteners, hair waving and straightening chemicals), industrial exposures (e.g., rubber manufacturing, petroleum products), mobile phones, electromagnetic fields, allergies/immunity, agricultural/farm animal exposures, handedness, birth weight/height, and various genetic polymorphisms. While the list is long, methodologic biases are believed to account for the bulk of observed associations. A comprehensive review of factors hypothesized to play a role in the etiology of brain tumors is beyond the intent of the current work and the reader is referred to several recent reviews on the topic (Ostrom and Barnholtz-Sloan 2011; Ohgaki 2009; Fisher et al 2007; Schwartzbaum et al 2006; Ohgaki and Kleihues 2005; Wrensch et al 2002). Rather, the aim of this section is to address the etiology of gliomas in the context of recent publications and current scientific debate on the topic.

3.1 Mobile phones

Mobile (cellular) phones initially appeared on the market in the late 1970's in Japan and soon thereafter were sold in Europe and the U.S. (Bellis 2011). The first commercial wireless call originating in the U.S. occurred on 13 October 1983 (Green 2008).

However, the widespread and frequent use of mobile phones on an affordable scale was not achieved until the earlier 2000's when unlimited usage service contracts became a viable option to "pay by the minute" billing plans. By the end of 2010 there were approximately 303 million mobile phone subscribers in the U.S., representing 9 times the number in 1995 (CTIA 2011). The World Health Organization estimates 4.6 billion subscribers globally in 2010 (WHO 2011).

The main challenge of epidemiologic studies on mobile phone risk has been the lack of long term, frequent use exposure data (NRPB 2003), especially among users who may be genetically predisposed to brain tumours (Wrensch et al 2009; Shete et al 2009). Population stratification and gene-environment interactions may mask the risk of mobile phone use in insufficiently powered studies. Compounding the situation, the average latency period for many cancers is measured in decades, sometimes as long as 50-60 years, and similarly long intervals may apply to brain tumours (Challis 2007). The flat or declining brain tumour incidence trends observed in the population during the same time period of increasing mobile phone use would seem incongruent if mobile phones are a significant cause of brain tumours (Inskip et al 2010). However, competing risks could explain the effect if brain tumours are caused by more than one factor.

The majority of epidemiologic studies to date generally do not support a causative association between mobile phone use and brain tumours (Ahlbom et al 2009). However, methodologic concerns point to a cumulative underestimation of risk (Kundi 2010). Downward bias may have affected studies that excluded deceased and terminally ill patients, if mobile phone use presumably increases the case fatality rate vis-à-vis enhanced tumor progression. Pre-diagnostic effects of brain tumours may have reduced cell phone use and differentially resulted in lower risk estimates, since referents would not have been affected (NRPB 2003). The use of interviews rather than mailed questionnaire data collection (where it is possible to verify mobile phone use by checking billing records) may have decreased risk estimates due to non-differential exposure misclassification from relying on proxy information. Furthermore, participants tend to underestimate the prevalence of mobile phone use by up to 15% compared with non-participants, leading to a differential reduction in risk estimates for mobile phone use, since participation rates among cases typically are higher than referents by 10-15% (Vrijheid et al 2009; The INTERPHONE Study Group 2010). Risk estimates below unity for brain tumours have been reported in several analyses of mobile phone use (The INTERPHONE Study Group 2010; Inskip et al 2001; Johansen et al 2001; Muscat et al 2000; Hepworth et al 2006). A biologic basis for the results, particularly reports of deceased risk for contralateral use, is ambiguous. In many cases, the inverse associations likely are explained by the aforementioned factors that bias risk estimates in the downward direction. On the other hand, studies in which the participants' status was blinded at interview tended to yield positive risk estimates compared with those who were not blinded (Myung et al 2008).

Two large recent studies have reported increased risks for mobile phone use, especially among heavy users. A multicentric study (13 countries) with 2708 glioma cases and matched referents (age within 5 years, sex, and region of residence within each study centre) observed a 1.40 odds ratio (OR) [95% confidence interval (CI)=1.03-1.89] for glioma among those in the highest mobile phone exposure category (cumulative call time≥1640 hours) compared with the lowest category (never a regular user) (The INTERPHONE Study Group 2010). A subset analysis of the concordance between tumour and preferred side of phone use similarly showed an increased estimated risk among those in the highest decile of cumulative call time (OR=1.55, 95%CI=1.24-1.99). Risk estimates were not reduced for the contralateral side, suggesting against potential reporting bias (Kundi et al 2009). A linear dose response pattern (i.e., consistently increasing risk estimates with dose) is a feature of many but not all known carcinogens and conveys greater weight for a causative association. An upward trend across deciles of cumulative call time was not observed in the above study.

However, in a second recently-conducted study of n=1251 maligant brain tumours (n=1148 gliomas) and n=1267 referents (aged 20-80 years at diagnosis), adjusted estimated risk (age, sex, socioeconomic index, and year of diagnosis) increased with cumulative hours (h) of mobile phone use (none, OR=1.0; 1-100 h, OR=1.2, 95%CI=0.98-1.4; 1001-2000 h, OR=1.5, 95%CI=11.1-2.1; >2000 h, OR=2.5, 95%CI=1.8-3.5) (Hardell et al 2011). Similarly, estimated risk (in the category with >74 hours cumulative use) increased with latency time [years (y) since first use of a cell phone until diagnosis] (none, OR=1.0; >1-5 y, OR=1.0, 95%CI=0.7-1.4; >5-10 y, OR=1.2, 95%CI=0.9-1.6; >10 y, OR=2.7, 95%CI=2.0-3.8), although the linear effect was less pronounce than for cumulative hours of exposure. A key advantage of this study was the use of a mailed questionnaire, which allowed participants to verify responses by checking telephone bills (Kundi 2010). Recall bias could have increased risk estimates in positive studies if more cases than referents believed mobile phone use to be the cause of their brain tumour (Sage and Carpenter 2009; Hepworth et al 2006).

Studies of mobile phone use have been difficult to compare and interpret due to methodologic differences and the paucity of rigorous design. Background levels of electromagnetic radiation (e.g., power lines, fluorescent lights, computer monitors, televisions, and mobile phone base stations) may have confounded studies that did not account for such effects. A recent case-referent study conducted in Japan found a dose-response pattern for increasing exposure to power-frequency magnetic fields (MF) measured in a child's bedroom and brain tumours (<0.1μT, OR=1.0; 0.1 to <0.2 μT, OR=0.74, 95%CI=0.17-3.18; 0.2 to <0.4 μT, OR=1.58, 95%CI=0.25-9.83; ≥0.4 μT, OR=10.9, 95%CI=1.05-113). The OR reported for bedroom MF levels above 0.3 μT, as opposed to above 0.4 μT, was 16 (95%CI=1.85-153). Mobile phones emit both radiofrequency and extremely-low frequency electromagnetic fields (Sage et al 2007). The level of near-field electromagnetic radiation typically emitted on a continuous basis by smart mobile phones ranges from 0.5-0.1 μT (spikes up to 93.5 μT have been recorded during send/receive mode operations), which is above the highest exposure category reported in the Japanese study (Sage et al 2007; Stevenson 2011). Measurements could have been influenced by near-field interference (Silva 2007; Jaffa and Herz 2007), however readings were generally consistent with other independent sources (Sage and Johansson 2007). A large pooled analysis of low-frequency MFs and childhood brain tumors did not observe a dose-response relationship (Kheifets et al 2010). However, inconsistent/imprecise exposure measurements and low participation rates (40%-80%) across studies may have biased results. Furthermore, the actual exposure levels in brain tissue may not necessarily reflect the levels radiated by the mobile phone due to anatomic details and variations in tissue conductivity/permittivity (Kouveliotis et al 2006; Kuster and Balzano 1992).

In March 2010, the Mobile Telecommunications and Health Research Programme (MTHR) initiated funding of a prospective cohort study that will follow approximately 250,000 mobile phone users across 5 European countries for up to 30 years (MTHR 2011; Stewart 2000). While MTHR concludes that short term (less than 10 years) exposure to mobile phone signals does not appear to be associated with an increase in brain and nervous system tumours, they emphasize that there remains "significant uncertainties that can only be resolved by monitoring the health of a large cohort of phone users over a long period of time (MTHR 2011)." Furthermore, the reactions of children to mobile phone emissions may be different and/or stronger than those of adults (as is the case for other environmental exposures such as lead, tobacco smoke, ultraviolet radiation, and ionising radiation) and very little research has been conducted so far to determine whether this is the case (MTHR 2011). No studies on mobile phone use and risk of brain tumours have been planned for the U.S. that are comparable in size and detail to the COSMOS.

The thermal radiation emitted during average mobile phone use is low and generally is not believed to cause direct DNA damage or any other significant deleterious biologic effects on the brain (Wainwright 2000; Johansen et al 2001; Sage and Carpenter 2009; NRPB 2003). However, questions remain regarding the non-thermal effects of non-ionising radiation from mobile phones. Using positron emission tomography (PET), a National Institutes of Health study of 47 participants demonstrated a 7% increase in brain glucose uptake (a measure of metabolic activity) in response to mobile phone signals, supposedly independent of any thermal effects (Volkow et al 2011). The increases in regional glucose metabolism induced by the mobile phone signals were similar in magnitude to those reported after suprathrehold transcranial magnetic stimulation of the sensorimotor cortex. The authors hypothesize that the non-thermal effects on neuronal activity may be mediated by changes in cell membrane permeability, calcium efflux, cell excitability, and/or neurotransmitter release. A significant change in cell proliferation in response to radiofrequency MFs, independent of thermal activity, has been reported in a cell culture experiment involving transformed human epithelial amnion cells (Velizarov et al 1999). Effects demonstrated in other studies include up-regulation of apoptosis genes, induction of reactive oxygen species, changes in protein conformation, the creation of stress proteins, and immune system disturbances (Zhao et al 2007; Sage and Carpenter 2009; NRPB 2003; Valentini et al 2007; Ruediger 2009). Caution is advised when interpreting these effects since numerous contradictory results are present in the literature.

The likelihood that mobile phone use has no impact on the brain is small. Yet, the exact biophysical/biologic mechanism(s), if any, underlying mobile phone effects on neuronal cells, especially in the context of cancer, remains to be confirmed. Additional research is needed to determine if mobile phone use specifically increases brain tumor risk, either independently or in combination with other potential risk factors. Until then, limiting exposure to potentially vulnerable populations (e.g., fetus, children) would seem to be prudent precautionary public health policy, especially given the unknown latency for the development of brain cancer (Kundi et al 2009; Sage and Carpenter 2009). Radiofrequency MF absorption rates are estimated to be two times higher in children than adults, due to the lower thickness of pinna, skin and skull of younger children (Wiart et al 2008). Accordingly, risk may be greater among individuals who use a mobile phone at younger ages, yet few studies have addressed this potential risk group as they age into adulthood. Based on an increased risk for glioma, the WHO/International Agency for Research on Cancer (IARC) has formally classified radiofrequency electromagnetic fields, such as those emitted by wireless communication devices, as "possibly carcinogic to humans (Group 2B) (WHO/IARC 2011)."

3.2 Atopic diseases and farm exposures

Several (Berg-Berkhoff et al 2009; Wigertz et al 2007; Schwartzbaum et al 2003; Hochberg et al 1990; Schlehofer et al 1992; Schlehofer et al 1999; Ryan et al 1992; Brenner et al 2002; Linos et al 2007; Wang and Diepgen 2005; Carrozzi and Viegi 2005) **but not all** (Hagströmer et al

2005; Turner et al 2005; Siegmund et al 2008; Eriksson et al 2005; Cicuttini et al 1997) epidemiologic studies of atopic diseases (e.g., asthma, allergies) have been negatively associated with glioma risk. The protective association has been suggested to reflect increased immune surveillance, although the exact biologic mechanism is unknown (Linos et al 2007; Carrozzi and Viegi 2005). Alterations of the immunological system can enhance the inflammatory response and promote tumor development (Carrozzi and Viegi 2005). The reduced association with allergies also may be due to reverse causality (i.e., immunosuppression induced by the tumor) (Wigertz et al 2007). Glioma patients are known to have an impaired immune system (Dix et al 1999). Interestingly, therapeutic immunity to intracranial tumors has been induced in the laboratory by peripheral immunization with interleukin-4 (IL-4) transduced glioma cells [Okada et al 2001; Benedetti et al 1998].

Farmers have been found to have an increased risk for brain cancer in some studies (Kristensen et al 1996; Reif et al 1989; Wingren et al 1992; Ahlbom et al 1986; Musicco et al 1982; Musicco et al 1988; Brownson et al 1990; Heineman et al 1995), although they generally are healthier than the population-at-large (Kristensen et al 1996; Bråbäck 2002; Population and Public Health Branch (PPHB) 1995; Blair et al 2005; Ronco et al 1992), live longer (Alavanja 1996), and die less frequently from cancer overall (Blair et al 1993). Being raised on a farm (Alfven et al 2006; Ege et al 2007; Riedler et al 2001; Braun-Fahrländer et al 1999; Riedler et al 2000; von Ehrenstein et al 2000; Kilpelainen et al 2000; Klintberg et al 2001; Ernst and Cormier 2000; Remes et al 2003; Leynaert et al 2001; Gassner-Bachmann and Wüthrich 2000; Vercelli 2008) or in a rural area (Godfrey 1975) has been shown to protect against asthma, hay fever, and atopic sensitization. Farm children are exposed to higher concentrations of airborne allergens, but paradoxically become sensitized less frequently and manifest a weaker sensitization response than non-farm controls (Gassner-Bachmann and Wüthrich 2000). The protective effect may be due to a form of "tolerance" that conceivably develops early in life, following repeated exposure to high levels of allergens (e.g., organic dusts, fungi, and endotoxins). Component lipopolysaccharides have been shown to excite Th1 responses and suppress the development of immunoglobulin-E (IgE)-antibodies (Klintberg et al 2001; Bråbäck 2002).

Specific determinants of asthma and atopy in the farm setting remain largely unknown. Any relationship with glioma risk likely is complex and must be interpreted in light of substantial heterogeneity in the protective ability of farming environments and differences in farming practices, especially with respect to microbial exposures (Alfven et al 2006; Ege et al 2007; Vercelli 2008). By self-selection, those who manifest allergies may choose a career path other than farming (i.e., healthy worker effect) (Bråbäck 2002). Farmers represent a diverse group (e.g., dairy, field crop, hog, beef cattle, poultry, fish, marijuana, cotton, and organic), and brain cancer risk, or lack thereof, for farmers could reflect differences in activities and the type, magnitude, and seasonality of exposures. In one report, marijuana smoking was associated with glioma risk, but the study did not specifically examine marijuana farming (Efird et al 2004). Farmers and their families have greater contact with seasonal elements. Season of birth has been associated with adult (Brenner et al 2004; Koch et al 2006; Mainio et al 2006; Efird 2009) and childhood brain tumours (Makino et al 2011; McNally et al 2002; Heuch et al 1998; Yamakawa et al 1979; Hoffman et al 2007; Halperin et al 2004), but the period of greatest risk has varied between studies.

Differences in the definition and the lack of objective measures of atopy should be considered when interpreting the above studies (Wang and Diepgen 2005; Schoemaker et al 2006). Furthermore, there is no definitive trend toward a decreasing risk for glioma with younger ages at onset of the allergic condition, arguing against an immunologic cause for glioma (Schoemaker et al 2006). Paradoxically, increased risk for glioma has been observed in patients with AIDS-related immuno-suppression (Goedert et al 1998; Frisch et al 2001; Grulich et al 1999), but not in those with iatrogenic immuno-suppression (Schiff 2004). Many farm chemicals are classified as probable or likely human carcinogens by the US Environmental Protection Agency (EPA) (e.g., acephate, dichlorvos, dimethoate, lindane, parathion, phosmet, and tetrachlorvinphos) and these agents acting alone or in parallel with decreased atopic sensitization conceivably may increase glioma risk (US Environmental Protection Agency 2003).

3.3 Infectious agents

Polyomaviruses have been detected in the cancerous brain tissue of some patients diagnosed with gliomas (Rollison et al 2003). Polyomaviruses manifest a strong tropism for glial cells in vivo, possibly due to the interaction of glial transcription factors such as Tst-1/Ict6/SCIP with viral promoter sequences (Vasilyera et al 2004). The inoculation of immunologic immature neonate mice with human polyomavirus has been shown to readily cause tumor formation at multiple sites including the brain; older mice do not develop tumors in response to polyoma virus either in the laboratory or by natural infection (Nagashima et al 1984; Zu Rhein and Varakis 1979; London et al 1978; London et al 1983, Sanders 1977; Nagashima et al 1984; Zu Rhein and Varakis, 1979). Similarly, owl and squirrel monkeys injected (intracerebral, subcutaneous, or intravenous) with human JC polyomavirus have developed astrocytomas and glioblastomas (London et al 1978; London et al 1983). Recently, two new members of the *Polyomaviridae family,Karolinska Institutet* Virus (KIPyV) and *Washington Univerisity* virus (WUPyV), have been detected in samples from children with lower respiratory tract disease (Foulongne et al 2008).

Paradoxically, animals are not a permissive host for human JC virus replication, even though integrated JC viral DNA has been identified in the tumors of animals induced with the virus (White et al. 2005; Miller et al, 1984). Though monkeys themselves are not affected, simian virus (SV)-40 (extracted from monkey kidneys) gives cancer to hamsters (Rosenfeld 1962). Human adenovirus type 12 and Rous sarcoma virus are examples of other neuro-oncogenic viruses capable of causing gliomas under laboratory conditions (Zimmerman 1975). Yet, adenovirus in the worst case only causes respiratory disease in humans (Rosenfeld 1962). Some tumor viruses must be injected in animals on the first day of life to be effective, although they may not cause cancer until years later (Bailar and Gurian 1964).

Analogous to human and simian polyomaviruses causing brain tumours in non-permissive rodents, animal polyomaviruses conceivably may cause brain tumours in humans, yet little is understood about the latter topic. Polyomavirus are ubiquous among animals (e.g., cattle, birds, rodents,) (Ashok and Atwood 2006). For example, mouse polyomaviruses (*Mus musculus*) are capable of inducing a wide array of mesenchymal and epithelial cell type cancers in mice (Dawe et al 1987). Exposure to farm animals has been associated in some studies with childhood brain tumours (Efird et al 2003; Bunin et al 1994) but not adult brain tumors (Ménégoz et al 2002).

Epidemiologic evidence in support of a viral/pathogenic etiology for brain tumors remains controversial. In adults, *Toxoplasma gondii* infection has been associated with an increased prevalence of astrocytomas (Schuman et al 1967), while decreased glioma risk has been associated with a history of infections/colds (Schlehofer et al 1999), and chicken pox

(Wrensch et al 2005; Wrensch et al 2001). On the other hand, increased risk for childhood brain tumors has been associated with a history of chicken pox (Bithell et al 1973), influenza (Dickinson et al 2002; Linos et al 1998), measles (Dickinson et al 2002), general viral infections (Fear et al 2001; Linet et al 1996), and neonatal urinary tract infections (Linet et al 1996). A 7.5-fold OR (95% CI=1.3-44.9) for low grade astrocytoma has been observed for neonatal urinary tract infections (Linet et al 1996).

A recent cohort study of 20,132 workers in poultry slaughtering and processing plants, a group with high potential exposures to avian leukosis/sarcoma, reticuloendothesliosis, and Marek's disease viruses, were observed to have a significant excess of brain cancer, compared with the U.S. population (standardized mortality ratio=1.7, 95% CI=1.1-2.4). Although the aforementioned poultry viruses are well established carcinogens in their natural species, it is not known if they cause cancer in humans (Johnson et al 2000).

An infectious etiology for brain tumors is complicated by many factors (Naumova 2006). The same infectious agent may present a different pattern of incidence depending on the host location. A peak evident in the general population may not behave uniformly within certain subpopulations. Temperature, humidity, precipitation, and indoor air quality are among the mitigating factors that may affect the survival and transmissibility of a pathogen. Other factors include poor nutrition, population density, travel, hygiene practices, cultural practices in food consumption/preparation, changes in herd immunity, or evolution of the infectious agent over time. Furthermore, seasonal variation in immune function may increase host susceptibility to infections at certain times of the year (Melnikov et al 1987; Carandente et al 1988).

4. Discussion

The vast majority of glioma cases are idiopathic in origin. Demographic differences in incidence by race, sex, and country suggests that genetics, hormones, and environmental risk factors may play a role in some gliomas. However, study bias (e.g., participation, information, survival), variations in health care access/utilization, residual confounding, and other yet-to-be realized influences may explain the differences in glioma incidence. Complicating matters, the etiology of glioma may be multifactor in nature. That is, several factors operating in unison may cumulatively increase/decrease risk or mask the effect of individual factors when examined in isolation. Additionally, gene-environment and gene-gene interactions may modify underlying risk. Future epidemiologic studies will benefit by improved measures of environmental exposures, more precise statistical methods for detecting interaction effects, and larger multicentre collaborations aimed at better understanding the impact of population stratification.

5. Acknowledgements

Katherine T. Jones (ECU) and Avima Ruder (CDC/NIOSH/DSHEFS) offered valuable comments during the writing of this manuscript. The author also thanks Tamara Sachs for research assistance.

6. References

Ahlbom A, Feychting M, Green A, Kheifets L, Savitz D, Swerdlow A, and ICNIRP (International Commission for Non-Ionizing Radiation Protection) Standing

Committee on Epidemiology. Epidemiology evidence on mobile phones and tumor risk - a review. *Epidemiology* 2009;20:639-652.

Ahlbom A, Navier I, Norell S, Olin R, Spännare R. Nonoccupational risk indicators for astrocytomas in adults. *Am J Epidemiol* 1986;124:334-337.

Alavanja M, Sandler D, McMaster S, Zahm S, McDonnell C, Lynch C, Pennybacker M, Rothman N, Dosemeci M, Bond A, Blair A. The Agricultural Health Study. *Environ Health Perspect* 1996;104:362-369.

Alfven T, Braun-Fahrländer C, Brunekreef B, von Mutius E, Riedler J, Scheynius A, van Hage M, Wickman M, Benz M, Buddle J, Michels K, Schram D, Ublagger E, Waser M, Pershagen G, the PARSIFAL study group. Allergic diseases and atopic sensitization in children related to farming and anthroposophic lifestyle - the PARSIFAL study. *Allergy* 2006;61:414-421.

Altekruse S, Kosary C, Krapcho M, Neyman N, Aminou R, Waldron W, Ruhl J, Howlader N, Tatalovich Z, Cho H, Mariotto A, Eisner M, Lewis D, Cronin K, Chen H, Feuer E, Stinchcomb D, Edwards B (eds). *SEER Cancer Statistics Review, 1975-2007*, National Cancer Institute. Bethesda, MD, http://seer.cancer.gov/csr/1975_2007/, based on November 2009 SEER data submission, posted to the SEER web site, 2010.

Ashok A, Atwood A. Virus receptors and tropism. In: Ahsan N (ed), Polyomaviruses and Human Diseases (Advances in Experimental Medicine and Biology, vol. 577). New York: Springer+Business Media; 2006.

Bailar J, Gurian J. Month of birth and cancer mortality. *J Natl Cancer Inst* 1964;33:237-242.

Berg-Berkhoff G, Schüz J, Blettner M, Münster E, Schlaefer K, Wahrendorf J, Schlehofer B. History of allergic disease and epilepsy and risk of glioma and meningioma (INTERPHONE study group, Germany). *Eur J Epidemiol* 2009;24:433-440.

Bellis M. Selling the cell phone. Part 1: History of cellular phones. http://inventors.about.com/library/weekly/aa070899. Accessed April 2011.

Benedetti S, Di Meco F, Cirenei N, Bruzzone M, Pollo B, Florio N, Caposio L, Colombo M, Cattaneo E, Finocchiaro G. IL-4 gene transfer for the treatment of experimental gliomas. *Adv Exp Med Biol* 1998;451:315-321.

Bithell J, Draper G, Gorbach P. Association between malignant disease in children and maternal virus infections. *Br Med J* 1973;24:706-708.

Blair A, Dosemeci M, Heineman E. Cancer and other causes of death among male and female farmers from twenty-three states. *Am J Ind Med* 1993;23:729-742.

Blair A, Sandler D, Tarone R, Lubin J, Thomas K, Hoppin J, Samanic C, Coble J, Kamel F, Knott C, Dosemeci M, Zahm S, Lynch C, Rothman N, Alavanja M. Mortality among participants in the agricultural health study. *Ann Epidemiol* 2005;15: 279-285.

Bondy M, Wrensch M. Epidemiology of primary malignant brain tumours. Baillieres *Clin Neurol* 1996;5:251-270.

Bråbäck L. Does farming provide protection from asthma and allergies? *Acta Paediatr* 2002;91:1147-1149.

Braun-Fahrländer C, Gassner M, Grize L, Neu U, Sennhauser F, Varonier H, Vuille J, Wäthrich B, and The SCARPOL Team. Prevalence of hay fever and allergic sensitization in farmer's children and their peers living in the same rural community. *Clin Exp Allergy* 1999;29:28-34.

Brenner A, Linet M, Fine H, Shapiro W, Selker R, Black P, Inskip P. History of allergies and autoimmune diseases and risk of brain tumors in adults. *Int J Cancer* 2002;99:252-259.

Brenner A, Linet M, Shapiro W, Selker R, Fine H, Black P, Inskip P. Season of birth and risk of brain tumors in adults. *Neurology* 2004;63:276-281.

Brownson R, Reif J, Chang J, Davis J. An analysis of occupational risks for brain cancer. *Am J Public Health* 1990;80:169-172.

Bunin G, Buckley J, Boesel C, Rorke L, Meadows A. Risk factors for astrocytic glioma and primitive neuroectodermal tumors of the brain in young children: a report from the Children's Cancer Group. *Cancer Epidemiol Biomarkers Prev* 1994;3:197-204.

Carandente F, Angeli A, De Vechi A, Dammacco F, Halberg F. Multifrequency rhythms of immunologic functions. *Chronobiologia* 1988;15:7-23.

Carrozzi L, Viegi G. Allergy and cancer: a biological and epidemiological rebus. *Allergy* 2005;60:1095-1097.

CBTRUS (2011). CBTRUS Statistical Report: Primary Brain and Central Nervous System Tumours Diagnosed in the United States in 2004-2007. Source: Central Brain Tumour Registry of the United States, Hinsdale, IL. website: www.cbtrus.org.

Challis L (Chairperson). Mobile Telecommunications and Health Research Programme Report 2007. MTHR Programme Management Committee. http://www.mthr.org.uk/documents/MTHR_report_2007.pdf. Accessed April 2011.

Cicuttini F, Hurley S, Forbes A, Donnan G, Salzberg M, Giles G, McNeil J. Association of adult glioma with medical conditions, family and reproductive history. *Int J Cancer* 1997;71:203-207.

CTIA (Cellular Telephone Industry Association). Background on CTIA's semi-annual wireless industry survey. http://files.ctia.org/pdf/CTIA_Survey_Year_End_2010_Graphics.pdf . Accessed April 2011.

Dawe C, Freund R, Mandel G, Baller-Hofer K, Talmage D, Benjamin T. Variations in polyoma virus genotype in relation to tumor induction in ,mice-characterization of wild type strains with widely differing profiles. *Am J Pathol* 1987;127:243-261.

Dickinson H, Nyari T, Parker L. Childhood solid tumours in relation to infections in the community in Cumbria during pregnancy and around the time of birth. *Br J Cancer* 2002;87:746-750.

Dix A, Brooks W, Roszman T, Morford L. Immune defects observed in patients with primary malignant brain tumors. *J Neuroimmunol* 1999;100:216-232.

Efird J. Season of birth and risk for adult gliomas (abstract). Brain Tumor Epidemiology Consortium Annual Meeting Abstract Session, The Houstonian Hotel, Houston, Texas, 4-6 April, 2009, Abstract #2.

Efird J, Friedman G, Sidney S, Klatsky A, Habel L. The risk for malignant primary adult-onset glioma ia a large, multiethnic, managed-care cohort: cigarette smoking and other lifestyle behaviors. *J Neuro-Oncol* 2004;68:57-69.

Efird J, Holly E, Preston-Martin S, Mueller B, Lubin F, Filippini G, Peris-Bonet R, McCredie M, Cordier S, Arslan A, Bracci P. Farm-related exposures and childhood brain tumours in seven countries: results from the SEARCH International Brain Tumour Study. *Paediatr Perinat Epidemiol* 2003;17:201-211.

Ege M, Frei R, Bieli C, Schram-Bijkerk D, Waser M, Benz M, Weiss G, Nyberg F, van Hage M, Pershagen G, Brunekreef B, Riedler J, Lauener R, Braun-Fahrländer C, von Mutius E, and the PASIFAL Study team. Not all farming environments protect against the development of asthma and wheeze in children. *J Allergy Clin Immunol* 2007;119: 1140-1147.

Eriksson N, Mikoczy Z, Hagmar L. Cancer incidence in 13811 patients skin tested for allergy. J *Investig Allergol Clin Immunol* 2005;15:161-166.

Ernst P, Cormier Y. Relative scarcity of asthma and atopy among rural adolescents raised on a farm. *Am J Respir Crit Care Med* 2000,161,1563-1566.

Fear N, Roman E, Ansell P, Bull D. Malignant neoplasms of the brain during childhood: the role of prenatal and neonatal factors (United Kindom). *Cancer Causes Control* 2001;12:443-449.

Fisher J, Schwartzbaum J, Wrensch M, Wiemels J. Epidemiology of Brain tumors. *Neurol Clin* 2007;25:867-890.

Foulongne V, Brieu N, Jeziorski E, Chatain A, Rodière M, Segondy M. KI and WU polyomaviruses in children, France. *Emer Infect Dis* 2008;14:523-525.

Frisch M, Bigger R, Engels E, Goedert J, for the AIDS-Cancer Match Registry Study Group. Association of cancer with AIDS-related immunosuppression in adults. *JAMA* 2001;285:1736-1745.

Fritz A, Percy C, Jack A, Shanmugaratnam K, Sobin L, Perkin DM, Whelan S (eds). International Classification of Diseases for Oncology, Third edition. Geneva: World Health Organization; 2000.

Gassner-Bachmann M, Wüthrich B. Farmers' children suffer less from hay fever and asthma. *Dtsch Med Wochenschr* 2000;125:924-931.

Godfrey R. Asthma and IgE levels in rural and urban communities of The Gambia. *Clin Allergy* 1975;5:201-207.

Goedert J, Coté T, Virgo P, Scoppa S, Kingma D, Gail M, Jaffe E, Biggar R, for the AIDS-Cancer Match Study Group. Spectrum of AIDS-associated malignant disorders. *Lancet* 1998;351:1833-1839.

Green E. After just 25 years, cell phones own us. http://www.post-gazette.com/pg/08287/919578-96.stm?cmpid=news.xml. Accessed April 2011.

Grulich A, Wan X, Law M, Coates M, Kaldor J. Risk of cancer in people with AIDS. *AIDS* 1999;13:839-843.

Hagströmer L, Ye W, Nyrén O, Emtestam L. Incidence of cancer among patients with atopic dermatitis. *Arch Dermatol* 2005;141:1123-1127.

Halperin E, Miranda M, Watson D, George S, Stanberry M. Medulloblastoma and birth date: evaluation of 3 U.S. datasets. *Arch Environ Health* 2004;59:26-30.

Hardell L, Carlberg M, Mild K. Pooled analysis of case-control studies on malignant brain tumours and the use of mobile and cordless phones including living and deceased subjects. *Int J Oncol* 2011;38:1465-1474.

Hardell L, Carlberg M, Mild K. Pooled analysis of two case-control studies on use of cellular and cordless telephones and the risk for malignant brain tumours diagnosed in 1997-2003. *Int Arch Occup Environ Health* 2006;79:630-639.

Hawaii Department of Human Services. Hawaii Med-QUEST Quality Strategy 2010. http://www.med-quest.us/PDFs/Quality%20Strategy/HI%20MQD%20 Quality%20Strategy%20Approved.pdf. Assessed April 2011.

Heineman E, Gao Y, Dosemeci M, McLaughlin J. Occupational risk factors for brain tumors among women in Shanghai, China. *J Occup Environ Med* 1995;37:288-293.

Hepworth S, Schoemaker M, Muir K, Swerdlow A, van Tongeren M, McKinney P. *BMJ* 2006;332:883-887.

Heuch J, Heuch I, Akslen L, Kvåle G. Risk of primary childhood brain tumors related to birth characteristics: a Norwegian prospective study. *Int J Cancer* 1998;77:498-503.

Hochberg F, Toniolo P, Cole P. Nonoccupational risk indicators of glioblastoma in adults. *J Neurooncol* 1990;8:55-60.

Hoffman S, Schellinger K, Propp J, McCarthy B, Campbell R, Davis F. Seasonal variation in incidence of pediatric medulloblastoma in the United States, 1995-2001. *Neuroepidemiology* 2007;29:89-95.

Inskip P, Hoover R, Devesa S. Brain cancer incidence trends in relation to cellular telephone use in the United States. *Neuro Oncol* 2010;12:1147-1151.

Inskip P, Tarone R, Hatch E, Wilcosky T, Shapiro W, Selker R, Fine H, Black P, Loeffler J, Linet M. Cellular-telephone use and brain tumors. *N Engl J Med* 2001;344:79-86.

Jaffa K, Herz M. Measuring ELF fields produced by mobile phones and personal digital assistants (PDAs). *Bioelectromagnetics* 2007;28:583-584.

Johansson O. Disturbance of the immune system by electromagnetic fields—a potentially underlying cause for cellular damage and tissue repair reduction which could lead to disease and impairment. *Pathophysiology* 2009;16:157-177.

Johansen C, Boice J, McLaughlin, Olsen J. Cellular telephones and cancer - a nationwide cohort study in Denmark. *JNCI* 2001;93:203-207.

Johnson E, Ndetan H, Lo K. Cancer mortality in poultry slaughtering/processing plant workers belonging to a union pension fund. Environ Res 2010;110:588-594.

Kanu O, Hughes B, Di C, Lin, Fu J, Bigner D, Yan H, Adamson C. Glioblastoma multiforme oncogenomics and signaling pathways. *Clin Med Oncol* 2009;3:39-52.

Kheifets L, Ahlbom A, Crespi C, Feychting M, Johansen C, Monroe J, Murphy M, Oksuzyan S, Preston-Martin S, Roman E, Saito T, Savitz D, Schüz J, Simpson J, Swanson J, Tynes T, Verkasalo P, Mezei G. A Pooled Analysis Of Extremely Low-Frequency Magnetic Fields And Childhood Brain Tumors. *Am J Epidemiol* 2010;172:752-761.

Kilpelainen M, Terho E, Helenius H, Koskenvuo M. Farm environment in childhood prevents the development of allergies. *Clin Exp Allergy* 2000;30:201-208.

Kliehues P, Burger P, Scheithauer B. The new WHO classification of brain tumours. *Brain Pathol* 1993;3:255-268.

Kleihues P, Cavenee W. *World Health Organization Classification of Tumours. Pathology and genetics of tumours of the nervous system.* IARC: Lyon, 2000.

Klintberg B, Berglung N, Lilga G, Wickman M, van Hage-Hamsten M. Fewer allergic respiratory disorders among farmers' children in a closed birth cohort from Sweden. *Eur Respir J* 2001;17:1151-1157.

Kristensen P, Andersen A, Irgens L, Laake P, Bye A. Incidence and risk factors of cancer among men and women in Norwegian agriculture. *Scand J Work Environ Health* 1996;22:14-26.

Koch H, Klinkhammer-Schalke M, Hofstädter F, Bogdahn U, Hau P. Seasonal patterns of births in patients with glioblastoma. *Chronobiol Int* 2006;23:1047-1052.

Kouveliotis N, Panagiotou S, Varlamos P, Capsalis C. Theoretical approach of the interaction between a human head model and a mobile handset helical antenna using numerical methods. *Progress In Electromagnetics Research, PIER* 2006;65:309-327

Kundi M. Mobile phone use and brain cancer: is the association biased? *Neuroepidemiology* 2010;35:115-116.

Kundi M, Hardell L, Sage C, Sobel E. Electromagnetic fields and the precautionary principle. *Environ Health Perspect* 2009;117:A484-A485.

Kuster N, Balzano Q. Energy absorption mechanisms by biological bodies in the near field of dipole antennas above 300 MHz. *IEEE Trans Vehicle Technol* 1992;41:174-181.

Lee C, Jung K, Yoo H, Park S, Lee S. Epidemiology of primary brain and central nervous system tumours in Korea. *J Korean Neurosurg* 2010;48:145-152.

Leynaert B, Neukirch C, Jarvis D, Chinn S, Burney P, Neukirch F, on behalf of the European Community Respiratory Health Survey. Does living on a farm during childhood protect against asthma, allergic rhinitis, and atopy in adulthood? *Am J Respir Crit Care Med* 2001;164:1829-1834.

Linet M, Gridley G, Cnattingius S, Nicholson H, Martinsson U, Glimelius B, Adami H, Zack M. Maternal and perinatal risk factors for childhood brain tumors (Sweden). *Cancer Causes Control* 1996;7:437-448.

Linos A, Kardara M, Kosmidis H, Katriou D, Hatzis C, Kontzoglou M, Koumandakis E, Tzartzatou-Stathopoulou F. Reported influenza in pregnancy and childhood tumour. *Eur J Epidemiol* 1998;14:471-475.

Linos E, Raine T, Alonso A, Michaud D. Atopy and risk of brain tumors: a meta-analysis. J *Natl Cancer Inst* 2007; 99:1544-1550.

London W, Houff S, Madden D, Fuccillo D, Gravell M, Wallen W, Palmer A, Sever J, Padgett B, Walker D, Zu Rhein G, Ohashi T. Brain tumors in owl monkeys inoculated with a human polyomavirus (JC virus). *Science* 1978;201:1246-1249.

London W, Houff S, McKeever P, Wallen W, Sever J, Padgett B, Walker D. Viral-induced astrocytomas in squirrel monkeys. In: Sever J, Madden (eds), Polyomaviruses and Human Neurological Diseases. New York: Alan R. Liss Inc; 1983.

Louis DN, Ohgaki H, Wiestler O, Cavanee W, Burger P, Jouvet A, Scheithauer B, Kleihues P. The 2007 WHO Classification of Tumours of the Central Nervous System. *Acta Neuropa*thol 2007;114:97-109.

Makino K, Nakamura H, Hide T, Kuratsu J. Risks of primary childhood brain tumors related to season of birth in Kumamoto Prefecture, Japan. *Childs Nerv Syst* 2011;27:75-78.

Mainio A, Hakko H, Koivukangas J, Niemelä A, Räsänen P. Winter birth in association with a risk of brain tumor among a Finnish patient population. *Neuroepidemiology* 2006;27:57-60.

Ménégoz F, Little J, Colonna M, Arslan A, Preston-Martin S, Schlehofer B, Blettner M, Howe G, Ryan P, Giles G, Rodvall Y, Choi W. Contacts with animals and humans as risk factors for adult brain tumours. An international case-control study. *Eur J Cancer* 2002;38:696-704.

National Cancer Institute (NCI). State Cancer Profiles. http://statecancerprofiles.cancer.gov. Accessed April 2011.

Matsuda T, Marugame T, Kamo K, Katanoda K, Ajiki W, Sobue T; The Japan Cancer Surveillance Research Group. Cancer Incidence and Incidence Rates in Japan in 2005: Based on Data from 12 Population-based Cancer Registries in the Monitoring of Cancer Incidence in Japan (MCIJ) Project. *Japan J Clin Oncol* 2011;41:139-47.

McNally R, Cairns D, Eden O, Alexander F, Taylor G, Kelsey G, Birch J. An infectious aetiology for childhood brain tumours? Evidence from space-time clustering and seasonality analyses. *Br J Cancer* 2002;86:1070-1077.

Melnikov O, Nikolsky I, Dugovskaya L, Balitskaya N, Kravchuk G. Seasonal aspects of immunological reactivity of human and animal organism. *J Hyg Epidemiol Microbiol. Immunol.* 1987;31:225-230.

Miller N, McKeever P, London W, Padgett B, Walker D, Wallen W. Brain tumors of owl monkeys inoculated with JC virus contain the JC virus genome. *J Virol* 1984;49:848-856.

Mobile Telecommunications and Health Research (MTHR) Programme. Cohort study of mobile phone use and health (COSMOS). http://www.ukcosmos.org/index.html. Accessed April 2011.

Muscat J, Malkin M, Thompson S, Shore R, Stellman S, McRee D, Neugut A, Wynder E. Handheld cellular telephone use and risk of brain cancer. *JAMA* 2000;284:3001-3007.

Musicco M, Filippini G, Bordo B, Melotto A, Morello G, Berrino F. Gliomas and occupational exposure to carcinogens: case-control study. *Am J Epidemiol* 1982;116: 782-790.

Musicco M, Sant M, Molinari S, Filippini G, Gatta G, Berrino F. A case-control study of brain gliomas and occupational exposure to chemical carcinogens: the risk to farmers. *Am J Epidemiol* 1988;128:778-785.

Myung S, Ju W, McDonnell D, Lee Y, Kazinets G, Cheng C, Moskowitz J. Mobile phone use and risk of tumors: a meta-analysis. *J Clin Oncol* 2009;27:5565-5572.

Nagashima K, Yasui K, Kimura J, Washizu M, Yamaguchi K, Mori W. Induction of brain tumors by a newly isolated JC virus (Tokyo-1 strain). *Am J Pathol* 1984;116:455-463.

National Cancer Institute (NCI) Surveillance Epidemiology and End Results (SEER). Stat Fact Sheets: Brain and Other Nervous System. http://seer.cancer.gov/statfacts/html/brain.html#survival. Accessed April 2011.

National Radiological Protection Board (NRPB). Health effects from radiofrequency electromagnetic fields. Report of an independent advisory group on non-ionising radiation. 2003;14(2):5-177. http://www.hpa.org.uk/web/HPAweb&HPAwebStandard/HPAweb_C/1254510602951. Accessed April 2011.

Naumova E. Mystery of seasonality: getting the rhythm of nature. *J Public Health Policy* 2006;27:2-12.

Ohgaki H. Epidemiology of brain tumors. In: Verma M, (ed), Methods of Molecular Biology, Cancer Epidemiology, vol. 472. New Jersey: Humana Press; 2009.

Ohgaki H, Kleihues P. Genetic profile of astrocytic and oligodendrogial gliomas. Brain Tumor Pathol [Epub ahead of print] DOI 10.1007.s10014-001-0029-1.

Ohgaki H, Kleihues P. Epidemiology and etiology of gliomas. *Acta Neuropathol* 2005;109:93-108.

Okada H, Villa L, Attanucci J, Erff M, Fellows W, Lotze M, Pollack I, Chambers W. Cytokine gene therapy of gliomas: effective induction of therapeutic immunity to intracranial tumors by peripheral immunization with interleukin-4 transduced glioma cells. *Gene Ther* 2001;8:1157-1166.

Ostrom Q, Barnholtz-Sloan J. Current state of our knowledge on brain tumor epidemiology. *Curr Neurol Neurosci Rep* 2011;11:329-335.

Parkin D, Bray F, Ferlay B, Pisani P. Global cancer statistics, 2002. *CA Cancer J Clin* 2005;55:74-108.

Population and Public Health Branch (PPHB), Health Canada. Farmers at lower risks for many diseases. *Farm Family Health* 1995;3:1-3

Porter K, McCarthy B, Freels S, Kim Y. Prevalence estimates for primary brain tumors in the United States by age, gender, behavior, and histology. *Neuro-Oncology* 2010;12:520-527.

Porter K, McCarthy B, Berbaum M, Davis F. Conditional survival of all primary brain tumor patients by age, behavior, and histology. Neuroepidemiology 2011;36:230-239.

Reif J, Pearce, N, Fraser J. Occupational risks for brain cancer: a New Zealand cancer registry-based study. *J Occup Med* 1989;31:863-867.

Riedler J, Braun-Fahrländer C, Eder W, Schreuer M, Waser M, Maisch S, Carr D, Schierl R, Nowak D, von Mutius E, and the ALEX Study Team. Exposure to farming in early life and development of asthma and allergy: a cross-sectional survey. *Lancet* 2001;358:1129-1133.

Riedler J, Eder W, Oberfeld G, Schreuer M. Austrian children living on a farm have less hay fever, asthma and allergic sensitization. *Clin Exp Allergy* 2000;30:194-200.

Remes S, Iivanainen K, Koskela H, Pekkanen J. Which factors explain the lower prevalence of atopy amongst farmers' children? *Clin Exp Allergy* 2003;33:427-434.

Rollison D, Helzlsouer K, Alberg A, Hoffman S, Hou J, Daniel R, Shah K, Major E. Serum antibodies to JC virus, BK virus, simian 40 virus, and the risk of incident adult astrocytic brain tumors. *Cancer Epidemiol Biomarkers Prev* 2003;12: 460-463.

Ronco G, Costa G, Lynge E. Cancer risk among Danish and Italian farmers. *Br J Ind Med* 1992;49:220-225.

Rosenfeld A. New evidence that cancer maybe infectious. Life Magazine 1962 (June 22);53:2-98.

Ruediger H. Genotoxic effects of radiofrequency electromagnetic fields. *Pathophysiology* 2009;16:89-102.

Ryan P, Lee M, North B, McMichael A. Risk factors for tumors of the brain and meninges: results from the Adelaide Adult Brain Tumor Study. *Int J Cancer* 1992;51:20-27.

Sage C, Carpenter D. Public health implications of wireless technologies. *Pathophysiology* 2009;16:233-246.

Sage C, Johansson O, Sage S. Personel digital assistant (PDA) cell phone units produce elevated extremely-low frequency electromagnetic field emissions. Bioelectromagnetics 2007;28:386-392.

Sage C, Johansson O. Response to comment on "personel digital assistant (PDA) cell phone units produce elevated extremely-low frequency electromagnetic field emissions." *Bioelectromagnetics* 2007;28:581-582.

Sanders F. Experimental carcinogenesis: Induction of multiple tumors by viruses. *Cancer* 1977;40:1841-1844.

Schiff D. Gliomas following organ transplantation: analysis of the contents of a tumor registry. *J Neurosurg* 2004;101:932-934.

Schlehofer B, Blettner M, Preston-Martin S, Niehoff D, Wahrendorf J, Arslan A, Ahlbom A, Choi W, Giles G, Howe G, Little J, Ménégoz F, Ryan P. Role of medical history in brain tumour development. Results from the international adult brain tumour study. *Int J Cancer* 1999;82:155-160.

Schlehofer B, Blettner M, Becker N, Martinsohn C, Wahrendorf J. Medical risk factors and the development of brain tumors. *Cancer* 1992;69:2541-2547.

Schoemaker M, Swerdlow A, Hepworth S, van Tongeren M, Muir K, McKinney P. History of allergies and risk of glioma in adults. *Int J Cancer* 2006;119:2165-2172.

Schuman L, Choi N, Gullen W. Relationship of central nervous system neoplasms to Toxoplasma gondii infection. *Am J Public Health Nations Health* 1967;57:848-856.

Schüz J, Böhler E, Berg G, Schlehofer B, Hettinger I, Schlaefer K, Wahrendorf J, Kunna-Grass K, Blettner M. *Am J Epidemiol* 2006;163:512-520.

Schwartzbaum J, Fisher J, Aldape K, Wrensch M. Epidemiology and molecular pathology of glioma. *Nat Clin Pract Neurol* 2006;2:494-503.

Schwartzbaum J, Jonsson F, Ahlbom A, Preston-Martin S, Lönn S, Söderberg K, Feychting M. Cohort studies of association between self-reported allergic conditions, immune-related diagnoses and glioma and meningioma risk. *Int J Cancer* 2003;106:423-428.

Shete S, Hosking F, Robertson L, Dobbins S, Sanson M, Malmer B, Simon M, Marie Y, Boisselier B, Delattre J, Delattre J, Hoang-Xuan K, El Hallani S, Idbaih A, Zelenika D, Andersson U, Henriksson R, Bergenheim AT, Feychting M, Lönn S, Ahlbom A, Schramm J, Linnebank M, Hemminki K, Kumar R, Hepworth S, Price A, Armstrong G, Liu Y, Gu X, Yu R, Lau C, Schoemaker M, Muir K, Swerdlow A, Lathrop M, Bondy M,Houlston R. Genome-wide association study identifies five susceptibility loci for glioma. *Nat Genet* 2009;41:899-904

Siegmund B, Schlehofer B, Wahrendorf J. Investigation on primary brain tumours and the co-morbidity with diabetes mellitus and atopic diseases in frame of the EPIC study. Brain Tumor Epidemiology Consortium Annual Meeting Abstract Session, German Cancer Research Center, Heidelberg, Germany, 5-7 April 2008, Abstract #5.

Silva M. Measuring ELF fields produced by mobile phones and personal digital assistants (PDAs). *Bioelectromagnetics* 2007;28:580-581.

Stevenson R. Electromagnetic radiation emitted by smart phones. Direct communication 18 April 2011.

Stewart W (Chairperson). Mobile Phones and Health. UK Independent Expert Group on Mobile Phones - 2000.
http://www.iegmp.org.uk/report/text.htm. Accessed April 2011.

The INTERPHONE Study Group. Brain tumour risk in relation to mobile telephone use: results of the INTERPHONE international case-control study. *Int J Epidemiol* 2010;39:675-694.

Tseng J, Merchant E, Tseng M. Effects of socioeconomic and geographic variations on survival for adult glioma in England and Wales. *Surg Neurol* 2006;66:258-263.

Turner M, Chen Y, Krewski D, Ghadirian P, Thun M, Calle E. Cancer mortality among US men and women with asthma and hay fever. *Am J Epidemiol* 2005;162:212-221.

US Environmental Protection Agency. April 2003. Chemicals evaluated for carcinogenic potential. Washington, DC, US Environmental Protection Agency, Office of Pesticide Programs, Health Effects Division.

Valentini E, Curcio G, Moroni F, Ferrara M, De Gennaro L, Bertini M. Neurophysiological effects of mobile phone electromagnetic fields on humans: a comprehensive review. *Bioelectromagnetics* 2007;28:415-432.

Vasilyeva I, Shamaev M, Glavatskiy A, Chopick N, Olexenko N, Tsyubko O, Galanta E, Malisheva T. Detection of polyomavirus DNA in human brain tumors. *Exp Oncol* 2004;26:78-80.

Velizarov S, Raskmark P, Kwee S. The effects of radiofrequency fields on cell proliferation are non-thermal. *Bioelectrochem Bioener* 1999;48:177-180.

Vercelli D. Advances in asthma and allergy genetics in 2007. *J Allergy Clin Immunol* 2008;122:267-271.

Volkow N, Tomasi D, Wang G, Vaska P, Fowler J, Telany F, Alexoff D, Logan J, Wong C. Effects of cell phone radiofrequency signal exposure on brain glucose metabolism. *JAMA* 2011;305:808-813.

von Ehrenstein O, von Mutius E, IIli S, Baumann I, Böhm B, von Kries R. Reduced risk of hay fever and asthma among children of farmers. *Clin Exp Allergy* 2000;30:187-193.

Vrijheid M, Richardson L, Armstrong B, Auvinen A, Berg G, Carroll M, Chetrit A, Deltour I, Feychting M, Giles G, Hours M, Iavarone I, Lagorio S, Lönn S, Mcbride M, Parent M, Sadetzki S, Salminen S, Sanchez M, Schlehofer B, Schüz J, Siemiatycki J, Tynes T,

Woodward A, Yamaguchi N, Cardis E. Quantifying the Impact of Selection Bias Caused by Nonparticipation in a Case-Control Study of Mobile Phone Use. *Ann Epidemiol* 2009;19:33–42.

Wainwright P. Thermal effects of radiation from cellular telephones. *Phys Med Biol* 2000;45:2363-2372.

Wang H, Diepgen T. Is atopy a protective or a risk factor for cancer? A review of epidemiological studies. *Allergy* 2005;60:1098-1111.

White M, Gordon J, Reiss K, Del Valle L, Croul S, Giordano A, Darbinyan A, Khalilu K. Human polyomaviruses and brain tumors. *Brain Res Rev* 2005;50:69-85.

WHO/International Agency for Research on Cancer (IARC). IARC Classifies Radiofrequency Electromagnetic fields as Possible Carcinogenic to Humans. Press Release No. 208, 31 May. IARC: Lyon, France.

Wiart J, Hadjem A, Wong M, Bloch I. Analysis of RF exposure in the head tissues of children and adults. *Phys Med Biol* 2008;53:3681-3695.

Wigertz A, Lönn S, Schwartzbaum J, Hall P, Auvinen A, Christensen H, Johansen C, Klæboe L, Salminen T, Schoemaker M, Swerdlow A, Tynes T, Feychting M. Allergic condition and brain tumor risk. *Am J Epidemiol* 2007;166:941-950.

Wingren G, Axelson O. Cluster of brain cancers spuriously suggesting occupational risk among glassworkers. *Scand J Work Environ Health* 1992;18:85-89.

Wrensch M, Jenkins R, Chang J, Yeh R, Xiao Y, Decker P,Ballman K, Berger M, Buckner J, Chang S, Giannini C, Halder C, Kollmeyer T, Kosel M, LaChance D, McCoy L, O'Neill B, Patoka J, Pico A, Prados M, Quesenberry C, Rice T, Rynearson A, Smirnov I, Tihan T, Wiemels J, Yang P, Wiencke J.Variants in the CDKN2B and RTEL1 regions are associated with high-grade glioma susceptibility. *Nat Genet* 2009;41:905–908

Wrensch M, Minn Y, Chew T, Bondy M, Berger M. Epidemiology of primary brain tumors: current concepts and review of the literature. *Neuro-Oncology* 2002;4:278-299.

Wrensch M, Weinberg A, Wiencke J, Miike R, Barger G, Kelsey K. Prevalence of antibodies to four herpesviruses among adults with glioma and controls. *Am J Epidemiol* 2001;154:161-165.

Wrensch M, Weinberg A, Wiencke J, Miike R, Sison J, Wiemels J, Barger G, DeLorenze G, Aldape K, Kelsey K. History of chickenpox and shingles and prevalence of antibodies to varicella-zoster virus and three other herpesviruses among adults with glioma and controls. *Am J Epidemiol* 2005;161:929-938.

World Health Organization (WHO). Electromagnetic fields and public health: mobile phones. http://www.who.int/mediacentre/factsheets/fs193/en/index.html. Accessed April 2011.

Yamakawa Y, Fukui M, Kinoshita K, Ohgami S, Kitamura K. Seasonal variation in incidence of cerebellar medulloblastoma by month of birth. *Fukuoka Igaku Zasshi* 1979; 70:295-300.

Zhao T, Zou S, Knapp P. Exposure to cell phone radiation up-regulates apoptosis genes in primary cultures of neurons and astrocytes. *Neurosci Lett* 2007;412:34-38.

Zimmerman H. The significance of experimental gliomas for human disease. In: Gliomas Current Concepts in Biology, Diagnosis, and Therapy, Hekmatpanah J (eds). New York: Springer-Verlag; 1975, pp. 6-19.

Zu Rhein G, Varakis J. Perinatal induction of medulloblastomas in Syrian golden hamsters by a human polyoma virus (JC). *Natl Cancer Inst Monogr* 1979;51:205-208,1979.

2

Molecular Etiology of Glioblastomas: Implication of Genomic Profiling From the Cancer Genome Atlas Project

Kimberly Ng.[1], Santosh Kesari[2], Bob Carter[3,4] and Clark C. Chen[1,5]
[1]*Department of Radiation Oncology, Dana-Farber Cancer Institute, Boston, MA*
[2]*Department of Neurology, Moores UCSD Cancer Center, UCSD,*
[3]*Center for Theoretic and Applied Neuro-Oncology,*
University of California San Diego, San Diego, CA
[4]*Department of Surgery, Division of Neurosurgery,*
University of California San Dieog, San Diego, CA
[5]*Division of Neurosurgery, Beth Israel Deaconess Medical Center, Boston, MA*
USA

1. Introduction

In the landmark review by Hanahan and Weinberg[1], the authors distilled the essence of cancer into six distinct phenotypes, including evasion of apoptosis, self-sufficiency in growth signals, insensitivity to anti-growth signals, tissue invasion and metastasis, limitless replicative potentials, and sustained angiogenesis. The widely accepted paradigm suggests that cancer arises as a result of mutations or epigenetic events, which alter function of genes critical for attaining these phenotypes. These gene functions are intimately linked to the regulation of developmental processes[2], their aberrant function in tumor inevitably lead to cell states that resemble stages during normal development. These cell states can be captured using genomic technologies to define distinct molecular subtypes. With the advent of The Genome Cancer Atlas project for glioblastoma[3,4], we now have a glimpse of the genetic events underlying glioblastoma pathogenesis as well as distinct molecular subtypes. In this review, the genomic profiles of glioblastoma will be reviewed in the context of the properties described by Hanahan and Weinberg. Molecular subtypes of glioblastoma will be discussed in the context of developmental biology and the cell of origin.

2. Glioblastoma

Glioblastoma is the most common form of primary brain tumor, with dismal prognosis. The incidence of this tumor is fairly low, with 2-3 cases per 100,000 people in Europe and North America. Despite its rarity, overall mortality related to glioblastoma is comparable to the more prevalent tumors[5]. This is, in large part, due to the near uniform fatality of the afflicted patients. Indeed, glioblastoma is one of the most aggressive of the malignant tumors. Without treatment, the median survival is approximately 3 months[6]. The current standard of treatment involves maximal surgical resection followed by concurrent radiation therapy and

chemotherapy with the DNA alkylating agent, temozolomide[7]. With this regimen, the median survival is approximately 14 months. For nearly all affected, the treatments available remain palliative.
Studies carried out over the past three decades suggest that glioblastomas, like other cancers, arise secondary to the accumulation of genetic alterations. These alterations can take the form of epigenetic modifications, point mutations, translocations, amplifications, or deletions, and modify gene function in ways that deregulate cellular signaling pathways leading to the cancer phenotype[1]. The exact number and nature of genetic alterations and deregulated signaling pathways required for tumorogenesis remains an issue of debate[8], although it is now clear that CNS carcinogenesis requires multiple disruptions to the normal cellular circuitry[3, 4].

3. The Cancer Genome Atlas (TCGA) project

The Cancer Genome Atlas (TCGA) is a comprehensive and coordinated effort to catalogue the genetic and epigenetic changes in the cancer genome, with goals of identifying those responsible for carcinogenesis. The project constitutes a joint effort of the National Human Genome Research Institute (NHGRI), National Cancer Institute (NCI), and the U.S. Department of Health and Human Services, and collects tumor specimen from major cancer centers spanning across the continental U.S. The project aims to provide the genomic profile of 500 specimens of various cancer types using state-of-the-art platforms for sequencing, microRNA, mRNA, single-nucleotide polymorphisms, and methylation profiling.
TCGA started as a pilot project in 2006 with focus on glioblastoma as the first cancer type for study. With the success of the pilot project, TCGA plans to expand its efforts to aggressively pursue 20 or more additional cancers. This article will review the major insights derived from the TCGA in the context of the cancer phenotypes proposed by Hanahan and Weinberg[1].

4. The cancer phenotype

The aggregate of cancer research investigation spanning the past three decades suggest that cancer is a genetic disease characterized by mutations or epigenetic events that abrogate or compromise regulatory circuitry governing cell proliferation and homeostasis[8]. In the landmark review by Hanahan and Weinberg[1], the authors distilled the essence of these regulatory circuits into six distinct phenotypes, including evading apoptosis, self-sufficiency in growth signals, insensitivity to anti-growth signals, tissue invasion and metastasis, limitless replicative potentials, and sustained angiogenesis. The following section will review the TCGA findings pertinent to these phenotypes.

4.1 Self-sufficiency in growth signals – The Receptor Tyrosine Kinase (RTK)/PhosphoInosital 3 Kinase (PI3K) signaling cascade

Active cellular proliferation in normal cells requires signals from its environment. These signals typically involve the binding of a transmembrane receptor to growth factors, extracellular matrix components, or cell surface components. This mitogenic signaling process is under stringent regulation in normal cells. Typically, multiple ligand-receptor interactions in a permissive cellular state are required before cellular proliferation can take place. This regulation minimizes the probability of dysregulated, autonomous cell growth[1,9]. The importance of growth factors in biology was recognized by a Nobel Prize in Physiology or Medicine to Stanley Cohen and Rita Levi-Montalcini in 1986. Subsequent identification that many oncogenes participate in cellular signaling related to growth factor function was also awarded a Nobel Prize in Physiology or Medicine (to Michael Bishop and Harold Varmus in 1989).

To abridge this stringent growth regulation, tumors often mutate the transmembrane receptors or their downstream effectors in ways that constitutively activate the pathway. The pathway most commonly mutated to achieve this end in glioblastoma involves the RTK-PI3K pathway[9,10]. RTKs are cell surface receptors that are normally activated only in response to growth factor binding[9]. Results from the TCGA revealed that nearly all glioblastomas harbor activating mutations or amplifications in genes required for this signaling cascade[3,4,11,12]. Epidermal Growth Factor Receptor (EGFR) and Platelet Derived Growth Factor Receptor (PDGFR) are two prototypical members of RTK[3, 4, 12].

For EGFR and PDGFR, binding of the growth factor to the ligand leads to homo- or hetero-dimerization of the receptor. This dimerization facilitates autophosphorylation of the cytoplasmic domains of the dimerized receptor at select tyrosine residues[9]. The phosphorylated tyrosine residue, in turn, recruits and binds to other signaling proteins to the cell membrane. In some cases, the phospho-tyrosine bound proteins serve as a platform for the recruitment of other effector proteins. In other cases, the bound protein undergoes a conformational change upon binding to the RTK and becomes activated in the process[9].

One of the critical cellular kinases that become activated upon binding to RTK is PI3K[13]. PI3Ks catalyze the phosphorylation of a critical component of the cell surface, phosphatidylinositol-4,5-isphosphate (PI(4,5)P2). This phosphorylation generates phosphatidylinositol-1,4,5-isphosphate (PI(1,4,5)P3), which in turn serves as a docking site for pro-proliferative down-stream effector proteins [10]. Thus, RTK activation transforms the cell membrane into a catalytic surface populated with a high density of pro-mitotic signaling molecules, ultimately leading to cell proliferation.

Expectedly, gene functions that inhibit the generation of this pro-proliferative "catalytic surface" function as tumor suppressors. For instance, the hydrolysis of (PI(1,4,5)P3) into (PI(4,5)P2) is catalyzed by a phosphatase termed Phosphatase and Tensin Homology (PTEN). PTEN inactivating mutations have been identified in up to 50% of tumor specimens [14]. Similarly, one of the effector proteins recruited to a phosphorylated RTK is Ras. Ras encodes a monomeric G-protein that cycles between an active form bound to GTP and an inactive form that binds to GDP[15]. It functions as a critical component of the pro-proliferative "catalytic surface". Through a series of protein-protein interactions, RTK activation catalyzes the exchange of GDP for GTP in Ras, initiating signals required for cellular proliferation. The protein encoded by neurofibromatosis 1 (NF1) functions to catalyze the exchange of GTP for GDP in Ras, consequently preventing cell proliferation. In this context, it is not surprising that NF1 patients are predisposed to gliomagenesis [16]. The TCGA results showed that approximately 20% of glioblastomas harbor loss of function mutations in NF1[3,4]. TCGA additionally revealed gain of function mutations in K-ras have also been identified in glioblastoma specimens [3].

4.2 Insensitivity to anti-growth signals – The RB axis

In addition to receiving pro-growth signals from their environment, cells also receive multiple anti-proliferative signals to prevent cell growth. These anti-growth signals, like

their pro-mitotic counterparts, are sensed by the binding of transmembrane receptors to soluble factors, extracellular matrix components, or cell surface components.
Most of these anti-proliferative signals operate at the G1 phase of the cell cycle to trigger either 1) entry into a transient quiescent (G0) state or 2) entry into a post-mitotic, differentiated state. The importance of cell cycle regulation in biology was recognized by a Nobel Prize in Physiology or Medicine to Leland Hartwell, Tim Hunt, and Sir Paul Nurse in 2001.
At the molecular level, nearly all of these signals converge at the retinoblastoma protein (RB) [1]. In quiescent cells, the RB protein is hyper-phosphorylated. This form of RB binds and sequesters the E2F family of transcription factors[17]. The genes transcribed by these transcription factors are essential for the G1-S transition of the cell cycle[18]. Phosphorylation of RB releases the sequestered E2F transcription factors and allows for cell growth. During normal cell cycle progression, induction of cyclin D1 and its associated cyclin-dependent kinases, CDK4 and CDK6, at the G1-S transition is responsible for the phosphorylation of RB. The kinase activity of the CDK4/6-cyclin D complex is under complex regulation, including the critical negative regulators CDKN2A ($p16^{Ink4a}$), CDKN2B, and CDKN2C. TCGA results showed that mutations and gene amplifications disrupting RB function are found in approximately 80% of glioblastomas, suggesting the critical importance of escaping anti-growth signals[3,4]. Additionally, single nucleotide polymorphisms in the *CDKN2A* and *CDKN2B* have been identified as risk factors for glioma development[19,20].

4.3 Evading apoptosis – The p53 axis

Apoptotic programs are inherent in all normal cells. These programs are activated by a number of physiologic signals during development and/or in response to cellular stress. Since the tumor state is associated with cellular stress capable of activating apoptosis (e.g. increased oxidative stress, increased DNA damage accumulation), inactivation of these programs constitute a critical step during carcinogenesis. The importance of apoptosis as a fundamental biologic process was recognized by a Nobel Prize in Physiology or Medicine awarded to Sydney Brenner, Robert Horvitz, and John Sulston in 2002.
The regulation of apoptotic pathways is highly complex[21]. Broadly speaking, there are two pathways of apoptosis that converge on the activation of effector proteases (termed caspases), which ultimately trigger the pathognomonic DNA fragmentation, cell shrinkage, and membrane blebbing. The intrinsic cell death pathway (often termed the mitochondrial apoptotic pathway) involves the release of cytochrome c from the mitochondrial membrane space[22]. Binding of cytochrome c to a protein termed apoptosis protease-activating factor 1 (APAF-1), in turn, initiates the caspase cascade. In contrast, the extrinsic apoptotic pathway operates independently of mitochondria and is activated by direct signaling from cell surface receptors to the effector caspase[23].
Both intrinsic and extrinsic apoptotic programs are profoundly influenced by the p53 tumor suppressor protein[24]. *TP53* encodes a transcription factor that regulates gene sets critical for cell cycle progression and apoptosis. Under normal conditions, p53 is a short-lived protein[25]. In response to cellular stress (for instance, DNA damage or oncogene expression), p53 undergoes post-translational modifications and protein-protein interactions that enhance its stability and transcriptional activity[25]. Key among the transcripts regulated by p53 are pro-apoptotic genes (including BAX and Puma) that facilitate both the intrinsic and extrinsic pathway[24]. Additionally, p53 interact with a number of anti-apoptotic proteins to inhibit their function[24].

There are several lines of evidence that point to the importance of the p53 axis in glioblastoma pathogenesis. In the TCGA database, mutations that inactivate this axis are found in greater than 70% of glioblastoma specimens[3,4]. Patients harboring germ-line mutations in *TP53* are afflicted with cancer predisposition including increased risk for glioblastoma[26]. Finally, inactivation of p53 is required for glioma formation in genetically defined murine models[27].

4.4 Replicative potential

The definition of cancer as a continuous growing entity implies that normal cells exhibit a limited capacity for proliferation. Indeed, estimates based on tissue culture work suggest that most normal cells have the capacity for 50 doublings [28]. Studies over the past three decades suggest that the main reason for this limited life span involve progressive shortening of chromosomes due to loss of telomeres. Telomeres consist of thousands of six base pair sequence element of repeats that are located at the ends of every chromosome. Because of the inability of DNA polymerases to replicate the 3′ ends of chromosomal DNA, approximately 60 base pairs of the telomeric sequence is lost with each replicative cycle[29]. With progressive erosion of the telomeric sequence, the unprotected chromosomal ends participate in aberrant fusion events that inevitably result in cell death[30].

To overcome this inherent limitation, most cancer cells activate an enzyme called telomerase. Telomerase is a reverse transcriptase capable of elongating telomeres[31]. Various mechanisms are employed by tumors to activate telomerase in order to sustain continued cell growth. Elizabeth Balckburn, Carol Greider, and Jack Szostak were awarded the Nobel Prize in Physiology or Medicine in 2009 for their discovery of telomerase.

With regards to glioblastomas, single nucleotide polymorphisms in two genes encoding components of the telomerase (*RTEL1* and *TERT*) have been identified as risk factors for glioma development[19, 20]. Additionally, elevated expression level of *TERT* in glioblastoma is associated with decreased patient survival [32]. These studies suggest a critical importance of telomeric biology in glioblastoma growth and survival.

Angiogenesis. The intense proliferation of cancer cells require continued supply of oxygen and nutrients. Due to inherent limitations on the distance that oxygen and macromolecules can travel, virtually all cells in a tissue reside with 100 um of a capillary. In xenograft model systems, solid tumors can only proliferate up to a size of 1-2 mm without development of new blood supply[33]. Thus, angiogenesis necessarily constitutes a pre-requisite during solid tumor progression.

One way by which cancer cells signal angiogenesis is by secretion of soluble factors that bind to receptors present on the surface endothelial cells. A key soluble factor that functions in such capacity is the Vascular Endothelial Growth Factor (VEGF). VEGF binds to RTKs on the surface of endothelial cells to facilitate their proliferation - leading to angiogenesis[34]. In normal cells, transcription of VEGF and other pro-angiogenic signaling factors are under strict regulation. The induction of Hypoxia Inducible Factor I (HIF1) is a pivotal element in this regulatory network[35]. HIF1 encodes a dimeric transcription factor consisting of two subunits: HIF1α and HIF1β. HIF1β is constitutively expressed irrespective of oxygen concentration, whereas HIF1α levels increase dramatically in response to hypoxia. The underlying mechanism for this regulation is that HIF1α is hydroxylated by HIF Prolyl-4-Hydroxylase (HPH) in the presence of di-oxygen (O2), iron, and α-ketoglutarate. The hydroxylated HIF1α is targeted for proteasome degradation. Without molecular oxygen,

HIF1α is not hydroxylated and is free to dimerize with HIF1β to activate the transcription of downstream pro-angiogenetic factors.

Integrated analysis of genomic data in glioblastoma revealed recurrent mutations in the R132 residue of isocitrate dehydrogenase 1 (IDH1)[4], a gene largely responsible for the production of α-ketoglutarate. The TCGA data revealed that the IDH1 mutation is predominantly found in one particular molecular subtype of glioblastoma[12, 36] (see following section on **molecular subtypes**). The wildtype IDH1 normally functions as a homodimer that converts isocitrate to α-ketoglutarate[37]. Biochemical characterization of the R132 mutated IDH1 revealed that it functions in a dominantly negative fashion to inhibit the process. Expectedly, glioblastoma harboring the *R132 IDH1* mutation harbor decreased levels of α -ketoglutarate. Given the importance of α -ketoglutarate in HIF1α degradation, one would anticipate increased HIF1α accumulation and increased VEGF secretion in glioblastoma harboring the *IDH1* mutation. These observations were confirmed in a panel of primary glioblastoma specimens[38]. Thus, the *IDH1* mutation constitutes an example of how glioblastoma subverts the endogenous molecular circuit to facilitate angiogenesis. It should be noted that the effect of the *IDH1* mutation appears pleiotropic. Another study revealed that the R132 mutant IDH1 proteins exhibits a gain-of-function phenotype by generating R(-)-2-hydroxyglutarate, a carcinogenic metabolite[39].

In glioblastomas without *IDH1* mutation, alternate mechanisms are utilized to facilitate angiogenesis. It is somewhat intuitive that during normal development, periods of cellular proliferation must be coordinated with angioogenesis. Indeed, a large body of work suggests that gene functions that facilitate cell-autonomous growth or insensitivity to growth inhibition and apoptosis also tend to facilitate angiogenesis[40, 41]. It is likely that most glioblastoma cells attain angiogenesis by aberrant activation of such coordinated developmental programs. For instance, EGFR activation has been shown to up-regulate VEGF in both HIF dependent and independent manner[42]. Inactivation of Rb increases VEGF expression and angiogenesis *in vivo*[40]. Similarly, p53 normally up-regulates thrombospondin 1, an inhibitor of angiogenesis[43]; inactivation of p53 can facilitate angiogenesis by ablation of this up-regulation.

4.5 Invasion and metastasis

The ability to invade and metastasize constitutes the fundamental distinction between benign and malignant tumors. It is important to note that invasion refers not just to distortion of normal tissue secondary to tumor growth. Instead, it refers to a coordinated set of cellular activities to destroy and migrate into the surrounding normal tissue. Metastasis refers to the capacity to travel via circulation to a distant tissue site[33]. Glioblastoma is unique in that while it is one of the most invasive of cancers, it rarely metastasizes outside of the central nervous system.

It is a truism that cancer cells generally retain some general properties of the cell of origin. Since glioblastoma originates from astrocytes, which normally possess significant migratory capacity, the invasive nature of glioblastoma would be anticipated. During normal development, astrocytes migrate in a centripetal manner to establish a scaffold for neuroblasts[44]. Additionally, in response to injury, astrocytes migrate to the affected region to form a gliotic scar[45]. This migratory capacity is the phenotypic expression of carefully orchestrated interactions between cellular cytoskeletal proteins, cell adhesion molecules, and extracellular matrix[33].

To date, the TCGA has not uncovered gain of function mutations in these proteins. However, enhanced invasive properties have been associated with mutations establishing autonomous growth or suppressing apoptosis. For instance, aberrant EGFR activation results in increased expression and phosphorylation of cell adhesion molecules that ultimately lead to increased invasiveness[46]. Similarly, the p53 mutation drives cancer invasiveness by facilitating the recycling of integrin, a class of cell surface receptor that interacts with extracellular matrix during cell migration[47].

The aggregate of the data suggest that both angiogenesis and cell migratory properties are intimately integrated into a master circuitry controlled by critical proteins that dictate cellular response to growth or apoptotic signals. In this context, mutations facilitating self-autonomous growth or suppression of apoptosis also contribute to angiogenesis and cell invasion.

4.6 Cross-talk between canonical pathways

The conceptualization of distinct pathways contributing to the various critical phenotypes constitutes a simplification aimed to consolidate distinct biological concepts. The reality is that pathways mediating the cancer phenotype exhibit high degrees of cross-talk and functional redundancy. For instance, EGFR hyperactivation is associated with increased tumor growth (replicative potential), angiogenesis, and increased tumor motility [48]. Similarly, many genes mediating cell motility, telomere function, and angiogenesis are under transcriptional regulation by p53 and RB associated E2Fs[49].

5. Pathway of glioblastoma progression

It was previously thought that glioblastoma arises from the acquisition of a defined set of mutations that occur in a particular temporal order. This model is largely grounded on the framework established in colon cancer, where a series of genetic alterations characterizes different phases of neoplastic progression[50]. The framework is supported by the observation that Grade II astrocytomas typically harbor mutations in p53; Grade III astrocytomas harbor activating mutations/amplifications of CDKN2A ($p16^{Ink4a}$); and Grade IV astrocytomas harbor mutations in PTEN and EGFR[51]. This data was interpreted to mean that glioblastoma results from sequential inactivation of the p53, RB, and RTK/PI3K axes.

While such a paradigm may hold true for a subset of the secondary glioblastomas, the picture emerging from the genomic characterization of primary glioblastomas reveals a much more dynamic process[3,4]. The profile of somatic mutations in different glioblastomas is highly variable. These results suggest that most glioblastomas evolve along a multitude of pathways in response to differing selective pressures to achieve the phenotypes described by Hanahan and Weinberg[52]. This somewhat stochastic model of cancer progression further implies that mutations critical at one juncture in the neoplastic process may lose relevance as additional mutations are acquired. Thus, while a mutational profile constitutes an archeological profile of the history of the neoplasm, extrapolating therapeutic targets from such a profile may be challenging.

6. Molecular subtypes

Genome-scale gene expression profiling using microarray technology have revealed distinct molecular subtypes within tumors previously classified as glioblastomas [12, 53-55]. The number of subtypes varies depending on the study, however, three subtypes consistently appear across independent studies and reflect distinct biologic and clinical behaviors [12, 55, 56]. Importantly, the transcript signature parallels those obtained during distinct stages in neural development, suggesting the tumor may have arisen from different stages of neurogenesis[55].

The first subtype is termed pro-neural. The transcript signature resembles those of neuro-blasts and oligodendrocytes derived from fetal and adult brain[55]. This subtype harbors molecular and clinical features that closely mirror those previously classified as secondary glioblastomas. Molecularly, pro-neural glioblastomas harbor mutations classically associated with the secondary subtype, including p53 and PDGFR[12]. Accordingly, grade II and III gliomas harbor molecular signatures most reminiscent of the pro-neural subtype[55]. Clinically, this subtype typically affects younger patients, is associated with improved overall survival[55], and responds poorly to concurrent radiation/temozolomide treatment upon disease progression[12]. Interestingly, mutations in the isocitrate **deh**ydrogenase 1 gene (*IDH1*), a metabolic protein required for conversion of isocitrate to a-ketoglutamate during the citric acid cycle, is frequently observed in pro-neural glioblastomas (see section on glioblastoma predisposition syndromes). The molecular basis of how this mutation contributes to the cancer phenotype remains an active area of investigation.

Classical (also termed proliferative by some authors) constitutes the second molecular subtype. Transcript signature in the classical subtype resembles those observed in transit amplifying neural progenitor cells[55] and murine astrocytes[12]. This subtype is exclusively found in WHO grade IV tumors and constitutes a form of primary glioblastoma[57]. Molecularly, this subtype is characterized by amplification of (or activating mutations in) EGFR and CDKN2A ($p16^{Ink4a}$). Genes involved in pathways highly active in neural stem and progenitor cells (including the Notch and Sonic hedgehog pathway) are highly expressed in the classical subtype).[58] The patients afflicted are typically older than those with the pro-neural subtype. Relative to the other subtype, patients afflicted with the classical subtype exhibit the worst prognosis, but the best therapeutic response to concurrent radiation/temozolomide treatment.

The mesenchymal subtype makes up the final category. The transcript signature in the mesenchymal subtype mirrors those observed in the neural stem cells of the forebrain[55] and cultured astroglial cells[59]. Most cultured glioblastoma cell lines exhibit transcript signatures that fall into this subtype. Molecularly, the subtype is characterized by inactivating NF1 and PTEN mutations[12]. This subgroup also has the highest expression of angiogenesis markers including VEGF (Vascular Epithelial Growth Factor) transcripts and highest density of microvascular proliferation[12]. The patients afflicted are typically older than those with the pro-neural subtype. Relative to the other subtypes, mesenchymal glioblastomas exhibit clinical response similar to the classical subtype, and a trend toward slightly improved prognosis and response to radiation/temozolomide therapy[12].

There is significant debate with regards to the origin of the distinct molecular subtypes. On one extreme is the thought that the subtypes originate from the same cell type with differences driven by distinct signaling pathways. The other extreme suggests that subtypes are determined by the same signaling pathways activated in a different cell of origin. The observation that the same canonical pathways are altered irrespective of subtype would tend to support the latter hypothesis. However, it is conceivable that different genes thought to participate in the same canonical pathway may modulate processes distinct of that pathway. Such functions may contribute to the distinct molecular subtypes. Still, it is conceivable that differences in signaling and cell of origin both contribute to subtype formation. This critical debate awaits experimental resolution.

7. Summary

The past three decades of work in cancer research has generated a sophisticated conceptual framework for the process of neoplastic transformation. The framework suggests that genetic and epigenetic events inactivating critical pathways that regulate several key aspects of cellular function are an etiology. These cellular functions can be categorized as self-sufficiency in growth signaling, evasion of apoptosis, insensitivity to anti-growth signals, tissue invasion, and limitless replicative potential and angiogenesis. This framework has largely been validated by a large scale, high-throughput characterization of the genomic and epigenomic landscape in glioblastomas. The picture emerging from these analyses suggests that most glioblastomas evolve along a multitude of pathways in response to differing selective pressures to achieve the cancer phenotypes. Transcript based analysis revealed distinct subtypes with potential implications with regards to the cell of origin. The dynamic interplay of growth dysregulation and the cell of origin during the neoplastic transformation process harbors vital implications with regards to therapeutic development.

8. References

[1] Hanahan D, Weinberg RA. The hallmarks of cancer. *Cell.* Jan 7 2000;100(1):57-70.

[2] Zelenka PS. Proto-oncogenes in cell differentiation. *Bioessays.* Jan 1990;12(1):22-26.

[3] TCGA. Comprehensive genomic characterization defines human glioblastoma genes and core pathways. *Nature.* Oct 23 2008;455(7216):1061-1068.

[4] Parsons DW, Jones S, Zhang X, et al. An integrated genomic analysis of human glioblastoma multiforme. *Science.* Sep 26 2008;321(5897):1807-1812.

[5] Wen PY, Kesari S. Malignant gliomas in adults. *N Engl J Med.* Jul 31 2008;359(5):492-507.

[6] Walker MD, Alexander E, Jr., Hunt WE, et al. Evaluation of BCNU and/or radiotherapy in the treatment of anaplastic gliomas. A cooperative clinical trial. *J Neurosurg.* Sep 1978;49(3):333-343.

[7] Stupp R, Mason WP, van den Bent MJ, et al. Radiotherapy plus concomitant and adjuvant temozolomide for glioblastoma. *N Engl J Med.* Mar 10 2005;352(10):987-996.

[8] Stratton MR, Campbell PJ, Futreal PA. The cancer genome. *Nature.* Apr 9 2009;458(7239):719-724.

[9] Schlessinger J. Cell signaling by receptor tyrosine kinases. *Cell.* Oct 13 2000;103(2):211-225.

[10] Hennessy BT, Smith DL, Ram PT, Lu Y, Mills GB. Exploiting the PI3K/AKT pathway for cancer drug discovery. *Nat Rev Drug Discov.* Dec 2005;4(12):988-1004.

[11] Stommel JM, Kimmelman AC, Ying H, et al. Coactivation of receptor tyrosine kinases affects the response of tumor cells to targeted therapies. *Science.* Oct 12 2007;318(5848):287-290.

[12] Verhaak RGW, Hoadley KA, Purdom E, et al. Integrated genomic analysis identifies clinically relevant subtypes of glioblastoma characterized by abnormalities in PDGFRA, IDH1, EGFR, and NF1. *Cancer Cell.* Jan 19 2010;17(1):98-110.

[13] Cantley LC. The phosphoinositide 3-kinase pathway. *Science.* May 31 2002;296(5573):1655-1657.

[14] Li J, Yen C, Liaw D, et al. PTEN, a putative protein tyrosine phosphatase gene mutated in human brain, breast, and prostate cancer. *Science.* Mar 28 1997;275(5308):1943-1947.

[15] Downward J. Targeting RAS signalling pathways in cancer therapy. *Nat Rev Cancer.* Jan 2003;3(1):11-22.

[16] Walker L, Thompson D, Easton D, et al. A prospective study of neurofibromatosis type 1 cancer incidence in the UK. *Br J Cancer.* Jul 17 2006;95(2):233-238.

[17] Knudsen ES, Wang JY. Targeting the RB-pathway in cancer therapy. *Clin Cancer Res.* Feb 15 2010;16(4):1094-1099.

[18] Buchkovich K, Duffy LA, Harlow E. The retinoblastoma protein is phosphorylated during specific phases of the cell cycle. *Cell.* Sep 22 1989;58(6):1097-1105.

[19] Shete S, Hosking FJ, Robertson LB, et al. Genome-wide association study identifies five susceptibility loci for glioma. *Nat Genet.* Aug 2009;41(8):899-904.

[20] Wrensch M, Jenkins RB, Chang JS, et al. Variants in the CDKN2B and RTEL1 regions are associated with high-grade glioma susceptibility. *Nat Genet.* Aug 2009;41(8):905-908.

[21] Fan TJ, Han LH, Cong RS, Liang J. Caspase family proteases and apoptosis. *Acta Biochim Biophys Sin (Shanghai).* Nov 2005;37(11):719-727.

[22] Lowe SW, Cepero E, Evan G. Intrinsic tumour suppression. *Nature.* Nov 18 2004;432(7015):307-315.

[23] Ashkenazi A, Dixit VM. Apoptosis control by death and decoy receptors. *Curr Opin Cell Biol.* Apr 1999;11(2):255-260.

[24] Haupt S, Berger M, Goldberg Z, Haupt Y. Apoptosis - the p53 network. *J Cell Sci.* Oct 15 2003;116(Pt 20):4077-4085.

[25] Harris CC. p53 tumor suppressor gene: from the basic research laboratory to the clinic--an abridged historical perspective. *Carcinogenesis.* Jun 1996;17(6):1187-1198.

[26] Li FP, Fraumeni JF, Jr. Soft-tissue sarcomas, breast cancer, and other neoplasms. A familial syndrome? *Ann Intern Med.* Oct 1969;71(4):747-752.

[27] Holland EC. Gliomagenesis: genetic alterations and mouse models. *Nat Rev Genet.* Feb 2001;2(2):120-129.

[28] Hayflick L. The Limited in Vitro Lifetime of Human Diploid Cell Strains. *Exp Cell Res.* Mar 1965;37:614-636.

[29] Zhang X, Mar V, Zhou W, Harrington L, Robinson MO. Telomere shortening and apoptosis in telomerase-inhibited human tumor cells. *Genes Dev.* Sep 15 1999;13(18):2388-2399.

[30] Artandi SE, Chang S, Lee SL, et al. Telomere dysfunction promotes non-reciprocal translocations and epithelial cancers in mice. *Nature.* Aug 10 2000;406(6796):641-645.

[31] Cohen SB, Graham ME, Lovrecz GO, Bache N, Robinson PJ, Reddel RR. Protein composition of catalytically active human telomerase from immortal cells. *Science.* Mar 30 2007;315(5820):1850-1853.

[32] Alonso MM, Fueyo J, Shay JW, et al. Expression of transcription factor E2F1 and telomerase in glioblastomas: mechanistic linkage and prognostic significance. *J Natl Cancer Inst.* Nov 2 2005;97(21):1589-1600.

[33] Leber MF, Efferth T. Molecular principles of cancer invasion and metastasis (review). *Int J Oncol.* Apr 2009;34(4):881-895.

[34] Veikkola T, Alitalo K. VEGFs, receptors and angiogenesis. *Semin Cancer Biol.* Jun 1999;9(3):211-220.

[35] Sharp FR, Bernaudin M. HIF1 and oxygen sensing in the brain. *Nat Rev Neurosci.* Jun 2004;5(6):437-448.

[36] Yan H, Parsons DW, Jin G, et al. IDH1 and IDH2 mutations in gliomas. *N Engl J Med.* Feb 19 2009;360(8):765-773.

[37] Yan H, Bigner DD, Velculescu V, Parsons DW. Mutant metabolic enzymes are at the origin of gliomas. *Cancer Res.* Dec 15 2009;69(24):9157-9159.

[38] Zhao S, Lin Y, Xu W, et al. Glioma-derived mutations in IDH1 dominantly inhibit IDH1 catalytic activity and induce HIF-1alpha. *Science.* Apr 10 2009;324(5924):261-265.

[39] Dang L, White DW, Gross S, et al. Cancer-associated IDH1 mutations produce 2-hydroxyglutarate. *Nature.* Dec 10 2009;462(7274):739-744.

[40] Gabellini C, Del Bufalo D, Zupi G. Involvement of RB gene family in tumor angiogenesis. *Oncogene.* Aug 28 2006;25(38):5326-5332.

[41] Hoeben A, Landuyt B, Highley MS, Wildiers H, Van Oosterom AT, De Bruijn EA. Vascular endothelial growth factor and angiogenesis. *Pharmacol Rev.* Dec 2004;56(4):549-580.

[42] Haley JD, Gullick WJ, eds. *EGFR Signaling Networks in Cancer Therapy.* New York: Humana Press; 2008.

[43] Rak J, Mitsuhashi Y, Sheehan C, et al. Oncogenes and tumor angiogenesis: differential modes of vascular endothelial growth factor up-regulation in ras-transformed epithelial cells and fibroblasts. *Cancer Res.* Jan 15 2000;60(2):490-498.

[44] Jacobsen CT, Miller RH. Control of astrocyte migration in the developing cerebral cortex. *Dev Neurosci.* Mar-Aug 2003;25(2-4):207-216.

[45] Ridet JL, Malhotra SK, Privat A, Gage FH. Reactive astrocytes: cellular and molecular cues to biological function. *Trends Neurosci.* Dec 1997;20(12):570-577.

[46] Micallef J, Taccone M, Mukherjee J, et al. Epidermal growth factor receptor variant III-induced glioma invasion is mediated through myristoylated alanine-rich protein kinase C substrate overexpression. *Cancer Res.* Oct 1 2009;69(19):7548-7556.

[47] Muller PA, Caswell PT, Doyle B, et al. Mutant p53 drives invasion by promoting integrin recycling. *Cell.* Dec 24 2009;139(7):1327-1341.

[48] Nakamura JL. The epidermal growth factor receptor in malignant gliomas: pathogenesis and therapeutic implications. *Expert Opin Ther Targets.* Apr 2007;11(4):463-472.

[49] Sherr CJ, McCormick F. The RB and p53 pathways in cancer. *Cancer Cell.* Aug 2002;2(2):103-112.

[50] Vogelstein B, Fearon ER, Hamilton SR, et al. Genetic alterations during colorectal-tumor development. *N Engl J Med.* Sep 1 1988;319(9):525-532.

[51] Gladson CL, Prayson RA, Liu WM. The pathobiology of glioma tumors. *Annu Rev Pathol.* 2010;5:33-50.

[52] Salk JJ, Fox EJ, Loeb LA. Mutational heterogeneity in human cancers: origin and consequences. *Annu Rev Pathol.* 2010;5:51-75.

[53] Nutt CL, Mani DR, Betensky RA, et al. Gene expression-based classification of malignant gliomas correlates better with survival than histological classification. *Cancer Res.* Apr 1 2003;63(7):1602-1607.
[54] Liang Y, Diehn M, Watson N, et al. Gene expression profiling reveals molecularly and clinically distinct subtypes of glioblastoma multiforme. *Proc Natl Acad Sci U S A.* Apr 19 2005;102(16):5814-5819.
[55] Phillips HS, Kharbanda S, Chen R, et al. Molecular subclasses of high-grade glioma predict prognosis, delineate a pattern of disease progression, and resemble stages in neurogenesis. *Cancer Cell.* Mar 2006;9(3):157-173.
[56] Brennan C, Momota H, Hambardzumyan D, et al. Glioblastoma subclasses can be defined by activity among signal transduction pathways and associated genomic alterations. *PLoS One.* 2009;4(11):e7752.
[57] Mischel PS, Shai R, Shi T, et al. Identification of molecular subtypes of glioblastoma by gene expression profiling. *Oncogene.* Apr 17 2003;22(15):2361-2373.
[58] Bar EE, Chaudhry A, Lin A, et al. Cyclopamine-mediated hedgehog pathway inhibition depletes stem-like cancer cells in glioblastoma. *Stem Cells.* Oct 2007;25(10):2524-2533.
[59] Gunther HS, Schmidt NO, Phillips HS, et al. Glioblastoma-derived stem cell-enriched cultures form distinct subgroups according to molecular and phenotypic criteria. *Oncogene.* May 1 2008;27(20):2897-2909.

3

Biological Markers of Recurrence and Survival of High-Grade Gliomas: The Role of Hepatocyte Growth Factor

Roberto García-Navarrete[1,2,3], Esperanza García Mendoza[1], Alfonso Marhx-Bracho[2] and Julio Sotelo[1]
[1]*Neuroimmunology Unit, Instituto Nacional de Neurología y Neurocirugía*
[2]*Neurosurgery Department, Instituto Nacional de Pediatría*
[3]*Hospital General Naval de Alta Especialidad, Armada de México*
México

1. Introduction

Malignant gliomas - the most frequent glial tumor of Central Nervous System (CNS) anaplasic astrocytoma and glioblastoma multiforme, are regarded by the World Health Organization as the form of cancer with the worst prognosis in humans. Its biological behavior and severity are associated with increased concentrations of various growth factors, like fibroblastic growth factor (FGF), vascular endothelial growth factor (VEGF), platelet-derived growth factor (PDGF) and hepatocyte growth factor (HGF).

Hepatocyte growth factor (HGF) is a pleomorphic protein with several properties. It was described in 1996 as a protein related to cell proliferation and motility in the rat liver. It has also been associated with morphogenesis of the central nervous system in mammals. HGF has been associated with proliferation of several cell lines, for example carcinoma of colon, stomach, gallbladder, pancreas, and breast. In human gliomas high intratumoral concentrations of HGF and its receptor c-met are associated with poor prognosis; it has also been associated with long-time recurrence of meningioma. In vitro, transfer of the HGF gene increases tumorigenicity, growth, and angiogenesis; interestingly, inhibition of this gene reduces growth rate and malignancy in experimentally induced-glioma in rats.

Human studies have shown that HGF contents in blood (Wen et al. 2011) are closely related with malignancy of glioma; low-grade glioma shows a lower intratumoral concentration of HGF than high-grade glioma.

Recently, we have found HGF directly related in human gliomas to increased angiogenesis, cellular proliferation, resistance to apoptosis induced by gamma radiation, and invasion of healthy tissue along white matter tracts. All of these features are characteristic of malignancy.

In the clinical setting, high HGF levels in cerebrospinal fluid predict mortality and a short disease-free time in patients with malignant glioma, and helps to explain the great variance observed on survival of patients with malignant glioma, suggesting that HGF inhibition strategies could be a useful means of improving survival and disease-free time among glioma patients.

Thus, experimental and clinical findings suggest that HGF is a good target for therapeutic strategies with pharmacogenomic methods and could be useful as a biological marker for monitoring malignant gliomas activity.

2. Malignant glioma

Intracranial neoplasms include a great diversity of tumors with different histopathologic origins, prognoses and treatments: Malignant gliomas such as anaplasic astrocytoma (AA) and glioblastoma multiforme (GM) are the most frequent glial tumors: their incidence is 4/100,000, and they account for 2% of all malignant tumors in adults. Malignant gliomas are associated with poor prognosis; the mean survival time of patients with GM is one year, this gloomy picture has not changed significantly for the last three decades. Similarly, the survival for patients with AA is minor than three years. Therefore, it is of paramount importance to understand the pathophysiology of malignant glial tumors and identify prognostic factors. Both GM and AA have high proliferation and intense vascularity, features closely related with malignant cell growth.

Malignant conditions are related to ability of malignant cells to produce growth factors such as vascular endothelial growth factor (VEGF), platelet derived growth factor (PDGF), and fibroblastic growth factor (FGF) (Arrieta et al., 2002).

Due to their invasive nature, glioblastomas cannot be resected completely by surgery and, despite the progress of neurosurgical techniques and radio/chemotherapy, less than a half of patients survive more than a year, aged subjects have the most significant adverse prognostic factor.

Glioblastoma is the most frequent malignant tumor of the brain, it account for approximately 12–15% of all intracranial neoplasms and 60-75% of astrocytic tumors (Lantos et al., 2002; Lois et al., 2007). In most European and North American countries, the yearly incidence is in the range of 3-4 new cases per 100 000 population (Lois et al., 2007).

2.1 Prognostic factors

Despite progress in surgery, radiotherapy and chemotherapy of brain tumors, the overall survival of patients with glioblastoma remains dismal. Population-based studies from Switzerland and Canada have shown that less than 20% of patients survive more than one year after diagnosis and less than 3% lived longer than 3 years (Lantos et al., 2002; Ohgaki et al., 2007). Clinical trials show a slightly better prognosis, with median survival rates of approximately 12 month; however, they have strong bias toward the recruitment of younger patients and those with higher preoperative Karnofsky performance scores, both are strong predictors of a more favorable clinical outcome.

Virtually all therapy trials have shown that younger glioblastoma patients (<50 years at diagnosis) have a significantly better prognosis (Lois et al., 2007). In a large population-based study, age was the most significant prognostic factor; persisting through all age groups in a linear manner (Ohgaki et al., 2007). Patients with secondary glioblastoma survived significantly longer than those with primary glioblastoma, but this is likely due to their age rather than a reflection of a different biological behavior.

The prognostic value of TP53 mutations in glioblastomas is controversial, it either shows no association or the presence of TP53 mutations was a favorable prognostic factor. In a large population-based study, the presence of TP53 mutations was predictive of longer survival but this was not significant when adjusted for younger age.

There is no consistent correlation of epidermal growth factor receptor (EGFR) amplification with survival largely irrespective of the age at first clinical manifestation. LOH 10 (Lois et al., 2007) is the most frequent genetic alteration in glioblastoma and is associated with reduced survival. The presence of PTEN mutations is not associated with prognosis of glioblastoma patients (Lois et al., 2007).
Since the initial histological description of astrocytic neoplasms, several efforts have been made to identify biomarkers that could predict the biological behavior of the tumor. However, to date only few peptides been identified substances that show a weak association with prognosis.

3. Biological markers of glioblastoma activity

The following paragraphs describe some substances that have been reported as candidates for surveillances of tumor activity by measuring their contents in serum.
A molecular event determining the development of malignancy is the activation of b-catenin, a protein necessary for the alignment and maintenance of epithelial cells by regulating cell growth and cell adhesion. The coexpression of α-catenin reduces the cellular growth and migration induced by EGF on human glioma cells (Ji et al., 2010).
A secreted protein of unknown function, YKL-40 (chitinase-3-like-1), is overexpressed in glioblastoma [4], its presence is associated with LOH 10q (Lois et al., 2007), poorer radiation response, shorter time to tumor progression and reduced overall survival (Ohgaki et al., 2004). It is typically coexpressed with matrix metalloproteinase-9 (MMP-9), and its detection in serum has been used to monitor patients with recurrent tumor growth (Pelloski et al., 2005). One report showed that increased expression of GD3 synthase mRNA, in combination with decreased GalNAcT, correlate with an increased survival of patients with glioblastoma (Hormingo et al. 2006).

3.1 Growth factors

The expression of growth factors and their receptors are associated with glioma malignancy. Thus, their potential therapeutic importance has been demonstrated using specific inhibitors of growth factors in experimental and clinical studies. However, recent results have shown that glioma cells are resistant to this treatment and illustrate the therapeutic difficulties in malignant gliomas.

3.2 Vascular endothelial growth factor

Vascular endothelial growth factor (VEGF) is a signal protein that stimulates vasculogenesis and angiogenesis; VEGF's normal function is to induce growth of vessels during early developmental stages, after injury, at muscle following exercise, and to generate new vessels to bypass blocked arteries. When VEGF is overexpressed, it can contribute to malignant glioma progression. Cancers that express VEGF grow and metastasize, VEGF belongs to platelet-derived growth factor family. They are involved in both, vasculogenesis, the novo, and angiogenesis (Mentlein et al., 2004; Reux et al., 2006).
Within the major growth factors related to angiogenesis, VEGF is one of the most important. In several tumors, VEGF plays a pivotal role for vascularization necessary to supply the malignant tissue with oxygen and nutrients. Human glioma cells are characterized by high production of VEGF, however, functional and autocrine growth stimulatory effects on glioma cells are minor (Reux et al., 2006).

In recurrent GBM trials with temozolomide shown a poor therapeutic response where as VEGF inhibitors as bevacizumab, improve the response rate by 25% to 74%, and the period-free of symptoms increases by 32% to 64%, which is superior to the rate reported for temozolomide alone (Pope et al., 2006; Guiu et al., 2008; Narayana et al., 2009; Nghiemphu et al., 2009; Poulsen et al., 2009; Zuniga et al., 2009). The main effect of VEGF inhibitors is centered on rapid reduction in peritumoral edema, improving corticosteroid use. These studies also indicated that bevacizumab treatment is well tolerated and the risk of intratumoral hemorrhage is low. Toxicity related to bevacizumab therapy in patients with malignant glioma includes hypertension, proteinuria, fatigue, thromboembolic events, and wound-healing delay.

3.2.1 Epidermal growth factor

Epidermal growth factor (EGF), is a prototype member of the EGF-family of peptides which have highly similar structural and functional characteristics. Other peptides include: Transforming Growth Factor-α (TGF-α), amphiregulin, epiregulin, and neuregulin 1-4, all of them related to tyrosine kinase activity which initiates a signal transduction cascade that result in several changes: rise in intracellular calcium contents, increased glycolysis, protein synthesis, DNA synthesis and cell proliferation (Fallon et al., 1984).

EGF is overexpressed in various cancers; malignant glioma, breast, pancreas and liver carcinoma, indicating its main role in malignant cell transformation, tumor occurrence and growth by promoting cell division (Xian et al., 2001). Recent reports show that +61G polymorphism of EGF gene increase the risk for glioma development in European subjects but are a protective factor in Chinese subjects (Tan et al., 2010).

The Epidermal growth factor receptor (EGFR) gene is amplified and overexpressed in approximately 40% of patients with primary GBMs. Increased EGFR signaling drives tumor cell proliferation, invasiveness, motility, angiogenesis, and inhibition of apoptosis. Attempts to identify biomarkers to help predict response to EGFR inhibitors have yielded conflicting results. Currently, there is no convincing evidence of a correlation between EGFR expression in tumoral tissue and prognosis (Van Meir et al., 2010).

3.2.2 Hepatocyte growth factor

Hepatocyte growth factor (HGF), also called scatter factor, is a multifunction protein with strong mitogenic effect on hepatocytes. It was initially isolated as a peptide related to hepatic regeneration. It is considered a reliable indicator of hepatic function alter hepatectomy. This protein is constituted by a heavy chain (60 kD) with four domains and a Light chain (32 kD); it binds through its tirosine-kinase receptor, a product of the proto-oncogene c-Met. Hepatocyte growth factor, secreted by mesenchymal cells, acts as a paracrine effector on different epithelial cells inducing mitogenesis and stimulating cellular motility. It is also a powerful angiogenic factor for endothelial cells in vitro and in vivo. In the liver and kidney, it may have a role as antiapoptotic (Xiao et al., 2001). It is also necessary for embriogenesis as regulator of cell migration and growth. Hepatocyte growth factor is also produced by other cells, such as osteoclasts, participating in the regulation of bone remodeling; its production by monocytes has a role in the regulation of hematopoyesis by stimulation of growth and differentiation of erythroid precursors (Arrieta et al., 2002).

Knockout mice for the HGF gene develop severe abnormalities in the liver, placenta, and nervous system causing fetal death. A direct genetic relation between HGF and cancer has also been recently proposed due to mutations in the catalytic domain of c-Met from patients with renal carcinoma. Overexpression of HGF is present in various cells lines of leukemia and lymphoma and in solid tumors of the breast, prostate, colon, liver, kidney, uterine cervix, endometrium, and bladder (Arrieta et al., 2002). Hepatocyte growth factor also promotes adhesion and migration of cancer cells, due to the high affinity of integrins to their ligands, a phenomenon related to the metastatic tendency of carcinomas (Trussolino et al., 2000; Arrieta et al., 2002).

Normal human astrocytes express HGF and its receptor c-Met (Yamada et al, 1994). Met is a proto-oncogene that when mutated can transform a variety of cell types; the Met receptor is a heterodimer consisting of an extracellular alpha chain and a trans-membrane beta chain, which is a tyrosine kinase, it is widely expressed by epithelial and endothelial cells as well as melanocytes, chondrocytes, skeletal muscle, hematopoietic, lymphoid, and neural cells. The activation of Met by HGF binding is linked to cell growth and survival, including the avoidance of anoikis which is apoptosis induced by insufficient association with cell-matrix, through activation of both the PI3-kinase/PDK/Akt and the Ras/Raf/MEK/ERK pathways and to cell mobility and cytoskeletal organization via activation of the Rho-GTPases, Rho, Rac and CDC (Arrieta et al., 2002).

Activation of Met tyrosine kinase also activates phospholipase C, resulting in the elevation of intracellular calcium and activation of conventional and novel protein kinase C pathways. HGF and Met have been associated with progression, invasiveness and metastasis in a number of neoplasms. Met is expressed in a wide variety of carcinomas, musculoskeletal tumors, soft tissue sarcomas, glioblastoma, astrosarcoma, and several hematopoietic malignancies. HGF Met signaling is a major potential target for the development of cancer therapeutics.

3.2.2.1 Hepatocyte growth factor and malignant gliomas

As HGF, its receptor c-met has been implicated in the genesis, malignant progression, and chemo/radioresistance of multiple human malignancies, including gliomas (Peruzzi et al, 2006; Carapancea et al, 2009; Hadjipanayis et al, 2009a, 2009b). Experimental studies using transient expression of anti-SF/HGF and anti-c-met U1snRNA/ribozymes suppress SF/HGF and c-met expression, c-met receptor activation, tumor cell migration, and anchorage-independent colony formation in vitro. The delivery of U1snRNA/ribozymes to established subcutaneous glioma xenografts via liposome-DNA complexes significantly inhibited tumor growth as well as tumor SF/HGF and c-met expression levels. Histological analysis of tumors treated showed a significant decrease in blood vessel density, increase in activation of the pro-apoptotic enzyme caspase-3, and increase in tumor cell apoptosis. Treatment of animals bearing intracranial glioma xenografts with anti-SF/HGF and anti-c-met U1snRNA/ribozymes substantially inhibited tumor growth and promoted animal survival (Abounander et al, 1999, 2002; Kim et al, 2006).

The use of monoclonal antibodies against the NK23 and NK422 domains of the HGF reduce tumor growth and mitotic rate (Bhargava et al., 1992; Boros et al., 1995; Kimura et al., 1995; Miwa et al., 1997; Neaud et al., 1997; Takeuchi et al 1997; Stella et al., 1999; Grierson et al., 2000; Cao et al, 2001; Brockmann et al, 2003; Burgess et al, 2006); Also, viral transgenes against HGF-RNA reduce invasion of white matter tracts, improving response to radiotherapy (Lal et al, 2005; Chu et al, 2006).

The therapeutic efficacy of SGX523 has recently been proven in human brain tumors. It seems that SGX523 inhibits c-Met, AKT and MAPK phosphorylation, cell proliferation, cell cycle progression, migration and invasion in different human glioblastoma cell lines, glioblastoma primary cells, glioblastoma stem cells and medulloblastoma cell lines. Importantly, oral administration of SGX523 to mice bearing intracranial human glioma xenografts led to inhibition of tumor growth in vivo. This experimental data suggests that c-Met kinase inhibition is a feasible and promising approach for brain tumor therapy (Guessous et al., 2010).

4. HGF and gliomas on clinical setting

Hepatocyte growth factor and its receptor (c-Met) have been detected in normal astrocytes as well as in human gliomas, and other malignant tumors (Koochekpour et al., 1995; Nabeshima et al., 1997; Hirose et al., 1998). In human cultured glioma cells, HGF and c-Met are simultaneously expressed, with an autocrinous effect inducing cell proliferation and migration.

Recent findings suggest that HGF contributes to glioma progression, inducing angiogenesis and expression of additional angiogenic autocrine factors such as VEGF (Laterra et al., 1997; Lamszus et al., 1999; Moriyama et al., 1999; Schmidt et al., 1999). The overexpression of HGF and its receptor c-Met increases cell motility and proliferation of human glioma cells in vitro (Koochekpour et al., 1995).

Intratumoral concentration of HGF in malignant gliomas is greatly increased in comparison with other intracranial tumors and nontumoral brain tissue (Arrieta et al., 2002); it is also related to cell proliferation and peritumoral edema, showing its participation in the pathogenesis of these tumors.

A common cause of failure of treatment of malignant gliomas is resistance to radiotherapy and chemotherapy; the mechanism by which the cell survives to therapeutic attempts involves the production of growth factors that regulate DNA repair and apoptosis. In vitro and in vivo, HGF inhibits drug-induced cytotoxicity and apoptosis in experimental neoplasms treated by radiation, cisplatin, and camptothencin (Bowers et al., 2000); this effect might decrease the therapeutic response of patients with high intratumoral contents of HGF.

There is intense infiltration by microglia in gliomas, which may enhance malignancy by secretion of epidermal growth factor and by inhibition of cytotoxic lymphocytes (Wood et al., 1983); in vitro HGF stimulates the microglial infiltration of gliomas, favoring their growth (Badie et al., 1999).

The direct correlation of cell proliferation with the presence of HGF supports its participation in the promotion of tumoral growth of glioma, as has been shown for other tumors such as breast carcinoma (Lamszus et al., 1997).

The mechanism by which HGF stimulates cell proliferation seems to be related to the tirosine kinase activity of its receptor, which involves Ras and mitosis activation proteins (Arrieta et al., 2002). Such effects can be antagonized by tirosine kinase inhibitors. However, not all HGF effects require phosphorylation of its receptor; for instance, its antiapoptotic effect is independent, suggesting that it could also participate in the genesis of the tumor. The insertion of the HGF gene in human glioma cells increases proliferation of independent colonies in vitro and tumorigenesis in vivo (Laterra et al., 1997).

There are some histological features of malignant glioma associated with prognosis, such as the extent of necrosis or vascular density (Barker et al., 1996). Hepatocyte growth factor is a strong inductor of angiogenesis; its effects are synergistic with other growth factors such as VEGF and bFGF. Intratumoral concentration of HGF shows a direct relation with peritumoral edema, independent of vascular density. Previous studies have shown that HGF increases the permeability of the hematoencephalic barrier, independently of VEGF expression, possibly by the induction of endothelial fenestrations and by the tumoral expression of proteases such as urokinase and extracellular matrix metalloproteinases (Book et al., 1999).

A paracrine loop for HGF effects related with migration of tumor cells along white matter has been described. The increase of HGF in CSF observed may therefore reflect either the transport of HGF from brain parenchyma to the ventricular system or the diffusion of HGF along the subarachnoid space (Garcia-Navarrete et al., 2010).

HGF concentration is closely related with malignancy of glioma; low-grade glioma shows a lower intratumoral concentration of HGF than high-grade glioma. CSF concentrations of HGF greater than 850 pg/ml prior to surgery was predictive of a shorter disease-free time among malignant glioma patients than was observed for patients with a lower concentration (6 ± 0.6 months (95% [CI], 5–7) vs. 9 ± 0.5 months (95% [CI], 8–10), respectively, $p< 0.001$), besides total-gross resection surgery (Garcia-Navarrete et al., 2010). CSF concentration of HGF shows a negative correlation with survival of patients with malignant glioma and explains with high certainty the variance for survival. This suggests that HGF could be a good target candidate for molecular therapy such as RNA interference, by silencing the specific gene for HGF.

Although HGF seems a good target for therapeutic attempts, a phase II study reported the use of a monoclonal antibody against HGF (AMD 102). This study was conducted in patients with histopathologically confirmed diagnosis of GBM, gliosarcoma and history of more than 3 relapses; increases up to 10 times the basal levels of HGF in patients during treatment with AMD did not induce changes in survival time or clinical status as compared with controls (Wen et al., 2011)

5.Conclusions

To date, there is no biological marker that can accurately discern the activity of malignant gliomas. The scientific evidence obtained from experimental studies suggests that Hepatocyte Growth Factor plays a crucial role in the pathophysiology of high-grade gliomas. Findings from clinical studies suggest that HGF may be considered a distinguishing marker of biological activity of malignant gliomas, as it has been consistently demonstrated that the intratumoral, cerebrospinal fluid and serum concentrations are directly associated with prognosis and survival. The results of clinical trials aimed to evaluate the role of inhibitors of HGF or its receptor c-Met have shown disappointing therapeutic results. However, scientific advances in molecular biology could improve the response to treatment with specific inhibitors of HGF metabolism through ingenious genomic manipulations in patients with malignant gliomas.

6. References

Abounader R, Lal B, Luddy C, Koe G, Davidson B, Rosen EM, Laterra J (2002) In vivo targeting of SF/HGF and c-met expression via U1snRNA/ribozymes inhibits glioma growth and angiogenesis and promotes apoptosis. FASEB J. Vol. 16, No. 1, pp. 108–10. PMID - 11729097

Abounader R, Ranganathan S, Lal B, Fielding K, Book A, Dietz H, Burger P, Laterra J (1999). Reversion of human glioblastoma malignancy by U1 small nuclear RNA/ribozyme targeting of scatter factor/hepatocyte growth factor and c-met expression. *J Natl Cancer Inst.* Vol. 91, No. 18, pp. 1548–56. PMID - 10491431

Arrieta O, Garcia E, Guevara P, Garcia-Navarrete R, Ondarza R, Rembao D, Sotelo J. (2002). Hepatocyte growth factor is associated with poor prognosis of malignant gliomas and is a predictor for recurrence of meningioma. *Cancer.* Vol. 15, No. 94, 3210-8. PMID- 12115353

Badie B, Schartner J, Klaver J, Vorphal J. (1999). In vitro modulation of microglia by glioma cells is mediated by hepatocyte growth factor/scatter factor. *Neurosurgery.* Vol. 44, No. 5, pp. 1077–82. PMID - 10232541

Barker FG 2nd, Davis RL, Chang SM, Prados MD. (1996). Necrosis as a prognostic factor in glioblastoma multiforme. *Cancer.* Vol. 77, No. 6, pp. 1161–66. PMID - 8635139

Bhargava M, Joseph A, Knesel J, Halaban R, Li Y, Pang S, Goldberg I, Setter E, Donovan MA, Zarnegar R, Michalopoulos GA, Nakamura T, Faletto D, Rosen EM.. (1992). Scatter factor and hepatocyte growth factor: activities, properties and mechanism. *Cell Growth Differ.* Vol. 3, No. 1, pp.11–20. PMID - 1534687

Boros P, Miller CM. Hepatocyte growth factor: a multifunctional cytokine. *Lancet.* Vol. 345, No. 8945, pp. 293–95. PMID - 7837864

Bowers DC, Fan S, Walter KA, Abounader R, Williams JA, Rosen EM, Laterra J. (2000). Scatter factor/hepatocyte growth factor protects against cytotoxic death in human glioblastoma via phosphatidylinositol 3-kinase- and AKT-dependent pathways. *Cancer Res.* Vol. 60, No. 15, pp. 4277–83. PMID - 10945642

Brockmann MA, Papadimitriou A, Brandt M, Fillbrandt R, Westphal M, Lamszus K (2003) Inhibition of intracerebral glioblastoma growth by local treatment with the scatter factor/hepatocyte growth factor-antagonist NK4. *Clin Cancer Res.* Vol. 9, No.12, pp. 4578–85. PMID - 14555533

Burgess T, Coxon A, Meyer S, Sun J, Rex K, Tsuruda T, Chen Q, Ho SY, Li L, Kaufman S, McDorman K, Cattley RC, Sun J, Elliott G, Zhang K, Feng X, Jia XC, Green L, Radinsky R, Kendall R (2006). Fully human monoclonal antibodies to hepatocyte growth factor with therapeutic potential against hepatocyte growth factor/c-Met-dependent human tumors. *Cancer Res.* Vol. 66, No. 3, pp. 1721–29. PMID - 16452232

Bussolino F, Di Renzo MF, Ziche M, et al. Hepatocyte growth factor is a potent angiogenic factor which stimulated endothelial cell motility and growth. *J Cell Biol.* Vol. 119, No. 2, pp. 629–41. PMID - 1383237

Cao B, Su Y, Oskarsson M, Zhao P, Kort EJ, Fisher RJ, Wang LM, Vande Woude GF (2001). Neutralizing monoclonal antibodies to hepatocyte growth factor/scatter factor (HGF/SF) display antitumor activity in animal models. *Proc Natl Acad Sci USA.* Vol. 98, No. 13, pp. 7443–48. PMID - 11416216

Carapancea M, Alexandru O, Fetea AS, Dragutescu L, Castro J, Georgescu A, Popa-Wagner A, Bäcklund ML, Lewensohn R, Dricu A. (2009). Growth factor receptors signaling in glioblastoma cells: therapeutic implications. *J Neurooncol.* Vol. 92, No. 2, pp. 137-47. PMID - 19043776

Chu SH, Zhu ZA, Yuan XH, Li ZQ, Jiang PC (2006). In vitro and in vivo potentiating the cytotoxic effect of radiation on human U251 gliomas by the c-Met antisense oligodeoxynucleotides. *J Neurooncol.* Vol. 80, No. 2, pp. 143–9. PMID - 16648987

Dreux AC, Lamb DJ, Modjtahedi H, Ferns GA (2006). The epidermal growth factor receptors and their family of ligands: their putative role in atherogenesis. *Atherosclerosis*. Vol. 186, No. 1, pp. 38–53. PMID - 15072443

Fallon JH, Seroogy KB, Loughlin SE, Morrison RS, Bradshaw RA, Knaver DJ, Cunningham DD (1984). Epidermal growth factor immunoreactive material in the central nervous system: location and development. *Science*. Vol. 224, No. 4653, pp. 1107–9. PMID - 6144184

Grierson I, Heathcote L, Hiscott P, Hogg P, Briggs M, Hagan S. (2000). Hepatocyte growth factor/scatter factor in the eye. *Prog Retin Eye Res*. Vol. 19, No. 6, pp. 779–802. PMID - 11029554

Guessous F, Zhang Y, diPierro C, Marcinkiewicz L, Sarkaria J, Schiff D, Buchanan S, Abounader R. (2010). An orally bioavailable c-Met kinase inhibitor potently inhibits brain tumor malignancy and growth. *Anticancer Agents Med Chem*. Vol. 10, No. 1, pp. 28-35. PMID - 20015006

Guiu S, Taillibert S, Chinot O, Taillandier L, Honnorat J, Dietrich PY, Maire JP, Guillamo JS, Guiu B, Catry-Thomas I, Capelle F, Thiebaut A, Cartalat-Carel S, Deville C, Fumoleau P, Desjardins A, Xuan KH, Chauffert B. (2008). Bevacizumab/irinotecan. An active treatment for recurrent high-grade gliomas: preliminary results of an ANOCEF multi-center study. *Rev Neurol (Paris)*. Vol. 164, No. 7, pp. 588–94. PMID - 1856535

Hadjipanayis CG, Van Meir EG. (2009a). Brain cancer propagating cells: biology, genetics and targeted therapies. *Trends Mol Med*. Vol. 14, No. 11, pp. 519–30. PMID - 19889578

Hadjipanayis CG, Van Meir EG. (2009b). Tumor initiating cells in malignant gliomas: biology and implications for therapy. *J Mol Med*. Vol. 87, No. 4, pp. 363–74. PMID - 19189072

Hirose Y, Kojima M, Sagoh M, Murakami H, Yoshida K, Shimazaki K, Kawase T. (1998). Immunohistochemical examination of c-Met protein expression in astrocytic tumors. *Acta Neuropathol (Berl)*. Vol. 95, No. 4, pp. 345–51. PMID - 9560011

Hormigo A, Gu B, Karimi S, Riedel E, Panageas KS, Edgar MA, Tanwar MK, Rao JS, Fleisher M, DeAngelis LM, Holland EC (2006). YKL-40 and matrix metalloproteinase-9 as potential serum biomarkers for patients with high-grade gliomas. *Clin Cancer Res* Vol. 12, No. 19, pp 5698-5704. PMID - 17020973

Ji H, Wang J, Fang B, Fang X, Lu Z. (2010). a-Catenin inhibits glioma cell migration, invasion, and proliferation by suppression of b-catenin transactivation. *J Neurooncol*. (Epub ahead of print). PMID - 20872274

Kim KJ, Wang L, Su YC, Gillespie GY, Salhotra A, Lal B, Laterra J (2006). Systemic anti-hepatocyte growth factor monoclonal antibody therapy induces the regression of intracraneal glioma xenografts. *Clin Cancer Res*. Vol. 12, No. 4, pp. 1292–98. PMID - 16489086

Kimura F, Miyazaki M, Suwa T, Kakizaki S, Itoh H, Kaiho T, Ambiru S, Shimizu H, Togawa A. (1996). Increased levels of human hepatocyte growth factor in serum and peritoneal fluid after partial hepatectomy. *Am J Gastroenterol*. Vol. 91, No. 1, pp. 116–21. PMID - 8561110

Koochekpour S, Jeffers M, Rulong S, Taylor G, Klineberg E, Hudson EA, Resau JH, Vande Woude GF. (1997). Met and hepatocyte growth factor/scatter factor expression in human gliomas. *Cancer Res.* Vol. 57, No. 23, pp. 5391–98. PMID - 9393765

Lal B, Xia S, Abounader R, Laterra J (2005). Targeting the c-Met pathway potentiates glioblastoma responses to gamma-radiation. *Clin Cancer Res.* Vol. 11, No. 12, pp. 4479–86. PMID - 15958633

Lamszus K, Jin L, Fuchs A, Shi E, Chowdhury S, Yao Y, Polverini PJ, Laterra J, Goldberg ID, Rosen EM. (1997). Scatter factor stimulates tumor growth and tumor angiogenesis in human breast cancers in the mammary fat pads of nude mice. *Lab Invest.* Vol. 76, No. 3, pp. 339–53. PMID - 9121117

Lamszus K, Laterra J, Westphal M, Rosen E. (1999). Scatter factor/ hepatocyte growth factor (SF/HGF) content and function in human gliomas. *Int J Dev Neurosci.* Vol. 17, No. 5-6, pp. 517–30. PMID - 10571413

Lantos PL, Louis DN, Rosenblum MK, Kleihues P (2002). Tumours of the Nervous System. *Oxford University Press*: London.

Laterra J, Rosen E, Nam M, Ranganathan S, Fielding K, Johnston P. (1997). Scatter factor/hepatocyte growth factor expression enhances human glioma tumorigenicity and growth. *Biochem Biophys Res Commun.* Vol. 235, No. 3, pp. 743–7. PMID - 9207232

Louis D.N., Ohgaki H., Wiestler O.D., Cavenee W.K. (2007) WHO Classification of Tumours of the Central Nervous System. *IARC*: Lyon 2007.

Mentlein R, Forstreuter F, Mehdorn HM, Held-Feindt J. (2004). Functional significance of vascular endothelial growth factor receptor expression on human glioma cells. *J Neurooncol.* Vol. 67, No. 1-2, pp. 9-18. PMID - 15072443

Miwa Y, Harrison PM, Farzaneh F, Langley PG, Williams R, Hudges RD. Plasma levels and hepatic mRNA expression of transforming factor-beta 1 in patients with hepatic fulminant failure. *J Hepatol.* Vol. 27, No. 5, pp. 780–88. PMID - 9382963

Moriyama T, Kataoka H, Koono M, Wakaisaka S. (1999). Expression of hepatocyte growth factor/scatter factor and its receptor c-Met in brain tumors: evidence for a role in progression of astrocytic tumors. *Int J Mol Med.* Vol. 3, No. 5, pp. 531–36. PMID - 10202187

Nabeshima K, Shimao Y, Sato S, Kataoka H, Moriyama T, Kawano H, Wakisaka S, Koono M. (1997). Expression of c-Met correlates with grade of malignancy in human astrocytic tumours: an immunohistochemical study. *Histopathology.* Vol. 31, No. 5, pp. 436–43. PMID - 9416484

Narayana A, Kelly P, Golfinos J, Parker E, Johnson G, Knopp E, Zagzag D, Fischer I, Raza S, Medabalmi P, Eagan P, Gruber ML. (2009). Antiangiogenic therapy using bevacizumab in recurrent high-grade glioma: impact on local control and patient survival. *J Neurosurg.* Vol. 110, No. 1, pp. 173–180. PMID - 18834263

Neaud V, Faouzi S, Guirouilh J, Le Bail B, Balabaud C, Bioulac-Sage P, Rosenbaum J. (1997). Human hepatic myofibroblast increase invasiveness of hepatocellular carcinoma cells: evidence for a role of hepatocyte growth factor. *Hepatology.* Vol. 26, No. 6, pp. 1458–66. PMID - 9397985

Nghiemphu PL, Liu W, Lee Y, Than T, Graham C, Lai A, Green RM, Pope WB, Liau LM, Mischel PS, Nelson SF, Elashoff R, Cloughesy TF. (2009). Bevacizumab and chemotherapy for recurrent glioblastoma: a single-institution experience. *Neurology*. Vol. 72, No. 14, pp. 1217–22. PMID - 19349600

Oblinger JL, Pearl DK, Boardman CL, Saqr H, Prior TW, Scheithauer BW, Jenkins RB, Burger PC, Yates AJ (2006). Diagnostic and prognostic value of glycosyltransferase mRNA in glioblastoma multiforme patients. *Neuropathol Appl Neurobiol*. Vol. 32, No. 4, pp. 410-18. PMID - 16866986

Ohgaki H, Dessen P, Jourde B, Horstmann S, Nishikawa T, Di Patre PL, Burkhard C, Schuler D, Probst-Hensch NM, Maiorka PC, Baeza N, Pisani P, Yonekawa Y, Yasargil MG, Lutolf UM, Kleihues P (2004). Genetic pathways to glioblastoma: a population-based study. *Cancer Res*, Vol. 64, No. 19, pp. 6892-99. PMID - 15466178

Ohgaki H, Kleihues P (2007). Genetic pathways to primary and secondary glioblastoma. *Am J Pathol*, Vol. 170, No. 5, pp 1445-53. PMID - 17456751

Pelloski CE, Mahajan A, Maor M, Chang EL, Woo S, Gilbert M, Colman h, Yang H, Ledoux A, Blair H, Passe S, Jenkins RB, Aldape KD (2005). YKL-40 expression is associated with poorer response to radiation and shorter overall survival in glioblastoma. *Clin Cancer Res*. Vol. 11, No. 9, pp. 3326-34. PMID - 15867231

Peruzzi, B. and Bottaro, D.P. (2006). Targeting the c-Met signaling pathway in cancer. *Clin. Cancer Res*. Vol. 12, No. 12, pp. 3657-60. PMID - 16778093

Pope WB, Lai A, Nghiemphu P, Mischel P, Cloughesy TF. (2006). MRI in patients with high-grade gliomas treated with bevacizumab and chemotherapy. *Neurology*. Vol. 66, No. 8, pp. 1258–60. PMID - 16636248

Poulsen HS, Grunnet K, Sorensen M, Olsen P, Hasselbalch B, Nelausen K, Kosteljanetz M, Lassen U. (2009). Bevacizumab plus irinotecan in the treatment patients with progressive recurrent malignant brain tumours. *Acta Oncol*. Vol. 48, No. 1, pp. 52–58. PMID - 19031176

Schmidt NO, Westphal M, Hagel C, Ergün S, Stavrou D, Rosen EM, Lamszus K. (1999). Levels of vascular endothelial growth factor, hepatocyte growth factor/scatter factor and basic fibroblast growth factor in human gliomas and their relation to angiogenesis. *Int J Cancer*. Vol. 84, No. 1, pp. 10-18. PMID - 9988225

Stella MC, Comoglio PM. (1999). HGF: a multifunctional growth factor controlling cell scattering. *Int J Biochem Cell Biol*. Vol. 31, No. 12, pp. 1357–62. PMID - 10641789

Takeuchi E, Nimura Y, Nagino M, Kurumiya Y, Maeda A, Kamiya J, Kondo S, Kanai M, Miyachi M, Uesaka K, Yoshida S. (1997). Human hepatocyte growth factor in bile: an indicator of posthepatectomy liver function in patients with biliary tract carcinoma. *Hepatology*. Vol. 26, No. 5, pp. 1092–99. PMID - 9362347

Tan D, Xu J, Li Y, Lai R. (2010). Association between +61G polymorphism of the EGF gene and glioma risk in different ethnicities: a meta-analysis. *Tohoku J Exp Med*. Vol. 222, No. 4, pp. 229-35. PMID – 21123997

Trusolino L, Cavassa S, Angelini P, Andó M, Bertotti A, Comoglio PM, Boccaccio C. (2000). HGF/scatter factor selectively promotes cell invasion by increasing integrin avidity. *FASEB J*. Vol. 14, No. 11, pp. 1629–40. PMID - 10928998

Van Meir EG, Hadjipanayis CG, Norden AD, Shu HK, Wen PY, Olson JJ.. (2010). Exciting New Advances in Neuro-Oncology: The Avenue to a Cure for Malignant Glioma. *CA Cancer J Clin*. Vol. 60, No. 3, pp 166–193. PMID - 20445000

Wen PY, Schiff D, Cloughesy TF, Raizer JJ, Laterra J, Smitt M, Wolf M, Oliner KS, Anderson A, Zhu M, Loh E, Reardon DA. (2011). A phase II study evaluating the efficacy and safety of AMG 102 (rilotumumab) in patients with recurrent glioblastoma. *Neuro Oncol.* Vol. 13, No. 4, pp. 437-46. PMID - 21297127

Wood GW, Morantz RA. (1983). Depressed T lymphocyte function in brain tumor patients: monocytes as suppressor cells. *J Neurooncol.* Vol. 1, No. 2, pp. 87–94. PMID - 6236289

Xian CJ, Li L, Deng YS, Zhao SP, Zhou XF. (2001). Lack of effects of transforming growth factor-alpha gene knockout on peripheral nerve regeneration may result from compensatory mechanisms. *Exp Neurol.* Vol. 172, No. 1, pp. 182-8. PMID - 11681850

Xiao G, Jeffers M, Bellacosa A, Mitsuuchi Y, Vande Woude G, Testa J. (2001). Anti-apoptotic signaling by hepatocyte growth factor/Met via the phosphatidylinositol 3-kinase/Akt and mitogen activated protein kinase pathways. Proc Natl Acad Sci. Vol.98, No. 1, pp. 247–52. PMID - 11134526

Yamada T, Tsubouchi H, Daikuhara Y, Prat M, Comoglio PM, McGeer PL, McGeer (1994). Immunohistochemistry with antibodies to hepatocyte growth factor and its receptor protein (c-Met) in human brain tissues. *Brain Res.* Vol. 637, No. 1-2, pp. 308–12. PMID - 8180811

Zuniga RM, Torcuator R, Jain R, Anderson J, Doyle T, Ellika S, Schultz L, Mikkelsen T.. (2009). Efficacy, safety and patterns of response and recurrence in patients with recurrent high-grade gliomas treated with bevacizumab plus irinotecan.*J Neurooncol.* Vol. 91, No. 3, pp. 329–36. PMID - 18953493

4

Biomarker Discovery, Validation and Clinical Application for Patients Diagnosed with Glioma

Kerrie L. McDonald
Cure For Life Neuro-oncology Group, University of NSW
Australia

1. Introduction

Combined radiotherapy and chemotherapy with the alkylating agent, temozolomide plus an additional six cycles of temozolomide has been the mainstay of treatment for patients diagnosed with glioblastoma for the past 6 years. Clinically, high variability in the response to this treatment is typically observed, with some patients enjoying progression free survival for longer than others. However, tumour relapse is inevitable in the majority of patients. Local tumour recurrence, occurring within 2-3cm of the original resection cavity (the area exposed to radiation treatment) is most frequently observed. *Relapsed glioblastomas are typically unmanageable with median survival after recurrence of only a few months (Brandes et al. 2001).* Numerous chemotherapeutic agents have been trialled in patients with recurrent glioblastomas and include enzastaurin (Wick et al. 2010), immunotherapeutic targeting of EGFRvIII (Sampson et al. 2011), cilengitide (trial ongoing) (Reardon et al. 2011), NovoTTF-100A (trial ongoing), gefitinib (Uhm et al. 2010), imatinib (Dresemann et al. 2010), bevacizumab plus irinotecan (Vredenburgh et al. 2007). Only bevacizumab has shown promise for the treatment of recurrent glioblastoma, although the benefits of such a drug are still debatable. The Food and Drug Administration (FDA) in the USA approved bevacizumab for GBM under its accelerated approval process. However in Europe, the Committee for Medicinal Products for Human Use (CHMP) adopted a negative opinion.

As new therapeutic regimes are developed, it is paramount that we develop a strategy for identifying the patients that will show a positive response to treatment. The recognition and validation of biomarkers of clinical response is important for several reasons: to avoid unnecessary toxicity in patients that fail to respond to the particular treatment; to reduce the colossal cost to healthcare which is typically associated with targeted therapy and most importantly, to better understand drug resistance. This improved knowledge could lead to new strategies to overcome the initial resistance and identify synergistic drug combinations.

1.1 Prognostic and predictive biomarkers

Hopes for progressing curative treatment programs for cancer patients centre on the development and successful implementation of personalised medicine. Personalised medicine hinges on biomarkers which are highly sensitive and highly specific in revealling information that is relevant for diagnosis, prognosis and therapy. The most sought after biomarkers are the ones that can identify which patients are at high risk of tumour relapse and developing cytotoxicity to specific chemotherapeutic agents. The use of biomarkers to identify patients who don't respond to treatment early could confer enormous benefits for patients diagnosed with glioblastoma, especially considering the short survival time. Many biomarkers have shown excellent utility in survival prognostication but not necessarily at the level of influencing an oncologist's decision to administer a specific drug or alter the treatment schedule (Figure 1). In addition, another challenge in oncology is the translation of prospective biomarkers from the lab into validated diagnostic tests.

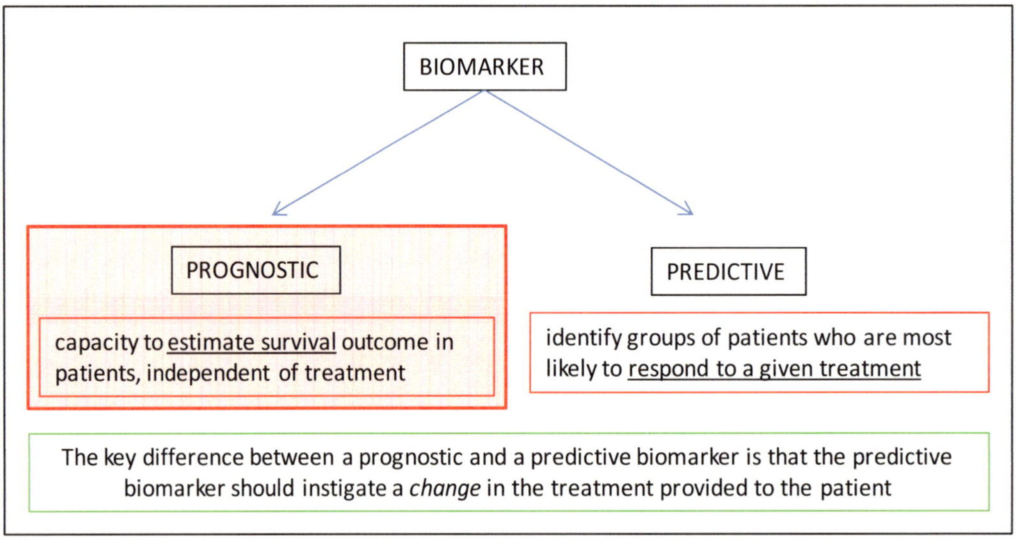

Fig. 1. Schematic overview of the key difference between biomarkers with prognostic and predictive qualities. Prognostic markers are more common in glioblastoma.

Most biomarkers often have both prognostic and predictive value. There is no strict rule when it comes to what constitutes a biomarker. A marker can consist of genomic and proteomic patterns, single genes or proteins, chromosomal abnormalities, epigenetic signatures, aberrant microRNA as well as imaging changes observed on a MRI or PET scan. A **prognostic marker** has the capacity to **estimate survival** outcome in patients, independent of treatment. The genetic profiling of large tumour cohorts with comprehensive clinical and survival data have promoted the discovery of novel molecular biomarkers associated with survival, in addition to traditional clinical and morphological features. Examples of biomarkers with prognostic significance include amplification of Epithelial Growth Factor Receptor (EGFR) (Shinojima et al. 2003; Layfield et al. 2006; Kaloshi et al. 2007; Gan et al. 2009; Inda et al. 2010), over-expression of chitinase-3-like-1 (CH3L1 or YKL-40) (Hormigo et al. 2006; Pelloski et al. 2007), osteopontin (Sreekanthreddy et al. 2010), loss of phosphatase and tensin homolog (PTEN) (Hill et al. 2003; Parsa et al. 2007) and mutations in the tumour suppressor protein, p53 (Shiraishi et al. 2002; Ruano et al. 2009). Prognostic biomarkers have great utility in the clinic. Not only do these markers present as potential therapeutic targets but they can be used to pool groups of glioma with similar genetic profile. This enrichment of the test population leads to increased homogeneity and a much more uniform response to treatment (Figure 2).

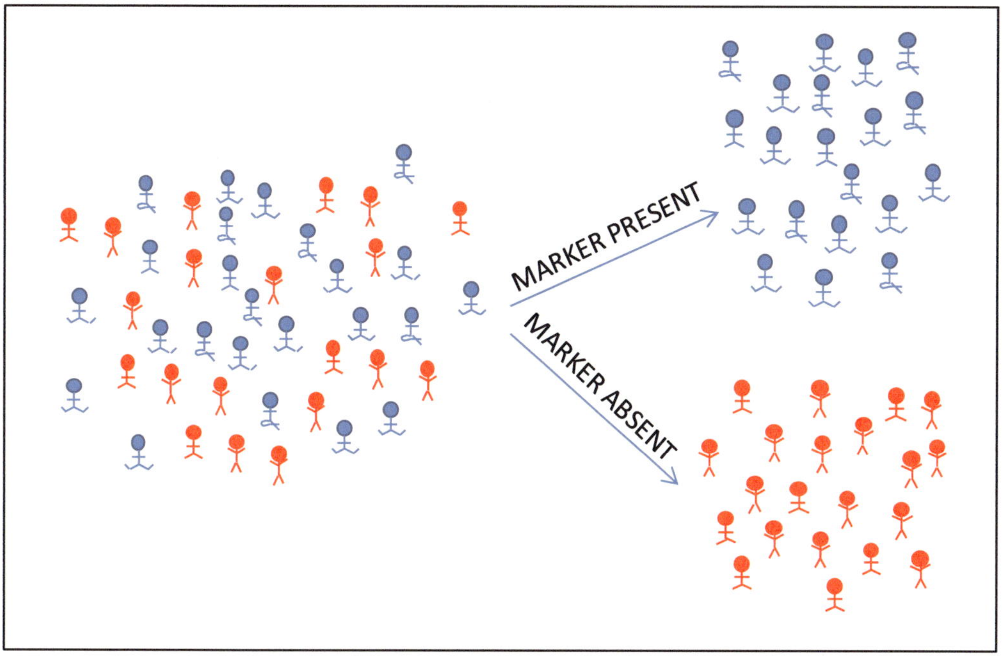

Fig. 2. Molecular diagnostics allows for the identification of GBM subgroups with similar genetic profile. This enrichment allows for a more uniform tumour response.

Much more difficult to identify are biomarkers with **predictive power** in the context of a specific therapy. Predictive biomarkers are markers which can be used to identify groups of patients who are most likely to respond to a given treatment. The key difference between a prognostic and a predictive biomarker is that the predictive biomarker should instigate a *change* in the treatment provided to the patient (Figure 1). Estrogen Receptor (ER) status in patients with breast cancer strongly predicts treatment response to tamoxifen (Kurokawa et al. 2000; Hu&Mokbel 2001). Additionally, patients with variant forms of the gene CYP2D6 (also called simply 2D6) may not receive full benefit from tamoxifen because of the slow metabolism of the tamoxifen prodrug into its active metabolite 4-hydroxytamoxifen (Goetz 2010; Stingl et al. 2010; de Souza&Olopade 2011). Approximately 60% of malignant melanomas harbour the BRAF mutation. Although patients with the damaged BRAF are non-responsive to the KRAS/BRAF inhibitor, sorafenib, response to the second-generation drug called PLX4720 is favourable (Whittaker et al. 2010). Improved outcomes have also been reported in patients with non-small cell lung cancer (NSCLC) harbouring EGFR mutations treated with the tyrosine kinase inhibitors (TKI) erlotinib and gefitinib (Kim et al. 2008; Paz-Ares et al. 2010).
In a highly heterogeneous tumour such as glioblastoma, the search for predictive markers to treatment for use in clinical trials and in every day clinic has been disappointing.

1.2 Molecular subtypes of glioblastoma

Most centres around the world use the World Health Organisation (WHO) grading of tumours of the central nervous system (Fuller&Scheithauer 2007). Glioma grade is defined by the presence or absence of histopathological features, namely: nuclear pleomorphism, mitoses, proliferative index and necrosis and/or microvascular proliferation. A significant limitation to this histopathology-based analysis is its inability to detect functional differences occurring on the subcellular level. This is evidenced by the high variability observed in the clinical outcomes in patients with the same diagnosis and differences in response to therapy. To advance survival times and clinical treatment of these patients with an, on average, dismal prognosis molecular markers with capacity to take into consideration the high molecular heterogeneity are needed in the clinic.

The wide spectrum of molecular difference in glioblastoma is evident from global expression studies, in particular, the molecular cataloguing project: The Cancer Genome Atlas (TCGA) (2008). Surveying the mutational environment of glioblastoma revealed that aberrations occur most commonly in genes whose protein products regulate the core cell growth signalling pathways that are already known to be important such as EGFR, PTEN, p53 and CDKN2A. What this survey did reveal was the extent of genomic complexity. Each tumour harbours different mutations. In addition, we are beginning to appreciate that the core pathways of cancer are not linear, rather complex and interacting. Given this complexity, it is very unlikely that a single genetic change will predict treatment response.

Gene expression profiling has provided an opportunity to further define prognostic and predictive factors (Settle&Sulman 2011). Gene signatures have successfully categorised glioblastomas that histologically appear indistinguishable, into molecular subgroups which often have very different clinical outcomes (Colman et al. 2010; Verhaak et al. 2010). Based on survival associated genes, 76 high grade gliomas were classified into the broad genotology groups; proneural, mesenchymal and proliferative (Phillips et al. 2006). The use of larger and multiple datasets have refined these subtypes into two broad groups, proneural and mesenchymal angiogenic (Colman et al. 2010). Overexpression of a mesenchymal gene expression signature and loss of a proneural signature are associated with a poor prognosis group. By subtyping glioblastoma into mesenchymal and proneural subtypes, the sameness of patient populations is improved. In addition, the genes belonging to each group provides biologists hints for therapeutic targeting. For example, the mesenchymal subtype of glioblastoma is over-represented by genes involved in angiogenesis and invasion (Colman et al. 2010). This subgroup of patients is more responsive to bevacizumab. Mutation in the isocitrate dehydrogenase 1 (IDH1) gene is strongly associated with the proneural subtype of glioblastoma and a much better prognosis (Noushmehr et al. 2010). Increasing evidence suggests that proneural glioblastomas have a different histogenic origin which is further supported by the recent discovery of a glioma-CpG island methylator phenotype (G-CIMP) (Noushmehr et al. 2010). Both IDH1mt and the G-CIMP have a higher incidence in secondary GBMs which arise from a prior, lower grade lesion. MGMT promoter methylation, G-CIMP and mutations in IDH1 are all prognostic. Although a correlation between proneural GBM subtypes and specific treatment has not been determined, it has been suggested by a few studies that chemotherapy agents such as temozolomide and others targeted at cell growth may not be as effective for this group as previously thought (Verhaak&Valk 2010).

2. Prognostic biomarkers in glioma

Molecular markers identified to hold prognostic significance in glioma include loss of heterozygosity of the chromosomal arms 1p and 19q (LOH 1p/19q), methylguanine methyltransferase (MGMT) promoter methylation, mutations in the isocitrate dehydrogenase 1 (IDH1) gene, mutations in TP53, loss of PTEN activity, amplification of

EGFR, presence of the EGFR delta variant (EGFRvIII) and overexpression of chitinase 3-like 1 (YKL40). Gene profiling and cross validation in multiple independent datasets has resulted in the separation of glioblastoma into two major subgroupings: proneural and mesenchymal. The proneural tumours have a much better survival outlook and can be further characterised by the presence of a glioma CpG island methylation phenotype (gCIMP).

Extensive reviews of EGFR, PTEN and TP53 are covered elsewhere. This discussion will focus on LOH 1p/19q, MGMT promoter methylation and mutations in IDH.

2.1. Loss of heterozygosity 1p and 19q

A hallmark of oligodendroglial tumours is the co-deletion of the chromosomal arms 1p and 19q corresponding to an unbalanced translocation t(1;19) (q10;p10). This can be readily detected using Fluorescence In situ hybridisation (FISH) (Figure 3). LOH at 1p19q is observed in up to 69% of grade II and grade III (anaplastic) oligodendrogliomas and is far more common in 'pure' oligodendroglioma than astrocytoma and mixed oligoastrocytoma (Barbashina et al. 2005). LOH of 1p19q confers a clear survival advantage in anaplastic oligodendroglioma and mixed oligoastrocytoma however the survival advantage conferred for grade II lesions is less clear (Laigle-Donadey et al. 2005; Jenkins et al. 2006; Walker et al. 2006) . Whether the co-deletion mediates a prognostic advantage or results in a heightened sensitivity to radiation and chemotherapy is unknown. In general, oligodendrogliomas with LOH at 1p19q represent a group of highly chemosensitive gliomas, especially to the combination of procarbazine, lomustine (CCNU), and vincristine (PCV).

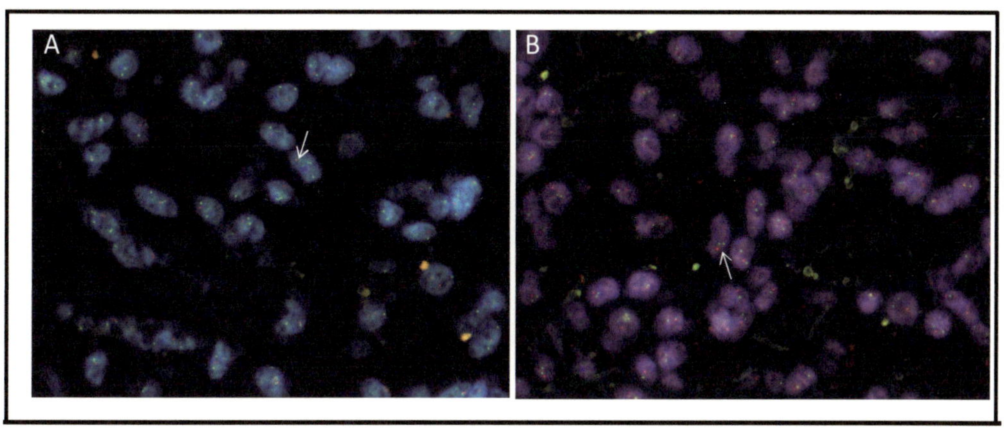

Fig. 3. Representative photomicrographs of loss of 1p (A) and loss of 19q (B) chromosomal arms detected using FISH. Arrow indicates only one chromosome copy instead of the expected two. Photomicrographs were kindly donated by Dr Michael Buckland, Department of Neuropathology, University of Sydney.

The standard treatment for anaplastic oligodendrogliomas consists of complete surgical removal where possible followed by radiation therapy and chemotherapy, typically with temozolomide because it is well tolerated. It is generally accepted that chemotherapy is of value in the treatment of patients with anaplastic oligodendrogliomas (Mokhtari et al. 2011).

Because of the potential toxicity to the CNS, many clinicians have suggested that radiotherapy treatment may be better reserved for progressive disease. Treatment with temozolomide is now favoured over PVC treatment because of its low toxicity. Studies treating anaplastic oligodendroglioma patients with temozolomide have also found that the presence of LOH at 1p/19q is a favourable predictive marker (Brandes et al. 2006; Mikkelsen et al. 2009; Ramirez et al. 2010). This could also be because the majority of oligodendrogliomas harbouring LOH at 1p/19q also show methylation in the promoter region of MGMT. Clinical studies have been designed to establish whether combining or adding chemotherapy to radiotherapy is of benefit to oligodendroglioma patients or whether these patients could benefit from upfront chemotherapy (without radiotherapy).

Two large prospective trials have shown little benefit for adding adjuvant PVC before radiotherapy (Cairncross et al. 2006) or after radiotherapy (van den Bent et al. 2006). To address whether treatment of oligodendrogliomas with chemotherapy alone is feasible and safe, the NOA-04 Phase III trial compared radiotherapy versus chemotherapy with either PCV or temozolomide as initial therapy in 318 patients with anaplastic gliomas (WHO grade 3) (randomly assigned 2:1:1 to receive radiotherapy (arm A) or chemotherapy with either PCV (arm B1) or temozolomide (arm B2)) (Wick et al. 2009). The clinical relevance of 1p/19q codeletion, O^6-methylguanine DNA-methyltransferase (*MGMT*) promoter methylation, and *IDH1* mutations in codon 132 in these tumours were also measured and analysed. This important trial confirmed that there was no survival difference in administering initial radiotherapy or initial chemotherapy (Wick et al. 2009). One very important finding to emerge from the study was the presence of mutations in IDH1 provided the best prognostic model. An ongoing EORCT 26081 Phase III trial of radiotherapy, temozolomide and concomitant and adjuvant temozolomide in patients with anaplastic oligodendrogliomas with 1p/19q codeletions will further confirm what the optimal treatment for these tumours is (more information below).

The gene products that are affected as a result of LOH remain under investigation and may include mediators of cytotoxic resistance or may represent an early oncogenic lesion still retaining sensitivity to genotoxic agents or insults. Microarray technology has been used to profile gene expression in oligodendrogliomas to look for putative tumour suppressor gene candidates and genes which could mediate the observed chemosensitivity using a variety of microarray platforms (Mukasa et al. 2002; Nutt et al. 2003; Mukasa et al. 2004; Tews et al. 2006; Tews et al. 2007; Ducray et al. 2008). These studies have identified some interesting gene candidates located on the 1p and 19q chromosomal arms however none have gone on to be validated prospectively. Interestingly, these profiling experiments identified a proneural signature associated with 1p19q codeleted oligodendrogliomas and a better survival outcome (Phillips et al. 2006). In contrast, the mesenchymal signature is more commonly associated with glioblastoma (discussed in more detail below). Noteworthy is the absence of EGFR amplifications in the proneural group. Ducray and colleagues compared 1p19q codeleted gliomas to EGFR-amplified gliomas and found that the proneural gene internexin (INA) which encodes neurofilament-interacting protein was significantly differentially expressed (Ducray et al. 2009). The prognostic significance of INA was further assessed and confirmed in the prospective, randomized EORTC 26951 trial of adjuvant PVC (Mokhtari et al. 2011). INA strongly correlated with 1p19q codeletion, mutated IDH1 and MGMT promoter methylation.

2.2 MGMT

The O^6-methylguanine-DNA methyltransferase gene, *MGMT*, located on chromosome 10q26.1 encodes a DNA repair protein that restores mutagenic O^6-alkylguanine to normal guanine within genomic DNA. O^6-alkylguanines can pair erroneously with thymine during DNA replication, resulting in G:C>A:T transitions, as well as causing cross-links between adjacent strands of DNA, both of which can lead to neoplastic transformation (Gerson 2004). MGMT thus protects cells from the toxic and carcinogenic effects of alkylating agents and is absent in many types of human malignancy. Loss of MGMT protein expression is frequently associated with transcriptional silencing of the MGMT gene by methylation of its CpG island promoter in various neoplasia, (Esteller et al. 1999) as exemplified by 35-55% of gliomas (Silber et al. 1998; Esteller et al. 2000; Nakamura et al. 2001; Kamiryo et al. 2004; Paz et al. 2004; Brell et al. 2005; Hegi et al. 2005). However, several large studies of glioma have shown the correlation between immunohistochemical loss of MGMT and promoter methylation is not always correlative (Preusser et al. 2008; Cao et al. 2009; Hawkins et al. 2009; Mellai et al. 2009).

Alkylating drugs such as temozolomide are used in chemotherapy for the targeted cell death of rapidly-replicating neoplastic cells and MGMT expression is a key factor in conferring resistance to these agents. In 2005, a new treatment regime was developed and tested in a randomised, phase III clinical trial whereby the alkylating agent, temozolomide was combined with radiotherapy (RT) in concurrent treatment followed by an additional 6 cycles of Temozolomide for newly diagnosed glioblastoma (Stupp et al. 2005). This was the first trial to achieve a clinically meaningful and statistically significant overall median survival benefit of 2.5 months when compared to radiotherapy alone. More compelling were the two-year survival rates with 26% of patients treated with concurrent treatment still alive after two years compared with just 10.4% for patients treated with radiotherapy alone. These survival benefits were still apparent after 5 years of follow-up (Stupp et al. 2009).

The molecular basis for the differential response of glioblastoma patients to temozolomide has been recognized. Temozolomide is an oral alkylating chemotherapy which is spontaneously converted into its active metabolite and readily crosses the blood-brain barrier. The primary mode of action of temozolomide is to damage the DNA by introducing alkyl adducts. These cause genetic mutations as well as cross-links between DNA strands that inhibit DNA replication and thereby trigger cell death. Thus alkylating agents target rapidly replicating neoplastic cells. However, while temozolomide introduces alkyl adducts into DNA, MGMT reverses them. Thus tumour cells expressing MGMT are chemoresistant to this class of drugs (Pegg 1990). In a companion laboratory study to the phase III trial combining radiotherapy with temozolomide, Hegi et al. demonstrated a pronounced positive survival response in patients whose tumours had lost MGMT by promoter methylation. Strikingly, patients whose tumours were MGMT-methylated demonstrated extended overall and progression-free survival compared to those whose tumours were unmethylated, and therefore MGMT methylation was postulated to be a positive predictor of patient response to alkylating agents (Esteller et al. 2000; Hegi et al. 2005). Since these seminal reports in 2005, the standard of care for patients diagnosed with glioblastoma has comprised surgery with maximal feasible resection and radiotherapy with concurrent and adjuvant temozolomide. Yet widespread adoption of MGMT methylation as a marker of response to temozolomide in clinical practice has not transpired.

2.2.1 Routine testing for MGMT methylation

While MGMT methylation could be routinely used as a prognostic/predictive marker in glioblastoma, there is so far no consensus on the method to be applied. Assessment of MGMT promoter methylation is difficult due to the complex nature of the techniques involved. To detect methylation, bisulfite treatment of the DNA is required, a process that may result in degradation of DNA and subsequent low success rates in PCR. This is further compounded by the fact that the most commonly available tissue for assessment is formalin fixed paraffin embedded (FFPE), and the DNA subsequently extracted from this tissue is usually fragmented, again making PCR more difficult.

Promoter methylation analysis by qualitative methyl-specific polymerase chain reaction (MSP) or semi-quantitative methyl-specific polymerase chain reaction (SQ-MSP), especially from FPPE tissue is technically demanding. MSP is the more limited because the methylation status of only a few CpG sites (i.e., those interfering with the PCR primer binding) can be interrogated at once. The technique also has the drawback of providing only a qualitative indication of the methylation status of the sites. Karayan-Tapon (Karayan-Tapon et al. 2010) evaluated MGMT promoter methylation using MSP, SQ-MSP and pyrosequencing. The best predictive value for overall survival was obtained by *pyrosequencing*. Pyrosequencing technology is a technique that generates a quantitative measure of methylation and automatically calculates and reports percent methylation for each CpG site in the studied sequence, thus allowing detection of partially methylated CpG sites.

There are other methodologies for assessing the promoter methylation of MGMT. The testing needs to be resolved for MGMT to be used routinely in the clinic and perhaps a surrogate marker of MGMT such as another protein product readily visualised by immunohistochemistry or a polymorphism detected in blood may be the way forward.

2.2.2 Strategies to overcome MGMT activity

With the recognition that an unmethylated MGMT promoter is associated with a poorer response to temozolomide, strategies have evolved to circumvent the resistance that MGMT confers. Combination therapy with multiple chemotherapeutic drugs known to deplete MGMT (specifically procarbazine and temozolomide) has been successfully assessed in a Phase I trial (Newlands et al. 2003) but as yet has not been shown to confer a benefit in survival. O^6 benzylguanine (O^6BG), a substrate for MGMT, has also been used to decrease MGMT levels. However, systemic administration of O^6BG has been associated with significant toxicity, thereby necessitating a reduction in chemotherapy dose (Quinn et al. 2002; Quinn et al. 2005). A recent case report of local administration of O^6BG, allowing the systemic effects to be avoided, shows some promise (Koch et al. 2007).

Alteration of temozolomide dosing regimens from the usual method of 5 days of treatment every 28 days to more frequent, lower-dose treatment has been evaluated. Protracted temozolomide exposure may reduce MGMT activity. Brock and colleagues demonstrated safety of a low dose of temozolomide for up to 49 consecutive days, however the efficacy of this lower dose is unclear (Brock et al. 1998). Depletion of peripheral mononuclear MGMT has been demonstrated with more prolonged dosing regimens and unfortunately this has been associated with profound lymphocytopaenia and opportunistic infections (Tolcher et al. 2003; Wick et al. 2004; Wick&Weller 2005). More recent evidence suggest that daily dosing may be associated with improved outcome (Buttolo et al. 2006). Additionally, a dosing regimen of 14 days of treatment out of every 28 days has not only been shown to

lead to a progression free survival benefit, outcome with this treatment regimen was not significantly associated with MGMT promoter methylation (Wick et al. 2007).
Treating patients with continuous 50mg/m^2 at relapse after a standard temozolomide schedule of 150-200mg/m^2 resulted in a PFS6 of 47-57% (Perry et al. 2008). The efficacy and safety of this continuous dose-intense temozolomide schedule for recurrent GBM was tested in a multicenter, phase II study, RESCUE. Overall, PFS6 in 116 patients with recurrent GBM was 24% (Perry et al. 2010). Not surprisingly, the best responding patients were those who were treated with conventional chemoradiotherapy. However, what was interesting was the similar benefit to treatment recorded in the patients who experienced early progression on standard therapy (Perry et al. 2010).

2.3 IDH mutations

The Cancer Genome Atlas (TCGA) efforts made the initial breakthrough discovery that 11% of glioblastomas harbour point mutations in cytoplasmic and mitochondrial NADP+-dependent isocitrate dehydrogenases 1 and 2 (IDH1 and IDH2) (Balss et al. 2008; Parsons et al. 2008; Dang et al. 2009). The normal function of the IDH enzymes is to convert isocitrate into α-ketoglutarate. Mutations, specifically at the arginine 132 (R132) codon, are more frequently observed in low grade and anaplastic gliomas and secondary glioblastomas (50-93%) than mutations found in IDH2 [arginine 172 (R172) codon] (3-5%). No gliomas have been found to have point mutations in both IDH1 and IDH2 (Yan et al. 2009).

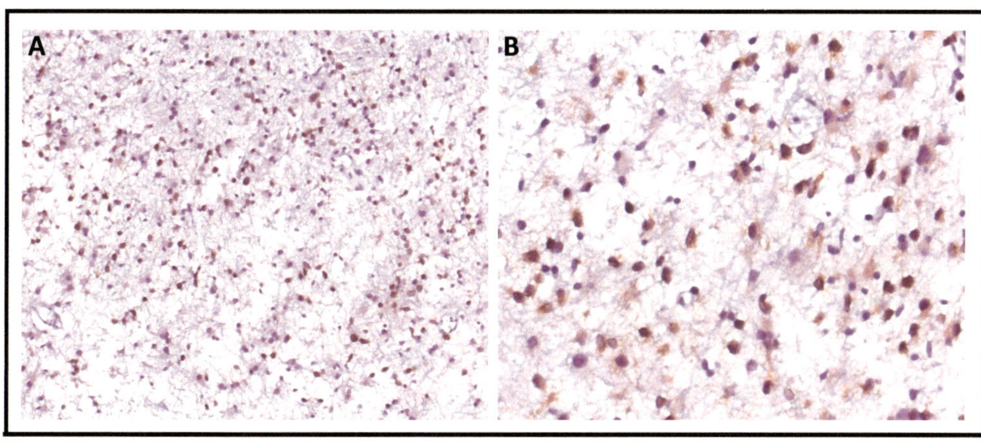

Fig. 4. Representative photomicrographs of IDH1 mutations detected with the Anti-Human IDH1 R132H Mouse Monoclonal Antibody (DIA-H09M) at x20 magnification (A) and x40 (B) Photomicrographs were kindly donated by Dr Michael Buckland, Department of Neuropathology, University of Sydney.

Hartmann and colleagues used an antibody which specifically detected the R132 mutation in IDH1 allowing assessment with simple immunohistochemistry (Hartmann et al. 2010). (Figure 4). The mutation was detected in 72% low grade astrocytomas (AII; n=227); 64% anaplastic astrocytomas (AA; n=228); 82% low grade oligodendroglioma (OII; n=128); 70% anaplastic oligodendroglioma (AO; n=174); 82% low grade oligoastrocytomas (OAII; n=76); 66% anaplastic oligoastrocytoma (AOA; n=177) and 9% glioblastoma (GBM; n=521). What was most significant about this study was the progression free and overall survival curves.

In order of most favourable to poor survival: (1) AA with IDH1 mutation, (2) GBM with IDH1 mutation, (3) AA with IDH1 wild type and (4) GBM with IDH1 wild type. Routine testing for IDH1 mutations will have clinical ramifications regarding histological diagnosis and treatment schemes. The IDH1 mutation is of greater prognostic relevance than histopathological diagnosis according to the World Health Organisation (WHO) classification system (Hartmann et al. 2010). Subsidised treatment schemes approved for glioblastoma such as concomitant radiotherapy and temozolomide and bevacizumab (USA only) may need to be revised to allow anaplastic gliomas with IDH1 wild type status to be treated.

Mutations of the codons in IDH1 and 2 lead to a loss in the production of α-ketoglutarate and a gain of the catalytic activity to produce 2-hydroxyglutarate (2-HG) (Xu et al. 2011). 2-HG levels are highly elevated in IDH-mutated cancers and lead to genome wide histone and DNA methylation alterations (Xu et al., 2011; Dang et al., 2009). Hypermethylation at a large number of loci have been associated with IDH-mutated glioma suggesting that IDH mutation is associated with a distinct DNA methylation phenotype (Noushmehr et al. 2010; Christensen et al. 2011). GoldenGate array methylation data was obtained from 131 glioma patients (all types and histological grades) to interrogate methylation patterns associated with IDH mutation and survival. IDH1 mutations were present in 60% of tumours. Distinct differences between the numbers of significantly differentially hypermethylated loci were noted in IDH mutant tumours compared to IDH wild type tumours. Specific to IDH mutant tumours, cellular signalling pathways were hypermethylated whilst metabolism and biosynthesis pathways were hypermethylated (Christensen et al. 2011). This might be compensatory for the metabolic stress related to the mutation.

In a series of elegant *in vitro*-based experiments, Yan's group transformed human oligodendroglial (HOG) cells with IDH1-R132 or treated cells with 2-HG (Yan et al. 2009). They noted changes in gene expression common to both IDH1-R132 cells and 2-HG-treated cells when compared to IDH1-wildtype and untreated cells, implying that these changes were the result of increased 2HG (Reitman et al. 2010; Reitman&Yan 2010). However, reductions in glutamate and several glutamate-related metabolites were observed exclusively in the IDH1-R132 cells. Particular attention was paid to reduced levels of a common dipeptide in the brain, N-acetyl-aspartyl-glutamate (NAAG), however its contribution to pathogenesis remains unclear (Reitman et al. 2011).

Recently, IDH mutations have been shown to be tightly associated with the presence of a glioma CpG island methylator phenotype (gCIMP) (Noushmehr et al. 2010). CIMPs are characterised by highly concordant DNA methylation of a subset of loci. Improved survival was observed in gliomas with IDH1 mutation and positive for gCIMP suggesting that there are molecular features within gCIMP gliomas that encourage a less aggressive phenotype. CIMP positive colon cancers also have a better prognosis. It is not known whether glioma cells acquire the mutation in IDH1 which then leads to genome histone and DNA methylation patterns, reflected by the presence of a gCIMP or that transcriptional silencing of gCIMP targets may provide the optimal environment for gliomas to acquire the mutation (genomic instability) (Noushmehr et al. 2010).

Gliomas with IDH1 mutations as well as the presence of gCIMP displayed significantly better overall survival (median survival: 2.9 years) compared to all other patients (median survival: 1.04 years). The favourable survival observed in IDH1 mutation-gCIMP positive gliomas may be because these tumours are highly represented in the proneural subset of gliomas. Clinically, the prognostic utility of IDH1 mutations emerged in the NOA-04 trial.

IDH1 mutations conferred a significantly longer time to treatment failure (TTF) which was independent of histology, treatment, codeletion of 1p and 19q and MGMT promoter methylation status (Wick et al. 2009). IDH1 mutations as well as the gCIMP represent a significant breakthrough in how we diagnose patients. Testing for IDH1 mutations has quickly translated into routine diagnostic use. No doubt, IDH1 mutations and perhaps the gCIMP will be used to stratify patients for future clinical trials. Attention has shifted to examining therapeutic targets for IDH1 as well as the possibility of inducing mutations in IDH1 in GBMs that don't possess the mutation.

3. Use as predictive biomarkers

Biomarkers which can foretell whether patients are resistant to a certain treatment and predict drug sensitivity are urgently needed. The success rate of matching biomarkers with treatments has been less than satisfactory. Fewer than 100 biomarkers have been validated for routine clinical practice, despite the publication of more than 150,000 claimed biomarkers. Impeding the successful translation of biomarkers into the clinical setting is non-standardised biological specimen and clinical data collection, particularly clinical information pertaining to drug sensitivity and progression free survival. In addition, far greater numbers of tumour specimens from patients treated uniformly may be needed to be analysed than what we previously assumed.

The only biomarker with reported predictive value is MGMT promoter methylation. As discussed earlier in the MGMT section, the role of MGMT is to protect cells from alkylating damage specifically by removing the alkyl adducts from the O^6 position of guanine and the O^4 position of thymine and effectively restoring the DNA bases and prevent TMZ-induced cell death. However, the present NOA-04 trial does not support the suggestion that *MGMT* promoter methylation is simply predictive for response to alkylating chemotherapy (Wick et al. 2009). NOA-04 showed a striking difference in PFS between patients with versus without *MGMT* promoter methylation who were treated with radiotherapy alone. Thus *MGMT* promoter hypermethylation in anaplastic gliomas may be regarded as (1) a prognostic marker for good outcome in patients treated with radiotherapy or (2) predictive for response to radiotherapy itself.

The most significant issue with implementing MGMT promoter methylation as a predictive test for TMZ therapy is that there is currently no alternative treatment strategy available for those patients with unmethylated MGMT tumours. Until alternative treatments are available and the MGMT test is more reliable and robust, will clinicians consider MGMT promoter methylation as a predictive test.

4. Use of biomarkers in clinical trials

Co-deletion of the chromosomal arms 1p and 19q is a requirement for entry of anaplastic gliomas into the CODEL study which is assessing the role of concomitant and adjuvant temozolomide added to standard radiotherapy and has temozolomide monotherapy in an observation arm. A phase III randomized sister study to CODEL, CATNON, examines radiotherapy with or without concurrent and/or adjuvant temozolomide in patients with non-1p/19q deleted anaplastic gliomas (Figure 5). This type of dual study design allows for the patient populations to be enriched in a specific marker, yet it doesn't exclude either tumour types (codeleted and nondeleted 1p/19q). All specimens will also be tested for MGMT promoter methylation.

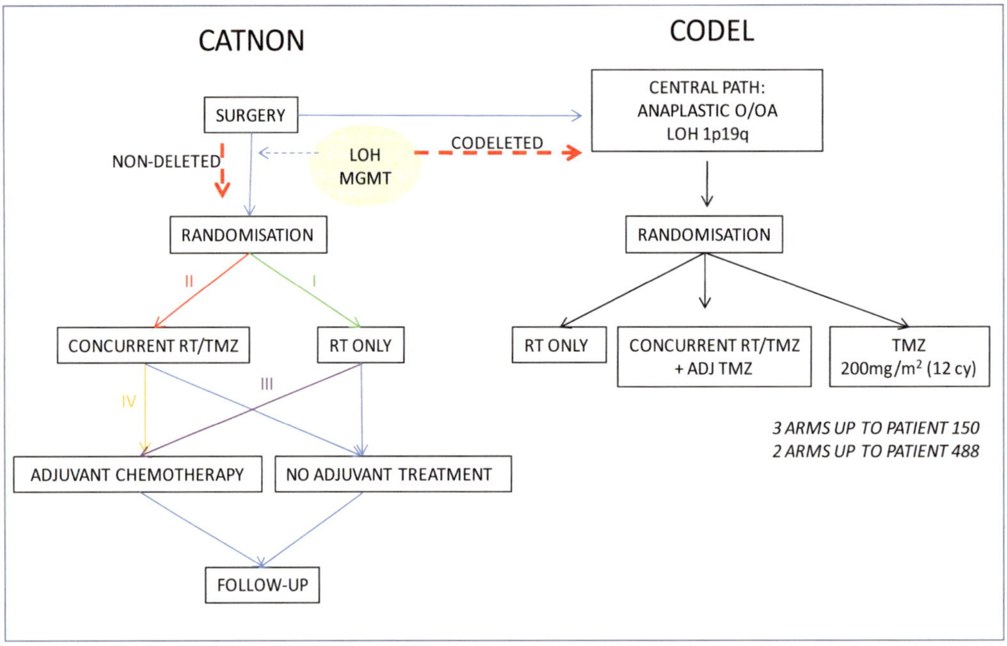

Fig. 5. Overview of the CATNON and CODEL trials

A phase I/IIa trial examined the effectiveness of adding cilengitide to concurrent chemoradiotherapy (Stupp et al. 2010). This study demonstrated the effectiveness of cilengitide but also showed that there was a clear survival benefit in the patients with MGMT promoter methylation (Stupp et al. 2010). The phase III CENTRIC trial (recruitment closed in Feb, 2011) restricted recruitment to newly diagnosed GBM patients with confirmed MGMT methylation. An additional two phase II trials sponsored by the pharmaceutical company, EMD Serono, are designed to treat patients with unmethylated MGMT: CORE (Cilengitide, Temozolomide, and Radiation Therapy in Treating Patients with Newly Diagnosed Glioblastoma and Unmethylated Gene Promoter Status) and ExCentric. CORE (trial still open; May 2011) examines the efficacy of increasing the dose schedule of cilengitide (2000mg twice weekly and 2000mg five times per week) versus standard concurrent chemoradiotherapy (without cilengitide). The ExCentric trial (recruitment open, May 2011) has taken a much different approach. In this trial, procarbazine is added to the concurrent schedule of radiotherapy, TMZ, cilengitide and patients will be treated adjuvantly for an additional 6 cycles with the triple cocktail of cilengitide, TMZ and procarbazine. The patients have so far shown excellent toleration of this combination.

The RTOG-0825 examines the effect of bevacizumab administered with radiotherapy compared to conventional concurrent chemoradiotherapy (TMZ) in primary GBM. All patients enrolled in this study will be tested for MGMT promoter methylation. Unique to this study, however, all samples will be prospectively tested with the nine-gene profile which separates the proneural GBM from the mesenchymal-angiogenic GBM (Colman et al. 2010). It is becoming mandatory for future trial design to incorporate molecular inclusion criteria to identify the poorly responding patients from the patients who benefit.

5. Targeted therapies for glioblastoma

Molecular targeted therapies specifically inhibit amplified or aberrant proteins that drive tumour cell growth. The key to targeted therapy is identifying a target whose *inhibition will stop the growth of the tumour cell*. Whilst this field has rapidly developed, our understanding at the molecular level of the precise role that potential targets have in tumorigenesis and the survival dependence that tumours have on these components has not progressed at the same rate. Unlike melanoma, lung and breast cancer, glioblastoma lacks significant driver mutations which are present in ample abundance and in all tumours. The TCGA analysis revealed a wide spectrum of molecular variation in glioblastoma. TCGA used global gene expression analysis to show aberrations occurred more commonly in genes whose protein products regulated the core cell growth signalling pathways that were already known to be important such as EGFR, PTEN, p53 and CDKN2A. One pathway which is frequently dysregulated is the receptor tyrosine kinase (RTK)/phosphatidylinositol 3-kinase (PI3K)/Akt/mammalian target of rapamycin (mTOR) cascade. Approximately 86% of clinical samples analysed by the TCGA with both copy number and sequencing data had a genetic alteration in the RTK/PI3K pathway (Parsons et al. 2008). In addition, genetic alterations in two other core pathways; RB (87%) and TP53 (78%) were documented. At the time (3 years ago now) it was reasonable to suggest that all tumours be sequenced and the genetic aberrations be documented before selecting the targeted therapy. For example, for tumours with alterations in CDKN2A or CDKN2C or amplifications in CDK4 or CDK6, a CDK inhibitor should be recommended. Unfortunately, we underestimated the extent of genomic complexity and it is very doubtful that therapies targeted to a single genetic change will ever be effective. A range of molecular targeted drugs applied in combination or in addition to each other is needed (Jansen et al. 2010). In clinical practice, the multi-drug approach is currently limited by intellectual property. Most likely the efficacy of two drugs may require two competing pharmaceutical companies to work together.
To understand why our current single targeted therapies are ineffective, it is useful to examine the earlier clinical studies with EGFR- and VEGF-targeted drugs. We can also glean value from trials using targeted therapy in other cancers. Even when the target of interest is much more prominent such as KRAS or BRAF, valuable lessons can still be learnt.

5.1 Targeting the RTK/PI3K pathway

In a study of 49 patients with recurrent glioblastoma, tumour shrinkage was evident in 9 patients (25%) (Mellinghoff et al. 2005). Logically, it was of great interest to better understand the underlying molecular biology of these 9 responders. Pre-treatment tissue was only available for 7 of the responding patients and 19 patients who did not respond. The authors found coexpression of EGFRvIII and PTEN sensitised glioblastoma to erlotinib and correctly validated this finding in tissue samples from different institutions undergoing similar treatment (n=33) (Mellinghoff et al. 2005). Unfortunately, the relationship between EGFRvIII and intact PTEN co-expression did not translate to the subsequent prospective phase I/II trials (Brown et al. 2008; van den Bent et al. 2009). No relationship between aberrations in the RTK core and the EGFR inhibitor, lapatinib (Thiessen et al. 2010) or addition of erlotinib with the mTOR inhibitor, sirolimus (Reardon et al. 2010) were linked with response.

5.2 Targeting angiogenesis

The development of anti-angiogenic agents for glioblastoma have been promising and include bevacizumab (Vascular endothelial growth factor [VEGF] antibody), cediranib (VEGF receptor antagonist), cilengitide (mentioned previously; integrin antagonist) and Enzastaurin (Protein Kinase-C-β-antagonist).

The preclinical and clinical data for cediranib treatment in glioblastoma looked very promising (Dietrich et al. 2009; Gerstner et al. 2011). Unfortunately, the International Multicentre Phase III trial, REGAL was negative. The REGAL study compared the use of cediranib alone, cediranib in combination with lomustine and lomustine plus placebo. In the 325 patients with recurrent GBM studied, only 16% treated with cediranib monotherapy were alive and progression free at 6 months (APF6) compared to 34.5% in the combination group and 24.5% in the lomustine plus placebo group (results reported by T. Batchelor at the Society of Neuro-oncology Annual Meeting, 2010; (Ahluwalia 2011)). Akin to cediranib, preclinical and studies of enzastaurin showed good anti-glioma activity but failed to show any significant benefits when trialled in a phase III study comparing enzastaurin to lomustine. Although less toxicity was observed with enzastaurin, no significant differences in median progression free survival and overall survival were observed (Wick et al. 2011).

The humanized antibody, Bevacizumab (Avastin), has received the most attention, with Food and Drug Administration (FDA) approval for use in recurrent GBM in the USA. No such approvals have been obtained in Europe and Australia. This is predominantly because there is only a modest overall survival benefit of 7.8-9.2 months suggesting a further improvement of efficacy is needed. Numerous phase II studies have shown modest survival benefits with bevacizumab either as a monotherapy or in combination with irinotecan (Chinot et al. 2011; Jakobsen et al. 2011; Lai et al. 2011; Prados et al. 2011; Reardon et al. 2011). Consistent to all trials examining bevacizumab efficacy is the reduction of steroids for patients and valuable palliation with preservation of key performance status (KPS), supporting a role for bevacizumab as a therapy in late stage disease (Hofer et al. 2011). Whether bevacizumab results in true glioma cell destruction or is it merely its ability to control the perivascular leak, resulting in better symptom control (associated with improvement of gadolinium MRI) needs to be elucidated.

An issue consistent with all trials of cediranib, enzastaurin and bevacizumab is their testing on recurrent glioblastoma as opposed to primary glioblastoma. Recurrent glioblastoma are already highly refractory to treatment and the potential benefits of these drugs may be missed. New studies are investigating bevacizumab up front with standard radiation therapy and temozolomide. This has shown to be well tolerated (Vredenburgh et al. 2011) and it is a strategy that the RTOG-0825 trial has incorporated (discussed previously).

With all of these targeted therapies, it would seem obvious that the more target present, the more efficacious the drug. Unfortunately, this has not been the case. For example, why patients with high expression of VEGF have not shown strong response to bevacizumab? These issues pertaining to biomarkers in targeted therapy trials will be discussed in turn below:

5.3 Many retrospective analyses of single arm investigations are performed in small and often heterogeneous cohorts of patients

The co-expression of EGFRvIII and PTEN was first discovered in an initial test set consisting of 49 recurrent GBM treated with either gefitinib (n=37) or erlotinib (n=12). 26 patients with clear-cut evidence of a response or tumour progression had sufficient tissue for molecular analysis. Hence, just over half of the originally small cohort was analysed for molecular biomarkers. The validation study used a different tissue type entirely as only paraffin-embedded slides were available. Again, this material was untreated tumour tissue, not the recurrent lesion. The validation set was extremely underpowered (n=33) with only 8 responders identified in this dataset. It is imperative that collaborations between different institutes and countries work together to increase the power of these biomarker studies.

5.3.1 A lack of standardisation in the methods used for marker measurement

Assays for biomarkers need to be reliable. The assay needs to give identical results if repeated in the same or in another laboratory. The result needs to be the same, even when different methodologies are used. And finally, we need to ask whether the test provides added value to clinical practice. This has often been a strong criticism of studies incorporating MGMT promoter methylation (as discussed previously) and unfortunately the same issues surround biomarkers for targeted therapies. The original study by Mellinghoff and colleagues used immunohistochemistry (IHC) to assess PTEN expression (Mellinghoff et al. 2005). The problem with this approach is the antibody used does not detect the full length PTEN protein. Should mutations arise in the C-terminal end of the protein, these would go undiscovered using IHC assay. IHC for EGFR is also contentious. EGFR overexpression in GBM is generally driven by EGFR amplification. The scoring of EGFR IHC can be variable and different antibodies have different specificities to the EGFR protein. Amplification of EGFR or more specifically gain of copy number is most commonly detected by fluorescence *in situ* hybridization (FISH) and can be routinely performed in most histopathological laboratories. What is puzzling is the lack of sequencing of both EGFR and PTEN genes in the subsequent phase I/II clinical trials assessing TKIs. The most frequent mutant form of EGFR is EGFR Variant III (EGFRvIII or EGFR delta) which is missing the ligand -binding domain resulting in the constitutive activation of the EGFR-phosphoinositide 3-kinase pathway. IHC specific to the EGFRvIII mutant form is highly specific as too is the commonly used RT-PCR method. However, there are additional missense mutations encoding extracellular EGFR that have been shown to drive oncogenesis *in vitro* and can be inhibited by small-molecular tyrosine kinase inhibitors.

The original pre-clinical/clinical study sequenced all exons and flanking intronic sequences for EGFR (kinase domain), the HER2/neu (kinase domain) and all exons of PTEN. FISH was also performed to detect EGFR amplification and RT-PCR was used to amplify EGFR (1044-bp product) and EGFRvIII (243-bp product). In addition, EGFR and PTEN were examined with IHC (Mellinghoff et al. 2005). 26 of the 49 patients underwent sequencing, which included 6 patients who showed a response to erlotinib. No mutations were found. Van den Bent and colleagues assessed the benefits of erlotinib compared to temozolomide or cumustine in recurrent GBM in a randomized phase II study (van den Bent et al. 2009). Obtaining full data for all patients in this study was problematic. From 100 patients, PTEN expression could be determined in 82 patient cases and pAKT in 64 patients. Like the Mellinghoff study, no mutations in EGFR were detected, however only exons 19 to 21 were assessed. Although an association between EGFRvIII and EGFR amplification with poor overall survival was shown, no correlation between response and the co-expression of PTEN and EGFR was measured (van den Bent et al. 2009). In fact, no significant activity of erlotinib was observed. In another study of 65 patients, erlotinib efficacy was assessed in combination with temozolomide (Prados et al. 2009). Again no association with EGFRvIII and PTEN and response was measured, however in this study, MGMT promoter methylation was associated with better response. EGFR was measured with FISH and IHC, PTEN and EGFRvIII were analysed by IHC. No mutational analysis of EGFR was undertaken. Reardon and colleagues assessed the combination of erlotinib with a mTOR inhibitor, sirolimus in recurrent GBM (Reardon et al. 2010). Again, EGFR, EGFRvIII, PTEN, PI3K and pS6 were assessed by IHC and no association for these markers with clinical response was found. Mutational analysis was not conducted. Moreover, the general methodologies did not differ in the studies addressing erlotinib and response and the Phase II studies could not validate the findings of Mellinghoff et al.

Elegant biomarker studies have been associated with the anti-angiogenic drugs. Attention has focused predominantly on secreted factors and imaging modalities. Interleukin 6 (IL-6) is over-expressed in the majority of gliomas and functions as an immune regulator and an autocrine growth factor (Saidi et al. 2009). High starting levels of IL-6 may influence the efficacy of bevacizumab as it provides redundancy for the VEGF/VEGFR pathway and promotes an immune response that stimulates angiogenesis by non-VEGF mechanisms. Sorenson et al. reported the combination of MRI imaging (measured changes in vascular permeability/flow [K^{trans}] and changes in microvessel volume) and circulating collagen IV levels in plasma to be predictive of outcome in glioblastoma patients treated with cediranib (Sorensen et al. 2009). The level of circulating endothelial progenitor cells (cEPCs) and viable circulating endothelial cells (cECs) has also been shown to correlate with response (Sorensen et al. 2009). The ability to identify changes in a tumour's perfusion offers the potential to predict growth or regression. Dynamic susceptibility-weighted contrast-enhanced (DSC) MR imaging can be used to measure relative cerebral blood volume (rCBV) as a surrogate marker of perfusion. A pilot study of 16 patients with recurrent glioblastoma and treatment with bevacizumab found that MR perfusion imaging showed a significantly improved correlation with time to progression (Sawlani et al. 2011). Studies from Tsien (Tsien et al. 2011) and Server (Server et al. 2011)- both show positive results for this scan in patients with PsPD. Only changes in the hypoxia inducing factor (HIF) 2 alpha [HIF2α] have been shown to be promising surrogates of response to anti-angiogenic therapies (Mao et al. 2011).

5.3.2 Methodologies chosen in the study may not represent a comprehensive analysis of multiple components of a specific pathway

None of the studies examining erlotinib have comprehensively analysed the downstream components involved in EGFR signalling. Additional testing of PI3K and PS6 were added in some studies. It is very common for glioblastomas to have dysregulated signalling cascades downstream of EGFR, particular the negative feedback loops. Several growth factor pathways are also triggered. It's not economically feasible in most instances to assess all aspects of the RTK/PI3K/AKT/mTOR signalling cascade. However, a new system of testing drugs and identifying which subtypes of glioblastoma are susceptible to the drug could be to use human glioblastoma xenograft panels serially passaged in nude mice. This model allows tumour burden to be monitored non-invasively and rapid assessment of biological pathways (Prasad et al. 2011).

Feedback mechanisms also pose an issue with targeted therapies blocking angiogenesis. Tumours frequently recur after treatment with cediranib and bevacizumab and are refractory to further treatments. There have been different theories postulated as to why this "rebound" effect occurs. Tumours may switch to VEGF-independent angiogenic pathways or vessel co-option. A commonly held theory is that recurrent glioblastomas switch their growth pattern after anti-VEGF treatment (di Tomaso et al. 2011). The tumour cells are exposed to an increased hypoxic environment leading to increased migration, invasion, heightened glycolysis and increased PI3K pathway activation. Combining bevacizumab with anti-glycolytic agents or PI3K inhibitors might be more effective. Tumour-initiating CD133+ve cells are radio-resistant and can self renew to reform tumours, suggesting that these cells are responsible for tumour relapse (Liu et al. 2009). More significantly, exposure to bevacizumab inhibited the maturation of tumour endothelial progenitors into the endothelium but not the differentiation of CD133+ cells into progenitor cells (Wang et al. 2011). This fundamental study showed that there is a dynamic balance between the CD133+ cell population and tumour cells and we need to target the endothelial transition as well as VEGF.

5.3.3 Not all mutations within a given gene are screened

In simplistic terms, the plethora of TKIs are designed to be effective on patients harbouring EGFR mutations. However, in the majority of studies exploring gefitinib and erlotinib, the EGFR gene is not fully sequenced to identify variants and mutations. TCGA analyses have identified a high diversity of genes mutated within glioblastoma. As prices drop with Next Generation sequencing, capabilities to better define precise genetic aberrations associated with response to a specific treatment will improve. Copy number aberrations (amplifications and deletions) and structural aberrations (intra-chromosomal rearrangements- inversions, inverted/tandem duplications) are not detected using traditional Sanger sequencing in the lab. Our ability to assess these aberrations must improve at the rate that new targeted therapies are flooding the market. BRAF is a commonly deleted gene in approximately 8% of solid tumours, however over 30 different mutations in the BRAF gene have been implicated in cancer (Dienstmann&Tabernero 2011; Puzanov et al. 2011).

5.3.4 A pathway-centric approach is needed

As eluded to in our discussion of multiple pathways and feedback loops in any given target, we need to develop ways to target multiple points of a pathway akin to attacking the Achilles heel of the tumour. Recent data suggest that miRNA expression is tightly coordinated, and that each miRNA may target numerous messages. Thus, a specific miRNA has the potential to regulate several members of an entire signalling pathway. miRNAs negatively regulate their targets by one of two mechanisms: either by near perfect binding to the mRNA target and induction of miRNA-associated, multiprotein RNA-induced-silencing complex (miRISC), which results in accelerated mRNA decay (Yekta 2004; Wu 2006) or by less perfect binding to the target mRNA 3′-UTR and inhibition of translation through a RISC complex similar to, or identical with, the complex recruited in RNA interference (RNAi) (Humphreys et al. 2005; Pillai et al. 2005; Esquela-Kerscher&Slack 2006).

miR-7 directly regulates the expression of EGFR in glioblastoma and has also been shown to directly attenuate the activation of AKT and ERK1/2 (extracellular signal-regulated kinase) indicating its ability to co-ordinately regulate EGFR signalling (Webster et al. 2009). We also showed that miR-124a attenuated glioblastoma migration and invasion at multiple points of the pathway (Fowler et al. 2011). New technologies are currently being developed to facilitate the use of miRNAs as a realistic therapeutic option. Until then, combination treatments and developing inhibitors which can affect a multiplicity of targets are critical.

5.3.5 Differing response criterion

The inability to accurately define endpoints from clinical trials makes the evaluation of new therapies subjective and significantly delays treatment development. At present overall survival (OS) and 6 month progression free survival (PFS6) are two defined end points accepted in most clinical trials testing for new GBM therapies. PFS6 relies on a combination of gadolinium enhanced MRI imaging and potentially subjective clinical evaluation. Seizures, depression and steroid induced myopathy can all influence clinical signs and symptoms. Since 1990, the MacDonald criterion has been used as an objective radiologic assessment of response in GBM. This two dimensional measurement has been mainstay for evaluating tumour response and is based upon measurements of the enhancing tumour area (the product of the maximal cross-sectional enhancing diameters) (Macdonald et al. 1990). With the advance of treatments administered to patients with GBM, the MacDonald Criteria has a number of important limitations. The MacDonald criteria does not discriminate measurable disease from non-measureable disease, cannot identify non-tumour related increases in enhancement and provides no use for the evaluation of anti-angiogenic drugs. Bevacizumab can cause accelerated regression of VEGF driven angiogenesis and rapid resolution of gadolinium MRI changes in responding patients. There is concern however as to whether anti-VEGF therapy results in true glioma cell destruction or their ability to control the perivascular leak, resulting in better symptom control (associated with improvement of gadolinium MRI).

An international working group was formed to review and improve the response assessment criteria for high grade gliomas, coined Response Assessment in Neuro-Oncology (RANO) (Wen et al. 2010). The guidelines have devised a better standardisation of how clinicians measure response, which will ultimately result in a more uniform assessment of disease status across different centres. Unfortunately, the new RANO guidelines do not address the persistent problem of the irregularity of gliomas and the difficulty of measuring tumours treated with anti-angiogenic drugs, suggesting that volumetric measurements that count all enhancing and non-enhancing voxels may prove more accurate in the future.The RANO working party acknowledges that an important area of future research is the need to *develop advanced novel MRI techniques.*

5.3.6 Inadequate tissue

Biobanks or biorepositories play a critical role in the evolution of biomarkers, targets and targeted therapies. Five years ago, the NCI announced their plans to enlist dozens of bio-repositories in the USA to provide large tumour numbers and use high-throughput DNA sequencing and computational biology to produce with new methods of detecting and treating cancers. Unfortunately sub-standard tissue and data collection provided a significant road block to the Cancer Genome Atlas effort. Biorepositories remain underfunded and unappreciated. Despite billions of dollars poured into cancer research, innovation in the field of biobanking is sadly lacking. Standard operating procedures (SOPs) are not consistent between sites, and sometimes differ within single institutes. Methodologies for preserving tissue vary and times between tumour removal and time of processing fluctuate. Significant genetic changes can occur between the time of tissue removal from the body and time of processing. The collection of tissue has to be taken seriously and investments need to be urgently made to promote basic, translational and clinical research as well as social gain in terms of improved cancer care and economic development.

Collection and storage of frozen tissue is critical for biomarker development. Many of our current biomarker assays are performed on Formalin Fixed Paraffin Embedded (FFPE) tissue. This type of tissue, whilst preserving morphology for diagnosis, induces problems for downstream molecular applications. High quality RNA is difficult to obtain from FFPE tissue and PCR amplification from FFPE DNA is limited to products of less than 200 base pairs. It is also difficult to control the processes leading up to tissue fixation. In a first class Neuro-oncology centre in Australia, FFPE blocks were being sent to Central Headquarters for MGMT methylation detection. Unfortunately, a sizeable batch of tissues were non-determinative (could not be amplified). Tissue from surgeries performed on a Friday were fixed in formalin, however the laboratory was unattended over the weekend, resulting in the tissue submerged in formalin for up to 72 hours (routinely, formalin should be removed after 24 hours).
Another issue that we are not taking into careful consideration are the molecular changes acquired in the tumour *after* treatment. Many biomarker studies are performed on tumour obtained at initial surgery event. This tissue has not been exposed to treatment. However, the majority of novel treatments are tested at the time of recurrence. Changes in chromosome aberrations and mismatch repair proteins have been detected in paired tumour specimens (primary and relapsed). Careful consideration of the tissue and its relevance to the clinical circumstance of the patient is required.

6. Future directions for biomarker development

To advance personalised medicine, a co-operative effort between cancer researchers and clinicians is urgently needed. There is very little collaboration between scientists working on targeted therapies such as the TKIs and anti-angiogenics...what worked, what didn't? Specific consideration needs to be paid to increasing sample sizes, sequencing entire genes, implementing robust methodologies and taking a holistic approach to understanding pathways. Cancer is multifaceted and we urgently need to unravel these complexities. Two prospective biomarker trials have been encouraging: the I-SPY 2 (investigation of serial studies to predict your therapeutic response with imaging and molecular analysis 2) for women with locally advanced breast cancer (Barker et al. 2009) and BATTLE (Biomarker Integrated Approaches of Targeted Therapy for Lung Cancer Elimination) for pre-treated patients with non-small cell lung cancer (NSLC) (Kim 2011). Both trials employ an adaptive phase II/III clinical trial design. The I-SPY 2 is performed as a neo-adjuvant trial. A core biopsy is provided and tested for Estrogen Receptor (ER), Progesterone Receptor (PR), Human Epidermal Growth Factor Receptor 2 (HER2) and MammaPrint status (a gene signature known to be predictive of outcome). Based upon the marker outcomes, the patients will be stratified into two arms of a standard neoadjuvant regime: paclitaxel (plus trastuzumab [Herceptin] for HER2+ patients followed by doxorubicin (Adriamycin) and cyclophosphamide (Cytoxan). Five new drugs will be trialled in the other arms (each being added to the standard therapy). Patients are currently being recruited. The BATTLE trial takes on a very similar adaptive design but differs in its examination of samples from post-treated NSLC. Key drugs and associated biomarkers (Erlotinib/EGFR; Vandetanib/VEGFR; Erlotinib + bexarotene/ Retinoid + EGFR and Sorafenib/ KRAS/BRAF) were tested both as an equal randomisation design and an adaptive randomisation design. This trial confirmed that tumours harbouring mutations in KRAS/BRAF showed a disease control of 79% when treated with sorafenib but only 14% of the patients responded to erlotinib. Conversely, sorafenib, although active against wild type or mutated KRAS, had worse disease control in patients with EGFR mutations. A limitation in applying these adaptive trial designs to glioblastoma will be adequate numbers. Additionally, the BATTLE trial identified that grouping mutations together were less predictive than individual markers. This may also impact on a highly heterogenous cancer such as glioblastoma. Nevertheless, these trials show that, with a highly integrated team of multidisciplinary investigators, better overall survival in glioblastoma is achievable.

7. Acknowledgements

I would like to acknowledge the support and financial assistance from the Cure For Life Foundation and the Cancer Institute NSW.

8. References

(2008). Comprehensive genomic characterization defines human glioblastoma genes and core pathways. *Nature*, Vol. 455, No. 7216, (Oct 23) pp. 1061-1068.

Ahluwalia, M. S. (2011). 2010 Society for Neuro-Oncology Annual Meeting: a report of selected studies. *Expert Rev Anticancer Ther*, Vol. 11, No. 2, (Feb) pp. 161-163.

Balss, J., et al. (2008). Analysis of the IDH1 codon 132 mutation in brain tumors. *Acta Neuropathol*, Vol. 116, No. 6, (Dec) pp. 597-602.

Barbashina, V., et al. (2005). Allelic losses at 1p36 and 19q13 in gliomas: correlation with histologic classification, definition of a 150-kb minimal deleted region on 1p36, and evaluation of CAMTA1 as a candidate tumor suppressor gene. *Clin Cancer Res*, Vol. 11, No. 3, (Feb 1) pp. 1119-1128.

Barker, A. D., et al. (2009). I-SPY 2: an adaptive breast cancer trial design in the setting of neoadjuvant chemotherapy. *Clin Pharmacol Ther*, Vol. 86, No. 1, (Jul) pp. 97-100.

Brandes, A. A., et al. (2001). Changing boundaries in the treatment of malignant gliomas. *Expert Rev Anticancer Ther*, Vol. 1, No. 3, (Oct) pp. 357-370.

Brandes, A. A., et al. (2006). Temozolomide 3 weeks on and 1 week off as first-line therapy for recurrent glioblastoma: phase II study from gruppo italiano cooperativo di neuro-oncologia (GICNO). *Br J Cancer*, Vol. 95, No. 9, (Nov 6) pp. 1155-1160.

Brell, M., et al. (2005). Prognostic significance of O6-methylguanine-DNA methyltransferase determined by promoter hypermethylation and immunohistochemical expression in anaplastic gliomas. *Clin Cancer Res*, Vol. 11, No. 14, (Jul 15) pp. 5167-5174.

Brock, C. S., et al. (1998). Phase I trial of temozolomide using an extended continuous oral schedule. *Cancer Research*, Vol. 58, No. 19, (Oct 1) pp. 4363-4367.

Brown, P. D., et al. (2008). Phase I/II trial of erlotinib and temozolomide with radiation therapy in the treatment of newly diagnosed glioblastoma multiforme: North Central Cancer Treatment Group Study N0177. *J Clin Oncol*, Vol. 26, No. 34, (Dec 1) pp. 5603-5609.

Buttolo, L., et al. (2006). Alternative schedules of adjuvant temozolomide in glioblastoma multiforme: A 6-year experience. *Journal Of Clinical Oncology*, Vol. 24, No. 18, (Jun 20) pp. 60S-60S.

Cairncross, G., et al. (2006). Phase III trial of chemotherapy plus radiotherapy compared with radiotherapy alone for pure and mixed anaplastic oligodendroglioma:

Intergroup Radiation Therapy Oncology Group Trial 9402. *J Clin Oncol*, Vol. 24, No. 18, (Jun 20) pp. 2707-2714.

Calin, G. A., et al. (2002). Frequent deletions and down-regulation of micro- RNA genes miR15 and miR16 at 13q14 in chronic lymphocytic leukemia. *Proc Natl Acad Sci U S A*, Vol. 99, No. 24, (Nov 26) pp. 15524-15529.

Cao, V. T., et al. (2009). The correlation and prognostic significance of MGMT promoter methylation and MGMT protein in glioblastomas. *Neurosurgery*, Vol. 65, No. 5, (Nov) pp. 866-875; discussion 875.

Chinot, O. L., et al. (2011). AVAglio: Phase 3 trial of bevacizumab plus temozolomide and radiotherapy in newly diagnosed glioblastoma multiforme. *Adv Ther*, Vol. 28, No. 4, (Apr) pp. 334-340.

Christensen, B. C., et al. (2011). DNA methylation, isocitrate dehydrogenase mutation, and survival in glioma. *J Natl Cancer Inst*, Vol. 103, No. 2, (Jan 19) pp. 143-153.

Colman, H., et al. (2010). A multigene predictor of outcome in glioblastoma. *Neuro Oncol*, Vol. 12, No. 1, (Jan) pp. 49-57.

Conti, A., et al. (2009). miR-21 and 221 upregulation and miR-181b downregulation in human grade II-IV astrocytic tumors. *J Neurooncol*, Vol. 93, No. 3, (Jul) pp. 325-332.

Dang, L., et al. (2009). Cancer-associated IDH1 mutations produce 2-hydroxyglutarate. *Nature*, Vol. 462, No. 7274, (Dec 10) pp. 739-744.

de Souza, J. A. and O. I. Olopade (2011). CYP2D6 genotyping and tamoxifen: an unfinished story in the quest for personalized medicine. *Semin Oncol*, Vol. 38, No. 2, (Apr) pp. 263-273.

di Tomaso, E., et al. (2011). Glioblastoma recurrence after cediranib therapy in patients: lack of "rebound" revascularization as mode of escape. *Cancer Res*, Vol. 71, No. 1, (Jan 1) pp. 19-28.

Dienstmann, R. and J. Tabernero (2011). BRAF as a Target for Cancer Therapy. *Anticancer Agents Med Chem*, Vol. 11, No. 3, (Mar 1) pp. 285-295.

Dietrich, J., et al. (2009). Cediranib: profile of a novel anti-angiogenic agent in patients with glioblastoma. *Expert Opin Investig Drugs*, Vol. 18, No. 10, (Oct) pp. 1549-1557.

Dresemann, G., et al. (2010). Imatinib in combination with hydroxyurea versus hydroxyurea alone as oral therapy in patients with progressive pretreated glioblastoma resistant to standard dose temozolomide. *J Neurooncol*, Vol. 96, No. 3, (Feb) pp. 393-402.

Ducray, F., et al. (2009). alpha-Internexin expression identifies 1p19q codeleted gliomas. *Neurology*, Vol. 72, No. 2, (Jan 13) pp. 156-161.

Ducray, F., et al. (2008). Anaplastic oligodendrogliomas with 1p19q codeletion have a proneural gene expression profile. *Mol Cancer*, Vol. 7, No., pp. 41.

Esquela-Kerscher, A. and F. J. Slack (2006). Oncomirs - microRNAs with a role in cancer. *Nat Rev Cancer*, Vol. 6, No. 4, (Apr) pp. 259-269.

Esteller, M., et al. (2000). Inactivation of the DNA-repair gene MGMT and the clinical response of gliomas to alkylating agents. *N Engl J Med*, Vol. 343, No. 19, (Nov 9) pp. 1350-1354.

Esteller, M., et al. (1999). Inactivation of the DNA repair gene O6-methylguanine-DNA methyltransferase by promoter hypermethylation is a common event in primary human neoplasia. *Cancer Res*, Vol. 59, No. 4, (Feb 15) pp. 793-797.

Fowler, A., et al. (2011). miR-124a is frequently down-regulated in glioblastoma and is involved in migration and invasion. *Eur J Cancer*, Vol. 47, No. 6, (Apr) pp. 953-963.

Fuller, G. N. and B. W. Scheithauer (2007). The 2007 Revised World Health Organization (WHO) Classification of Tumours of the Central Nervous System: newly codified entities. *Brain Pathol*, Vol. 17, No. 3, (Jul) pp. 304-307.

Gan, H. K., et al. (2009). The EGFRvIII variant in glioblastoma multiforme. *J Clin Neurosci*, Vol. 16, No. 6, (Jun) pp. 748-754.

Gerson, S. L. (2004). MGMT: its role in cancer aetiology and cancer therapeutics. *Nat Rev Cancer*, Vol. 4, No. 4, (Apr) pp. 296-307.

Gerstner, E. R., et al. (2011). Infiltrative patterns of glioblastoma spread detected via diffusion MRI after treatment with cediranib. *Neuro Oncol*, Vol. 12, No. 5, (May) pp. 466-472.

Goetz, M. P. (2010). Update on CYP2D6 and its impact on tamoxifen therapy. *Clin Adv Hematol Oncol*, Vol. 8, No. 8, (Aug) pp. 536-538.

Hartmann, C., et al. (2010). Patients with IDH1 wild type anaplastic astrocytomas exhibit worse prognosis than IDH1-mutated glioblastomas, and IDH1 mutation status accounts for the unfavorable prognostic effect of higher age: implications for classification of gliomas. *Acta Neuropathol*, Vol. 120, No. 6, (Dec) pp. 707-718.

Hawkins, N. J., et al. (2009). MGMT methylation is associated primarily with the germline C>T SNP (rs16906252) in colorectal cancer and normal colonic mucosa. *Mod Pathol*, Vol. 22, No. 12, (Dec) pp. 1588-1599.

Hegi, M. E., et al. (2005). MGMT gene silencing and benefit from temozolomide in glioblastoma. *N Engl J Med*, Vol. 352, No. 10, (Mar 10) pp. 997-1003.

Hill, C., et al. (2003). Genetic markers in glioblastoma: prognostic significance and future therapeutic implications. *Adv Anat Pathol*, Vol. 10, No. 4, (Jul) pp. 212-217.

Hofer, S., et al. (2011). Clinical outcome with bevacizumab in patients with recurrent high-grade glioma treated outside clinical trials. *Acta Oncol*, Vol. 50, No. 5, (Jun) pp. 630-635.

Hormigo, A., et al. (2006). YKL-40 and matrix metalloproteinase-9 as potential serum biomarkers for patients with high-grade gliomas. *Clin Cancer Res*, Vol. 12, No. 19, (Oct 1) pp. 5698-5704.

Hu, J. C. and K. Mokbel (2001). Does c-erbB2/HER2 overexpression predict adjuvant tamoxifen failure in patients with early breast cancer? *Eur J Surg Oncol*, Vol. 27, No. 4, (Jun) pp. 335-337.

Humphreys, D. T., et al. (2005). MicroRNAs control translation initiation by inhibiting eukaryotic initiation factor 4E/cap and poly(A) tail function. *Proc Natl Acad Sci U S A*, Vol. 102, No. 47, (Nov 22) pp. 16961-16966.

Inda, M. M., et al. (2010). Tumor heterogeneity is an active process maintained by a mutant EGFR-induced cytokine circuit in glioblastoma. *Genes Dev*, Vol. 24, No. 16, (Aug 15) pp. 1731-1745.

Jakobsen, J. N., et al. (2011). Irinotecan and bevacizumab in recurrent glioblastoma multiforme. *Expert Opin Pharmacother*, Vol. 12, No. 5, (Apr) pp. 825-833.

Jansen, M., et al. (2010). Molecular pathology in adult gliomas: diagnostic, prognostic, and predictive markers. *Lancet Neurol*, Vol. 9, No. 7, (Jul) pp. 717-726.

Jenkins, R. B., et al. (2006). A t(1;19)(q10;p10) mediates the combined deletions of 1p and 19q and predicts a better prognosis of patients with oligodendroglioma. *Cancer Res*, Vol. 66, No. 20, (Oct 15) pp. 9852-9861.

Ji, J., et al. (2009). MicroRNA expression, survival, and response to interferon in liver cancer. *N Engl J Med*, Vol. 361, No. 15, (Oct 8) pp. 1437-1447.

Kaloshi, G., et al. (2007). FABP7 expression in glioblastomas: relation to prognosis, invasion and EGFR status. *J Neurooncol*, Vol. 84, No. 3, (Sep) pp. 245-248.

Kamiryo, T., et al. (2004). Correlation between promoter hypermethylation of the O6-methylguanine-deoxyribonucleic acid methyltransferase gene and prognosis in patients with high-grade astrocytic tumors treated with surgery, radiotherapy, and 1-(4-amino-2-methyl-5-pyrimidinyl)methyl-3-(2-chloroethyl)-3-nitrosourea-b ased chemotherapy. *Neurosurgery*, Vol. 54, No. 2, (Feb) pp. 349-357; discussion 357.

Karayan-Tapon, L., et al. (2010). Prognostic value of O6-methylguanine-DNA methyltransferase status in glioblastoma patients, assessed by five different methods. *Journal of neuro-oncology*, Vol. 97, No. 3, pp. 311-322.

Kefas, B., et al. (2009). The neuronal microRNA miR-326 acts in a feedback loop with notch and has therapeutic potential against brain tumors. *J Neurosci*, Vol. 29, No. 48, (Dec 2) pp. 15161-15168.

Kim, E., Herbst RS, Wistuba II, Lee IJ, Blumenschein GR, Tsao A, Stewart DJ, Hicks ME, Erasmus J, Gupta S, Alden CM, Liu S, Tang X, Khuri FR, Tran HT, Johnson BE, Heymach JV, Mao L, Fossella F, Kies MS, Papadimitrakopoulou, David SE, Lippman SM, Hong WK (2011). The BATTLE Trial: Personalizing Therapy for Lung Cancer. *Cancer Discovery*, Vol. 1, No. 1, pp. 43.

Kim, H., et al. Integrative genome analysis reveals an oncomir/oncogene cluster regulating glioblastoma survivorship. *Proc Natl Acad Sci U S A*, Vol. 107, No. 5, (Feb 2) pp. 2183-2188.

Kim, H. P., et al. (2008). Combined lapatinib and cetuximab enhance cytotoxicity against gefitinib-resistant lung cancer cells. *Mol Cancer Ther*, Vol. 7, No. 3, (Mar) pp. 607-615.

Koch, D., et al. (2007). Local intracerebral administration of O(6)-benzylguanine combined with systemic chemotherapy with temozolomide of a patient suffering from a recurrent glioblastoma. *J Neurooncol*, Vol. 82, No. 1, (Mar) pp. 85-89.

Kurokawa, H., et al. (2000). Inhibition of HER2/neu (erbB-2) and mitogen-activated protein kinases enhances tamoxifen action against HER2-overexpressing, tamoxifen-resistant breast cancer cells. *Cancer Res*, Vol. 60, No. 20, (Oct 15) pp. 5887-5894.

Lai, A., et al. (2011). Phase II study of bevacizumab plus temozolomide during and after radiation therapy for patients with newly diagnosed glioblastoma multiforme. *J Clin Oncol*, Vol. 29, No. 2, (Jan 10) pp. 142-148.

Laigle-Donadey, F., et al. (2005). [Molecular biology of oligodendroglial tumors]. *Neurochirurgie*, Vol. 51, No. 3-4 Pt 2, (Sep) pp. 260-268.

Layfield, L. J., et al. (2006). Epidermal growth factor receptor gene amplification and protein expression in glioblastoma multiforme: prognostic significance and relationship to other prognostic factors. *Appl Immunohistochem Mol Morphol*, Vol. 14, No. 1, (Mar) pp. 91-96.

Li, Y., et al. (2009). MicroRNA-21 targets LRRFIP1 and contributes to VM-26 resistance in glioblastoma multiforme. *Brain Res*, Vol. 1286, No., (Aug 25) pp. 13-18.

Liu, Q., et al. (2009). Molecular properties of CD133+ glioblastoma stem cells derived from treatment-refractory recurrent brain tumors. *J Neurooncol*, Vol. 94, No. 1, (Aug) pp. 1-19.

Macdonald, D. R., et al. (1990). Response criteria for phase II studies of supratentorial malignant glioma. *J Clin Oncol*, Vol. 8, No. 7, (Jul) pp. 1277-1280.

Mao, X. G., et al. (2011). Overexpression of ZNF217 in glioblastoma contributes to the maintenance of glioma stem cells regulated by hypoxia-inducible factors. *Lab Invest*, Vol., No., (Apr 11).

Mellai, M., et al. (2009). MGMT promoter hypermethylation in a series of 104 glioblastomas. *Cancer Genomics Proteomics*, Vol. 6, No. 4, (Jul-Aug) pp. 219-227.

Mellinghoff, I. K., et al. (2005). Molecular determinants of the response of glioblastomas to EGFR kinase inhibitors. *N Engl J Med*, Vol. 353, No. 19, (Nov 10) pp. 2012-2024.

Mikkelsen, T., et al. (2009). Temozolomide single-agent chemotherapy for newly diagnosed anaplastic oligodendroglioma. *Journal of neuro-oncology*, Vol. 92, No. 1, pp. 57-63.

Mokhtari, K., et al. (2011). Alpha-internexin expression predicts outcome in anaplastic oligodendroglial tumors and may positively impact the efficacy of chemotherapy: European organization for research and treatment of cancer trial 26951. *Cancer*, Vol., No., (Jan 18).

Mukasa, A., et al. (2004). Selective expression of a subset of neuronal genes in oligodendroglioma with chromosome 1p loss. *Brain Pathol*, Vol. 14, No. 1, (Jan) pp. 34-42.

Mukasa, A., et al. (2002). Distinction in gene expression profiles of oligodendrogliomas with and without allelic loss of 1p. *Oncogene*, Vol. 21, No. 25, (Jun 6) pp. 3961-3968.

Nakamura, M., et al. (2001). Promoter methylation of the DNA repair gene MGMT in astrocytomas is frequently associated with G:C --> A:T mutations of the TP53 tumor suppressor gene. *Carcinogenesis*, Vol. 22, No. 10, (Oct) pp. 1715-1719.

Newlands, E. S., et al. (2003). Phase I study of temozolamide (TMZ) combined with procarbazine (PCB) in patients with gliomas. *Br J Cancer*, Vol. 89, No. 2, (Jul 21) pp. 248-251.

Noushmehr, H., et al. (2010). Identification of a CpG island methylator phenotype that defines a distinct subgroup of glioma. *Cancer Cell*, Vol. 17, No. 5, (May 18) pp. 510-522.

Nutt, C. L., et al. (2003). Gene expression-based classification of malignant gliomas correlates better with survival than histological classification. *Cancer Res*, Vol. 63, No. 7, (Apr 1) pp. 1602-1607.

Parsa, A. T., et al. (2007). Loss of tumor suppressor PTEN function increases B7-H1 expression and immunoresistance in glioma. *Nat Med*, Vol. 13, No. 1, (Jan) pp. 84-88.

Parsons, D. W., et al. (2008). An integrated genomic analysis of human glioblastoma multiforme. *Science*, Vol. 321, No. 5897, (Sep 26) pp. 1807-1812.

Paz-Ares, L., et al. (2010). Clinical outcomes in non-small-cell lung cancer patients with EGFR mutations: pooled analysis. *J Cell Mol Med*, Vol. 14, No. 1-2, (Jan) pp. 51-69.

Paz, M. F., et al. (2004). CpG island hypermethylation of the DNA repair enzyme methyltransferase predicts response to temozolomide in primary gliomas. *Clin Cancer Res*, Vol. 10, No. 15, (Aug 1) pp. 4933-4938.

Pegg, A. E. (1990). Mammalian O6-alkylguanine-DNA alkyltransferase: regulation and importance in response to alkylating carcinogenic and therapeutic agents. *Cancer Res*, Vol. 50, No. 19, (Oct 1) pp. 6119-6129.

Pelloski, C. E., et al. (2007). Epidermal growth factor receptor variant III status defines clinically distinct subtypes of glioblastoma. *J Clin Oncol*, Vol. 25, No. 16, (Jun 1) pp. 2288-2294.

Perry, J. R., et al. (2010). Phase II trial of continuous dose-intense temozolomide in recurrent malignant glioma: RESCUE study. *J Clin Oncol*, Vol. 28, No. 12, (Apr 20) pp. 2051-2057.

Perry, J. R., et al. (2008). Temozolomide rechallenge in recurrent malignant glioma by using a continuous temozolomide schedule: the "rescue" approach. *Cancer*, Vol. 113, No. 8, (Oct 15) pp. 2152-2157.

Phillips, H. S., et al. (2006). Molecular subclasses of high-grade glioma predict prognosis, delineate a pattern of disease progression, and resemble stages in neurogenesis. *Cancer Cell*, Vol. 9, No. 3, (Mar) pp. 157-173.

Pierson, J., et al. (2008). Regulation of cyclin dependent kinase 6 by microRNA 124 in medulloblastoma. *J Neurooncol*, Vol. 90, No. 1, (Oct) pp. 1-7.

Pillai, R. S., et al. (2005). Inhibition of translational initiation by Let-7 MicroRNA in human cells. *Science*, Vol. 309, No. 5740, (Sep 2) pp. 1573-1576.

Prados, M., et al. (2011). Response as a predictor of survival in patients with recurrent glioblastoma treated with bevacizumab. *Neuro Oncol*, Vol. 13, No. 1, (Jan) pp. 143-151.

Prados, M. D., et al. (2009). Phase II study of erlotinib plus temozolomide during and after radiation therapy in patients with newly diagnosed glioblastoma multiforme or gliosarcoma. *J Clin Oncol*, Vol. 27, No. 4, (Feb 1) pp. 579-584.

Prasad, G., et al. (2011). Inhibition of PI3K/mTOR pathways in glioblastoma and implications for combination therapy with temozolomide. *Neuro Oncol*, Vol. 13, No. 4, (Apr) pp. 384-392.

Preusser, M., et al. (2008). Anti-O6-methylguanine-methyltransferase (MGMT) immunohistochemistry in glioblastoma multiforme: observer variability and lack of association with patient survival impede its use as clinical biomarker. *Brain Pathol*, Vol. 18, No. 4, (Oct) pp. 520-532.

Puzanov, I., et al. (2011). Biological challenges of BRAF inhibitor therapy. *Mol Oncol*, Vol. 5, No. 2, (Apr) pp. 116-123.

Quinn, J. A., et al. (2005). Phase I trial of temozolomide plus O6-benzylguanine for patients with recurrent or progressive malignant glioma. *J Clin Oncol*, Vol. 23, No. 28, (Oct 1) pp. 7178-7187.

Quinn, J. A., et al. (2002). Phase II trial of carmustine plus O(6)-benzylguanine for patients with nitrosourea-resistant recurrent or progressive malignant glioma. *J Clin Oncol*, Vol. 20, No. 9, (May 1) pp. 2277-2283.

Ramirez, C., et al. (2010). Loss of 1p, 19q, and 10q heterozygosity prospectively predicts prognosis of oligodendroglial tumors--towards individualized tumor treatment? *Neuro-oncology*, Vol. 12, No. 5, pp. 490-499.

Reardon, D. A., et al. (2010). Phase 2 trial of erlotinib plus sirolimus in adults with recurrent glioblastoma. *J Neurooncol*, Vol. 96, No. 2, (Jan) pp. 219-230.

Reardon, D. A., et al. (2011). Cilengitide: an RGD pentapeptide alphanubeta3 and alphanubeta5 integrin inhibitor in development for glioblastoma and other malignancies. *Future Oncol*, Vol. 7, No. 3, (Mar) pp. 339-354.

Reitman, Z. J., et al. (2011). Profiling the effects of isocitrate dehydrogenase 1 and 2 mutations on the cellular metabolome. *Proc Natl Acad Sci U S A*, Vol. 108, No. 8, (Feb 22) pp. 3270-3275.

Reitman, Z. J., et al. (2010). IDH1 and IDH2: not your typical oncogenes. *Cancer Cell*, Vol. 17, No. 3, (Mar 16) pp. 215-216.

Reitman, Z. J. and H. Yan (2010). Isocitrate dehydrogenase 1 and 2 mutations in cancer: alterations at a crossroads of cellular metabolism. *J Natl Cancer Inst*, Vol. 102, No. 13, (Jul 7) pp. 932-941.

Ruano, Y., et al. (2009). Worse outcome in primary glioblastoma multiforme with concurrent epidermal growth factor receptor and p53 alteration. *Am J Clin Pathol*, Vol. 131, No. 2, (Feb) pp. 257-263.

Saidi, A., et al. (2009). Combined targeting of interleukin-6 and vascular endothelial growth factor potently inhibits glioma growth and invasiveness. *Int J Cancer*, Vol. 125, No. 5, (Sep 1) pp. 1054-1064.

Salter, K. H., et al. (2008). An integrated approach to the prediction of chemotherapeutic response in patients with breast cancer. *PLoS One*, Vol. 3, No. 4, pp. e1908.

Sampson, J. H., et al. (2011). Greater chemotherapy-induced lymphopenia enhances tumor-specific immune responses that eliminate EGFRvIII-expressing tumor cells in patients with glioblastoma. *Neuro Oncol*, Vol. 13, No. 3, (Mar) pp. 324-333.

Sasayama, T., et al. (2009). MicroRNA-10b is overexpressed in malignant glioma and associated with tumor invasive factors, uPAR and RhoC. *Int J Cancer*, Vol. 125, No. 6, (Sep 15) pp. 1407-1413.

Sawlani, R. N., et al. (2011). Glioblastoma: a method for predicting response to antiangiogenic chemotherapy by using MR perfusion imaging--pilot study. *Radiology*, Vol. 255, No. 2, (May) pp. 622-628.

Server, A., et al. (2011). Diagnostic examination performance by using microvascular leakage, cerebral blood volume, and blood flow derived from 3-T dynamic susceptibility-weighted contrast-enhanced perfusion MR imaging in the differentiation of glioblastoma multiforme and brain metastasis. *Neuroradiology*, Vol. 53, No. 5, (May) pp. 319-330.

Settle, S. H. and E. P. Sulman (2011). Tumor profiling: development of prognostic and predictive factors to guide brain tumor treatment. *Curr Oncol Rep*, Vol. 13, No. 1, (Feb) pp. 26-36.

Shi, L., et al. (2008). hsa-mir-181a and hsa-mir-181b function as tumor suppressors in human glioma cells. *Brain Res*, Vol. 1236, No., (Oct 21) pp. 185-193.

Shinojima, N., et al. (2003). Prognostic value of epidermal growth factor receptor in patients with glioblastoma multiforme. *Cancer Res*, Vol. 63, No. 20, (Oct 15) pp. 6962-6970.

Shiraishi, S., et al. (2002). Influence of p53 mutations on prognosis of patients with glioblastoma. *Cancer*, Vol. 95, No. 2, (Jul 15) pp. 249-257.

Silber, J., et al. (2008). miR-124 and miR-137 inhibit proliferation of glioblastoma multiforme cells and induce differentiation of brain tumor stem cells. *BMC Med*, Vol. 6, No., pp. 14.

Silber, J. R., et al. (1998). O6-methylguanine-DNA methyltransferase activity in adult gliomas: relation to patient and tumor characteristics. *Cancer Res*, Vol. 58, No. 5, (Mar 1) pp. 1068-1073.

Sorensen, A. G., et al. (2009). A "vascular normalization index" as potential mechanistic biomarker to predict survival after a single dose of cediranib in recurrent glioblastoma patients. *Cancer Res*, Vol. 69, No. 13, (Jul 1) pp. 5296-5300.

Sreekanthreddy, P., et al. (2010). Identification of potential serum biomarkers of glioblastoma: serum osteopontin levels correlate with poor prognosis. *Cancer Epidemiol Biomarkers Prev*, Vol. 19, No. 6, (Jun) pp. 1409-1422.

Stingl, J. C., et al. (2010). Impact of CYP2D6*4 genotype on progression free survival in tamoxifen breast cancer treatment. *Curr Med Res Opin*, Vol. 26, No. 11, (Nov) pp. 2535-2542.

Stupp, R., et al. (2009). Effects of radiotherapy with concomitant and adjuvant temozolomide versus radiotherapy alone on survival in glioblastoma in a randomised phase III study: 5-year analysis of the EORTC-NCIC trial. *Lancet Oncol*, Vol. 10, No. 5, (May) pp. 459-466.

Stupp, R., et al. (2010). Phase I/IIa study of cilengitide and temozolomide with concomitant radiotherapy followed by cilengitide and temozolomide maintenance therapy in patients with newly diagnosed glioblastoma. *J Clin Oncol*, Vol. 28, No. 16, (Jun 1) pp. 2712-2718.

Stupp, R., et al. (2005). Radiotherapy plus concomitant and adjuvant temozolomide for glioblastoma. *N Engl J Med*, Vol. 352, No. 10, (Mar 10) pp. 987-996.

Tews, B., et al. (2006). Identification of novel oligodendroglioma-associated candidate tumor suppressor genes in 1p36 and 19q13 using microarray-based expression profiling. *Int J Cancer*, Vol. 119, No. 4, (Aug 15) pp. 792-800.

Tews, B., et al. (2007). Hypermethylation and transcriptional downregulation of the CITED4 gene at 1p34.2 in oligodendroglial tumours with allelic losses on 1p and 19q. *Oncogene*, Vol. 26, No. 34, (Jul 26) pp. 5010-5016.

Thiessen, B., et al. (2010). A phase I/II trial of GW572016 (lapatinib) in recurrent glioblastoma multiforme: clinical outcomes, pharmacokinetics and molecular correlation. *Cancer Chemother Pharmacol*, Vol. 65, No. 2, (Jan) pp. 353-361.

Tolcher, A. W., et al. (2003). Marked inactivation of O-6-alkylguanine-DNA alkyltransferase activity with protracted temozolomide schedules. *British Journal Of Cancer*, Vol. 88, No. 7, (Apr 7) pp. 1004-1011.

Tsien, C., et al. (2011). Parametric response map as an imaging biomarker to distinguish progression from pseudoprogression in high-grade glioma. *J Clin Oncol*, Vol. 28, No. 13, (May 1) pp. 2293-2299.

Uhm, J. H., et al. (2010). Phase II Evaluation of Gefitinib in Patients with Newly Diagnosed Grade 4 Astrocytoma: Mayo/North Central Cancer Treatment Group Study N0074. *Int J Radiat Oncol Biol Phys*, Vol., No., (May 24).

van den Bent, M. J., et al. (2009). Randomized phase II trial of erlotinib versus temozolomide or carmustine in recurrent glioblastoma: EORTC brain tumor group study 26034. *J Clin Oncol*, Vol. 27, No. 8, (Mar 10) pp. 1268-1274.

van den Bent, M. J., et al. (2006). Adjuvant procarbazine, lomustine, and vincristine improves progression-free survival but not overall survival in newly diagnosed anaplastic oligodendrogliomas and oligoastrocytomas: a randomized European Organisation for Research and Treatment of Cancer phase III trial. *J Clin Oncol*, Vol. 24, No. 18, (Jun 20) pp. 2715-2722.

Verhaak, R. G., et al. (2010). Integrated genomic analysis identifies clinically relevant subtypes of glioblastoma characterized by abnormalities in PDGFRA, IDH1, EGFR, and NF1. *Cancer Cell*, Vol. 17, No. 1, (Jan 19) pp. 98-110.

Verhaak, R. G. and P. J. Valk (2010). Genes predictive of outcome and novel molecular classification schemes in adult acute myeloid leukemia. *Cancer Treat Res*, Vol. 145, No., pp. 67-83.

Vredenburgh, J. J., et al. (2007). Bevacizumab plus irinotecan in recurrent glioblastoma multiforme. *J Clin Oncol*, Vol. 25, No. 30, (Oct 20) pp. 4722-4729.

Vredenburgh, J. J., et al. (2011). The Addition of Bevacizumab to Standard Radiation Therapy and Temozolomide Followed by Bevacizumab, Temozolomide and Irinotecan for Newly Diagnosed Glioblastoma. *Clin Cancer Res*, Vol., No., (Apr 29).

Walker, C., et al. (2006). Clinical use of genotype to predict chemosensitivity in oligodendroglial tumors. *Neurology*, Vol. 66, No. 11, (Jun 13) pp. 1661-1667.

Wang, R., et al. (2011). Glioblastoma stem-like cells give rise to tumour endothelium. *Nature*, Vol. 468, No. 7325, (Dec 9) pp. 829-833.

Wang, S. and E. N. Olson (2009). AngiomiRs--key regulators of angiogenesis. *Curr Opin Genet Dev*, Vol. 19, No. 3, (Jun) pp. 205-211.

Webster, R. J., et al. (2009). Regulation of epidermal growth factor receptor signaling in human cancer cells by microRNA-7. *J Biol Chem*, Vol. 284, No. 9, (Feb 27) pp. 5731-5741.

Wen, P. Y., et al. (2010). Updated response assessment criteria for high-grade gliomas: response assessment in neuro-oncology working group. *J Clin Oncol*, Vol. 28, No. 11, (Apr 10) pp. 1963-1972.

Whittaker, S., et al. (2010). Gatekeeper mutations mediate resistance to BRAF-targeted therapies. *Sci Transl Med*, Vol. 2, No. 35, (Jun 9) pp. 35ra41.

Wick, A., et al. (2007). Efficacy and tolerability of temozolomide in an alternating weekly regimen in patients with recurrent glioma. *J Clin Oncol*, Vol. 25, No. 22, (Aug 1) pp. 3357-3361.

Wick, W., et al. (2009). NOA-04 randomized phase III trial of sequential radiochemotherapy of anaplastic glioma with procarbazine, lomustine, and vincristine or temozolomide. *J Clin Oncol*, Vol. 27, No. 35, (Dec 10) pp. 5874-5880.

Wick, W., et al. (2010). Phase III study of enzastaurin compared with lomustine in the treatment of recurrent intracranial glioblastoma. *J Clin Oncol*, Vol. 28, No. 7, (Mar 1) pp. 1168-1174.

Wick, W., et al. (2011). Phase III study of enzastaurin compared with lomustine in the treatment of recurrent intracranial glioblastoma. *J Clin Oncol*, Vol. 28, No. 7, (Mar 1) pp. 1168-1174.

Wick, W., et al. (2004). One week on/one week off regimen of temozolomide for recurrent glioblastoma: A phase III study. *Journal Of Clinical Oncology*, Vol. 22, No. 14, (Jul 15) pp. 116S-116S.

Wick, W. and M. Weller (2005). How lymphotoxic is dose-intensified temozolomide? The glioblastoma experience. *Journal Of Clinical Oncology*, Vol. 23, No. 18, (Jun 20) pp. 4235-4236.

Wu, L. e. a. (2006). MicroRNA direct rapid demethylation of mRNA. *PNAS*, Vol. 103, No., pp. 4034-4039.

Xu, W., et al. (2011). Oncometabolite 2-hydroxyglutarate is a competitive inhibitor of alpha-ketoglutarate-dependent dioxygenases. *Cancer Cell*, Vol. 19, No. 1, (Jan 18) pp. 17-30.

Yan, H., et al. (2009). IDH1 and IDH2 mutations in gliomas. *N Engl J Med*, Vol. 360, No. 8, (Feb 19) pp. 765-773.

Yekta, S. e. a. (2004). MicroRNA-directed cleavage of *HOXB8* mRNA. *Science*, Vol. 304, No., pp. 594-596.

Zhang, Y., et al. (2009). MicroRNA-128 inhibits glioma cells proliferation by targeting transcription factor E2F3a. *J Mol Med*, Vol. 87, No. 1, (Jan) pp. 43-51.

Part 2

Gliomagenesis

5

Genomic Abnormalities in Gliomas

Giovanny Pinto et al.*
*Federal University of Piauí, Parnaíba,
Brazil*

1. Introduction

In general, studies reveal that cancer arises through genetic and epigenetic alterations that affect specific genes within a given cell type. These changes involve a gain of function when the alterations involve oncogenes, a loss of function when the target genes are tumor suppressor genes. Thus, both genetic and epigenetic changes promote the instability of cellular homeostasis (Bello & Rey, 2006; Richardson, 2003; Sugimura & Ushijima, 2000). This lack of stability reflects the complexity of cancer because the loss of controlled cell growth occurs due to changes in one or more genes. These genetic and epigenetic events are followed by the growing accumulation of changes in hundreds, if not thousands, of genes. Over time, this accumulation causes the tumor to reach its highest degree of malignancy, which usually culminates in metastasis (Bartek & Lukas, 2001). However, in recent years, a subpopulation of tumor cells has been found to display a slow rate of cell division, high tumorigenic potential and characteristics similar to those of normal stem cells. This discovery has changed the concept of metastasis to one associated with strictly terminal states (Stiles & Rowitch, 2008).

Hanahan & Weinberg (2000) proposed that all tumor cells must acquire six essential alterations in cell physiology that collectively dictate malignant growth: (1) loss of normal signaling for cell proliferation arrest, (2) loss of signaling for cell differentiation, (3) autocrine signaling for cell division, (4) reduction in apoptosis, (5) ability to enter the basement membrane and other tissues and organs, and (6) induction of angiogenesis. All of these processes involve biochemical pathways that form a complex network of cell signaling. These processes are usually altered in tumors because the genes that compose them are changed, resulting in cell cycle dysregulation. Therefore, the identification and determination of oncogenes and tumor suppressor genes is essential for understanding both cancer biology and clinical applications, such as the identification of therapeutic targets, early detection, and prediction of the disease course. Studies concerning cell cycle control genes have served as a starting point for identifying genes related to tumorigenesis and their biochemical role in various pathways (Paige, 2003).

* France Yoshioka[1], Fábio Motta[1], Renata Canalle[1], Rommel Burbano[2], Juan Rey[3], Aline Custódio[4] and Cacilda Casartelli[4]
[1]*Federal University of Piauí, Parnaíba,Brazil*
[2]*Federal University of Pará, Belém, Brazil*
[3]*University Hospital La Paz, Madrid, Spain*
[4]*University of São Paulo, Ribeirão Preto, Brazil*

Changes in oncogenes can lead to constitutive activation, which involves activation under conditions in which an oncogene would normally be inactive. For this process to occur, a cell needs only one allele of an oncogene to be altered, resulting in a selective growth advantage. In contrast, changes in tumor suppressor genes often reduce the gene product and consequently its activity. For this reason, cells that develop a selective advantage with changes in tumor suppressor genes usually require inactivation of both alleles of the target gene. Conceptually, tumor suppressor genes can be subdivided into two categories: "gatekeepers" that directly inhibit tumor growth and thereby suppress tumor formation and "caretakers" that ensure DNA integrity by repairing damage or preventing genomic instability (Vogelstein & Kinzler, 2004).

Studies of hereditary and sporadic forms of tumors, particularly retinoblastoma, culminated in the formulation of Knudson's "two events" model in 1971. In hereditary tumors, the first mutation occurs in one allele in the germline and results in a predisposition to develop tumors. Throughout development, a second change (mutation or loss of heterozygosity) inactivates the other allele and silences the altered gene. In contrast, sporadic tumors acquire the two allelic alterations that lead to gene silencing throughout the organism's development (Knudson, 1971). Over time, the neoplastic transformation and metabolic-phenotype of the cell can evolve. Ultimately, these changes result in a cancer in which clonal expansion of modified somatic cells destroys the adjacent normal tissue (Bartek & Lukas, 2001).

For many years, research in cancer genetics has prioritized understanding the role of genetic alterations in carcinogenesis. Studies revealed that base deletions, insertions, recombination and amplification in oncogenes and tumor suppressor genes were related to metastasis and invasion. These changes were also closely related to tumorigenesis and tumor progression. For this reason, the scientific community accepted that genetic changes almost exclusively explained the process of carcinogenesis (Sugimura & Ushijima, 2000). However, studies also indicated that embryogenesis and differentiation, which are characterized by specific patterns of gene expression in tissues and organs, can occur without changes in the DNA sequence. This notion has interested the scientific community in potential epigenetic mechanisms of carcinogenesis (Jones & Buckley, 1990; Rush & Plass, 2002).

An epigenetic phenomenon is defined as a change in gene function that is heritable through mitosis or meiosis but cannot be explained by changes in the DNA sequence. Aberrant epigenetic mechanisms, such as promoter hypermethylation, histone modifications, or non-coding RNA expression, are known to be important for tumor formation and comprise the "third pathway" in Knudson's model. These mechanisms result in transcriptional repression equivalent to that observed with the mutations and deletions proposed in Knudson's model (Jones & Baylin, 2007).

DNA methylation, the main epigenetic modification studied, occurs at cytosine residues in the cytosine-guanine sequences (CpG) of DNA through the action of an enzyme family called DNA methyltransferases (DNMT). In humans, approximately 70% of CpG sites, which are generally located in repetitive DNA sequences, are methylated. Clusters of unmethylated CpG sites are present in the genome as well, and these clusters are referred to as CpG islands. Approximately 60% of genes have CpG islands in the promoter regions and in the first exon. CpG islands are often dimethylated when associated with housekeeping genes. Moreover, CpG islands are tissue specific and are generally methylated except in those tissues where the associated gene is expressed (Cross & Bird, 1995; Gonzalez-Gomez et al., 2003). A recent genome-wide analysis revealed that CpG islands are also found in non-promoter regions. In addition, epigenetic abnormalities causing loss of gene function are more frequent than genetic abnormalities in cancer cells (Schuebel et al., 2007). Thus, cellular epigenetic inheritance mediated by aberrant DNA methylation resulting in gene silencing, gene imprinting, and/or activation of cancer-associated genes is now accepted as an important factor defining the transformed phenotype (Natsume et al., 2010)

2. Tumors of the central nervous system

Tumors of the central nervous system (CNS) are relatively rare and represent approximately 5-9% of all cancers, with an estimated incidence of 4.2 to 5.4 per 100,000 people/year. Moreover, tumors of the CNS carry a very poor prognosis and are associated with considerable morbidity and mortality. They are a leading cause of childhood cancer deaths, the second leading cause of cancer-related death in men aged 20–39, and the fifth leading cause of cancer-related death in women aged 20-39 (Ohgaki & Kleihues, 2005).

Although the incidence of CNS tumors is small compared with the incidence of other cancers, CNS tumors are among the most serious human malignancies because they affect the organ responsible for the coordination and integration of all biological activities. Moreover, as each region of the brain has a vital function, therapies used to treat other cancers (e.g., total surgical removal of an organ or tumor with a generous margin of normal tissue) cannot be applied to brain tumors. The inability to use these therapies hinders quality of life and patient survival (Louis et al., 2002).

In CNS tumors, the histopathological classifications are extensive and based primarily on descriptive morphology. Because the histogenesis of these tumors is unique and heterogeneous, it is difficult to characterize several of the tumor subtypes, which is reflected in the difficulties encountered in tumor diagnosis (Gilbertson, 2002).

In contrast with the first World Health Organization (WHO) classifications for CNS tumors (Kleihues et al., 1993; Zülch, 1979), the third edition by Kleihues & Cavenee (2000) incorporated genetic profiles as additional aids in defining brain tumors. The fourth edition of the WHO classifications for CNS tumors, which was published in 2007, lists several new characteristics. The fourth edition is based on consensus from an international working group of 25 pathologists and geneticists, as well as contributions from more than 70 international experts. Currently, this edition is the standard for defining brain tumors for clinical oncology and cancer research communities world-wide (Louis et al., 2007).

3. Gliomas

Gliomas are the most common tumors of the CNS. However, in spite of marked progress in characterizing the molecular pathogenesis of gliomas, these tumors remain incurable. In most cases, gliomas are also refractory to treatment because of their molecular heterogeneity. Gliomas rarely metastasize outside of the brain but instead infiltrate extensively into the surrounding normal brain. Therefore, surgery is not curative but can establish the diagnosis and relieve symptoms by decompressing the brain, which is located in the rigid intracranial cavity. Radiation therapy and chemotherapy increase survival; however, disease recurrence is frequently inevitable (Park & Rich, 2009).

The following four degrees of malignancy are recognized by the WHO: grades I and II (low-grade), which are biologically less aggressive and grades III and IV (high-grade), which are the most aggressive. The histological criteria for grading malignancies are not uniform for all subtypes of gliomas. Thus, all tumors should be classified before the degree of malignancy is determined. This classification is made according to the cell type thought to be responsible for the tumor and based on the characteristics exhibited by astrocytes, oligodendrocytes, ependymal cells, or their neuronal progenitors (Louis et al., 2007). Table 1 shows the heterogeneous WHO classification for gliomas according to the degree of malignancy.

	WHO Grade						**WHO Grade**			
Astrocytic tumors	**I**	**II**	**III**	**IV**		**Ependymal tumors**	**I**	**II**	**III**	**IV**
Subependymal giant cell astrocytoma	•					Subependymoma	•			
Pilocytic astrocytoma	•					Myxopapillary ependymoma	•			
Pilomyxoid astrocytoma		•				Ependymoma		•		
Diffuse astrocytoma		•				Anaplastic ependymoma			•	
Pleomorphic xanthoastrocytoma		•								
Anaplastic astrocytoma			•			**Choroid plexus tumors**				
Glioblastoma				•		Choroid plexus papilloma	•			
Giant cell glioblastoma				•		Atypical choroid plexus papilloma		•		
Gliosarcoma				•		Choroid plexus carcinoma			•	
Oligodendroglial tumors						**Other neuroepithelial tumors**				
Oligodendroglioma		•				Angiocentric glioma	•			
Anaplastic oligodendroglioma			•			Chordoid glioma of the third ventricle		•		
Oligoastrocytic tumors										
Oligoastrocytoma		•								
Anaplastic oligoastrocytoma			•							

Table 1. WHO grading of gliomas (Louis et al., 2007).

Gliomas of astrocytic, oligodendroglial, and ependymal origin account for 80% of CNS tumors. For this reason, some morphological and genetic characteristics of these tumors are discussed below.

3.1 Astrocytomas

Astrocytomas represent the vast majority of gliomas and account for 70% of the total gliomas seen in patients. Astrocytomas can be further characterized as pilocytic astrocytomas (WHO grade I) or diffuse astrocytomas, including low-grade astrocytomas (WHO grade II), anaplastic astrocytomas (WHO grade III) and glioblastomas (WHO grade IV) (Kleihues et al., 2002).

Pilocytic astrocytomas are more commonly seen in children and carry a good prognosis because of their biology. Patients with neurofibromatosis type 1, a familial syndrome caused by germline mutations in the gene *NF1* (neurofibromin 1), have an increased incidence of pilocytic astrocytomas. These tumors are usually not aggressive and stand out among astrocytomas because they have maintained their WHO grade I status for years and even decades, in contrast to diffuse astrocytic tumors (WHO grades II-IV). However, some cases can progress to a higher degree of malignancy, though such a progression is rare (Listernick et al., 1999).

More than 100 cases of pilocytic astrocytomas were analyzed by cytogenetics and many others were used for comparative genomic hybridization (CGH); however, the vast majority of the results indicated normal patterns (Bigner et al., 1997; Sanoudou et al., 2000; Zattara-Cannoni et al., 1998). In adults, genetic changes were more frequent but were still rare. The few molecular genetics studies on these tumors indicated allelic loss of both gene loci *TP53* (tumor protein p53) and *NF1* in regions 17p and 17q, respectively. In sporadic tumors, few mutations were reported in the *TP53* locus and none in *NF1* (Gutmann et al., 2000; Kluwe et al., 2001).

The relevance of a malignancy-grading scheme based on histopathology is indicated by the correlation with patient survival. Patients with low-grade astrocytomas (WHO grade II) have a median survival of approximately seven years, whereas patients with anaplastic astrocytomas (WHO grade III) have a mean survival of half that time (McCormack et al., 1992). Patients with glioblastomas have a median survival time of 9 to 11 months (Simpson et al., 1993).

Unlike pilocytic astrocytomas, diffuse astrocytic tumors are often seen in adults. Low-grade astrocytomas have a peak incidence between 25 and 50 years of age, whereas glioblastomas have a peak incidence between 45 and 50 years (Colins, 2004).

Ng & Lam (1998) suggested dividing glioblastomas into two distinct molecular and clinical entities: primary or de novo glioblastomas, which occur in elderly patients and are clinically very aggressive and secondary glioblastomas, which develop from low-grade astrocytomas and have a more prolonged clinical course.

Many mechanisms are involved in the initiation and progression of secondary glioblastomas, including the loss of *NF1* and *TP53* genes and the activation of signal transduction pathways, such as *PDGF* (platelet-derived growth factor) and its receptor *PDGFR* (PDGF receptor). These pathways are involved in the induction of low-grade tumors (e.g., pilocytic astrocytomas), which can progress to high-grade tumors (e.g., anaplastic astrocytomas and secondary glioblastoma). This progression is associated with the lack of a functional *RB1* (retinoblastoma 1) because of the loss of *RB1* or gene amplification/overexpression of *CDK4* (cyclin-dependent kinase 4) (Fig. 1a). In primary glioblastomas, the same genetic pathways are disrupted but by different mechanisms. For example, reduction of the *TP53* pathway generally occurs through the loss of the gene *ARF4* (ADP-ribosylation factor 4) or less frequently through amplification of the gene *MDM2* (transformed 3T3 cell double minute 2). The lack of *RB1* also occurs via a loss of the gene *CDKN2A* (cyclin-dependent kinase inhibitor 2A). In primary glioblastomas, amplification and/or mutation of *EGFR* (epidermal growth factor receptor) and loss of *PTEN* (phosphatase and tensin homolog) are the most frequently observed genetic defects (Fig. 1b) (Zu & Parada, 2002).

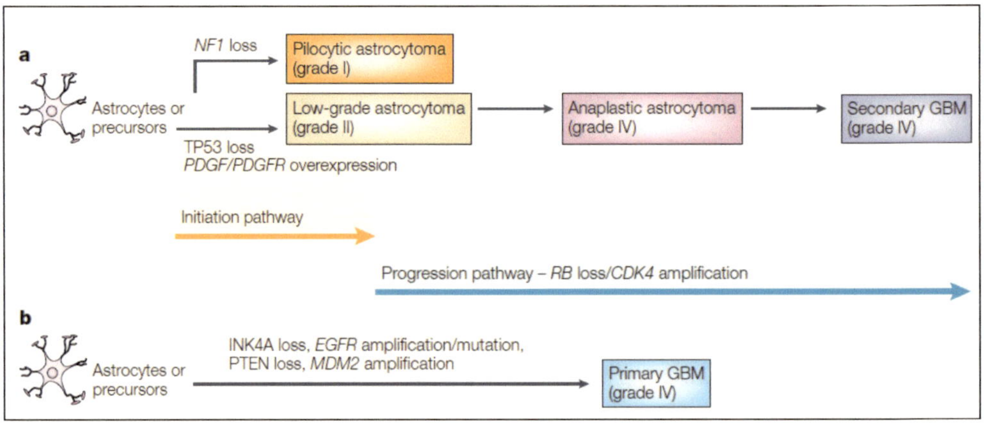

Fig. 1. Genetic pathways involved in the development of (a) primary and (b) secondary glioblastomas (Zhu & Parada, 2000).

Sequencing of the genome recently identified mutations in the *IDH1/IDH2* genes (isocitrate dehydrogenase 1 and 2 genes) that occur in the majority of WHO grade II–III gliomas and secondary glioblastomas (Hartmann et al., 2009; Yan et al., 2009), all of which harbor a better prognosis compared with the wild-type cases (Sanson et al., 2009). However, pilocytic astrocytomas (WHO grade I) that are potentially curable by complete resection rarely harbor *IDH* mutations. *IDH* appears to function as a tumor suppressor when inactivated through mutation, rendering the IDH enzyme unable to catalyze conversion of isocitrate to alphaketoglutarate. This process also induces HIF1-alpha (hypoxia-inducible factor), which triggers the angiogenic process. However, the precise mechanism of its effect on tumor biology remains unclear (Dang et al., 2009).

Aberrant activation of the *BRAF* proto-oncogene (v-raf murine sarcoma viral oncogene homolog B1) at 7q34, which is most commonly caused by gene duplication and fusion or less frequently by point mutation, has only recently been identified as the characteristic genetic aberration in pilocytic astrocytomas. *BRAF* abnormalities occur in 60–80% of pilocytic astrocytomas but almost never in diffuse, infiltrating astrocytomas (Jones et al., 2009). Thus, testing for *BRAF* gene alterations might be helpful for differentiating during diagnosis between pilocytic astrocytomas and low-grade, diffuse astrocytomas (Korshunov et al., 2009).

The importance of silencing DNA repair pathways, especially the DNA-repair enzyme AGAT (O6-alkylguanine DNA alkyltransferase), which is encoded by the gene *MGMT* (O6-methylguanine-DNA-methyltransferase), has been the subject of substantial debate in recent years (Hofer & Lassman, 2010). The *MGMT* gene is frequently silenced by promoter hypermethylation in diffuse gliomas, and this hypermethylation has been pinpointed as an epigenetic mechanism that reduces *MGMT* expression levels. There are 97 CpG islands in the *MGMT* promoter, and these CpG islands are further divided into two hypermethylated regions (Nakagawachi et al., 2003). Because of its critical role in DNA repair, the epigenetic silencing of *MGMT* is associated with an increased number of mutations and with a poorer outcome in glioblastomas. Thus, *MGMT* silencing is considered to be a biomarker for poor prognosis (Komine et al., 2003). However, an association between *MGMT* promoter methylation and the response of malignant gliomas to alkylating chemotherapy using nitrosourea compounds, temozolomide, or a combination of both has been observed (Esteller et al., 2000; Herrlinger et al., 2006). Furthermore, Hegi et al. (2005) reported that patients treated with radiotherapy and temozolomide, and whose tumors had a methylated *MGMT* promoter (which is seen in approximately 40% of primary glioblastomas), survived significantly longer than did patients whose tumors lacked *MGMT* promoter methylation. Rivera et al. (2010) recently reported that *MGMT* promoter methylation in anaplastic gliomas (WHO grade III) is also predictive of the response to radiotherapy and linked to longer survival in the absence of adjuvant chemotherapy. The use of temozolomide based on *MGMT* methylation status highlights the importance of understanding epigenetic changes in glioblastomas for the discovery of novel therapies and prognostic factors for the treatment of this deadly cancer (Komine et al., 2003; Nakagawachi et al., 2003)

3.2 Oligodendrogliomas

Oligodendrogliomas represent approximately 10-15% of gliomas, are more common in adults, and can be divided into two histological subtypes: low-grade (WHO grade II) and anaplastic (WHO grade III) (Kleihues et al., 2002).

Low-grade oligodendrogliomas are less biologically aggressive than are astrocytic tumors. Therefore, the prognosis is quite favorable and survival beyond 15 years is achieved in up to 90% of cases that receive a complete surgical resection. There is potential for malignancy, but even the aggressive tumors respond well to additional treatments (e.g., radiation and chemotherapy). Anaplastic oligodendrogliomas have a more aggressive course; however, survival is still five to eight years longer than that observed with anaplastic astrocytomas (Reifenberger & Louis, 2003).

In 1990, the PCV chemotherapy regimen (procarbazine, carmustine, and vincristine) was shown to result in a dramatic tumor response in oligodendrogliomas. Since that time, the identification of all forms of gliomas with oligodendroglial components became crucial (Macdonald et al., 1990). Importantly, these studies indicated that the prognostic power of oligodendroglial components was independent of whether radiotherapy, chemotherapy or combined radio-chemotherapy was used (Wick et al., 2009). This phenomenon is likely due to oligodendrogliomas exhibiting specific genetic abnormalities that distinguish them from other gliomas. Reifenberger et al. (1994), after a thorough analysis of the genome, reported a loss of genetic information in the 1p and 19q loci in oligodendrogliomas, the so-called chromosome 1p/19q co-deletion. This loss was later linked with a good response to PCV and provided the first molecular indicator of treatment response in brain tumors (Cairncross et al., 1998; Reifenberger et al., 2003). Further studies corroborated these findings, and it is now known that the chromosomal loss results from an unbalanced translocation (Franco-Hernandez et al., 2009; Jenkins et al., 2006). Approximately 85% of low-grade oligodendrogliomas and 65% of anaplastic oligodendrogliomas present with 1p/19q co-deletions (Smith et al., 2000).

Low-grade oligodendrogliomas and astrocytomas present a loss of *ARF4* expression and overexpression of *EGFR* and PDGF signaling. Malignant progression is associated with additional genetic abnormalities that are similar to those described above for astrocytomas, including a lack of the *RB1* pathway, loss of *RB1,* or gene amplification/overexpression of the *CDK4* gene (Franco-Hernandez et al., 2007; Reifenberger & Louis, 2003).

3.3 Ependymomas

Ependymomas arise in or near the ependymal surface, and these tumors can occur anywhere in the ventricular system, spinal cord and even occasionally at extraneural sites. The most common location is in the fourth ventricle, followed by the spinal cord, the lateral ventricles and the third ventricle. These tumors are more common in children but can also occur in adults (Ebert et al., 1999).

WHO classification identifies four major subtypes of ependymomas: subependymomas (WHO grade I), myxopapillary ependymomas (WHO grade I), low-grade ependymomas (WHO grade II) and anaplastic ependymomas (WHO grade III). Subependymomas are intraventricular in location, while myxopapillary ependymomas are commonly found in the cauda equina. The low-grade ependymomas can be differentiated from their anaplastic counterparts based on the low rate of mitosis and the low level of nuclear polymorphism; however, the distinction between the two tumors remains poorly defined (Kleihues et al., 2002).

In ependymomas, chromosomal abnormalities detected by classic cytogenetics and CGH involve chromosomes 1, 6, 7, 9, 10, 13, 17, 19 and 22. Deletions are the most commonly observed changes, and chromosome 22 losses are common in adults (50%) but rare in pediatric ependymomas (Kraus et al., 2001; Lamszus et al., 2001; von Haken et al., 1996). The target genes, located in regions of chromosomal gain or loss, are unknown, with the exception of cases in which both copies of the wild-type *NF2* gene (neurofibromin 2) are lost in intramedullary ependymomas (Alonso et al., 2002). Isolated cases of *MEN1* gene (multiple endocrine neoplasia I) loss have also been reported (Urioste et al., 2002). Germline mutations in *TP53* are uncommon, in contrast with those seen in diffuse astrocytomas (Nozaki et al., 1998).

When reviewed together, the data on genetic and epigenetic abnormalities presented above allow us to define four molecular biomarkers: *MGMT* hypermethylation in glioblastomas and anaplastic gliomas, *IDH1* and *IDH2* mutations in diffuse gliomas, *BRAF* aberrations in pilocytic astrocytomas, and combined deletions of chromosome arms 1p and 19q in oligodendroglial tumors. These biomarkers and their clinical significance are summarized in Table 2.

4. Single nucleotide polymorphisms and gliomas

A single nucleotide polymorphism (SNP) is generally defined as a stable replacement of only one DNA base, with a frequency greater than 1% in at least one population (Taylor et al., 2001). In human genetics studies, SNPs are simply referred to as bi-allelic markers because tri-and tetra-allelic markers are rare (Brookes, 1999).

Initially, only a few thousand SNPs were thought to exist in the entire genome. However, since 2000, that number has increased about one thousand-fold. In 2001, an international consortium on mapping SNPs described 1.42 million polymorphic loci. More important than this large number is the precision of their placement in the genome; there is approximately one polymorphism every 1.91 Kb. Therefore, 90% of sequences greater than 20 Kb in length have at least one SNP, and this density can be higher in genic regions. Of the known genes, 93% contain SNPs and 98% are at least 5 Kb away from a SNP. Soon, almost all genes or gene regions will be marked by one of these variable sequences (Sachidanandam et al., 2001).

Molecular marker	Clinical significance
IDH1/IDH2 mutation	• Diagnostic marker for diffuse WHO grade II and III gliomas, as well as secondary glioblastomas, and associated with a better prognosis in these tumors • Rare in primary glioblastomas, but when present, it is associated with a more favorable outcome • Not predictive for response to a particular type of therapy
BRAF duplication/fusion	• Diagnostic marker for pilocytic astrocytomas and helpful in distinguishing these tumors from diffuse astrocytomas • Prognostic significance within the group of pilocytic astrocytoma patients is unknown
MGMT promoter methylation	• Predictive for response of glioblastomas to alkylating chemotherapy • Associated with longer survival in glioblastoma patients treated with radiotherapy combined with concurrent and adjuvant temozolomide • Prognostic in anaplastic glioma patients treated with radiotherapy and/or alkylating chemotherapy
1p/19q co-deletion	• Associated with improved prognosis in oligodendroglial tumor patients receiving adjuvant radiotherapy and/or chemotherapy • Not predictive for response to a particular type of therapy

Table 2. The four most relevant markers for the molecular diagnosis of gliomas (Hofer & Lassman, 2010; Riemenschneider et al., 2010).

Because they are found throughout the genome, some alleles containing SNPs produce functional or physiologically relevant gene products. For example, SNPs in a coding region can affect the coded protein. When located in an intron, SNPs can influence the splicing mechanism, and when located in the promoter, SNPs can alter gene transcription (Krawczak et al., 1992). For this reason, SNPs are recognized as important tools in human genetics and medicine and have been widely used in genetic association studies of various complex diseases, including cancer. In humans, several reviews of SNPs have been carried out in an attempt to determine the patterns of SNP haplotypes in different populations (Conrad et al., 2006; Gonzalez-Neira et al., 2006; Jakobsson et al., 2008; Nothnagel & Rohde, 2005; Salisbury et al., 2003). Data from these tests are extremely useful for studying the genetic basis of cancer. For this reason, several research groups have focused on elucidating the role of SNPs in different genes related to the initiation and progression of gliomas in different populations. We performed association studies between SNPs, the risk of developing gliomas, and the prognosis for gliomas in a Brazilian population. Brazilians form one of the most heterogeneous populations in the world, which is the result of five centuries of interethnic crosses of peoples from three continents: the European colonizers who are mainly represented by the Portuguese, the African slaves, and the autochthonous Amerindians (Parra et al., 2003).

Until recently, we were the only laboratory investigating the association between *WRN* Cys1367Arg, the risk for brain tumor development, and the prognosis of brain tumors, especially with regard to gliomas (Pinto et al., 2008a). Werner syndrome (WS) is a premature aging disorder characterized by early onset of symptoms related to normal aging and is caused by inherited, recessive mutations in the *WRN* gene. The *WRN* gene encodes a member of the RecQ family of helicases involved in DNA replication and in maintaining the integrity of the genome (Harrigan et al., 2006). The cells of WS patients exhibit a high level of chromosomal translocations and deletions, and these patients present an increased predisposition to various types of cancer, including CNS tumors (Kobayashi et al., 1980). However, despite its putative tumor suppressor function, little is known about the contribution of the WRN protein to sporadic human malignancies. Taking into account that almost all cancers occur in the elderly and that mutations in the *WRN* gene lead to accelerated aging, it has been suggested that polymorphisms of the *WRN* gene, similar to Cys1367Arg, might be associated with age-related pathologies and cancer predisposition. However, our data indicate that neither glioma risk (OR = 1.38; 95% CI, 0.78-2.43; P = 0.334) nor patient survival (overall and disease-free survival, P = 0.396 and P = 0.843, respectively) was associated with variant alleles.

Similar results were found when we evaluated the genotype distribution of *TP53* Pro47Ser and Arg72Pro SNPs for their involvement in susceptibility to gliomas and in determining the oncologic prognosis of patients (Pinto et al., 2008b). A critical site in the TP53 protein for apoptosis signaling is a proline-rich region located between codons 64 and 92. Dumont et al. (2003) reported that the homozygous Arg72 allele induces apoptosis at a rate that is 15-fold higher than the Pro72 allele. According to Leu et al. (2004), the apoptosis-inducing ability of the Arg72 allele is in part due to its mitochondrial location, which makes it possible for TP53 to directly interact with the pro-apoptotic protein, BAK. However, the *TP53* Pro47Ser SNP resulted in a significantly decreased ability of the TP53 protein to induce apoptosis. A critical event in TP53-induced apoptosis is phosphorylation of the serine residue at codon 46. This region is where allele Pro47 acts as a substrate for proline-directed kinases such as the MAPK1 protein. Li et al. (2005) reported that the Ser47 allele, which is a poor substrate for MAPK1, has an apoptosis-inducing ability that is 5-fold lower than that of the wild-type Pro47 allele. However, our data again indicated that neither glioma susceptibility nor patient survival was associated with the *TP53* Arg72Pro or Pro47Ser alleles in the Brazilian population.

In 2009, we investigated the role of *EGF* +61 A>G as a potential risk factor and/or prognostic marker for gliomas in the Brazilian population. The *EGF* gene encodes a ligand for EGFR that activates a cascade of events responsible for promoting cell proliferation, inhibition of apoptosis, and differentiation. Alterations in the EGF/EGFR signaling pathway are associated with tumor progression in a variety of human cancers. Therefore, high expression of EGF may play a key role in glioma development and progression (Salomon et al., 1995). Shahbazi et al. (2002) first reported that the +61 A>G SNP in the 5'-UTR region of *EGF* is associated with increased EGF production and risk of malignant melanoma. Since that discovery, other research groups have obtained conflicting findings regarding the relationship of this functional SNP with different human cancers, including gliomas (Bao et al., 2010; Bhowmick et al., 2004; Costa et al., 2007; Liu et al., 2009; Vauleon et al., 2007; Wang et al., 2010). In our results, the genotype and allele frequencies between cases and controls were similar, indicating no significant association with glioma risk ($P = 0.94$ and $P = 0.887$, respectively) and suggesting that *EGF* +61 A>G may not significantly contribute to the susceptibility to gliomas in the Brazilian population. This result is consistent with that of Vauleon et al. (2007) and Liu et al. (2009) in French and Chinese populations, respectively. However, we found that the major +61G allele (frequency among controls, 0.51) was associated with a shorter overall survival in patients ($P = 0.023$). Thus, with regard to patient survival, our results corroborate those of Bhowmick et al. (2004) in a population of North American patients.

We have also studied the *GSTP1* gene, which encodes a protein accounting for approximately 90% of the enzymatic activity of the glutathione S-transferase (GST) family (Custodio et al., 2010). GSTs constitute a superfamily of ubiquitous, multifunctional enzymes that are involved in cellular detoxification of a large number of endogenous and exogenous chemical agents that possess electrophilic functional groups (Ryberg et al., 1997). The GSTP1 protein is a pi-class enzyme and *GSTP1* structure has been extensively examined in association with the risk of cancer (White et al., 2008). The influence of the *GSTP1* Ile105Val SNP on cancer has been reported with inconsistent results from different parts of the world (Syamala et al., 2008). Our results demonstrate that the Val105 allele was more frequent in a population of cancer patients than in a healthy population (0.29 and 0.06, respectively; $P < 0.001$) and that the presence of this genotype may increase the risk of developing astrocytomas and glioblastomas (OR = 8.60; 95% CI, 4.14-17.87; $P < 0.001$). However, we did not find an association between the *GSTP1* Ile105Val SNP and patient survival.

Recently, we began studying SNPs in DNA repair genes and we performed association analysis of SNPs in genes for the *XRCC* (X-ray cross-complementing) family, *XRCC1* and *XRCC3*, in a series of gliomas (unpublished data). Human tumors may develop through alterations to the DNA repair system, which is crucially important for cellular life (Kawabata et al., 2005). To ensure the integrity of the genome, a complex system of DNA repair was developed. Base excision repair is the first defense mechanism of cells against DNA damage and a major means for preventing mutagenesis (Hu et al., 2005). Repair genes may play an important role in maintaining genomic stability through different pathways mediating base excision repair (Sreeja et al., 2008). For this reason, much attention has been given to the study of SNPs in *XRCCs* and their involvement in different types of cancer, including gliomas. We performed analysis of the Arg194Trp and Arg399Gln SNPs in *XRCC1* and the Thr241Met SNP in *XRCC3* to assess their roles in the risk and prognosis for gliomas in Brazilians. Our results provide evidence that the *XRCC*1 Arg194Trp SNP may contribute to the etiology of human gliomas because the Trp194 allele was strongly associated with risk and the Gln399 allele revealed a small, increased risk for tumor development. In regard to the *XRCC3* Thr241Met SNP, we also found evidence that *XRRC3* Thr241Met may contribute to the etiology of human gliomas. However, when the Arg194Trp and Arg399Gln SNPs in *XRCC1* and the Thr241Met SNP in *XRCC3* were considered together, we did not find statistical difference between genotypes and patient survival.

Around the globe, other groups have analyzed the association between SNPs found in *XRCCs* genes and the risk of developing gliomas. Kiuru et al. (2003) evaluated the association between the *XRCC1* Arg194Trp, Arg280His, and Arg399Gln SNPS, the *XRCC3*

Thr241Met SNP, and glioma risk in a prospective, population-based, case-control study conducted in Denmark, Finland, Sweden, and the UK. They found no significant association with gliomas for any of the SNPs when examined individually. However, the results indicated possible associations between combinations of *XRCC1* and *XRCC3* SNPs and the risk of glioma development, as carriers of both homozygous variant genotypes, i.e., *XRCC1* Gln399Gln and *XRCC3* Met241Met were associated with a three-fold increased risk of glioma (OR = 3.18; 95% CI, 1.26-8.04). In a haplotype-based approach in a Chinese population, Liu et al. (2007) investigated the role of 22 tagging SNPs (tSNPs) of *XRCC5*, *XRCC6* and *XRCC7*. They found that glioma risk was significantly associated with three of the *XRCC5* tSNPs (rs828704, rs3770502 and rs9288516, P = 0.005, 0.042 and 0.003, respectively), one *XRCC6* tSNP (rs6519265, P = 0.044), and none of the *XPCC7* tSNPs in a single-locus analysis. Haplotype-based association analysis revealed that glioma risk was significantly associated with one protective *XRCC5* haplotype "CAGTT," which accounted for a 40% reduction (OR = 0.60, 95% CI, 0.43-0.85) in glioma risk. In a study of North Americans, Wang et al. (2004) found that the variant XRCC7T allele of the *XRCC7* G6721T SNP was significantly more common in the glioma cases than in the controls (P = 0.045). The *XRCC7* genotype frequency was also significant when comparing the cases and controls (P = 0.040). Likewise, the difference in distribution of the combined T-variant genotype (GT + TT) between the cases and controls was also statistically significant (P = 0.012), suggesting that the T allele may be a risk factor for glioma.

In addition to the studies mentioned above, several others were published indicating the results of associations, positive or negative, of genomic variations with the risk of developing gliomas. However, the ethnic variations, methodological variations, and the presence of responsible, functionally unknown SNPs in linkage disequilibrium with those SNPs analyzed have contributed to the dissemination of conflicting results in different parts of the world. Gu et al. (2009) presented a review including a list of eight literature-defined, putative, functional, SNPs associated with gliomas in at least two populations from case-control studies. A summary of this list is presented in Table 3.

Gene selection for association studies has previously been based on studies reporting the role of genes and their SNPs in the regulation of cellular functions. However, after the completion of the human genome project and the development of analytical platforms capable of parallel genotype processing, which resulted in new selection strategies for identifying susceptibility genes in many complex genetic disorders, gene selection is currently based on genome-wide association (GWA) studies.

The two glioma GWA studies performed so far were published in 2010 in the same issue of Nature Genetics. In the first pages, Shete et al. (2009) presented the results of a meta-analysis of two GWA studies that involved the genotyping of 454,576 tSNPs in a total of 1,878 glioma cases and 3,670 controls, with posterior validation in three additional independent series totaling 2,545 cases and 2,953 controls. The authors identified five risk loci for glioma at 5p15.33 (*TERT* rs2736100), 8q24.21 (*CCDC26* rs4295627), 9p21.3 (*CDKN2A-CDKN2B* rs4977756), 11q23.3 (*PHLDB1* rs498872), and 20q13.33 (*RTEL1* rs6010620). In the second study, Wrensch et al. (2009) analyzed 275,895 SNPs in 692 adult patients with high-grade glioma and 3,992 controls, with a replication series of 176 high-grade glioma cases and 174 controls. That analysis provided further evidence to implicate 9p21 (*CDKN2B* rs1412829) and 20q13.3 (*RTEL1* rs6010620) in glioma risk.

Main paths, genes	Associated SNPs	Effect	OR (95% CI)
DNA repair			
XRCC7	G6721T	Risk	GG vs. TT, 1.82 (1.13-2.93)[1]
			GG vs. TT, 1.44 (1.13-1.84)[2]
XRCC1	Arg399Gln	Risk	AA vs. GG, 1.23 (0.96-1.57)[2]
			AA vs. GG, 1.32 (0.97-1.81)[3]
			GA/AA vs. GG, 1.44 (1.05-1.92)[4]
PARP1	Val762ala	Protective	CT/CC vs. TT, 0.80 (0.67-0.95)[2]
			CT/CC vs. TT, 0.71 (0.52-0.97)[4]
ERCC1	A8092C	Risk	AA/AC vs. CC, 4.41 (1.6-12.2)[5]
			AA/AC vs. CC, 1.67 (0.93-3.02)[6]
ERCC2	Gln751Lys	Risk	CC vs. AA, 1.19 (0.93-1.52)[2]
			AA vs. AC/CC, 1.66 (1.01-2.72)[6]
MGMT	Phe84Leu	Protective or risk?	CT/TT vs. CC, 0.66 (0.45-0.94)[4]
			CT/TT vs. CC, 1.26 (0.90-1.75)[7]
Cell cycle, *EGF*	+61 A>G	Risk	$P = 0.032$[8]
			AG/GG vs. AA, 1.52 (1.03-2.23)[9]
Inflammation: *IL13*	Arg130Gln	Protective	AG vs. GG, 0.75 (0.48-1.17)[10]
			TT vs. CC/CT, 0.39 (0.16-0.93)[11]

Table 3. Selected glioma susceptibility genes and SNPs observed in at least two studies. [1]Wang et al. (2004); [2]McKean-Cowdin et al. (2009); [3]Kiuru et al. (2008); [4]Liu et al. (2009); [5]Chen et al. (2000); [6]Wrensch et al. (2005); [7]Felini et al. (2007); [8]Bhowmick et al. (2004); [9]Costa et al. (2007); [10]Schwartzbaum et al. (2005); [11]Amirian et al. (2010).

5. Cancer stem cells

Both the invasive nature of the tumor and its heterogeneity probably contribute to the poor response to the treatment regimens available today. Tumor heterogeneity is traditionally attributed to the accumulation of regional variations in the tumor microenvironment and the diversity of subpopulations of cancer cells, which result from random genetic changes (Reya et al., 2001).

The majority tumors consist of a heterogeneous population of cells with different proliferative potential, as well as the ability to re-form the tumor upon transplantation into immunodeficient mice (Visvader & Lindeman, 2008). Recently, evidence has accumulated that tumors contain a population with characteristics similar to normal stem cells called cancer stem cells, which are also multipotent cells. This subpopulation has the ability to repair itself and is believed to control tumor initiation, a process that is responsible for tumor recurrence and the resistance to therapy observed in different tumor types, including gliomas (Bao et al., 2006). The observation that normal stem cells and cancer stem cells share common features (e.g., undifferentiated state and unlimited capacity for self-regeneration) led to the hypothesis of cancer stem cells (Park & Rich, 2009).

A practical component of the cancer stem cell hypothesis is directed to the matter of intrinsic resistance to radiation and chemotherapy. Cancer stem cells are predicted to be difficult targets for tumor therapy because they exhibit a slowed cell cycle and high levels of drug export. Furthermore, these cells may not express or may not be dependent on the oncoproteins that are targeted by the most recent generation of cancer drugs (Cheng et al., 2010).

Cancer stem cells, similar to normal stem cells, are dependent on the microenvironment in which they are located. This microenvironment, formed by cells and extracellular matrix, controls the maintenance of organ functions. Therefore, disturbance of the local microenvironment in neoplastic processes can trigger tumor development (Barcellos-Hoff et al., 2009). In glioma, for example, studies have shown that the microenvironment is surrounded by blood vessels, which provide access to signaling molecules, nutrition, and possibly to the use of the nascent vasculature for migration, which provides direct cell contact and secreted factors that are responsible for maintaining the state of quiescence of cancer stem cells, regulating their self-renewal and multipotency (Gilbertson & Rich, 2007; Jandial et al., 2008). Thus, one can say that cancer stem cells and the microenvironment are parts of the tumor. Therefore, knowledge of the associated characteristics will lead to a new understanding of tumor biology and the development of new therapeutic strategies against these cells. For this reason, it is extremely important to characterize the different subpopulations of cancer stem cells that contribute to tumor formation (Denysenko et al., 2010).

6. Conclusion

The development and progression of gliomas may likely be due to a multistep process that involves the functional inactivation of tumor suppressor genes and DNA repair genes, as well as the activation of oncogenes. Given the limitations of current therapies, understanding the pathways that lead to tumor progression should remain a high priority in cancer research. If the mechanisms that culminate in metastasis are fully understood, the development of new diagnostic and therapeutic methods may allow for a substantial improvement in the quality of life of affected patients and a better means of predicting patient prognosis. Genetic and epigenetic studies involving large cohorts of glioma patients in different populations have provided important information for understanding the role of key genes in the development and risk of gliomas. Because it is considered a work in progress, the WHO classification for brain tumors may soon incorporate molecular data to refine the classification of these diseases, which are complex from a therapeutic standpoint.

SNPs have become increasingly popular in the genetic study of gliomas because of the quick, inexpensive and accurate analysis of SNPs. The identification of SNPs as risk factors for different glioma subtypes can be important for prevention, diagnosis and prognosis. Variations in the genomic sequence contribute to phenotypic diversity and susceptibility to or protection against many complex diseases. Thus, it is estimated that the risk of gliomas may be strongly influenced by the patterns of SNPs in certain key susceptibility genes; these SNPs are still being identified. The same reasoning can be applied to inter-individual variations in genetic responses to medications, which is a field of great interest to the pharmaceutical industry. The benefit of having a SNP map of different populations is that it allows for coverage of the entire genome so that researchers can compare the patterns and frequencies of SNPs in their patients and associate these patterns with the disease concerned. The GWA studies with significant numbers and carefully matched controls have become a powerful tool in identifying genes involved in common genetic diseases, including gliomas. The identification of susceptibility alleles provides a greater understanding of gliomagenesis and provides target genes for potential therapeutic intervention. Unlike environmental exposure, SNPs do not change during the process of tumorigenesis. Therefore, SNPs may be useful as indicators of risk.

The main features of normal stem cells are the capacity for self-regeneration and differentiation to different cell types. These characteristics are heavily regulated by the local microenvironment. Because studies have shown that cancer stem cells behave like normal stem cells, understanding the regulatory mechanisms of cancer stem cells and their microenvironment has changed our understanding of the biology of gliomas and has precipitated a reassessment of current therapies. The cure of glioma will require the elimination of all tumor cells, including cancer stem cells. Therefore, further studies to provide a better understanding of the origin of cancer stem cells and their interactions with the microenvironment are needed. These findings hold great promise for the development of new therapies that can help us improve the results achieved with current therapies and thereby prolong patient survival.

7. References

Alonso, M.E., Bello, M.J., Arjona, D., Gonzalez-Gomez, P., Lomas, J., de Campos, J.M., Kusak, M.E., Isla, A. & Rey, J.A. (2002). Analysis of the NF2 gene in oligodendrogliomas and ependymomas. *Cancer Genet Cytogenet*, Vol.134, No.1, pp. 1-5

Amirian, E., Liu, Y., Scheurer, M.E., El-Zein, R., Gilbert, M.R. & Bondy, M.L. (2010). Genetic variants in inflammation pathway genes and asthma in glioma susceptibility. *Neuro Oncol*, Vol.12, No.5, pp. 444-452

Bao, G., Wang, M., Guo, S., Han, Y. & Xu, G. (2010). Association between epidermal growth factor +61 G/A polymorphism and glioma risk in a Chinese Han population. *J Int Med Res*, Vol.38, No.5, pp. 1645-1652

Bao, S., Wu, Q., McLendon, R.E., Hao, Y., Shi, Q., Hjelmeland, A.B., Dewhirst, M.W., Bigner, D.D. & Rich, J.N. (2006). Glioma stem cells promote radioresistance by preferential activation of the DNA damage response. *Nature*, Vol.444, No.7120, pp. 756-760

Barcellos-Hoff, M.H., Newcomb, E.W., Zagzag, D. & Narayana, A. (2009). Therapeutic targets in malignant glioblastoma microenvironment. *Semin Radiat Oncol*, Vol.19, No.3, pp. 163-170

Bartek, J. & Lukas, J. (2001). Are all cancer genes equal? *Nature*, Vol.411, No.6841, pp. 1001-1002

Bello, M.J. & Rey, J.A. (2006). The p53/Mdm2/p14ARF cell cycle control pathway genes may be inactivated by genetic and epigenetic mechanisms in gliomas. *Cancer Genet Cytogenet*, Vol.164, No.2, pp. 172-173

Bhowmick, D.A., Zhuang, Z., Wait, S.D. & Weil, R.J. (2004). A functional polymorphism in the EGF gene is found with increased frequency in glioblastoma multiforme patients and is associated with more aggressive disease. *Cancer Res*, Vol.64, No.4, pp. 1220-1223

Bigner, S.H., McLendon, R.E., Fuchs, H., McKeever, P.E. & Friedman, H.S. (1997). Chromosomal characteristics of childhood brain tumors. *Cancer Genet Cytogenet*, Vol.97, No.2, pp. 125-134

Brookes, A.J. (1999). The essence of SNPs. *Gene*, Vol.234, No.2, pp. 177-186

Cairncross, J.G., Ueki, K., Zlatescu, M.C., Lisle, D.K., Finkelstein, D.M., Hammond, R.R., Silver, J.S., Stark, P.C., Macdonald, D.R., Ino, Y., Ramsay, D.A. & Louis, D.N. (1998). Specific genetic predictors of chemotherapeutic response and survival in patients with anaplastic oligodendrogliomas. *J Natl Cancer Inst*, Vol.90, No.19, pp. 1473-1479

Chen, P., Wiencke, J., Aldape, K., Kesler-Diaz, A., Miike, R., Kelsey, K., Lee, M., Liu, J. & Wrensch, M. (2000). Association of an ERCC1 polymorphism with adult-onset glioma. *Cancer Epidemiol Biomarkers Prev*, Vol.9, No.8, pp. 843-847

Cheng, L., Bao, S. & Rich, J.N. (2010). Potential therapeutic implications of cancer stem cells in glioblastoma. *Biochem Pharmacol*, Vol.80, No.5, pp. 654-665

Collins, V.P. (2004). Brain tumours: classification and genes. *J Neurol Neurosurg Psychiatry*, Vol.75 Suppl 2, pp. ii2-11

Conrad, D.F., Jakobsson, M., Coop, G., Wen, X., Wall, J.D., Rosenberg, N.A. & Pritchard, J.K. (2006). A worldwide survey of haplotype variation and linkage disequilibrium in the human genome. *Nat Genet*, Vol.38, No.11, pp. 1251-1260

Costa, B.M., Ferreira, P., Costa, S., Canedo, P., Oliveira, P., Silva, A., Pardal, F., Suriano, G., Machado, J.C., Lopes, J.M. & Reis, R.M. (2007). Association between functional EGF+61 polymorphism and glioma risk. *Clin Cancer Res*, Vol.13, No.9, pp. 2621-2626

Cross, S.H. & Bird, A.P. (1995). CpG islands and genes. *Curr Opin Genet Dev*, Vol.5, No.3, pp. 309-314

Custodio, A.C., Almeida, L.O., Pinto, G.R., Santos, M.J., Almeida, J.R., Clara, C.A., Rey, J.A. & Casartelli, C. (2010). GSTP1 Ile105Val polymorphism in astrocytomas and glioblastomas. *Genet Mol Res*, Vol.9, No.4, pp. 2328-2334

Dang, L., White, D.W., Gross, S., Bennett, B.D., Bittinger, M.A., Driggers, E.M., Fantin, V.R., Jang, H.G., Jin, S., Keenan, M.C., Marks, K.M., Prins, R.M., Ward, P.S., Yen, K.E., Liau, L.M., Rabinowitz, J.D., Cantley, L.C., Thompson, C.B., Vander Heiden, M.G. & Su, S.M. (2009). Cancer-associated IDH1 mutations produce 2-hydroxyglutarate. *Nature*, Vol.462, No.7274, pp. 739-744

Denysenko, T., Gennero, L., Roos, M.A., Melcarne, A., Juenemann, C., Faccani, G., Morra, I., Cavallo, G., Reguzzi, S., Pescarmona, G. & Ponzetto, A. (2010). Glioblastoma cancer stem cells: heterogeneity, microenvironment and related therapeutic strategies. *Cell Biochem Funct*, Vol.28, No.5, pp. 343-351

Dumont, P., Leu, J.I., Della Pietra, A.C., 3rd, George, D.L. & Murphy, M. (2003). The codon 72 polymorphic variants of p53 have markedly different apoptotic potential. *Nat Genet*, Vol.33, No.3, pp. 357-365

Ebert, C., von Haken, M., Meyer-Puttlitz, B., Wiestler, O.D., Reifenberger, G., Pietsch, T. & von Deimling, A. (1999). Molecular genetic analysis of ependymal tumors. NF2 mutations and chromosome 22q loss occur preferentially in intramedullary spinal ependymomas. *Am J Pathol*, Vol.155, No.2, pp. 627-632

Esteller, M., Garcia-Foncillas, J., Andion, E., Goodman, S.N., Hidalgo, O.F., Vanaclocha, V., Baylin, S.B. & Herman, J.G. (2000). Inactivation of the DNA-repair gene MGMT and the clinical response of gliomas to alkylating agents. *N Engl J Med*, Vol.343, No.19, pp. 1350-1354

Franco-Hernandez, C., Martinez-Glez, V., Alonso, M.E., De Campos, J.M., Isla, A., Vaquero, J., Gutierrez, M. & Rey, J.A. (2007). Gene dosage and mutational analyses of EGFR in oligodendrogliomas. *Int J Oncol*, Vol.30, No.1, pp. 209-215

Franco-Hernandez, C., Martinez-Glez, V., de Campos, J.M., Isla, A., Vaquero, J., Gutierrez, M., Casartelli, C. & Rey, J.A. (2009). Allelic status of 1p and 19q in oligodendrogliomas and glioblastomas: multiplex ligation-dependent probe amplification versus loss of heterozygosity. *Cancer Genet Cytogenet*, Vol.190, No.2, pp. 93-96

Felini, M.J., Olshan, A.F., Schroeder, J.C., North, K.E., Carozza, S.E., Kelsey, K.T., Liu, M., Rice, T., Wiencke, J.K. & Wrensch, M.R. (2007). DNA repair polymorphisms XRCC1 and MGMT and risk of adult gliomas. *Neuroepidemiology*, Vol.29, No.1-2, pp. 55-58

Gilbertson, R. (2002). Paediatric embryonic brain tumours. biological and clinical relevance of molecular genetic abnormalities. *Eur J Cancer*, Vol.38, No.5, pp. 675-685

Gilbertson, R.J. & Rich, J.N. (2007). Making a tumour's bed: glioblastoma stem cells and the vascular niche. Nat Rev Cancer, Vol.7, No.10, pp. 733-736

Gonzalez-Gomez, P., Bello, M.J., Arjona, D., Lomas, J., Alonso, M.E., De Campos, J.M., Vaquero, J., Isla, A., Gutierrez, M. & Rey, J.A. (2003). Promoter hypermethylation of multiple genes in astrocytic gliomas. Int J Oncol, Vol.22, No.3, pp. 601-608

Gonzalez-Neira, A., Ke, X., Lao, O., Calafell, F., Navarro, A., Comas, D., Cann, H., Bumpstead, S., Ghori, J., Hunt, S., Deloukas, P., Dunham, I., Cardon, L.R. & Bertranpetit, J. (2006). The portability of tagSNPs across populations: a worldwide survey. *Genome Res*, Vol.16, No.3, pp. 323-330

Gu, J., Liu, Y., Kyritsis, A.P. & Bondy, M.L. (2009). Molecular epidemiology of primary brain tumors. *Neurotherapeutics*, Vol.6, No.3, pp. 427-435

Gutmann, D.H., Donahoe, J., Brown, T., James, C.D. & Perry, A. (2000). Loss of neurofibromatosis 1 (NF1) gene expression in NF1-associated pilocytic astrocytomas. *Neuropathol Appl Neurobiol*, Vol.26, No.4, pp. 361-367

Hanahan, D. & Weinberg, R.A. (2000). The hallmarks of cancer. *Cell*, Vol.100, No.1, pp. 57-70

Harrigan, J.A., Wilson, D.M., 3rd, Prasad, R., Opresko, P.L., Beck, G., May, A., Wilson, S.H. & Bohr, V.A. (2006). The Werner syndrome protein operates in base excision repair and cooperates with DNA polymerase beta. *Nucleic Acids Res*, Vol.34, No.2, pp. 745-754

Hartmann, C., Meyer, J., Balss, J., Capper, D., Mueller, W., Christians, A., Felsberg, J., Wolter, M., Mawrin, C., Wick, W., Weller, M., Herold-Mende, C., Unterberg, A.,

Jeuken, J.W., Wesseling, P., Reifenberger, G. & von Deimling, A. (2009). Type and frequency of IDH1 and IDH2 mutations are related to astrocytic and oligodendroglial differentiation and age: a study of 1,010 diffuse gliomas. *Acta Neuropathol*, Vol.118, No.4, pp. 469-474

Hegi, M.E., Diserens, A.C., Gorlia, T., Hamou, M.F., de Tribolet, N., Weller, M., Kros, J.M., Hainfellner, J.A., Mason, W., Mariani, L., Bromberg, J.E., Hau, P., Mirimanoff, R.O., Cairncross, J.G., Janzer, R.C. & Stupp, R. (2005). MGMT gene silencing and benefit from temozolomide in glioblastoma. *N Engl J Med*, Vol.352, No.10, pp. 997-1003

Herrlinger, U., Rieger, J., Koch, D., Loeser, S., Blaschke, B., Kortmann, R.D., Steinbach, J.P., Hundsberger, T., Wick, W., Meyermann, R., Tan, T.C., Sommer, C., Bamberg, M., Reifenberger, G. & Weller, M. (2006). Phase II trial of lomustine plus temozolomide chemotherapy in addition to radiotherapy in newly diagnosed glioblastoma: UKT-03. *J Clin Oncol*, Vol.24, No.27, pp. 4412-4417

Hofer, S. & Lassman, A.B. (2010). Molecular markers in gliomas: impact for the clinician. *Target Oncol*, Vol.5, No.3, pp. 201-210

Hu, Z., Ma, H., Chen, F., Wei, Q. & Shen, H. (2005). XRCC1 polymorphisms and cancer risk: a meta-analysis of 38 case-control studies. *Cancer Epidemiol Biomarkers Prev*, Vol.14, No.7, pp. 1810-1818

Jakobsson, M., Scholz, S.W., Scheet, P., Gibbs, J.R., VanLiere, J.M., Fung, H.C., Szpiech, Z.A., Degnan, J.H., Wang, K., Guerreiro, R., Bras, J.M., Schymick, J.C., Hernandez, D.G., Traynor, B.J., Simon-Sanchez, J., Matarin, M., Britton, A., van de Leemput, J., Rafferty, I., Bucan, M., Cann, H.M., Hardy, J.A., Rosenberg, N.A. & Singleton, A.B. (2008). Genotype, haplotype and copy-number variation in worldwide human populations. *Nature*, Vol.451, No.7181, pp. 998-1003

Jandial, R., U, H., Levy, M.L. & Snyder, E.Y. (2008). Brain tumor stem cells and the tumor microenvironmen. *Neurosurg Focus*, Vol.24, No.3-4, pp. E27

Jenkins, R.B., Blair, H., Ballman, K.V., Giannini, C., Arusell, R.M., Law, M., Flynn, H., Passe, S., Felten, S., Brown, P.D., Shaw, E.G. & Buckner, J.C. (2006). A t(1;19)(q10;p10) mediates the combined deletions of 1p and 19q and predicts a better prognosis of patients with oligodendroglioma. *Cancer Res*, Vol.66, No.20, pp. 9852-9861

Jones, D.T., Kocialkowski, S., Liu, L., Pearson, D.M., Ichimura, K. & Collins, V.P. (2009). Oncogenic RAF1 rearrangement and a novel BRAF mutation as alternatives to KIAA1549:BRAF fusion in activating the MAPK pathway in pilocytic astrocytoma. *Oncogene*, Vol.28, No.20, pp. 2119-2123

Jones, P.A. & Baylin, S.B. (2007). The epigenomics of cancer. *Cell*, Vol.128, No.4, pp. 683-692

Jones, P.A. & Buckley, J.D. (1990). The role of DNA methylation in cancer. *Adv Cancer Res*, Vol.54, pp. 1-23

Kawabata, M., Kawabata, T. & Nishibori, M. (2005). Role of recA/RAD51 family proteins in mammals. *Acta Med Okayama*, Vol.59, No.1, pp. 1-9

Kiuru, A., Lindholm, C., Heinavaara, S., Ilus, T., Jokinen, P., Haapasalo, H., Salminen, T., Christensen, H.C., Feychting, M., Johansen, C., Lonn, S., Malmer, B., Schoemaker, M.J., Swerdlow, A.J. & Auvinen, A. (2008). XRCC1 and XRCC3 variants and risk of glioma and meningioma. *J Neurooncol*, Vol.88, No.2, pp. 135-142

Kleihues, P. & Cavenee, W.K. (2000). World Health Organisation classification of tumours: Pathology and genetics of tumours of the nervous system. IARC Press, Lyon, France

Kleihues, P., Louis, D.N., Scheithauer, B.W., Rorke, L.B., Reifenberger, G., Burger, P.C. & Cavenee, W.K. (2002). The WHO classification of tumors of the nervous system. *J Neuropathol Exp Neurol*, Vol.61, No.3, pp. 215-225; discussion 226-219

Kleihues, P.; Burger, P.C. & Scheithauer, B.W. (1993). Histological typing of tumours of the central nervous system. World Health Organization international histological classification of tumours. Springer Verlag, Berlin, Heidelberg

Kluwe, L., Hagel, C., Tatagiba, M., Thomas, S., Stavrou, D., Ostertag, H., von Deimling, A. & Mautner, V.F. (2001). Loss of NF1 alleles distinguish sporadic from NF1-associated pilocytic astrocytomas. *J Neuropathol Exp Neurol*, Vol.60, No.9, pp. 917-920

Knudson, A.G., Jr. (1971). Mutation and cancer: statistical study of retinoblastoma. *Proc Natl Acad Sci U S A*, Vol.68, No.4, pp. 820-823

Kobayashi, S., Gibo, H., Sugita, K., Komiya, I. & Yamada, T. (1980). Werner's syndrome associated with meningioma. *Neurosurgery*, Vol.7, No.5, pp. 517-520

Komine, C., Watanabe, T., Katayama, Y., Yoshino, A., Yokoyama, T. & Fukushima, T. (2003). Promoter hypermethylation of the DNA repair gene O6-methylguanine-DNA methyltransferase is an independent predictor of shortened progression free survival in patients with low-grade diffuse astrocytomas. *Brain Pathol*, Vol.13, No.2, pp. 176-184

Korshunov, A., Meyer, J., Capper, D., Christians, A., Remke, M., Witt, H., Pfister, S., von Deimling, A. & Hartmann, C. (2009). Combined molecular analysis of BRAF and IDH1 distinguishes pilocytic astrocytoma from diffuse astrocytoma. *Acta Neuropathol*, Vol.118, No.3, pp. 401-405

Kraus, J.A., de Millas, W., Sorensen, N., Herbold, C., Schichor, C., Tonn, J.C., Wiestler, O.D., von Deimling, A. & Pietsch, T. (2001). Indications for a tumor suppressor gene at 22q11 involved in the pathogenesis of ependymal tumors and distinct from hSNF5/INI1. *Acta Neuropathol*, Vol.102, No.1, pp. 69-74

Krawczak, M., Reiss, J. & Cooper, D.N. (1992). The mutational spectrum of single base-pair substitutions in mRNA splice junctions of human genes: causes and consequences. *Hum Genet*, Vol.90, No.1-2, pp. 41-54

Lamszus, K., Lachenmayer, L., Heinemann, U., Kluwe, L., Finckh, U., Hoppner, W., Stavrou, D., Fillbrandt, R. & Westphal, M. (2001). Molecular genetic alterations on chromosomes 11 and 22 in ependymomas. *Int J Cancer*, Vol.91, No.6, pp. 803-808

Leu, J.I., Dumont, P., Hafey, M., Murphy, M.E. & George, D.L. (2004). Mitochondrial p53 activates Bak and causes disruption of a Bak-Mcl1 complex. *Nat Cell Biol*, Vol.6, No.5, pp. 443-450

Li, X., Dumont, P., Della Pietra, A., Shetler, C. & Murphy, M.E. (2005). The codon 47 polymorphism in p53 is functionally significant. *J Biol Chem*, Vol.280, No.25, pp. 24245-24251

Listernick, R., Charrow, J. & Gutmann, D.H. (1999). Intracranial gliomas in neurofibromatosis type 1. *Am J Med Genet*, Vol.89, No.1, pp. 38-44

Liu, Y., Scheurer, M.E., El-Zein, R., Cao, Y., Do, K.A., Gilbert, M., Aldape, K.D., Wei, Q., Etzel, C. & Bondy, M.L. (2009). Association and interactions between DNA repair gene polymorphisms and adult glioma. *Cancer Epidemiol Biomarkers Prev*, Vol.18, No.1, pp. 204-214

Liu, Y., Zhang, H., Zhou, K., Chen, L., Xu, Z., Zhong, Y., Liu, H., Li, R., Shugart, Y.Y., Wei, Q., Jin, L., Huang, F., Lu, D. & Zhou, L. (2007). Tagging SNPs in non-homologous end-joining pathway genes and risk of glioma. *Carcinogenesis*, Vol.28, No.9, pp. 1906-1913

Louis, D.N., Ohgaki, H., Wiestler, O.D., Cavenee, W.K., Burger, P.C., Jouvet, A., Scheithauer, B.W. & Kleihues, P. (2007). The 2007 WHO classification of tumours of the central nervous system. *Acta Neuropathol*, Vol.114, No.2, pp. 97-109

Louis, D.N., Pomeroy, S.L. & Cairncross, J.G. (2002). Focus on central nervous system neoplasia. *Cancer Cell*, Vol.1, No.2, pp. 125-128

Macdonald, D.R., Gaspar, L.E. & Cairncross, J.G. (1990). Successful chemotherapy for newly diagnosed aggressive oligodendroglioma. *Ann Neurol*, Vol.27, No.5, pp. 573-574

McCormack, B.M., Miller, D.C., Budzilovich, G.N., Voorhees, G.J. & Ransohoff, J. (1992). Treatment and survival of low-grade astrocytoma in adults--1977-1988. *Neurosurgery*, Vol.31, No.4, pp. 636-642; discussion 642

McKean-Cowdin, R., Barnholtz-Sloan, J., Inskip, P.D., Ruder, A.M., Butler, M., Rajaraman, P., Razavi, P., Patoka, J., Wiencke, J.K., Bondy, M.L. & Wrensch, M. (2009). Associations between polymorphisms in DNA repair genes and glioblastoma. *Cancer Epidemiol Biomarkers Prev*, Vol.18, No.4, pp. 1118-1126

Nakagawachi, T., Soejima, H., Urano, T., Zhao, W., Higashimoto, K., Satoh, Y., Matsukura, S., Kudo, S., Kitajima, Y., Harada, H., Furukawa, K., Matsuzaki, H., Emi, M., Nakabeppu, Y., Miyazaki, K., Sekiguchi, M. & Mukai, T. (2003). Silencing effect of CpG island hypermethylation and histone modifications on O6-methylguanine-DNA methyltransferase (MGMT) gene expression in human cancer. *Oncogene*, Vol.22, No.55, pp. 8835-8844

Natsume, A., Kondo, Y., Ito, M., Motomura, K., Wakabayashi, T. & Yoshida, J. (2010). Epigenetic aberrations and therapeutic implications in gliomas. *Cancer Sci*, Vol.101, No.6, pp. 1331-1336

Ng, H.K. & Lam, P.Y. (1998). The molecular genetics of central nervous system tumors. *Pathology*, Vol.30, No.2, pp. 196-202

Nothnagel, M. & Rohde, K. (2005). The effect of single-nucleotide polymorphism marker selection on patterns of haplotype blocks and haplotype frequency estimates. *Am J Hum Genet*, Vol.77, No.6, pp. 988-998

Nozaki, M., Tada, M., Matsumoto, R., Sawamura, Y., Abe, H. & Iggo, R.D. (1998). Rare occurrence of inactivating p53 gene mutations in primary non-astrocytic tumors of the central nervous system: reappraisal by yeast functional assay. *Acta Neuropathol*, Vol.95, No.3, pp. 291-296

Ohgaki, H. & Kleihues, P. (2005). Epidemiology and etiology of gliomas. *Acta Neuropathol*, Vol.109, No.1, pp. 93-108

Paige, A.J. (2003). Redefining tumour suppressor genes: exceptions to the two-hit hypothesis. *Cell Mol Life Sci*, Vol.60, No.10, pp. 2147-2163

Park, D.M. & Rich, J.N. (2009). Biology of glioma cancer stem cells. *Mol Cells*, Vol.28, No.1, pp. 7-12

Parra, F.C., Amado, R.C., Lambertucci, J.R., Rocha, J., Antunes, C.M. & Pena, S.D. (2003). Color and genomic ancestry in Brazilians. *Proc Natl Acad Sci U S A*, Vol.100, No.1, pp. 177-182

Pinto, G.R., Yoshioka, F.K., Clara, C.A., Santos, M.J., Almeida, J.R., Burbano, R.R., Rey, J.A. & Casartelli, C. (2008a). WRN Cys1367Arg SNP is not associated with risk and prognosis of gliomas in Southeast Brazil. *J Neurooncol*, Vol.90, No.3, pp. 253-258

Pinto, G.R., Yoshioka, F.K., Silva, R.L., Clara, C.A., Santos, M.J., Almeida, J.R., Burbano, R.R., Rey, J.A. & Casartelli, C. (2008b). Prognostic value of TP53 Pro47Ser and Arg72Pro single nucleotide polymorphisms and the susceptibility to gliomas in individuals from Southeast Brazil. *Genet Mol Res*, Vol.7, No.1, pp. 207-216

Reifenberger, G. & Louis, D.N. (2003). Oligodendroglioma: toward molecular definitions in diagnostic neuro-oncology. *J Neuropathol Exp Neurol*, Vol.62, No.2, pp. 111-126

Reifenberger, J., Reifenberger, G., Liu, L., James, C.D., Wechsler, W. & Collins, V.P. (1994). Molecular genetic analysis of oligodendroglial tumors shows preferential allelic deletions on 19q and 1p. *Am J Pathol*, Vol.145, No.5, pp. 1175-1190

Reya, T., Morrison, S.J., Clarke, M.F. & Weissman, I.L. (2001). Stem cells, cancer, and cancer stem cells. *Nature*, Vol.414, No.6859, pp. 105-111

Richardson, B. (2003). Impact of aging on DNA methylation. *Ageing Res Rev*, Vol.2, No.3, pp. 245-261

Riemenschneider, M.J., Jeuken, J.W., Wesseling, P. & Reifenberger, G. (2010). Molecular diagnostics of gliomas: state of the art. *Acta Neuropathol*, Vol.120, No.5, pp. 567-584

Rivera, A.L., Pelloski, C.E., Gilbert, M.R., Colman, H., De La Cruz, C., Sulman, E.P., Bekele, B.N. & Aldape, K.D. (2010). MGMT promoter methylation is predictive of response to radiotherapy and prognostic in the absence of adjuvant alkylating chemotherapy for glioblastoma. *Neuro Oncol*, Vol.12, No.2, pp. 116-121

Rush, L.J. & Plass, C. (2002). Alterations of DNA methylation in hematologic malignancies. *Cancer Lett*, Vol.185, No.1, pp. 1-12

Ryberg, D., Skaug, V., Hewer, A., Phillips, D.H., Harries, L.W., Wolf, C.R., Ogreid, D., Ulvik, A., Vu, P. & Haugen, A. (1997). Genotypes of glutathione transferase M1 and P1 and their significance for lung DNA adduct levels and cancer risk. *Carcinogenesis*, Vol.18, No.7, pp. 1285-1289

Sachidanandam, R., Weissman, D., Schmidt, S.C., Kakol, J.M., Stein, L.D., Marth, G., Sherry, S., Mullikin, J.C., Mortimore, B.J., Willey, D.L., Hunt, S.E., Cole, C.G., Coggill, P.C., Rice, C.M., Ning, Z., Rogers, J., Bentley, D.R., Kwok, P.Y., Mardis, E.R., Yeh, R.T., Schultz, B., Cook, L., Davenport, R., Dante, M., Fulton, L., Hillier, L., Waterston, R.H., McPherson, J.D., Gilman, B., Schaffner, S., Van Etten, W.J., Reich, D., Higgins, J., Daly, M.J., Blumenstiel, B., Baldwin, J., Stange-Thomann, N., Zody, M.C., Linton, L., Lander, E.S. & Altshuler, D. (2001). A map of human genome sequence variation containing 1.42 million single nucleotide polymorphisms. *Nature*, Vol.409, No.6822, pp. 928-933

Salisbury, B.A., Pungliya, M., Choi, J.Y., Jiang, R., Sun, X.J. & Stephens, J.C. (2003). SNP and haplotype variation in the human genome. *Mutat Res*, Vol.526, No.1-2, pp. 53-61

Salomon, D.S., Brandt, R., Ciardiello, F. & Normanno, N. (1995). Epidermal growth factor-related peptides and their receptors in human malignancies. *Crit Rev Oncol Hematol*, Vol.19, No.3, pp. 183-232

Sanoudou, D., Tingby, O., Ferguson-Smith, M.A., Collins, V.P. & Coleman, N. (2000). Analysis of pilocytic astrocytoma by comparative genomic hybridization. *Br J Cancer*, Vol.82, No.6, pp. 1218-1222

Sanson, M., Marie, Y., Paris, S., Idbaih, A., Laffaire, J., Ducray, F., El Hallani, S., Boisselier, B., Mokhtari, K., Hoang-Xuan, K. & Delattre, J.Y. (2009). Isocitrate dehydrogenase 1 codon 132 mutation is an important prognostic biomarker in gliomas. *J Clin Oncol*, Vol.27, No.25, pp. 4150-4154

Schuebel, K.E., Chen, W., Cope, L., Glockner, S.C., Suzuki, H., Yi, J.M., Chan, T.A., Van Neste, L., Van Criekinge, W., van den Bosch, S., van Engeland, M., Ting, A.H., Jair, K., Yu, W., Toyota, M., Imai, K., Ahuja, N., Herman, J.G. & Baylin, S.B. (2007). Comparing the DNA hypermethylome with gene mutations in human colorectal cancer. *PLoS Genet*, Vol.3, No.9, pp. 1709-1723

Schwartzbaum, J., Ahlbom, A., Malmer, B., Lonn, S., Brookes, A.J., Doss, H., Debinski, W., Henriksson, R. & Feychting, M. (2005). Polymorphisms associated with asthma are inversely related to glioblastoma multiforme. *Cancer Res*, Vol.65, No.14, pp. 6459-6465

Shahbazi, M., Pravica, V., Nasreen, N., Fakhoury, H., Fryer, A.A., Strange, R.C., Hutchinson, P.E., Osborne, J.E., Lear, J.T., Smith, A.G. & Hutchinson, I.V. (2002). Association between functional polymorphism in EGF gene and malignant melanoma. *Lancet*, Vol.359, No.9304, pp. 397-401

Shete, S., Hosking, F.J., Robertson, L.B., Dobbins, S.E., Sanson, M., Malmer, B., Simon, M., Marie, Y., Boisselier, B., Delattre, J.Y., Hoang-Xuan, K., El Hallani, S., Idbaih, A., Zelenika, D., Andersson, U., Henriksson, R., Bergenheim, A.T., Feychting, M., Lonn, S., Ahlbom, A., Schramm, J., Linnebank, M., Hemminki, K., Kumar, R., Hepworth, S.J., Price, A., Armstrong, G., Liu, Y., Gu, X., Yu, R., Lau, C., Schoemaker, M., Muir, K., Swerdlow, A., Lathrop, M., Bondy, M. & Houlston, R.S. (2009). Genome-wide association study identifies five susceptibility loci for glioma. *Nat Genet*, Vol.41, No.8, pp. 899-904

Simpson, J.R., Horton, J., Scott, C., Curran, W.J., Rubin, P., Fischbach, J., Isaacson, S., Rotman, M., Asbell, S.O., Nelson, J.S. & et al. (1993). Influence of location and extent of surgical resection on survival of patients with glioblastoma multiforme: results of three consecutive Radiation Therapy Oncology Group (RTOG) clinical trials. *Int J Radiat Oncol Biol Phys*, Vol.26, No.2, pp. 239-244

Smith, J.S., Perry, A., Borell, T.J., Lee, H.K., O'Fallon, J., Hosek, S.M., Kimmel, D., Yates, A., Burger, P.C., Scheithauer, B.W. & Jenkins, R.B. (2000). Alterations of chromosome arms 1p and 19q as predictors of survival in oligodendrogliomas, astrocytomas, and mixed oligoastrocytomas. *J Clin Oncol*, Vol.18, No.3, pp. 636-645

Sreeja, L., Syamala, V.S., Syamala, V., Hariharan, S., Raveendran, P.B., Vijayalekshmi, R.V., Madhavan, J. & Ankathil, R. (2008). Prognostic importance of DNA repair gene polymorphisms of XRCC1 Arg399Gln and XPD Lys751Gln in lung cancer patients from India. *J Cancer Res Clin Oncol*, Vol.134, No.6, pp. 645-652

Stiles, C.D. & Rowitch, D.H. (2008). Glioma stem cells: a midterm exam. *Neuron*, Vol.58, No.6, pp. 832-846

Sugimura, T. & Ushijima, T. (2000). Genetic and epigenetic alterations in carcinogenesis. *Mutat Res*, Vol.462, No.2-3, pp. 235-246

Syamala, V.S., Sreeja, L., Syamala, V., Raveendran, P.B., Balakrishnan, R., Kuttan, R. & Ankathil, R. (2008). Influence of germline polymorphisms of GSTT1, GSTM1, and GSTP1 in familial versus sporadic breast cancer susceptibility and survival. *Fam Cancer*, Vol.7, No.3, pp. 213-220

Taylor, J.G., Choi, E.H., Foster, C.B. & Chanock, S.J. (2001). Using genetic variation to study human disease. *Trends Mol Med*, Vol.7, No.11, pp. 507-512

Urioste, M., Martinez-Ramirez, A., Cigudosa, J.C., Colmenero, I., Madero, L., Robledo, M., Martinez-Delgado, B. & Benitez, J. (2002). Complex cytogenetic abnormalities including telomeric associations and MEN1 mutation in a pediatric ependymoma. *Cancer Genet Cytogenet*, Vol.138, No.2, pp. 107-110

Vauleon, E., Auger, N., Benouaich-Amiel, A., Laigle-Donadey, F., Kaloshi, G., Lejeune, J., Delattre, J.Y., Thillet, J. & Sanson, M. (2007). The 61 A/G EGF polymorphism is functional but is neither a prognostic marker nor a risk factor for glioblastoma. *Cancer Genet Cytogenet*, Vol.172, No.1, pp. 33-37

Visvader, J.E. & Lindeman, G.J. (2008). Cancer stem cells in solid tumours: accumulating evidence and unresolved questions. *Nat Rev Cancer*, Vol.8, No.10, pp. 755-768

Vogelstein, B. & Kinzler, K.W. (2004). Cancer genes and the pathways they control. *Nat Med*, Vol.10, No.8, pp. 789-799

von Haken, M.S., White, E.C., Daneshvar-Shyesther, L., Sih, S., Choi, E., Kalra, R. & Cogen, P.H. (1996). Molecular genetic analysis of chromosome arm 17p and chromosome arm 22q DNA sequences in sporadic pediatric ependymomas. *Genes Chromosomes Cancer*, Vol.17, No.1, pp. 37-44

Wang, L.E., Bondy, M.L., Shen, H., El-Zein, R., Aldape, K., Cao, Y., Pudavalli, V., Levin, V.A., Yung, W.K. & Wei, Q. (2004). Polymorphisms of DNA repair genes and risk of glioma. *Cancer Res*, Vol.64, No.16, pp. 5560-5563

Wang, S., Zhao, Y., Ruan, Z., Chen, H., Fan, W., Chen, J., Wu, Q., Qian, J., Zhang, T., Huang, Y. & Lu, D. (2010). Association between EGF +61 G/A and glioma risk in a Chinese population. *BMC Cancer*, Vol.10, pp. 221

White, D.L., Li, D., Nurgalieva, Z. & El-Serag, H.B. (2008). Genetic variants of glutathione S-transferase as possible risk factors for hepatocellular carcinoma: a HuGE systematic review and meta-analysis. *Am J Epidemiol*, Vol.167, No.4, pp. 377-389

Wick, W., Hartmann, C., Engel, C., Stoffels, M., Felsberg, J., Stockhammer, F., Sabel, M.C., Koeppen, S., Ketter, R., Meyermann, R., Rapp, M., Meisner, C., Kortmann, R.D., Pietsch, T., Wiestler, O.D., Ernemann, U., Bamberg, M., Reifenberger, G., von Deimling, A. & Weller, M. (2009). NOA-04 randomized phase III trial of sequential radiochemotherapy of anaplastic glioma with procarbazine, lomustine, and vincristine or temozolomide. *J Clin Oncol*, Vol.27, No.35, pp. 5874-5880

Wrensch, M., Jenkins, R.B., Chang, J.S., Yeh, R.F., Xiao, Y., Decker, P.A., Ballman, K.V., Berger, M., Buckner, J.C., Chang, S., Giannini, C., Halder, C., Kollmeyer, T.M., Kosel, M.L., LaChance, D.H., McCoy, L., O'Neill, B.P., Patoka, J., Pico, A.R., Prados, M., Quesenberry, C., Rice, T., Rynearson, A.L., Smirnov, I., Tihan, T., Wiemels, J., Yang, P. & Wiencke, J.K. (2009). Variants in the CDKN2B and RTEL1 regions are associated with high-grade glioma susceptibility. *Nat Genet*, Vol.41, No.8, pp. 905-908

Wrensch, M., Kelsey, K.T., Liu, M., Miike, R., Moghadassi, M., Sison, J.D., Aldape, K., McMillan, A., Wiemels, J. & Wiencke, J.K. (2005). ERCC1 and ERCC2 polymorphisms and adult glioma. *Neuro Oncol*, Vol.7, No.4, pp. 495-507

Yan, H., Parsons, D.W., Jin, G., McLendon, R., Rasheed, B.A., Yuan, W., Kos, I., Batinic-Haberle, I., Jones, S., Riggins, G.J., Friedman, H., Friedman, A., Reardon, D., Herndon, J., Kinzler, K.W., Velculescu, V.E., Vogelstein, B. & Bigner, D.D. (2009). IDH1 and IDH2 mutations in gliomas. *N Engl J Med*, Vol.360, No.8, pp. 765-773

Zattara-Cannoni, H., Gambarelli, D., Lena, G., Dufour, H., Choux, M., Grisoli, F. & Vagner-Capodano, A.M. (1998). Are juvenile pilocytic astrocytomas benign tumors? A cytogenetic study in 24 cases. *Cancer Genet Cytogenet*, Vol.104, No.2, pp. 157-160

Zhu, Y. & Parada, L.F. (2002). The molecular and genetic basis of neurological tumours. *Nat Rev Cancer*, Vol.2, No.8, pp. 616-626

Zülch, K.J. (1979). Histologic typing of tumours of the central nervous system. World Health Organization, Geneva, Switzerland

6

Genetic Diversity of Glioblastoma Multiforme: Impact on Future Therapies

Franz-Josef Klinz[1], Sergej Telentschak[1],
Roland Goldbrunner[2] and Klaus Addicks[1]
*[1]Department of Anatomy I,
University of Cologne,
[2]Department of Neurosurgery,
University of Cologne,
Germany*

1. Introduction

Glioblastoma multiforme (GBM; WHO grade IV) is the most malignant type of glioma and in addition the most abundant malignant cancer of the adult human brain. Despite progress in diagnosis, surgery and chemotherapy, the median survival time of patients suffering from GBM is approximately 15 months (Stupp et al., 2005). The five years survival time is less than 5% (CBTRUS, 2010). Because glioblastoma cells show a highly infiltrating growth into the brain tissue, a total resection is not possible. In addition, glioblastoma cells are remarkably resistant to chemotherapy and ionizing radiation. In addition, the association of a portion of these cells with hypoxic and necrotic areas within the tumor increases their resistance.

Gliobastoma multiforme tumors can be classified:

1. by histopathology (WHO) in conventional glioblastomas (93%), giant cell glioblastoma (5%) and gliosarcoma (2%);
2. by pathogenesis in primary GBM (90%) and secondary GBM (10%);
3. by gene expression analysis in (I) classical, (II) mesenchymal, (III) proneural or (IV) neural type of GBM;
4. by genomic analysis in subgroups harboring specific mutations and/or altered gene dosage/chromosome number.

Conventional glioblastomas constitute approximately 93% of all glioblastomas and can be divided into primary or secondary tumors: primary glioblastomas represent approximately 90% and develop de novo, whereas the incidence of secondary glioblastomas that arise from astroyctomas WHO grade II and III is in the range of 5 to 10%. Primary and secondary glioblastomas differ in their genetic defects: for example 39% of primary glioblastomas harbor an amplification of the EGF receptor (EGFR) locus, whereas in secondary glioblastomas no amplification was detected. Mutations within the p53 gene are more abundant in secondary glioblastomas. Unconventional glioblastomas include giant cell glioblastomas, gliosarcomas and other rare types (for details see section 4).

	Conventional Glioblastoma		Giant cell glioblastoma	Gliosarcoma
	Primary glioblastoma	Secondary glioblastoma		
Frequency	93%		5%	2%
	90%	10%		
Clinical onset	de novo	secondary	de novo	de novo
Preoperative history (mo)	1,7	>25	1,6	2
Age at diagnosis (yr)	55	39	42	56

Table 1. Clinical profile of the common histopathological glioblastoma subtypes according to WHO. Modified from Kleihues et al., 2007; Peraud et al., 1997; Peraud et al., 1999 and Reis et al., 2000.

2. Genetics of glioblastoma multiforme

2.1 Genetic defects in human cancer

For an introduction into the history of this field the reader is referred to the review of Bignold et al. (2006). Abnormalities of mitoses and chromosomes in cancer cells were described in late 1880s and Hansemann (1890) suggested that cancer cells develop from normal cells due to a tendency to maldistribute chromosomes during mitosis. The term somatic mutation was introduced into tumor biology by Tyzzer (1916). To explain the complexity of cancer phenomena "multi-hit" models (Knudson, 1971) increased in popularity over "single-hit" models of somatic mutation. In the multistep progression model of sporadic colorectal carcinoma five to ten genetic alterations seemed to be necessary for generation of the malignant phenotype (for review see: Fearon and Vogelstein, 1990). The onset and extent of genetic alterations in progression of sporadic colorectal tumors was studied in detail by Stoler et al. (1999). Their observation of about 10,000 genomic alterations occurring per cancer cell has brought into attention the issue of genetic instability in human cancer. Genetic and phenotypic instability are hallmarks of cancer cells and appear early in tumor progression; most cancers are of clonal origin, but individual cancer cells are highly heterogenous. There are three major forms of genetic instability in cancer: (1) aneuploidy, in which entire chromosomes are lost or gained; (2) intrachromosomal instability, distinguished by insertions, deletions, translocations or amplifications and (3) point mutations, which accumulate in certain forms of hereditary cancer as well as in a small portion of sporadic cancers. Stanbridge et al. (1981) reported that specific chromosome loss is associated with the expression of tumorigenicity in human cell hybrids. It was published by Duesberg et al. (1998) that genetic instability of cancer cells is proportional to their degree of aneuploidy. Aneuploidy, an abnormal number of chromosomes, is the result of asymmetrical segregation of chromosomes to daughter cells during mitosis. Once aneuploid, cells will continue to segregate chromosomes asymmetrically during subsequent rounds of mitosis, a process that has been termed "chromosome error propagation" (for review see: Holliday, 1989).

Unlike oncogenes, tumor suppressor genes generally follow the "two hit" model, which implies that both alleles of a particular tumor suppressor gene have to be inactivated before an effect is manifested. If only one allele is inactivated, the second correct allele can still produce the correct protein. Whereas mutant oncogene alleles are typically dominant, mutant tumor suppressor genes are usually recessive.

The mutational activation of oncogenes induces loss of heterozygosity and genomic instability in mammalian cells. These results have used to formulate the oncogene-induced replication stress model (for review see: Halazonetis et al., 2008). In precancerous lesions with intact p53 gene, the oncogene-induced DNA damage leads to p53-dependent apoptosis and/or senescence. After the function of p53 is lost, cells are able to escape its apoptotic and/or senescence effects, and the precancerous lesion is predestinated to become cancerous (Gorgoulis et al., 2005; Bartkova et al., 2005; Bartkova et al., 2006; Di Micco et al., 2006). DNA damage has an important role in promoting polyploidization. If cells with altered DNA enter mitosis, defects in chromosomal segregation and cytokinesis occur (for review see: Chow and Poon, 2010).

The gene for the tumor suppressor protein p53 is mutated in about half of human cancers. It was shown recently by several groups, that eliminating p53 function by mutation leads to dramatically increased reprogramming efficiency of differentiated cells into induced pluripotent stem cells. Important for the field of cancer biology is the report of Mizuno et al. (2010), demonstrating that breast and lung cancers harboring TP53 mutations exhibit stem cell-like transcriptional signatures. These data suggest a role for active p53 in preventing the emergence of cancerous stem-like cells during tumor progression. Since TP53 mutations often arise in a late stage of tumor progression, when many cancer cells with different genetic alterations coexist, some cancer cells may be susceptible to reprogramming to generate stem-like cancer cells, leading to further tumor progression and cellular heterogeneity.

2.2 Genetic diversity of glioblastoma multiforme

DNA sequencing and gene dosage analysis of GBM revealed a high number of shared as well as individual-specific mutations, deletions and amplifications of DNA sequences. A hallmark of many primary GBMs is the loss of one copy of chromosome 10 harboring the locus for the PTEN tumor suppressor gene and/or amplification of the EGF receptor locus at chromosome 7. As a consequence, the Akt signalling pathway is often overactivated in GBM. Array comparative genomic hybridization (CGH) analyses revealed, that primary glioblastomas can be divided into three major genetic subgroups, i.e. tumors with chromosome 7 gain and chromosome 10 loss, tumors with chromosome 10 loss and tumors without copy number changes in chromosomes 7 or 10 (Misra et al., 2005).

Parsons et al. (2008) sequenced 20661 genes coding for proteins in 22 GBM samples and 1 normal sample. They observed that 685 genes contained at least 1 non-silent somatic mutation. 94% of these alterations were single base substitutions that were uniformly distributed among the 21 GBM samples, resulting in an average of 47 mutations per GBM. About 15% of the missense mutations were predicted to have a significant effect on protein function. The same 22 GBM samples were analysed for copy number alterations through hybridization of DNA samples to single nucleotide polymorphism (SNP) arrays, leading to the identification of 147 amplifications and 134 homozygous deletions.

Parsons et al. (2008) next studied the probabilities that the mutations were either "driver" or "passenger". Driver mutations may provide a selective advantage to the cancer cell, whereas passenger mutations arise by the instability of the tumor genome and have no effect on tumor growth. Analysis of all data was used to identify GBM candidate cancer genes that were likely drivers, pointing to alterations in several signaling pathways: CDKN2A (altered in 50% of GBMs); TP53, EGFR, and PTEN (altered in 30 to 40%); NF1, CDK4, and RB1 (altered in 12 to 15%); and PIK3CA and PIK3R1 (altered in 8 to 10%). By analysing additional gene members within signaling pathways affected by these genes, the authors identified alterations of critical genes in the RB1 pathway (RB1, CDK4, and CDKN2A; altered in 68% of GBMs), TP53 pathway (TP53, MDM2, and MDM4; altered in 64%), and the PI3K/PTEN pathway (PIK3CA, PIK3R1, PTEN, and IRS1; altered in 50%). Mutations in the NF1 gene (coding for neurofibromatosis-related protein NF-1 or neurofibromin 1, a stimulator of GTPase activity of ras proteins) were observed in 16 of 105 GBMs (15%). Mutations in the IDH1 gene (coding for the citric acid cycle enzyme isocitrate dehydrogenase 1) were reported in 18 of 149 GBMs (12%).

The Cancer Genome Atlas Research Network (2008) study analysed 91 GBM samples and found 453 non-silent somatic mutations in 223 genes. Affected signaling pathways include TP53, PTEN, NF1, EGFR, ERBB2, RB1, NF1, PIK3R1, and PIK3CA. High-level amplifications were observed frequently for EGFR, CDK4, PDGFR, MDM2, and MDM4 genes, whereas homozygous deletion events were often associated with CDKN2A/B and PTEN genes. In this study, GBMs from patients treated with temozolomide and/or lomustine were analysed for mutations. Treatment with alkylating agents resulted in more than tenfold increase in the number of mutations, that was dependent on the methylation status of the gene for the DNA repair enzyme O^6-methylguanine-DNA methyltransferase (MGMT).

Bredel et al. (2009) published "A Network Model of a Cooperative Genetic Landscape in Brain Tumors". The authors demonstrate that a multigene risk scoring model based on gene dosis and expression of 7 landscape genes (POLD2, CYCS, MYC, AKR1C3, YME1L1, ANXA7, and PDCD4) is associated with the overall length of survival in 189 glioblastoma samples. Yadav et al. (2009) reported that loss of function of ANXA7 (annexin 7) stabilizes the EGFR protein and increases EGFR signaling in glioblastoma cells. ANXA7 haploinsuffiency doubles the tumorigenic potential of glioblastoma cells. The heterozygous loss of ANXA7 in about 75% of GBM in the Cancer Genome Atlas Research Network study (2008) plus the observed infrequent ANXA7 mutation in about 6% of GBM is indicative for its role as a haploinsuffiency gene. A multigene predictor model of outcome in GBM based on expression analysis of 9 genes was published by Colman et al. (2009).

Verhaak et al. (2010) used gene expression analysis to divide GBM into 4 subtypes: I. Classical, II. Mesenchymal, III. Proneural, and IV. Neural. The reproducibility of this classification was demonstrated in an independent validation set. To get insight into the genomic events, the authors used copy number and sequence data from the Cancer Genome Atlas Research Network (2008).

I. Classical subtype of GBM (21% of core samples):

Neural precursor and stem cell markers NES, as well as Notch and Sonic hedgehog signaling pathways were highly expressed in the Classical subtype. Chromosome 7 amplification paired with chromosome 10 loss was seen in 100% of the Classical subtype. High level EGF receptor (EGFR) gene amplification was observed in 97% of the Classical subtype and infrequently in other subtypes. Even though TP53 is the most frequently mutated gene in GBM (Cancer Genome Atlas Research Network, 2008), there was a distinct lack of TP53 mutations in the Classical subtype samples sequenced. Deletion events at 10q23 harboring the PTEN locus were observed in 100% of the Classical subtype. Focal 9p21.3 homozygous deletion targeting CDKN2A (encoding for both p16INK4A and p14 ARF) was frequent and co-occurred with EGFR amplification in 94% of the Classical subtype.

II. Mesenchymal subtype of GBM (32% of core samples):

The Mesenchymal subtype displayed expression of mesenchymal markers as described earlier (Phillips et al. 2006). Genes in the tumor necrosis super family pathway are highly expressed in this subtype. Focal hemizygous deletion of a region at 17q11.2, containing the gene NF1 (coding for neurofibromatosis-related protein NF-1 or neurofibromin 1, a stimulator of GTPase activity of ras proteins) occurred predominantly in the Mesenchymal subtype. NF1 mutations were found in 20 samples, 14 of which were classified as Mesenchymal subtype, resulting in 53% of samples with NF1 abnormalities.

Mutated Gene	Classical Subtype	Mesenchymal Subtype	Proneural Subtype	Neural Subtype	Approximate Overall Frequency
TP53	**0%**	32%	**54%**	21%	23%
PTEN	23%	32%	16%	21%	17%
NF1	5%	**37%**	5%	16%	13%
EGFR	32%	5%	16%	26%	13%
IDH1	0%	0%	**30%**	5%	8%
PIK3R	5%	0%	19%	11%	6%
RB1	0%	13%	3%	5%	5%
ERBB2	5%	3%	5%	16%	5%
EGFRvIII	**23%**	3%	3%	0%	5%
PIK3CA	5%	3%	8%	5%	4%
PDGFRA	0%	0%	**11%**	0%	3%

Table 2. Frequently mutated genes in Glioblastoma multiforme and their distribution among GBM subtypes according to Verhaak et al (2010). Outstanding frequencies are grayed out for comparison between subtypes. Modified from Verhaak et al. (2010).

III. Proneural subtype of GBM (31% of core samples):

The Proneural group showed high expression of oligodendrocytic genes, underlining its status as an atypical GBM subtype. The majority of TP53 mutations and TP53 loss of heterozygosity were found in Proneural samples. The classic GBM signature, chromosome 7 amplification associated with chromosome 10 loss was less prevalent and occurred in only 54% of the Proneural subtype. Focal amplifications of the locus at 4q12 harboring the PDGF Receptor A (PDGFRA) gene were seen in all subtypes of GBM but at a much higher rate

(35%) in Proneural samples. 11 of the 12 observed mutations in the isocitrate dehydrogenase 1 gene (IDH1) were found in this class.

IV. Neural subtype of GBM (16% of core samples):

The Neural subtype was typified by the expression of neuron markers. The two normal brain tissues samples examined in this data set were both classified as Neural subtype. Chomosome 7 amplification associated with chromosome 10 loss was prevalent in the Neural subtype.

		Known Cancer Gene in Region	Classical Subtype	Mesenchymal Subtype	Proneural Subtype	Neural Subtype
Amplification Events	7p11.2	EGFR	100%	95%	54%	96%
	7q21.2	CDK6	92%	89%	46%	96%
	7q31.2	MET	86%	91%	54%	92%
	7q34		86%	91%	52%	92%
	4q12	PDGFRA	5%	9%	35%	13%
Homo- and Hemizygous Deletion Events	17q11.2	NF1	5%	38%	6%	17%
	10q23	PTEN	100%	87%	69%	96%
	9p21.3	CDKN2A/CDKN2B	95%	67%	56%	71%
	13q14	RB1	16%	53%	52%	46%

Table 3. Frequency of copy number alterations in Glioblastoma subtypes according to gene expression. Modified from Verhaak et al. (2010).

2.2.1 Subtypes and clinical correlations

Three of four tumors classified as secondary GBMs were found in the Proneural group. The Proneural subtype was associated with younger age, PDGFRA abnormalities, IDH1 and TP53 mutations, all of which have been associated with secondary GBM in earlier studies (Arjona et al., 2006; Furnari et al., 2007; Kleihues and Ohgaki, 1999; Watanabe et al., 1996; Yan et al., 2009). Verhaak et al. (2010) concluded that tumors did not change class at recurrence, because recurrent tumors were found in all subtypes (Murat et al., 2008). Although statistically not significant, there was a trend towards longer survival for patients with a Proneural signature. Aggressive treatment significantly reduced mortality in Classical and Mesenchymal subtypes, had a less pronounced effect in the Neural subtype and did not alter survival in the Proneural subtype. There was no association of GBM subtype with methylation status of the DNA repair gene MGMT, which has been positively linked to therapy response (all data and conclusions from Verhaak et al., 2010).

Bredel et al. (2010) reported that NFKBIA (nuclear factor of κ-light polypeptide gene enhancer in B-cells inhibitor-α), an inhibitor of EGFR signaling pathway, is often deleted in GBM (Table 4). Most deletions occur in non-classical subtypes of GBM. Deletion and low expression of NFKBIA were reported to be associated with unfavorable outcomes. The authors present a two-gene model based on the expression of NFKBIA and MGMT that is strongly associated with the clinical course of GBM (Table 5).

Genetic Alteration	Classical Subtype	Nonclassical Glioblastomas		
		Mesenchymal Subtype	Proneural Subtype	Neural Subtype
NFKBIA deletion	**6**%	30%	39%	22%
EGFR amplification	**80**%	20%	11%	46%

Table 4. Relationship of four molecular subtypes of glioblastoma to gene-dosage profiles for NFKBIA and EGFR across 188 glioblastomas. NFKBIA deletions are rare in classical (6%) and more common in non-classical (32%) glioblastomas.

Irrespective of subtype a degree of mutual exclusivity between NFKBIA deletion and EGFR amplification was suggested: NFKBIA deletion or EGFR amplification were observed in 53%, whereas concomitant occurrence (NFKBIA deletion together with EGFR amplification) was observed only in 5%. All data and conclusions are from Bredel et al. (2010). Glioblastoma subtypes were classified according to Verhaak et al. (2010).

Risk Groups	NFKBIA and MGMT Expression	Median Survival	NFKBIA Expression and MGMT Promoter Methylation Status	Media Survival (Weeks)	With Radiotherapie and Temozolomide	
					NFKBIA Expression and MGMT Promoter Methylation Status	Median Survival (Weeks)
High-risk	Low NFKBIA, High MGMT	44	Low NFKBIA, Unmeth. MGMT	45	Low NFKBIA, Unmeth. MGMT	35
Inter-mediate-risk	Low NFKBIA, Low MGMT or High NFKBIA, High MGMT	59	Low NFKBIA, Meth. MGMT or High NFKBIA, Unmeth. MGMT	63	Low NFKBIA, Meth. MGMT or High NFKBIA, Unmeth. MGMT	71
Low-risk	High NFKBIA, Low MGMT	92	High NFKBIA, Meth. MGMT	91	High NFKBIA, Meth. MGMT	122

Table 5. The strong association of the clinical course of GBM with expression of NFKBIA and expression/methylation status of the promoter of O^6-methylguanine-DNA methyltransferase (MGMT). All data and conclusions are from Bredel et al. (2010).

To add an additional level of complexity, gene dosage analysis of separate tumor areas derived from one GBM revealed area-specific genomic imbalances (see chapter 5).

2.3 Correlation between genetic and histopathologic diversity in GBM

Glioblastomas are morphologically highly heterogeneous and in addition the histological features often vary in different areas of one tumor. Currently three distinct common histopathological variants of GBM are recognized by the actual World Health Organization classification scheme, including conventional glioblastoma, giant cell glioblastoma, and gliosarcoma.

Despite of lack of any histopathological difference, *primary* (de novo) and *secondary* (with an evidence of a lower-grade precursor) *conventional glioblastomas* harbor distinct molecular genetic abnormalities: Primary glioblastomas are characterized by relatively high frequencies of EGFR amplification, PTEN deletion, and CDKN2A (p16) loss, whereas secondary glioblastomas often contain TP53 mutations, especially those involving codons 248 and 273 or G:C->A:T mutations at CpG sites (Ohgaki et al., 2004).

Even within the conventional glioblastoma category, the cellular composition is heterogeneous and may include small or fibrillary, gemistocytic, granular, lipidized and occasional giant cells or oligodendroglial components. According to the predomination of one of these cell types indicating patterns of differentiation, the WHO distinguishes respective subtypes of glioblastoma such as small cell glioblastoma, glioblastoma with granular cell astrocytoma features, glioblastoma with lipidized cells; whereas giant cell glioblastoma is recognized as a distinct clinicopathologic entity (Kleihues et al., 2007; Miller and Perry, 2007).

Small cell astrocytoma is an aggressive histologic variant being often misdiagnosed as anaplastic oligodendroglioma because of considerable morphologic similarities. Despite of histological overlap clinicopathologic and genetic features are distinct: there are no small cell astrocytomas harboring 1p/19q codeletions, whereas vIII mutant form of EGFR, EGFR amplification and 10q deletions are present in 50%, 69% and 97% of small cell astrocytomas, respectively (Perry et al., 2004).

Once thought to represent a reactive component, *gemistocytes* have been found to harbor TP53 mutations and cytogenetic abnormalities (chromosome 7p gains and 10q losses); therefore, they are now thought to represent a true neoplastic component (Kros et al., 2000).

In rare cases *granular cells* may predominate and create the impression of a granular cell tumor. Similar to astrocytomas with non-granular cytology, these tumors may also harbor TP53 mutations, high-frequency loss of heterozygosity at 9p, 10q, and 17p, and less frequent loss of heterozygosity at 1p and 19q (Castellano-Sanchez et al., 2003). Brat et al. (2002) reported the largest series of such tumors to date (22 cases, including 4 grade II, 7 grade III, and 11 grade IV tumors) and found that these tumors were more aggressive than non-granular cell astrocytomas of the same grade.

Glioblastoma with oligodendroglioma component is an astrocytoma WHO-grade IV containing oligodendroglial areas varying in size and frequency (Kleihues et al., 2007). Despite of oligodendroglial component and in contrast to rather frequent codeletions in WHO grade III anaplastic oligodendroglioma (approximately 85%), deletion of either 1p (24%), 19q (43%), or combined 1p/19q (22%) is relatively infrequent in glioblastoma with oligodendroglioma component (Miller and Perry, 2007).

Giant cell glioblastoma is a rare variant that constitutes up to 5% of glioblastoma and is recognized as a distinct clinicopathologic entity in the WHO 2007 classification. Although occasional giant cells may be found in conventional glioblastoma, these cells are a predominating cytologic component in giant cell glioblastoma. As the name implies, the tumor cells are markedly enlarged and bizarre, often appear often multi-nucleated and

tumor masses are typically well-circumscribed. It occurs in younger patients (fifth decade) (Kleihues et al., 2007).
The molecular genetic features include relatively high frequencies of TP53 mutations (59% to 90%) and PTEN deletion (up to 33%), whereas EGFR amplification/overexpression and homozygous p16 deletion ($p16^{INK4a}$ gene at the CDKN2A locus, 9p21) are lacking in comparison to conventional glioblastoma (Meyer-Puttlitz et al., 1997; Peraud et al., 1997; Peraud et al. 1999; Temme et al. 2010). Therefore, giant cell glioblastomas contain clinical and molecular genetic features of both primary and secondary glioblastomas. Giant cell glioblastomas have an increased expression of Aurora Kinase B; combined with TP53 mutations this may be responsible in induce cytokinesis defects and the development of multinucleated cells (Temme et al., 2010).

	Gliosarcoma	Primary glioblastoma	Giant cell glioblastoma	Secondary glioblastoma
PTEN mutation	38%	32%	33%	4%
EGFR amplification	0%	39%	5%	0%
TP53 mutation	23%	11%	84%	67%
$p16^{INK4a}$ deletion	37%	36%	0%	4%
MDM2 amplification	5%	8%	0%	0%

Table 6. Genetic profile of the common histopathological glioblastoma subtypes. Similar tendencies are indicated by grayscale. Modified from Kleihues et al., 2007; Peraud et al., 1997; Peraud et al., 1999 and Reis et al., 2000.

Despite showing a very poor prognosis giant cell glioblastoma appears to carry a slightly better prognosis than conventional glioblastoma (Burger and Vollmer, 1980; Margetts and Kalyan-Raman, 1989; Shinojima et al., 2004), perhaps because of a less infiltrative behaviour.
Gliosarcoma constitutes roughly 2% of GBMs and is also recognized as a distinct clinico-pathologic entity in the WHO 2007 classification. These tumors are characterized by their well-circumscribed, biphasic tissue pattern with clearly distinguishable areas of glial and mesenchymal differentiation. The glial component of gliosarcoma may display any of the aforementioned cytologic attributes and is typically immunoreactive for GFAP. The mesenchymal component is GFAP-negative and may also carry a wide variety of morphologic appearances, with evidence of differentiation along fibroblastic, cartilaginous, osseous, smooth and striated muscle, and adipose lines (Kleihues et al., 2007). There is a cytogenetic and molecular evidence for a monoclonal origin of both components (Actor et al., 2002; Paulus et al., 1994; Reis et al., 2000).
Exept for the infrequent EGFR amplification, gliosarcomas are genetically similar to primary glioblastomas: they harbor likewise low frequency of TP53 mutations (up to 24%) and similar rates of PTEN deletions (38%) as well as deletions of $p16^{INK4a}$ gene (at the CDKN2A locus, 9p21) in roughly 37% (Actor et al., 2002; Reis et al., 2000).
Comparative genomic hybridization analysis in 20 gliosarcomas by Actor et al. (2002) revealed such common chromosomal imbalances as gains on chromosomes 7 (75%), X (20%), 9q and 20q (15% each) as well as losses on chromosomes 13q (15%), 10 and 9p (35% each).

2.4 Area-specific genomic Imbalances in glioblastoma multiforme

Using flow cytometry data analysis Hoshino et al. (1978) reported that different tumor regions of one glioblastoma showed a highly variable distribution of ploidy. By use of a DNA fingerprinting technique Misra et al. (2000) analysed genetic alterations within two or three tumor areas from seven glioblastomas. In all cases except one, different areas of one tumor displayed different fingerprints, indicating a striking extent of intratumoral genetic heterogeneity. Conventional comparative genomic hybridization (CGH) was used to study the intratumoral patterns of genomic imbalance in Glioblastoma multiforme (Harada et al., 1998; Jung et al., 1999). Array comparative genomic hybridization was utilized by Nobusawa et al. (2010) to study in detail tumor area-specific genomic imbalances. Genetic alterations common to all the areas analyzed within a single tumor included gains at chromosomes 1q32.1 (PIK3C2B, MDM4), 4q11-q12 (KIT, PDGFRA), 7p12.1-11.2 (EGFR), 12q13.3-12q14.1 (GLI1, CDK4), and 12q15 (MDM2), and loss of chromosomes at 9p21.1-24.3 ($p16^{INK4a}/p14^{ARF}$ = CDKN2a), 10p15.3-q26.3 (PTEN, etc.), and 13q12.11-q34 (SPRY2, RB1). These alterations are likely to be causative in the pathogenesis of glioblastomas (driver mutations). Additionally, the authors reported numerous tumor area-specific genomic imbalances, which may be either nonfunctional (passenger mutations) or functional, but constitute secondary events reflecting clonal selection and/or progressive genomic instability, a hallmark of glioblastomas. Area specific-evolution of genomic imbalances in GBM may be comparable to the genetic evolution and genomic instability of metastatic pancreas cancer that has been studied in detail recently (Campbell et al., 2010; Yachida et al., 2010).

Loeper et al. (2001) reported that frequent mitotic errors occur in genetically micro-heterogenous glioblastomas. The authors used fluorescent in situ hybridization (FISH) to study chromosome numbers in a series of 24 glioblastomas. All examined chromosomes showed mitotic instability indicated by numerical aberrations within significant amounts of tumor cells. For chromosomes 10 and 17 only monosomy was observed, whereas chromosome 7 showed trisomy/polysomy. In contrast to other chromosomes displaying monosomy as well as trisomy, copy number changes of chromosomes 7, 10 and 17 seem to be the result of selection in favor of the respective aberration (Loeper et al., 2001). In this context it is interesting to note that neural stem and progenitor cells in the subventricular zone of mouse postnatal brain are frequently aneuploid (Kaushal et al., 2003) and that chromosome segregation defects contribute to aneuploidy in normal neural progenitor cells of the mouse cerebral cortex (Yang et al., 2003). Studies in mice and human demonstrate that chromosomal mosaicism is a prominent feature of neural stem cells, whereas interchromosomal translocations or partial chromosomal deletions or insertions are extremely rare (for review see: Peterson et al., 2008). Glioblastoma stem cells share several properties with neural stem cells, i.e. the growth in floating spheres under serum-free conditions, the expression of the stem cell marker nestin and the differentiation into neural cells like astrocytes or neurons. This similarity in marker expression and behaviour has led to the hypothesis that glioblastoma stem cells may be derived from NSCs (Berger et al., 2004; Sanai et al., 2005).

Recent research makes clear that GBMs do not behave as a whole; local heterogeneity may arise because the tumor regionally adapts to the microenvironment. The influence of microenvironment-induced stimuli may be the force behind clonal selection and acquisition of area specific genomic imbalances in GBM. In addition, regional genomic alterations may be associated with the development of resistance to irradiation and/or chemotherapy, resulting in tumor recurrence and/or progression.

2.5 Mechanisms leading to genetic alterations in glioblastoma multiforme

Analysis of copy number alterations showed an average of 7 amplifications and 6 homozygous deletions per GBM. In addition, an average of 47 mutations was reported (Parsons et al., 2008).

A characteristic feature of GBM is a chromosomal instability (CIN) phenotype distinguished by the loss or gain of complete chromosomes, for example by the gain of chromosome 7 and/or loss of chromosome 10. These chromosome copy number changes can be explained by merotelic spindle attachment that is associated with bipolar but more often with multipolar mitosis. Multipolar spindle pole coalescence in cells with supernumerary centrosomes has been reported as a major source of chromosomal misattachment and chromosome missegregation in colorectal cancer cell lines (Silkworth et al., 2009). Obviously, specific chromosome aberrations may be associated with growth advantage for clonal populations of cancer cells (for example by the loss of tumor suppressor genes).

In addition to its well-defined role in signal transduction at the plasma membrane, recent results have identified PTEN as a new guardian of the genome (for review see: Yin and Shen, 2008). Pten-deficient mouse embryo fibroblasts revealed an increased frequency of mitotic centromere-associated chromosomal instability as well as spontaneous DNA double-strand breaks (Shen et al., 2007). Li Li et al. (2008) developed a mouse model by infecting PTEN-/- neural precursor cells with an EGFRvIII expressing retrovirus and found that EGFRvIII expression and PTEN loss synergistically induced chromosomal instability and glial tumors.

Interestingly, polyploidization of mammalian hepatocytes occurs through failed cytokinesis and is followed by a process that was called reductive mitoses (Duncan et al. 2010). The authors postulate a dynamic model of hepatocyte polyploidization, ploidy reversal and aneuploidy (ploidy conveyor) and propose that this mechanism evolved to generate genetic diversity and permits adaptation of hepatocytes to xenobiotic and nutritional injury.

Several studies point to a link between centrosome amplification, chromosomal instability and the development of cancer (for review see: D´Assoro et al., 2002). Cells in resected high grade gliomas and cultured glioblastoma cells have been reported to exhibit often centrosome amplifications (Loh et al., 2010) and the centrosomal protein γ-tubulin is over-expressed and shows altered subcellular localization in GBM (Katsetos et al., 2006; Loh et al., 2010). Multipolar mitoses were occasionally observed in time lapse recordings of cultured glioblastoma cells (Hegedüs et al., 2000). Our laboratory used long term life cell imaging to study mitoses in a newly established glioblastoma cell line and found that cytokinesis defects followed by multipolar mitosis may be an important mechanism that is used by glioblastoma cells to reduce ploidy and generate viable daughter cells (our unpublished results).

2.6 Epigenetics in glioblastoma multiforme

To add another level of complexity, many types of cancer cells carry aberrant epigenetic modifications. Changes in epigenetic marks (caused or not caused by genetic alterations) may have an fundamental impact on tumor development and/or tumor progression. Epigenetic markers in human gliomas have been reviewed by Hesson et al. (2008). Two groups have studied in detail DNA methylation profiles in GBM (Etcheverry et al. 2010; Nousmehr et al., 2010). Hypermethylation at a large number of genetic loci occurred in a subgroup (proneural group) of glioblastoma patients and was associated with improved outcome (Nousmehr et al., 2010).

Epigenetic mechanisms like methylation of DNA have already an impact on chemotheraypy of GBM. Temozolomide (TMZ, Temodal®) is an orally administered alkylating drug that is often used for chemotherapy of GBM. O^6-Methylguanine-DNA methyltransferase (MGMT) is a DNA repair enzyme that specifically removes promutagenic alkyl DNA adducts from the O^6 position of guanine residues in DNA which are induced by alkylating agents like temozolomide (Goth and Rajewsky, 1974; Margison and Kleihues, 1975). Loss of MGMT expression may be caused by transcriptional silencing through hypermethylation of its CpG islands (Esteller et al., 1999; Qian & Brent, 1997), is frequently (45% to 75%) present in glioblastomas (Bello et al., 2004; Kamiryo et al., 2004; Nakamura et al., 2001) and results in improved survival of glioblastoma patients treated with the alkylating agent temozolomide (Fukushima et al., 2009; Hegi et al, 2005; Hegi et al., 2008). On the other hand not all glioblastoma patients with MGMT promoter methylation respond to alkylating agents and in addition responding GBMs cannot avoid eventual recurrence (Fukushima et al., 2009; Hegi et al., 2008). MGMT promoter methylation appears to occur with a higher frequency in secondary than in primary glioblastoma (Bello et al., 2004; Nakamura et al., 2001) but there is no evidence about its correlation with other histopathologic subtypes.

However, prospective randomized studies of EORTC (European Organisation for Research and Treatment of Cancer) and NCIC (National Cancer Institute of Canada) trial have revealed a significant prolongation of progression free and overall survival for patients with newly diagnosed glioblastoma treated by the concomitant and adjuvant temozolomide and irradiation. By this means median survival has been increased over one year (Stupp et al., 2005, 2009).

The methylation status of the MGMT gene promoter is being used as a biomarker for the potential benefit of the addition of temozolomide to the therapy because its epigenetic silencing has been identified as a strong and independent predictive factor of treatment response for anaplastic glioma patients undergoing chemotherapy with alkylating agents (Hegi et al., 2005; Wick et al., 2009). 3 to 5% of the GBM patients survive for more than 3 years. MGMT hypermethylation was reported to be significantly more frequent in the long-term survivor group (Krex et al., 2007).

The assumption that DNA methylation of CpG island on the MGMT promoter represses consecutively transcriptional activity of the MGMT gene and expression of MGMT protein has been used to explain the correlation between the positive promoter methylation status and favorable treatment response after chemotherapy with temozolomide (Kaina et al., 2007).

However, studies that were performed to validate a relationship between MGMT promoter methylation and protein expression have yielded contradictory results in brain tumors as well as in other neoplasms (Brell et al., 2011). While some studies report a significant correlation between MGMT protein expression analyzed by immunohistochemistry (IHC) and MGMT promoter status measured by methylation-specific polymerase chain reaction (MSP) in glioblastoma and brain metastases of various origin (Ingold et al., 2009; Spiegl-Kreinecker et al., 2009; Tang et al., 2011), other studies failed to detect correlations between both parameters (Brell et al., 2005, 2011; Christmann et al., 2010; Preusser et al., 2008).

In addition, there is increasing evidence that MGMT mRNA expression, unlike MGMT protein expression, could be a better predictor for tumor sensitivity to alkylating agents than MGMT methylation status (Everhard et al., 2009; Kreth et al., 2011). Kreth et al. (2011) provide not only evidence that the degree of MGMT mRNA expression is highly correlated with the MGMT promoter methylation status, but also that low MGMT mRNA expression is strongly

predictive for prolonged time to progression, treatment response, and length of survival. Furthermore, the authors found that in case of discordance the patients with methylated tumors combined with high MGMT mRNA expression did significantly worse than those with low transcriptional activity or unmethylated tumors with low MGMT mRNA expression. Finally Kreth et al. (2011) assume methylation-independent pathways of MGMT expression regulation; however, the exact role of DNA-methyltransferases DNMT1 and DNMT3b that are likely to be involved in methylation of CpG islands of MGMT gene promoter remains unclear.
In the Cancer Genome Atlas Research Network (2008) study, GBMs from patients treated with temozolomide and/or lomustine were analysed for mutations. Treatment with alkylating agents resulted in a more than tenfold increase in the number of mutations that was dependent on the methylation status of the MGMT gene. This phenotype seems to be caused by mutations in the MSH6 gene (Cahill et al., 2007; Hunter et al., 2006; Yip et al., 2009) and other genes of the DNA mismatch repair pathway (Cancer Genome Atlas Research Network, 2008). The loss of the mismatch repair protein MSH6 in GBM is associated with tumor progression during temozolomide treatment (Cahill et al., 2007; Hunter et al., 2006; Yip et al., 2009).

2.7 Stem cells in glioblastoma multiforme

The cancer stem cell concept that is of importance for the genesis of many types of cancer receives increasing credit also in the field of GBM. A minor population of GBM cancer stem cells, which may be derived from genetically altered neural stem cells, is presumed to generate transit amplifying cells with high mitotic activity. Because these stem cells appear to have a low mitotic activity, they are difficult to target by radiotherapy and conventional chemotherapy.
For recent reviews on glioblastoma stem cells the reader is referred to Huang et al. (2010) and McLendon and Rich (2010). Ignatova et al. (2002) firstly described cells with stem-like properties in human cortical glial tumors. Singh et al. (2003) used the cell surface marker CD133 to isolate a clonogenic population of cells showing stem-like features in medullo-blastomas and pilocytic astrocytomas. These cells were declared as tumor stem cells based on their capabilities of self-renewal and multilineage differentiation. Galli et al. (2004) and Yuan et al. (2004) confirmed these findings for glioblastomas. Bao et al. (2006a) selected CD133+ cells from glioblastoma biopsies that were capable of forming tumorspheres in vitro, demonstrated self-renewal and multilineage differentiation and resulted in tumours after transplantation into nude mice. In contrast, CD133- cells did not form tumorspheres in vitro und were not tumorigenic in nude mice. CD133+ cells proved to be a minor population of cells in GBM biopsies. Clinical studies suggested that the percentage of CD133+ cells (Zhang et al., 2008; Zeppernick et al., 2008) or the rate of tumorsphere formation in vitro (Laks et al., 2009; Panosyan et al., 2010) can be used to predict overall survival time of patients. However, it should be noted, that contrary results also exist (Phi et al., 2009; Kim et al., 2011). In recurrent glioblastomas the percentage of CD133+ cells is increased strongly when compared with primary glioblastomas (Pallini et al., 2010). Surprisingly, the increase in expression of CD133 after tumor recurrence was associated significantly with longer survival. Thon et al. (2008) described a correlation between the amount of CD133+ cells within the tumor mass and the WHO grade of glioma (WHO grade II, III and IV). Bao et al. (2006a) demonstrated that CD133+ cells constitutively expressed DNA repair genes at much higher levels that CD133- cells, mediating resistance to X-irradiation in CD133+ cells.

Brain tumor stem cells seem to be localized in a perivascular niche (Bao et al., 2006b; Calabrese et al., 2007; Shen et al., 2008) and low oxygen tension (hypoxia) is associated with its undifferentiated state. In glioblastomas, cancer stem cells express much higher levels of VEGF than non-stem cancer cells and show increased angiogenic potential in vivo (Bao et al., 2006b; Li et al., 2009). Because VEGF expression is under control of transcription factors of the hypoxia inducible factor (HIF) family, one should note that expression of HIF2α is unique to glioma stem cells and correlated with poor patient survival, whereas HIF1α is found in all malignant cells (Li et al., 2009). It has been reported that different human cancers (GBM, colorectal carcinoma, and NSCL carcinoma) converge at the HIF2α oncogenic axis (Franovic et al., 2009). The authors propose that inhibition of HIF2α may be of broad clinical interest in the treatment of cancers with different genetic signatures. Hjelmeland et al. (2010) published recently that acidic stress promotes a glioma stem cell phenotype by induction of HIF2α and other glioma stem cell markers. The authors suggest that an increase in intratumoral pH may be of benefit for targeting the stem cell phenotype.

Three recent papers demonstrate that stem-like cells in GBM are able to differentiate into endothelial cells and may give rise to tumor endothelium (Ricci-Vitiani et al., 2010; Thon et al., 2008; Wang et al., 2010). These results define a novel mechanism for cancer vasculogenesis and may help to explain the failure of currently used inhibitors of angiogenesis. Glioma stem cells as targets for novel strategies of treatment have been recently reviewed (Dietrich et al., 2010; Gilbert & Ross, 2011).

2.8 Promising targets for chemotherapy of glioblastoma multiforme

GBMs are highly infiltrative tumors that show resistance to conventional chemotherapy. Many chemotherapeutic agents are not able to reach the tumor in sufficient doses, because the blood brain barrier is at least partially intact in these tumors.

Most mitotic inhibitors used in clinic impair the function of mitotic spindles by targeting tubulins that are basic components of microtubules. Because microtubules in non-mitotic cells are also affected, these compounds often exhibit significant side effects (for example neurotoxicity). Future therapies of GBM may involve small molecules that inhibit the activity of aurora kinases A or B, polo kinases or the mitotic kinesin Eg5, all proteins that have specific functions in different phases of mitosis (for review see: Kaestner and Bastians, 2010; Sudakin and Yen, 2007). Pharmaceutical companies are on the way to develop selective inhibitors that target these proteins. Phase I and II studies on different forms of solid cancers are currently underway to study newly developed mitosis inhibitors and may also open the way for a more efficient therapy of GBM. Interestingly, it has been reported that in glioblastoma expression of aurora kinases A (Barton et al., 2010) and B (Zeng et al., 2007) were both associated with poor prognosis and may be targets for therapy. Among several other proteins also histone deacetylases (HDACs) may be promising targets for future therapy of GBM (Argyriou and Kalofonos, 2009). ABC transporters play an important role in the development of multidrug resistance. The role of ABC transporters in the resistance network of glioblastoma was reviewed by Bleau et al. (2009).

The humanized monoclonal antibody against vascular endothelial growth factor (Bevacizumab, Avastin®) has been approved by the FDA for treatment of GBM. Although targeting the tumor vasculature with Bevacizumab reduced the number of cancer-like stem cells in orthotopic brain tumor xenografts (Calabrese et al., 2007), a recent phase II study indicates that bevacizumab does not affect median survival of patients with recurrent GBM (Pope et al, 2011).

Potential targets for directed therapy of GBM may include extracellular matrix proteins of the perivascular niche that influence proliferation and/or migration of cancer stem cells. Targeting integrin α6 has recently been shown to inhibit self-renewal, proliferation, and tumor formation capacity of glioblastoma stem cells (Lathia et al., 2010). Cilengitide (Impetreve®) is a cyclic pentapeptide harboring a RGD sequence. RGD sequences present on extracellular matrix proteins mediate the binding to integrins, a class of cell surface receptors. Cilengitide is a selective inhibitor of αvβ3/5 integrins and currently under study as an inhibitor of angiogenesis in several types of solid cancer. Cilengitide monotherapy was well tolerated and exhibited modest antitumor activity among patients with recurrent GBM in a randomized phase II study (Reardon et al., 2008). Also targeting glioma stem cells through the neural cell adhesion molecule L1CAM has been reported to suppress glioma growth (Bao et al., 2008). Glioblastoma cells display complex surface structures with numerous microvilli and filopodia that resist the actions of cytolytic effector lymphocytes (Hoa et al., 2010). It should also be noted that gliomas are accompanied by numerous microglia/macrophages. As was recently reported, inhibition of microglia/macrophage activation may represent a new and effective strategy to suppress proliferation of glioma cells (Zhai et al., 2011).

Subtypes of breast cancer or leukemia can be efficiently treated by inhibiting the one excessively activated signal transduction pathway that is linked to malignancy. For GBM a monocausal therapy by inhibition of a single overactivated signaling pathway seems to be less promising, because cells or even regions with different genetic defects coexist in one tumor. A personalized therapy based on analysis of the individual genetic defects is not yet in sight for GBM.

3. Summary and perspective

Many types of cancer cells evolve through a multistep process in which genetic aberrations accumulate and finally lead to cells exhibiting aberrant gene expression programs. GBM has been considered as a system/network disease (Fathallah-Shaykh, 2010), because its phenotypes appear to be generated by several interconnected aberrant signal transduction pathways as well as numerous molecular abnormalities, thereby resulting in uncontrolled mitosis and migration of GBM cancer cells. In GBM local heterogeneity arises as the tumor regionally adapts to microenvironmental cues. Future molecular therapies of GBM should target its Achilles' heels: the elimination of the small intratumoral subpopulation of cells that exert stem cell properties and the inhibition of mitosis within the population of transit amplifying cells, which is responsible for forming the tumor mass.

4. Acknowledgments

We thank the Maria-Pesch Stiftung and the Nolting-Stiftung for support.

5. References

Actor, B.; Cobbers, J.M., Buschges, R., Wolter, M., Knobbe, C.B., Lichter, P., Reifenberger, G. & Weber, R.G. (2002). Comprehensive analysis of genomic alterations in gliosarcoma and its two tissue components. *Genes Chromosomes Cancer,* Vol.34, No.4, (December 2002), pp. 416–427, ISSN 1045-2257

Argyriou, A.A. & Kalofonos, H.P. (2009). Molecularly targeted therapies for malignant gliomas. *Mol Med.* Vol.15, No.3-4, (March-April 2009), pp. 115-22, ISSN 1076-1551

Arjona, D.; Rey, J.A. & Taylor, S.M. (2006). Early genetic changes involved in low-grade astrocytic tumor development. *Curr Mol Med.,* Vol.6, No.6, (September 2006), pp. 645-50, ISSN 1566-5240

Bao, S.; Wu, Q., McLendon, R.E., Hao, Y., Shi, Q., Hjelmeland, A.B., Dewhirst, M.W., Bigner D.D. & Rich, J.N. (2006a). Glioma stem cells promote radioresistance by preferential activation of the DNA damage response. *Nature,* Vol.444, No.7120, (December 2006a), pp. 756-60, ISSN 0028-0836

Bao, S.; Wu, Q., Sathornsumetee, S., Hao, Y., Li, Z., Hjelmeland, A.B., Shi, Q., McLendon, R.E., Bigner, D.D. & Rich, J.N. (2006b). Stem cell-like glioma cells promote tumor angiogenesis through vascular endothelial growth factor. *Cancer Res.,* Vol.66, No.16, (August 2006b), pp. 7843-7848, ISSN 0008-5472

Bao, S.; Wu, Q., Li, Z., Sathornsumetee, S., Wang, H., McLendon, R.E., Hjelmeland, A.B. & Rich, J.N. (2008). Targeting cancer stem cells through L1CAM suppresses glioma growth. *Cancer Res.,* Vol.68, No.15, (August 2008), pp. 6043-6048, ISSN 0008-5472

Bartkova, J.; Horejsí, Z., Koed, K., Krämer, A., Tort, F., Zieger, K., Guldberg, P., Sehested, M., Nesland, J.M., Lukas, C., Ørntoft, T., Lukas, J. & Bartek, J. (2005). DNA damage response as a candidate anti-cancer barrier in early human tumorigenesis. *Nature,* Vol.434, No.7035, (April 2005), pp. 864-70, ISSN 0028-0836

Bartkova, J.; Rezaei, N., Liontos, M., Karakaidos, P., Kletsas, D., Issaeva, N., Vassiliou, L.V., Kolettas, E., Niforou, K., Zoumpourlis, V.C., Takaoka, M., Nakagawa, H., Tort, F., Fugger, K., Johansson, F., Sehested, M., Andersen, C.L., Dyrskjot, L., Ørntoft, T., Lukas, J., Kittas, C., Helleday, T., Halazonetis, T.D., Bartek, J. & Gorgoulis, V.G. (2006). Oncogene-induced senescence is part of the tumorigenesis barrier imposed by DNA damage checkpoints. *Nature,* Vol.444, No.7119, (November 2006), pp. 633-637, ISSN: 0028-0836

Barton, V.N.; Foreman, N.K., Donson, A.M., Birks, D.K., Handler, M.H. & Vibhakar, R. (2010). Aurora kinase A as a rational target for therapy in glioblastoma. *J Neurosurg Pediatr.,* Vol.6, No.1, (July 2010), pp. 98-105, ISSN 1933-0707

Bello, M.J.; Alonso, M.E., Amiñoso, C., Anselmo, N.P., Arjona, D., Gonzalez-Gomez, P., Lopez-Marin, I., de Campos, J.M., Gutierrez, M., Isla, A., Kusak, M.E., Lassaletta, L., Sarasa, J.L., Vaquero, J., Casartelli, C. & Rey, J.A. (2004). Hypermethylation of the DNA repair gene MGMT: association with TP53 G:C to A:T transitions in a series of 469 nervous system tumors. *Mutat Res.,* Vol.554, No.1-2, (October 2004), pp. 23-32, ISSN 0027-5107

Berger, F.; Gay, E., Pelletier, L., Tropel, P. & Wion, D. (2004). Development of gliomas: potential role of asymmetrical cell division of neural stem cells. *Lancet Oncol.,* Vol.5, No.8, (August 2004), pp. 511-514, ISSN 1470-2045

Bignold, L.P.; Coghlan, B.L. & Jersmann, H.P. (2006). Cancer morphology, carcinogenesis and genetic instability: a background. *EXS,* Vol.96, (2006), pp. 1-24, ISSN 1023-294X

Bleau, A.M.; Huse, J.T. & Holland, E.C. (2009). The ABCG2 resistance network of glioblastoma. *Cell Cycle,* Vol.8, No.18, (September 2009), pp. 2936-2944, ISSN 1538-4101

Brat, D.J.; Scheithauer, B.W., Medina-Flores, R., Rosenblum, M.K. & Burger, P.C. (2002). Infiltrative astrocytomas with granular cell features (granular cell astrocytomas): a study of histopathologic features, grading, and outcome. *Am J Surg Pathol.*, Vol.26, No.6, (June 2002), pp. 750-757, ISSN 0147-5185

Bredel, M.; Scholtens, D.M., Harsh, G.R., Bredel, C., Chandler, J.P., Renfrow, J.J., Yadav, A.K., Vogel, H., Scheck, A.C., Tibshirani, R. & Sikic, B.I. (2009). A network model of a cooperative genetic landscape in brain tumors. *JAMA*, Vol.302, No.3, (Juli 2009), pp. 261-75, ISSN 0098-7484

Bredel, M.; Scholtens, D.M., Yadav, A.K., Alvarez, A.A., Renfrow, J.J., Chandler, J.P., Yu, I.L., Carro, M.S., Dai, F., Tagge, M.J., Ferrarese, R., Bredel, C., Phillips, H.S., Lukac, P.J., Robe, P.A., Weyerbrock, A., Vogel, H., Dubner, S., Mobley, B., He, X., Scheck, A.C., Sikic, B.I., Aldape, K.D., Chakravarti, A. & Harsh, G.R. 4th. (2010). NFKBIA deletion in glioblastomas. *N Engl J Med.*, Vol.364, No.7, (February 2011), pp. 17627-17637, ISSN 0028-4793

Brell, M.; Ibáñez, J. & Tortosa, A. (2011). O6-Methylguanine-DNA methyltransferase protein expression by immunohistochemistry in brain and non-brain systemic tumours: systematic review and meta-analysis of correlation with methylation-specific polymerase chain reaction. *BMC Cancer,* Vol.11, No.1, (January 2011), pp. 35, ISSN 1471-2407

Brell, M.; Tortosa, A., Verger, E., Gil, J.M., Viñolas, N., Villà, S., Acebes, J.J., Caral Pons, J.J., Pujol, T., Ferrer, I., Ribalta, T. & Graus, F. (2005). Prognostic significance of O6 - Methilguanine DNA methyltransferase determined by promoter methylation and immunohistochemical expression in anaplastic gliomas. *Clin Cancer Res.*, Vol.11, No.14, (July 2005), pp. 5167-5174; ISSN 1078-0432

Burger, P.C. & Vollmer, R.T. (1980). Histologic factors of prognostic significance in the glioblastoma multiforme. *Cancer,* Vol.46, No.5, (September 1980), pp. 1179-1186, ISSN 1837-9664

Cahill, D.P.; Levine, K.K., Betensky, R.A., Codd, P.J., Romany, C.A., Reavie, L.B., Batchelor, T.T., Futreal, P.A., Stratton, M.R., Curry, W.T., Iafrate, A.J. & Louis, D.N. (2007). Loss of the mismatch repair protein MSH6 in human glioblastomas is associated with tumor progression during temozolomide treatment. *Clin Cancer Res.,* Vol.13, No.7, (April 2007), pp. 2038-2045, ISSN 1078-0432

Calabrese, C.; Poppleton, H., Kocak, M., Hogg, T.L., Fuller, C., Hamner, B., Oh, E.Y., Gaber, M.W., Finklestein, D., Allen, M., Frank, A., Bayazitov, I.T., Zakharenko, S.S., Gajjar, A., Davidoff, A. & Gilbertson R.J. (2007). A perivascular niche for brain tumor stem cells. *Cancer Cell,* Vol.11, No.1, (January 2007), pp. 69-82, ISSN 1535-6108

Campbell, P.J.; Yachida, S., Mudie, L.J., Stephens, P.J., Pleasance, E.D., Stebbings, L.A., Morsberger, L.A., Latimer, C., McLaren, S., Lin, M.L., McBride, D.J., Varela, I., Nik-Zainal, S.A., Leroy, C., Jia, M., Menzies, A., Butler, A.P., Teague, J.W., Griffin, C.A., Burton, J., Swerdlow, H., Quail, M.A., Stratton, M.R., Iacobuzio-Donahue, C. & Futreal, P.A. (2010). The patterns and dynamics of genomic instability in metastatic pancreatic cancer. *Nature,* Vol.467, No.7319, (October 2010), pp. 1109-1113, ISSN 0028-0836

Cancer Genome Atlas Research Network (2008). Comprehensive genomic characterization defines human glioblastoma genes and core pathways. *Nature,* Vol.455, No.7216, (October 2008), pp. 1061-1068, ISSN 0028-0836

Castellano-Sanchez, A.A.; Ohgaki, H., Yokoo, H., Scheithauer, B.W., Burger, P.C., Hamilton, R.L., Finkelstein, S.D. & Brat, D.J. (2003). Granular cell astrocytomas show a high frequency of allelic loss but are not a genetically defined subset. *Brain Pathol.,* Vol.13, No.2, (April 2003), pp. 185-194, ISSN 1015-6305

Central Brain Tumor Registry of the United States (2010) . Primary Brain and Central Nervous System Tumors Diagnosed in Unated States 2004-2006, In CBRUS Statistical Report (2010), 15.04.2011, Available from http://www.cbtrus.org/2010-NPCR-SEER/CBTRUS-WEBREPORT-Final-3-2-10.pdf

Chow, J. & Poon, R.Y. (2010). DNA damage and polyploidization. *Adv Exp Med Biol.,* Vol.676, (2010), pp. 57-71, ISSN 0065-2598

Colman, H.; Zhang, L., Sulman, E.P., McDonald, J.M., Shooshtari, N.L., Rivera, A., Popoff, S., Nutt, C.L., Louis, D.N., Cairncross, J.G., Gilbert M.R., Phillips, H.S., Mehta, M.P., Chakravarti, A., Pelloski, C.E., Bhat, K., Feuerstein, B.G., Jenkins, R.B. & Aldape, K. (2009). A multigene predictor of outcome in glioblastoma. *Neuro Oncol.,* Vol.12, No.1, (January 2010), pp. 49-57, ISSN 1522-8517

Christmann, M.; Nagel, G., Horn, S., Krahn, U., Wiewrodt, D., Sommer, C. & Kaina, B. (2010). MGMT activity, promoter methylation and immunohistochemistry of pretreatment and recurrent malignant gliomas: a comparative study on astrocytoma and glioblastoma. *Int J Cancer,* Vol.127, No.9, (November 2010), pp. 2106-2118, ISSN 0898-6924

D'Assoro, A.B.; Lingle, W.L. & Salisbury, J.L. (2002). Centrosome amplification and the development of cancer. *Oncogene,* Vol.21, No.40, (September 2002), pp. 6146-6153, ISSN 0950-9232

Di Micco, R.; Fumagalli, M., Cicalese, A., Piccinin, S., Gasparini, P., Luise, C., Schurra, C., Garre', M., Nuciforo, P.G., Bensimon A., Maestro, R., Pelicci, P.G. & d'Adda di Fagagna F. (2006). Oncogene-induced senescence is a DNA damage response triggered by DNA hyper-replication. *Nature.* Vol.444, No.7119, (November 2006), pp. 638-42, ISSN 0028-0836

Dietrich, J.; Diamond, E.L., & Kesari, S. (2010). Glioma stem cell signaling: therapeutic opportunities and challenges. *Expert Rev Anticancer Ther.,* Vol.10, No.5, (May 2010), pp. 709-22, ISSN 1473-7140

Duesberg, P.; Rausch, C., Rasnick, D. & Hehlmann, R. (1998). Genetic instability of cancer cells is proportional to their degree of aneuploidy. *Proc Natl Acad Sci U S A,* Vol.95, No.23, (November 1998), pp. 13692-13697, ISSN 0027-8424

Duncan, A.W.; Taylor, M.H., Hickey, R.D., Hanlon Newell, A.E., Lenzi, M.L., Olson, S.B., Finegold, M.J. & Grompe, M. (2010). The ploidy conveyor of mature hepatocytes as a source of genetic variation. *Nature,* Vol.467, No.7316, (October 2010), pp. 707-710, ISSN 0028-0836

Etcheverry, A.; Aubry, M., de Tayrac, M., Vauleon, E., Boniface, R., Guenot, F., Saikali, S., Hamlat, A., Riffaud, L., Menei, P., Quillien, V. & Mosser, J. (2010). DNA methylation in glioblastoma: impact on gene expression and clinical outcome. *BMC Genomics,* Vol.11, (December 2010), pp. 701, ISSN 1471-2164

Esteller, M.; Hamilton, S.R., Burger, P.C., Baylin, S.B. & Herman, J.G. (1999). Inactivation of the DNA repair gene O6-methylguanine-DNA methyltransferase by promoter hypermethylation is a common event in primary human neoplasia. *Cancer Res.*, Vol.59, No.4, (February 1999), pp. 793-797, ISSN 0008-5472

Everhard, S.; Tost, J., El Abdalaoui, H., Crinière, E., Busato, F., Marie, Y., Gut, I.G., Sanson, M., Mokhtari, K., Laigle-Donadey, F., Hoang-Xuan, K., Delattre, J.Y. & Thillet, J. (2009). Identification of regions correlating MGMT promoter methylation and gene expression in glioblastomas. *Neuro Oncol.*, Vol.11, (August 2009), pp. 348–356, ISSN 1522-8517

Fathallah-Shaykh, H.M. (2010). Malignant astrocytomas: a system disease. *Arch Neurol.*, Vol.67, No.3, (March 2010), pp. 353-355, ISSN 0003-9942

Fearon, E.R. & Vogelstein, B. (1990). A genetic model for colorectal tumorigenesis. *Cell*, Vol.61, No.5, (June 1990), pp. 759-767

Franovic, A.; Holterman, C.E., Payette, J. & Lee, S. (2009). Human cancers converge at the HIF-2alpha oncogenic axis. *Proc Natl Acad Sci U S A*, Vol.106, No.50, (December 2009), pp. 21306-21311, ISSN 0027-8424

Fukushima, T.; Takeshima, H. & Kataoka, H. (2009). Anti-glioma therapy with temozolomide and status of the DNA-repair gene MGMT. *Anticancer Res.*, Vol.29, No.11, (November 2009), pp. 4845-4854, ISSN 0250-7005

Furnari, F.B.; Fenton, T., Bachoo, R.M., Mukasa, A., Stommel, J.M., Stegh, A., Hahn, W.C., Ligon, K.L., Louis, D.N., Brennan, C., Chin, L., DePinho, R.A. & Cavenee, W.K. (2007). Malignant astrocytic glioma: genetics, biology, and paths to treatment. *Genes Dev.*, Vol.21, No.21, (November 2007), pp. 2683-2710, ISSN 0890-9369

Galli, R.; Binda, E., Orfanelli, U., Cipelletti, B., Gritti, A., De Vitis, S., Fiocco, R., Foroni C., Dimeco, F. & Vescovi, A. (2004). Isolation and characterization of tumorigenic, stem-like neural precursors from human glioblastoma. *Cancer Res.*, Vol.64, No.19, (October 2004), pp. 7011-7021, ISSN 0008-5472

Gilbert, C.A. and Ross A.H. (2011). Glioma Stem Cells: Cell Culture, Markers and Targets for New Combination Therapies, In: *Cancer Stem Cells Theories and Prac*tice, S. Shostak (Ed.), InTech, Retrieved from http://www.intechopen.com/articles /show/title/glioma-stem-cells-cell-culture-markers-and-targets-for-new-combination-therapies

Gorgoulis, V.G.; Vassiliou, L.V., Karakaidos, P., Zacharatos, P., Kotsinas, A., Liloglou, T., Venere, M., Ditullio, R.A.Jr., Kastrinakis, N.G., Levy, B., Kletsas, D., Yoneta, A., Herlyn, M., Kittas, C. & Halazonetis, T.D. (2005). Activation of the DNA damage checkpoint and genomic instability in human precancerous lesions. *Nature*, Vol. 434, No.7035, (April 2005), pp. 907-913, ISSN 0028-0836

Goth, R. & Rajewsky, M.F. (1974). Persistence of O6-ethylguanine in rat-brain DNA: correlation with nervous system-specific carcinogenesis by ethylnitrosourea. *Proc Natl Acad Sci U S A*. Vol.71, No.3, (March 1974), pp. 639-43, ISSN 0027-8424

Halazonetis, T.D.; Gorgoulis, V.G. & Bartek, J. (2008). An oncogene-induced DNA damage model for cancer development. *Science*, Vol.319, No.5868, (March 2008), pp. 1352-5, ISSN 0193-4511

Hansemann, D. (1890). Ueber asymmetrische Zellteilung in Epithelkrebsen und deren biologische Bedeutung [On the asymmetrical cell divisions in epithelial cancers and its biological significance]. *Arch Pathol Anat etc., Berlin (Virchow´s Arch),* Vol.119, (1890), pp. 299-326

Harada, K.; Nishizaki, T., Ozaki, S., Kubota, H., Ito, H. & Sasaki, K. (1998). Intratumoral cytogenetic heterogeneity detected by comparative genomic hybridization and laser scanning cytometry in human gliomas. *Cancer Res.* Vol.58, No.20, (October 1998), pp. 4694-700, ISSN 0008-5472

Hegedüs, B.; Czirók, A., Fazekas, I., B'abel, T., Madar'asz, E. & Vicsek, T. (2000). Locomotion and proliferation of glioblastoma cells in vitro: statistical evaluation of videomicroscopic observations. *J Neurosurg.,* Vol.92, No.3, (March 2000), pp. 428-34, ISSN 0022-3085

Hegi, M.E.; Diserens, A.C., Gorlia, T., Hamou, M.F., de Tribolet, N., Weller, M., Kros, J.M., Hainfellner, J.A., Mason, W., Mariani, L., Bromberg, J.E., Hau, P., Mirimanoff, R.O., Cairncross, J.G., Janzer, R.C. & Stupp, R. (2005). MGMT gene silencing and benefit from temozolomide in glioblastoma. *N Engl J Med.,* Vol.352, No.10, (March 2005),pp. 997-1003, ISSN 0028-4793

Hegi, M.E.; Liu, L., Herman, J.G., Stupp, R., Wick, W., Weller, M., Mehta, M.P. & Gilbert, M.R. (2008). Correlation of O6-methylguanine methyltransferase (MGMT) promoter methylation with clinical outcomes in glioblastoma and clinical strategies to modulate MGMT activity. *J Clin Oncol.,* Vol.26, No.25, (September 2008), pp. 4189-99 ISSN 0732-183X

Hesson, L.B. ; Krex, D. & Latif, F. (2008). Epigenetic markers in human gliomas: prospects for therapeutic intervention. *Expert Rev Neurother.,* Vol.8, No.10, (October 2008), pp. 1475-96, ISSN 1473-7175

Hjelmeland, A.B.; Wu, Q., Heddleston, J.M., Choudhary, G.S., Macswords, J., Lathia, J.D., McLendon, R., Lindner, D., Sloan, A. & Rich, J.N. (2010). Acidic stress promotes a glioma stem cell phenotype. *Cell Death Differ.,* [Epub ahead of print], ISSN 1476-5403

Hoa, N.; Ge, L., Kuznetsov, Y., McPherson, A., Cornforth, A.N., Pham, J.T., Myers, M.P., Ahmed, N., Salsman, V.S., Lamb, L.S.Jr., Bowersock, J.E., Hu, Y., Zhou, Y.H. & Jadus M.R. (2010). Glioma cells display complex cell surface topographies that resist the actions of cytolytic effector lymphocytes. *J Immunol.,* Vol.185, No.8, (October 2010), pp. 4793-803, ISSN 0022-1767

Holliday, R. (1989). Chromosome error propagation and cancer. *Trends Genet.* Vol.5, No.2, (February 1989), pp. 42-5, ISSN 0168-9525

Hoshino, T.; Nomura, K., Wilson, C.B., Knebel, K.D. & Gray, J.W. (1978). The distribution of nuclear DNA from human brain-tumor cells. *J Neurosurg.,* Vol.49, No.1, (July 1978), pp. 13-21, ISSN 0022-3085

Huang, Z.; Cheng, L., Guryanova, O.A., Wu, Q. & Bao, S. (2010). Cancer stem cells in glioblastoma-molecular signaling and therapeutic targeting. *Protein Cell,* Vol.1, No.7, (July 2010), pp. 638-55, ISSN 1674-800X

Hunter,C.; Smith, R., Cahill, D.P., Stephens, P., Stevens, C., Teague, J., Greenman, C., Edkins, S., Bignell, G., Davies, H., O'Meara, S., Parker, A., Avis, T., Barthorpe, S., Brackenbury, L., Buck, G., Butler, A., Clements, J., Cole, J., Dicks, E., Forbes, S., Gorton, M., Gray, K., Halliday, K., Harrison, R., Hills, K., Hinton, J., Jenkinson, A., Jones, D., Kosmidou, V., Laman, R., Lugg, R., Menzies, A., Perry, J., Petty, R., Raine,

K., Richardson, D., Shepherd, R., Small, A., Solomon, H., Tofts, C., Varian, J., West, S., Widaa, S., Yates, A., Easton, D.F., Riggins, G., Roy, J.E., Levine, K.K., Mueller, W., Batchelor, T.T., Louis, D.N., Stratton, M.R., Futreal, P.A. & Wooster R. (2006). A hypermutation phenotype and somatic MSH6 mutations in recurrent human malignant gliomas after alkylator chemotherapy. Cancer Res., Vol.66, No.8, (April 2006), pp. 3987-91, ISSN-0008-5472

Ignatova, T.N.; Kukekov, V.G., Laywell, E.D., Suslov, O.N., Vrionis, F.D. & Steindler, D.A. (2002). Human cortical glial tumors contain neural stem-like cells expressing astroglial and neuronal markers in vitro. *Glia,* Vol.39, No.3, (September 2002), pp. 193-206, ISSN 0894-1491

Ingold, B.; Schraml, P., Heppner, F.L. & Moch, H. (2009). Homogeneous MGMT immunoreactivity correlates with an unmethylated MGMT promoter status in brain metastases of various solid tumors. *PLoS ONE,* Vol.4, No.3, (March 2009), pp. e4775, ISSN 1932-6203

Jung, V.; Romeike, B.F., Henn, W., Feiden, W., Moringlane, J.R., Zang, K.D. & Urbschat, S. (1999). Evidence of focal genetic microheterogeneity in glioblastoma multiforme by area-specific CGH on microdissected tumor cells. *J Neuropathol Exp Neurol.,* Vol. 58, No.9, (September 1999), pp. 993-9, ISSN 0022-3069

Kaestner, P. & Bastians, H. (2010). Mitotic drug targets. *J Cell Biochem.,* Vol.111, No.2, (October 2010), pp. 258-65, ISSN 0730-2312

Kaina, B.; Christmann, M., Naumann, S. & Roos, W.P. (2007). MGMT: key node in the battle against genotoxicity, carcinogenicity and apoptosis induced by alkylating agents. *DNA Repair (Amst),* Vol.6, No.8, (August 2007), pp. 1079–1099, ISSN 1568-7864

Kamiryo, T.; Tada, K., Shiraishi, S., Shinojima, N., Kochi, M. & Ushio, Y. (2004). Correlation between promoter hypermethylation of the O6-methylguanine-deoxyribonucleic acid methyltransferase gene and prognosis in patients with high-grade astrocytic tumors treated with surgery, radiotherapy, and 1-(4-amino-2-methyl-5-pyrimidinyl)methyl-3-(2-chloroethyl)-3-nitrosourea-based chemotherapy. *Neurosurgery,* Vol.54, No.2, (February 2004), pp. 349-57, ISSN 0148-396X

Katsetos, C.D.; Reddy, G., Dráberová, E., Smejkalová, B., Del Valle, L., Ashraf, Q., Tadevosyan, A., Yelin, K., Maraziotis, T., Mishra, O.P., Mörk, S., Legido, A., Nissanov, J., Baas, P.W., de Chadarévian, J.P. & Dráber, P. (2006). Altered cellular distribution and subcellular sorting of gamma-tubulin in diffuse astrocytic gliomas and human glioblastoma cell lines. *J Neuropathol Exp Neurol.,* Vol.65, No.5, (May 2006), pp. 465-77, ISSN 0022-3069

Kaushal, D.; Contos, J.J., Treuner, K., Yang, A.H., Kingsbury, M.A., Rehen, S.K., McConnell M.J., Okabe, M., Barlow, C. & Chun, J. (2003). Alteration of gene expression by chromosome loss in the postnatal mouse brain. *J Neurosci.,* Vol.23, No.13, (July 2003), pp. 5599-606, ISSN 0270-6474

Kim, K.J.; Lee, K.H., Kim, H.S., Moon, K.S., Jung, T.Y., Jung, S. & Lee, M.C. (2011). The presence of stem cell marker-expressing cells is not prognostically significant in glioblastomas. *Neuropathology,* (January 2011), [Epub ahead of print], ISSN 0919-6544

Kleihues, P.; Burger, P.C., Aldape, K.D., Brat, D.J., Biernat, W., Bigner, D.D., Nakazato, Y., Plate, K.H., Giangaspero, F., von Deimling, A., Ohgaki, H., Cavenee, W.K. (2007).

Glioblastoma. In: *Classification of Tumors of the Central Nervous System*, Louis, D.N., Ohgaki, H., Wiestler, O.D., Cavenee, W.K., pp. 33-49, WHO, ISBN 978-92-832-2430-2, Lyon: IARC

Kleihues, P. & Ohgaki, H.(1999). Primary and secondary glioblastomas: from concept to clinical diagnosis. *Neuro Oncol.,* Vol.1, No.1, (January 1999), pp. 44-51, ISSN 1522-8517

Knudson, A. (1971). Mutation and cancer: statistical study of retinoblastoma. *Proc Natl Acad Sci U S A,* Vol.68, No.4, (April 1971), pp. 820–3, ISSN 0027-8424

Kreth, S.; Thon, N., Eigenbrod, S, Lutz, J., Ledderose, C., Egensperger, R., Tonn, J.C., Kretzschmar, H.A., Hinske, L.C. & Kreth, F.W. (2011). O-Methylguanine-DNA Methyltransferase (MGMT) mRNA Expression Predicts Outcome in Malignant Glioma Independent of MGMT Promoter Methylation. *PLoS One,* Vol.6, No.2, (February 2011), pp. e17156, ISSN 1932-6203

Krex, D.; Klink, B., Hartmann, C., von Deimling, A., Pietsch, T., Simon, M., Sabel, M., Steinbach, J.P., Heese, O., Reifenberger, G., Weller, M. & Schackert, G. (2007). German Glioma Network. Long-term survival with glioblastoma multiforme. *Brain,* Vol.130, No.10, (October 2007), pp. 2596-606, ISSN 0006-8950

Kros, J.M.; Waarsenburg, N., Hayes, D.P., Hop, W.C. & van Dekken, H. (2000). Cytogenetic analysis of gemistocytic cells in gliomas. *J Neuropathol Exp Neurol.,* Vol.59, No.8, (August 2000), pp. 679–686, ISSN 0022-3069

Laks, D.R.; Masterman-Smith, M., Visnyei, K., Angenieux, B., Orozco, N.M., Foran, I., Yong, W.H., Vinters, H.V., Liau, L.M., Lazareff, J.A., Mischel, P.S., Cloughesy, T.F., Horvath, S. & Kornblum, H.I. (2009). Neurosphere formation is an independent predictor of clinical outcome in malignant glioma. *Stem Cells,* Vol.27, No.4, (April 2009), pp. 980-7, ISSN 0250-6793

Lathia, J.D.; Gallagher, J., Heddleston, J.M., Wang, J., Eyler, C.E., Macswords, J., Wu, Q., Vasanji, A., McLendon, R.E., Hjelmeland, A.B. & Rich, J.N. (2010). Integrin alpha 6 regulates glioblastoma stem cells. *Cell Stem Cell,* Vol.6, No.5, (May 2010), pp. 421-32, ISSN 1934-5909

Li, Z.; Bao, S., Wu, Q., Wang, H., Eyler, C., Sathornsumetee, S., Shi, Q., Cao, Y., Lathia, J., McLendon, R.E., Hjelmeland, A.B. & Rich, J.N. (2009). Hypoxia-inducible factors regulate tumorigenic capacity of glioma stem cells. *Cancer Cell,* Vol.15, No.6, (June 2009), pp. 501-13, ISSN 1535-6108

Li, L.; Dutra, A., Pak, E., Labrie, J.E. 3rd, Gerstein, R.M., Pandolfi, P.P., Recht, L.D., Ross, A.H(2008). EGFRvIII expression and PTEN loss synergistically induce chromosomal instability and glial tumors. *Neuro Oncol.* Vol.11, No.1, (February 2009),pp. 9-21, ISSN 1522-8517

Loeper, S.; Romeike, B.F., Heckmann, N., Jung, V., Henn, W., Feiden, W., Zang, K.D. & Urbschat, S. (2001). Frequent mitotic errors in tumor cells of genetically micro-heterogeneous glioblastomas. *Cytogenet Cell Genet.,* Vol.94, No.1-2, (2001), pp. 1-8, ISSN 0301-0171

Loh, J.K.; Lieu, A.S., Chou, C.H., Lin, F.Y., Wu, C.H., Howng, S.L., Chio, C.C. & Hong, Y.R. (2010). Differential expression of centrosomal proteins at different stages of human glioma. *BMC Cancer,* Vol.10, (June 2010); pp. 268, ISSN 1471-2407

Margetts, J.C. & Kalyan-Raman, U.P. (1989). Giant-celled glioblastoma of brain. A clinico-pathological and radiological study of ten cases (including immunohistochemistry and ultrastructure). *Cancer*, Vol.63, No.3, (Feb 1989), pp. 524-31

Margison, G.P. & Kleihues, P. (1975). Chemical carcinogenesis in the nervous system. Preferential accumulation of O6-methylguanine in rat brain deoxyribonucleic acid during repetitive administration of N-methyl-N-nitrosourea. *Biochem J.*, Vol.148, No.3, (June 1975), pp. 521-5, ISSN 0264-6021

McLendon, R.E. & Rich, J.N. (2010). Glioblastoma Stem Cells: A Neuropathologist's View. *J Oncol.*, Vol.2011, (2011), pp. 397195, ISSN 1687-8450

Meyer-Puttlitz, B.; Hayashi, Y., Waha, A., Rollbrocker, B., Boström, J., Wiestler, O.D., Louis, D.N., Reifenberger, G., von Deimling, A. (1997). Molecular genetic analysis of giant cell glioblastomas. *Am J Pathol.*, Vol.151, No.3, (September 1997), pp. 853–857, ISSN 0002-9440

Miller, C.R. & Perry, A. (2007). Glioblastoma. Morphologic and Molecular Genetic Diversity. *Arch Pathol Lab Med.*, Vol.131, No.3, (March 2007), pp. 397-406, ISSN 0003-9985

Misra, A.; Chattopadhyay, P., Dinda, A.K., Sarkar, C., Mahapatra, A.K., Hasnain, S.E. & Sinha, S. (2000). Extensive intra-tumor heterogeneity in primary human glial tumors as a result of locus non-specific genomic alterations. *J Neurooncol.* Vol.48, No.1, (May 2000), pp. 1-12, ISSN 0167-594X

Misra, A.; Pellarin, M., Nigro, J., Smirnov, I., Moore, D., Lamborn, K.R., Pinkel, D., Albertson, D.G. & Feuerstein, B.G. (2005). Array comparative genomic hybridization identifies genetic subgroups in grade 4 human astrocytoma. *Clin Cancer Res.*, Vol.11, No.8, (April 2005), pp. 2907-18, ISSN 1078-0432

Mizuno, H.; Spike B.T., Wahl, G.M. & Levine, A.J. (2010). Inactivation of p53 in breast cancers correlates with stem cell transcriptional signatures. *Proc Natl Acad Sci U S A*, Vol.107, No.52, (December 2010), pp. 22745-50, ISSN 0027-8424

Murat, A.; Migliavacca, E., Gorlia, T., Lambiv, W.L., Shay, T., Hamou, M.F., de Tribolet, N., Regli, L., Wick, W., Kouwenhoven, M.C., Hainfellner, J.A., Heppner, F.L., Dietrich, P.Y., Zimmer, Y., Cairncross, J.G., Janzer, R.C., Domany, E., Delorenzi, M., Stupp, R. & Hegi, M.E. (2008). Stem cell-related "self-renewal" signature and high epidermal growth factor receptor expression associated with resistance to concomitant chemoradiotherapy in glioblastoma. *J Clin Oncol.*, Vol.26, No.18, (June 2008), pp. 3015-24, ISSN 0732-183X

Nakamura, M.; Watanabe, T., Yonekawa, Y., Kleihues, P. & Ohgaki, H. (2001). Promoter methylation of the DNA repair gene MGMT in astrocytomas is frequently associated with G:C --> A:T mutations of the TP53 tumor suppressor gene. *Carcinogenesis*, Vol.22, No.10, (October 2001), pp. 1715-9, ISSN 0143-3334

Nobusawa, S.; Lachuer, J., Wierinckx, A., Kim, Y.H., Huang, J., Legras, C., Kleihues, P. & Ohgaki, H. (2010). Intratumoral patterns of genomic imbalance in glioblastomas. *Brain Pathol.*, Vol.20, No.5, (September 2010), pp. 936-44, ISSN 1015-6305

Noushmehr, H.; Weisenberger, D.J., Diefes, K., Phillips, H.S., Pujara, K., Berman, B.P., Pan, F., Pelloski, C.E., Sulman, E.P., Bhat, K.P., Verhaak, R.G., Hoadley, K.A., Hayes, D.N., Perou, C.M., Schmidt, H.K., Ding, L., Wilson, R.K., Van Den Berg, D., Shen, H., Bengtsson, H., Neuvial, P., Cope, L.M., Buckley, J., Herman, J.G., Baylin, S.B., Laird, P.W. & Aldape, K. (2010). Cancer Genome Atlas Research Network.

Identification of a CpG island methylator phenotype that defines a distinct subgroup of glioma. *Cancer Cell,* Vol.17, No.5, (May 2010), pp. 510-22, ISSN 1535-6108

Ohgaki, H., Dessen, P., Jourde, B., Horstmann, S., Nishikawa, T., Di Patre, P.L., Burkhard, C., Schüler, D., Probst-Hensch, N.M., Maiorka, P.C., Baeza, N., Pisani, P., Yonekawa, Y., Yasargil, M.G., Lütolf, U.M. & Kleihues, P. (2004). Genetic pathways to glioblastoma: a population-based study. *Cancer Res.,* Vol.64, No.19, (October 2004), pp. 6892-9, ISSN 0008-5472

Pallini, R.; Ricci-Vitiani, L., Montano, N., Mollinari, C., Biffoni, M., Cenci, T., Pierconti, F., Martini, M., De Maria, R. & Larocca, L.M. (2010). Expression of the stem cell marker CD133 in recurrent glioblastoma and its value for prognosis. *Cancer,* Vol.117, No.1, (January 2011), pp. 162-74

Panosyan, E.H.; Laks, D.R., Masterman-Smith, M., Mottahedeh, J., Yong, W.H., Cloughesy, T.F., Lazareff, J.A., Mischel, P.S., Moore, T.B. & Kornblum, H.I. (2010). Clinical outcome in pediatric glial and embryonal brain tumors correlates with in vitro multi-passageable neurosphere formation. *Pediatr Blood Cancer,* Vol.55, No.4, (October 2010), pp. 644-51, ISSN 1545-5009

Parsons, D.W., Jones, S., Zhang, X., Lin, J.C., Leary, R.J., Angenendt, P., Mankoo, P., Carter, H., Siu, I.M., Gallia, G.L., Olivi, A., McLendon, R., Rasheed, B.A., Keir, S., Nikolskaya, T., Nikolsky, Y., Busam, D.A., Tekleab, H., Diaz, L.A.Jr., Hartigan, J., Smith, D.R., Strausberg, R.L., Marie, S.K., Shinjo, S.M., Yan, H., Riggins, G.J., Bigner, D.D., Karchin, R., Papadopoulos, N., Parmigiani, G., Vogelstein, B., Velculescu, V.E. & Kinzler, K.W. (2008). An integrated genomic analysis of human glioblastoma multiforme. *Science,* Vol.321, No.5897, (September 2008), pp. 1807-12, ISSN 0036-8075

Paulus, W.; Bayas, A., Ott, G. & Roggendorf, W. (1994). Interphase cytogenetics of glioblastoma and gliosarcoma. *Acta Neuropathol (Berl),* Vol.88, No.5, (1994), pp. 420–425, ISSN 0001-6322

Peraud, A.; Watanabe, K., Plate, K.H., Yonekawa, Y., Kleihues, P. & Ohgaki, H. (1997). p53 mutations versus EGF receptor expression in giant cell glioblastomas. *J Neuropathol Exp Neurol.,* Vol.56, No.11, (November 1997), pp. 1236-41, ISSN 0022-3069

Peraud, A.; Watanabe, K., Schwechheimer, K., Yonekawa, Y., Kleihues, P. & Ohgaki, H. (1999). Genetic profile of the giant cell glioblastoma. *Lab Invest,* Vol.79, No.2, (February 1999), pp. 123–129, ISSN 0023-6837

Perry, A.; Aldape, K.D., George, D.H. & Burger, P.C. (2004). Small cell astrocytoma: an aggressive variant that is clinicopathologically and genetically distinct from anaplastic oligodendroglioma. *Cancer,* Vol.101, No.10, (November 2004), pp. 2318-26

Peterson, S.E., Westra, J.W., Paczkowski, C.M. & Chun, J. (2008). Chromosomal mosaicism in neural stem cells. *Methods Mol Biol.* Vol.438, (2008), pp. 197-204, ISSN 1064-3745

Phi, J.H.; Park, S.H., Chung, C.K., Wang, K.C., Cho, B.K. & Kim, S.K. (2009). Atypical cell clusters expressing both neuronal and oligodendrocytic markers: novel histological pattern of glioneuronal tumors? *Pathol Int.,* Vol.59, No.10, (October 2009), pp. 735-43, ISSN 1320-5463

Phillips, H.S.; Kharbanda, S., Chen, R., Forrest, W.F., Soriano, R.H., Wu, T.D., Misra, A., Nigro, J.M., Colman, H., Soroceanu, L., Williams, P.M., Modrusan, Z., Feuerstein, B.G. & Aldape, K. (2006). Molecular subclasses of high-grade glioma predict prognosis, delineate a pattern of disease progression, and resemble stages in neurogenesis. *Cancer Cell,* Vol.9, No.3, (March 2006), pp. 157-73, ISSN 1535-6108

Pope, W.B.; Xia, Q., Paton, V.E., Das, A., Hambleton, J., Kim, H.J., Huo, J., Brown, M.S., Goldin, J. & Cloughesy, T. (2011). Patterns of progression in patients with recurrent glioblastoma treated with bevacizumab. *Neurology,* Vol.76, No.5, (February 2011), pp. 432-7, ISSN 028-3878

Preusser, M.; Charles, J.R., Felsberg, J., Reifenberger, G., Hamou, M.F., Diserens, A.C., Stupp, R., Gorlia, T., Marosi, C., Heinzl, H., Hainfellner, J.A. & Hegi, M. (2008). Anti-O6-methylguanine-methyltransferase (MGMT) immunohistochemistry in glioblastoma multiforme: observer variability and lack of association with patient survival impede its use as clinical biomarker. *Brain Pathol.,* Vo.18, No.4, (October 2008), pp. 520–532, ISSN 1015-6305

Qian, X.C. & Brent, T.P. (1997). Methylation hot spots in the 5' flanking region denote silencing of the O6-methylguanine-DNA methyltransferase gene. *Cancer Res.,* Vol.57, No.17, (September 1997), pp. 3672-7, ISSN 0008-5472

Reardon, D.A.; Fink, K.L., Mikkelsen, T., Cloughesy, T.F., O'Neill, A., Plotkin, S., Glantz, M., Ravin, P., Raizer, J.J., Rich, K.M., Schiff, D., Shapiro, W.R., Burdette-Radoux, S., Dropcho, E.J., Wittemer, S.M., Nippgen, J., Picard, M. & Nabors, L.B. (2008). Randomized phase II study of cilengitide, an integrin-targeting arginine-glycine-aspartic acid peptide, in recurrent glioblastoma multiforme. *J Clin Oncol.,* Vol.26, No.34, (December 2008), pp. 5610-7, ISSN 0732-183X

Reis, R.M.; Konu-Lebleblicioglu, D., Lopes, J.M., Kleihues, P. & Ohgaki, H. (2000). Genetic profile of gliosarcomas. *Am J Pathol.,* Vol.156, (2000), pp. 425–432

Ricci-Vitiani, L.; Pallini, R., Biffoni, M., Todaro, M., Invernici, G., Cenci, T., Maira, G., Parati, E.A., Stassi, G., Larocca, L.M. & De Maria, R. (2010). Tumour vascularization via endothelial differentiation of glioblastoma stem-like cells. *Nature,* Vol.468, No.7325, (December 2010), pp. 824-8, ISSN 0028-0836

Sanai, N.; Alvarez-Buylla, A. & Berger, M.S. (2005). Neural stem cells and the origin of gliomas. *N Engl J Med.,* Vol.353, No.8, (August 2005), pp. 811-22, ISSN 0028-4793

Shen, W.H.; Balajee, A,S., Wang, J., Wu, H., Eng, C., Pandolfi, P.P., Yin, Y (2007) Essential role for nuclear PTEN in maintaining chromosomal integrity. Cell. Vol.128, No.1, (January 2007), pp. 157-70, ISSN:0092-8674

Shen, Q.; Wang, Y., Kokovay, E., Lin, G., Chuang, SM., Goderie, S.K., Roysam, B. & Temple, S. (2008). Adult SVZ stem cells lie in a vascular niche: a quantitative analysis of niche cell-cell interactions. *Cell Stem Cell,* Vol.3, No.3, (September 2008), pp. 289-300, ISSN 1934-5909

Shinojima, N.; Kochi, M., Hamada, J., Nakamura, H., Yano, S., Makino, K., Tsuiki, H., Tada, K., Kuratsu, J., Ishimaru, Y. & Ushio, Y. (2004). The influence of sex and the presence of giant cells on postoperative long-term survival in adult patients with supratentorial glioblastoma multiforme. *J Neurosurg.,* Vol.101, (2004), pp. 219–226

Silkworth, W.T.; Nardi, I.K., Scholl, L.M. & Cimini, D. (2009). Multipolar spindle pole coalescence is a major source of kinetochore mis-attachment and chromosome mis-segregation in cancer cells. *PLoS One*, Vol.4, No.8, (August 2009), pp. e6564, ISSN 1932-6203

Singh, S.K.; Clarke, I.D., Terasaki, M., Bonn, V.E., Hawkins, C., Squire, J. & Dirks, P.B. (2003). Identification of a cancer stem cell in human brain tumors. *Cancer Res.*, Vol.63, No.18, (September 2003), pp. 5821-8, ISSN 0099-7013

Spiegl-Kreinecker, S.; Pirker, C., Filipits, M., Lötsch, D., Buchroithner, J., Pichler, J., Silye, R., Weis, S., Micksche, M., Fischer, J. & Berger, W. (2009). O6-Methylguanine DNA methyltransferase protein expression in tumor cells predicts outcome of temozolomide therapy in glioblastoma patients. *Neuro Oncol.,* Vol.12, No.1, (January 2010), pp. 28-36, ISSN 1522-8517

Stanbridge, E.J.; Flandermeyer, R.R., Daniels, D.W. & Nelson-Rees, W.A. (1981). Specific chromosome loss associated with the expression of tumorigenicity in human cell hybrids. *Somatic Cell Genet.,* Vol.7, No.6, (November 1981), pp. 699-712, ISSN 0098-0366

Stoler, D.L.; Chen, N., Basik, M., Kahlenberg, M.S., Rodriguez-Bigas, M.A., Petrelli, N.J. & Anderson, G.R. (1999). The onset and extent of genomic instability in sporadic colorectal tumor progression. *Proc Natl Acad Sci U S A,* Vol.96, No.26, (December 1999), pp. 15121-6, ISSN 0027-8424

Stupp, R.; Mason, W.P., van den Bent, M.J., Weller, M., Fisher, B., Taphoorn, M.J., Belanger, K., Brandes, A.A., Marosi, C., Bogdahn, U., Curschmann, J., Janzer, R.C., Ludwin, S.K., Gorlia, T., Allgeier, A., Lacombe, D., Cairncross, J.G., Eisenhauer, E. & Mirimanoff, R.O. (2005). Radiotherapy plus concomitant and adjuvant temozolomide for glioblastoma. *N Engl J Med,* Vol. 352, No.10, (March 2005), pp. 987–996, ISSN 0028-4793

Stupp, R.; Hegi, M.E., Mason, W.P., van den Bent, M.J., Taphoorn, M.J., Janzer R.C., Ludwin, S.K., Allgeier, A., Fisher, B., Belanger, K., Hau, P., Brandes, A.A., Gijtenbeek, J., Marosi, C., Vecht, C.J., Mokhtari, K., Wesseling, P., Villa, S., Eisenhauer, E., Gorlia, T., Weller, M., Lacombe, D., Cairncross, J.G., Mirimanoff, R.O., European Organisation for Research and Treatment of Cancer Brain Tumour and Radiation Oncology Groups & National Cancer Institute of Canada Clinical Trials Group. (2009). Effects of radiotherapy with concomitant and adjuvant temozolomide versus radiotherapy alone on survival in glioblastoma in a randomised phase III study: 5-year analysis of the EORTC-NCIC trial. *Lancet Oncol.*, Vol.10, No.5, (May 2009), pp. 459-66, ISSN 1470-2045

Sudakin, V. & Yen, T.J. (2007). Targeting mitosis for anti-cancer therapy. *BioDrugs*, Vol.21, No.4, (2007), pp. 225-33, ISSN 1173-8804

Tang, K.; Jin, Q., Yan, W., Zhang, W., You, G., Liu, Y. & Jiang, T. (2011). Clinical correlation of MGMT protein expression and promoter methylation in Chinese glioblastoma patients. *Med Oncol.,* (Mar 2011), [Epub ahead of print], ISSN 1357-0560

Temme, A.; Geiger, K.D., Wiedemuth, R., Conseur, K., Pietsch, T., Felsberg, J., Reifenberger, G., Tatsuka, M., Hagel, C., Westphal, M., Berger, H., Simon, M., Weller, M. & Schackert, G. (2010). Giant cell glioblastoma is associated with altered aurora b expression and concomitant p53 mutation. *J Neuropathol Exp Neurol.,* Vol.69, No.6, (June 2010), pp. 632-42, ISSN 0022-3069

Thon, N.; Damianoff, K., Hegermann, J., Grau, S., Krebs, B., Schnell, O., Tonn, J.C. & Goldbrunner, R. (2008). Presence of pluripotent CD133+ cells correlates with malignancy of gliomas. *Mol Cell Neurosci.,* Vol.43, No.1, (January 2010), pp. 51-9, ISSN 1044-7431

Tyzzer, E.E. (1916). Tumor immunity. *J Cancer Res.,* Vol.1, (1916), pp. 125-155

Verhaak, R.G.; Hoadley, K.A., Purdom, E., Wang, V., Qi, Y., Wilkerson, M.D., Miller, C.R., Ding, L., Golub, T., Mesirov, J.P., Alexe, G., Lawrence, M., O'Kelly, M., Tamayo, P., Weir, B.A., Gabriel, S., Winckler, W., Gupta, S., Jakkula, L., Feiler, H.S., Hodgson, J.G., James, C.D., Sarkaria, J.N., Brennan, C., Kahn, A., Spellman, P.T., Wilson, R.K., Speed, T.P., Gray, J.W., Meyerson, M., Getz, G., Perou, C.M., Hayes, D.N., Cancer Genome Atlas Research Network. (2010). Integrated genomic analysis identifies clinically relevant subtypes of glioblastoma characterized by abnormalities in PDGFRA, IDH1, EGFR, and NF1. *Cancer Cell,* Vol.17, No.1, (January 2010), pp. 98-110, ISSN 1535-6108

Wang, R.; Chadalavada, K., Wilshire, J., Kowalik, U., Hovinga, K.E., Geber, A., Fligelman, B., Leversha, M., Brennan, C. & Tabar, V. (2010). Glioblastoma stem-like cells give rise to tumour endothelium. *Nature,* Vol.468, No.7325, (December 2010), pp. 829-33, ISSN 0028-0836

Watanabe, K.; Tachibana, O., Sata, K., Yonekawa, Y., Kleihues, P. & Ohgaki, H. (1996). Overexpression of the EGF receptor and p53 mutations are mutually exclusive in the evolution of primary and secondary glioblastomas. *Brain Pathol.,* Vol.6, No.3, (July 1996), pp. 217-23, ISSN 1015-6305

Wick, W.; Hartmann, C., Engel, C., Stoffels, M., Felsberg, J., Stockhammer, F., Sabel, M.C., Koeppen, S., Ketter, R., Meyermann, R., Rapp, M., Meisner, C., Kortmann, R.D., Pietsch, T., Wiestler, O.D., Ernemann, U., Bamberg, M., Reifenberger, G., von Deimling, A. & Weller, M. (2009). NOA-04 randomized phase III trial of sequential radiochemotherapy of anaplastic glioma with procarbazine, lomustine, and vincristine or temozolomide. *J Clin Oncol,* Vol.27, No.35, (December 2009), pp. 5874-80, ISSN 0732-183X

Yachida, S.; Jones, S., Bozic, I., Antal, T., Leary, R., Fu, B., Kamiyama, M., Hruban, R.H., Eshleman, J.R., Nowak, M.A., Velculescu, V.E., Kinzler, K.W., Vogelstein, B. & Iacobuzio-Donahue, C.A. (2010). Distant metastasis occurs late during the genetic evolution of pancreatic cancer. *Nature,* Vol.467, No.7319, (October 2010), pp. 1114-7, ISSN 0028-0836

Yadav, A.K.; Renfrow, J.J., Scholtens, D.M., Xie, H., Duran, G.E., Bredel, C., Vogel, H., Chandler, J.P., Chakravarti, A., Robe, P.A., Das, S., Scheck, A.C., Kessler, J.A., Soares, M.B., Sikic, B.I., Harsh, G.R. & Bredel, M. (2009). Monosomy of chromosome 10 associated with dysregulation of epidermal growth factor signaling in glioblastomas. *JAMA,* Vol.302, No.3, (July 2009), pp. 276-89, ISSN 0098-7484

Yan, H.; Parsons, D.W., Jin, G., McLendon, R., Rasheed, B.A., Yuan, W., Kos, I., Batinic-Haberle, I., Jones, S., Riggins, G.J., Friedman, H., Friedman, A., Reardon, D., Herndon, J., Kinzler, K.W., Velculescu, V.E., Vogelstein, B. & Bigner, D.D. (2009). IDH1 and IDH2 mutations in gliomas. *N Engl J Med.,* Vol.360, No.8, (February 2009), pp. 765-73, ISSN 0028-4793

Yang, A.H.; Kaushal, D., Rehen, S.K., Kriedt, K., Kingsbury, M.A., McConnell, M.J. & Chun, J. (2003). Chromosome segregation defects contribute to aneuploidy in normal neural progenitor cells. *J Neurosci.*, Vol.23, No.32, (November 2003), pp. 10454-62, ISSN 0270-6474

Yin, Y & Shen, W.H. (2008). PTEN: a new guardian of the genome. Oncogene. Vol.27, No.41, (September 2008), pp. 5443-53, ISSN 0950-9232

Yip, S.; Miao, J., Cahill, D.P., Iafrate, A.J., Aldape, K., Nutt, C.L. & Louis, D.N. (2009). MSH6 mutations arise in glioblastomas during temozolomide therapy and mediate temozolomide resistance. *Clin Cancer Res.*, Vol.15, No.14, (July 2009), pp. 4622-9, ISSN 1078-0432

Yuan, X.; Curtin, J., Xiong, Y., Liu, G., Waschsmann-Hogiu, S., Farkas, D.L., Black, K.L. & Yu, J.S. (2004). Isolation of cancer stem cells from adult glioblastoma multiforme. *Oncogene*, Vol.23, No.58, (December 2004), pp. 9392-400, ISSN 0950-9232

Zeng, W.F.; Navaratne, K., Prayson, R.A. & Weil, R.J. (2007). Aurora B expression correlates with aggressive behaviour in glioblastoma multiforme. *J Clin Pathol.*, Vol.60, No.2, (February 2007), pp. 218-21, ISSN 0021-9746

Zeppernick, F.; Ahmadi, R., Campos, B., Dictus, C., Helmke, B.M., Becker, N., Lichter, P., Unterberg, A., Radlwimmer, B. & Herold-Mende, C.C. (2008). Stem cell marker CD133 affects clinical outcome in glioma patients. *Clin Cancer Res.*, Vol.14, No.1, (January 2008), pp. 123-9, ISSN 1078-0432

Zhai, H.; Heppner, F.L. & Tsirka, S.E. (2011). Microglia/macrophages promote glioma progression. *Glia*, Vol.59, No.3, (March 2011), pp. 472-85, ISSN 0894-1491

Zhang, M.; Song, T., Yang, L., Chen, R., Wu, L., Yang, Z. & Fang, J. (2008). Nestin and CD133: valuable stem cell-specific markers for determining clinical outcome of glioma patients. *J Exp Clin Cancer Res.*, Vol.27, (December 2008), pp. 85, ISSN 0392-9078

7

Role of the Centrosomal MARK4 Protein in Gliomagenesis

Ivana Magnani, Chiara Novielli and Lidia Larizza
Università degli Studi di Milano
Italy

1. Introduction

Human gliomas are the most frequent tumours of the central nervous system (Kleihues & Cavenee, 2000). They are of neuroectodermal origin and present as different histological types and malignancy grades (Louis et al., 2007).
According to the WHO (world health organization) system, astrocytoma, oligodendroglioma and mixed oligoastrocytoma are classified as differentiated gliomas, while anaplastic glioma and glioblastoma show increasing grades of malignancy (Box 1).

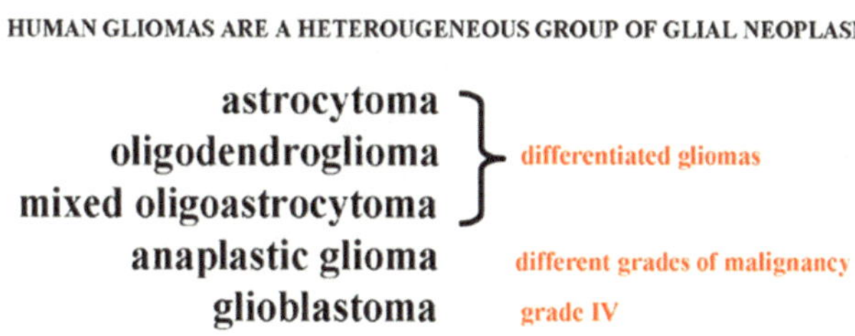

Box 1.

Gliomas are composed of different cell types displaying, even within low-grade tumours, a wide spectrum of heterogeneity regarding morphology, genotype, invasive potentiality, and treatment sensitivity (Noble & Dietrich, 2004). The development and progression of glioma malignancies is driven by accumulation of genomic alterations, including both mutations and chromosomal instability (CIN).

2. Chromosomal instability (CIN) in glioma

CIN refers to the rate of lost or gained chromosomes and/or structural chromosome anomalies and ploidy changes during cell divisions (Geigl et al., 2008; Lengauer et al., 1998). Structural chromosome anomalies (translocations, deletions, insertions, inversion and additions) may be balanced or unbalanced and involve one or more chromosomes (Bayani et al., 2007). Chromosomal instability in glioma is mainly characterized by aneuploidy (Bigner et al., 1988; Hecht et al., 1995; Jenkins et al., 1989; Lindstrom et al., 1991; Magnani et al., 1994; Park et al., 1995; Thiel et al., 1992) affecting in particular glioblastoma, the most malignant glioma. Gliomas frequently display near-diploid (2n+/-) and/or near-tri-tetraploid (3n+/-)/(4n+/-) karyotypes, implicating aberrant mitotic divisions, in addition to chromosomal rearrangements. Highly polyploid subpopulations and the presence of apoptotic nuclei are also reported (Figures 1a-d).

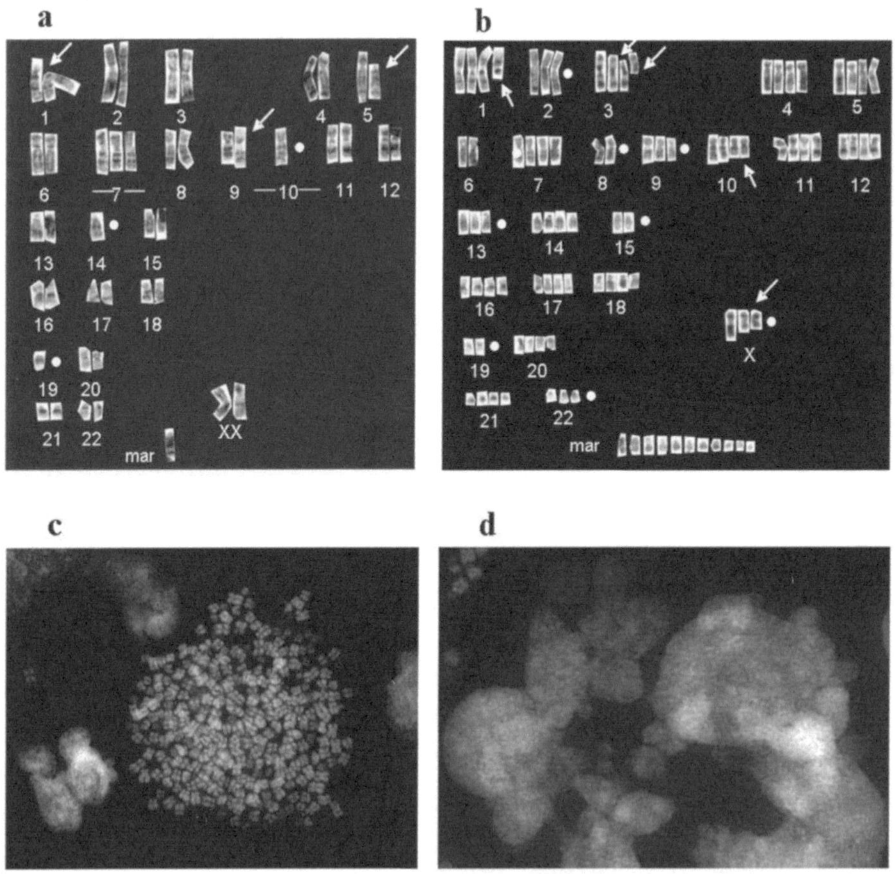

Fig. 1. (a) The G-banded, near diploid karyotype of MI-4 GBM (glioblastoma multiforme) cell line (Magnani et al., 1994), showing trisomy of chromosome 7, monosomy of chromosome 10 and a complex rearrangement involving chromosomes 1, 9 and 19. (b) The G-banded, near tetraploid karyotype of MI-4 cell line, displaying several chromosome losses and structural rearrangements including marker chromosomes. (c) Representative polyploid metaphase from MI-60 GBM cell line, characterized by a high frequency of hyperdiploid cells. (d) Apoptotic and large nuclei of MI-60 cell line.

Low-grade astrocytomas and oligodendrogliomas (WHO grades I-II) show a number of chromosome aberrations quite low. When present, they involve the gain of chromosome 7, the loss of chromosomes 10, 22 and one sex chromosome (see Figures 1a, b), while structural changes affect in particular 1p (Figure 2a) and 9p (Figure 2b) chromosome arms.

These chromosome abnormalities are qualitatively similar to those found in anaplastic astrocytoma (WHO grade III) and glioblastoma (WHO grade IV), but their frequency is increased in the latter and multiple chromosomal rearrangements are also present. The finding of common abnormalities associated to both low- and high-grade glioma has suggested a progressive chromosomal evolution during tumour growth (Bigner et al., 1988; Jenkins et al., 1989; Magnani et al., 1994; Thiel et al., 1992) even though it has been demonstrated that a subset of glioblastomas arises clonally *de novo*, further emphasizing the genetic heterogeneity of glioma (Kleihues & Ohgaki, 2000; von Deimling et al., 1993). Given that numerical CIN features many cancer cells, it has been hypothesized that it may have a primary role in tumorigenesis (Duesberg et al., 2006; Weaver et al., 2007). Recently it has been shown that the main pathway to aneuploidy in cancer cells is triggered by extra centrosomes that, increasing improper merotelic attachments of kinetochores to spindle microtubules, cause chromosome mis-segregation (Meraldi et al., 2002) (Figure 3) (see Box 3 for centrosomes and Box 4 for mitotic spindle).

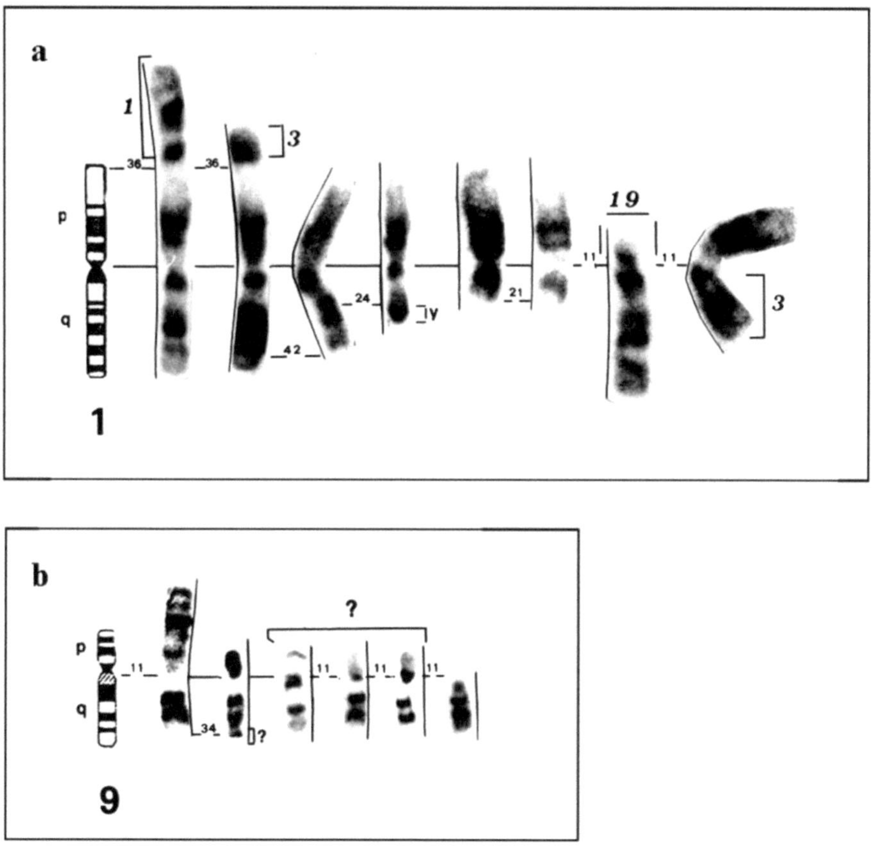

Fig. 2. (a) Chromosome 1 rearrangements of both p and q arms observed in different glioma cell lines by G-banding. (b) Rearrangements of chromosome 9p, sharing the loss of p21 band, observed in different glioblastoma cell lines by G-banding.

At early mitosis, the merotelic orientation escapes the spindle mitotic checkpoint thus representing the major mechanism of chromosome mis-segregation in non-cancer cells. Usually these errors are corrected before cells enter anaphase, to preserve genome stability (Cimini et al., 2004).

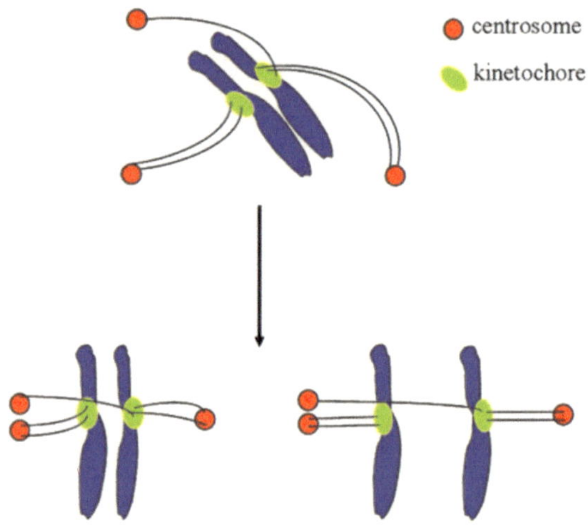

Fig. 3. Proposed events of lagging chromosomes in cancer cells with extra centrosomes through merotelic kinetochore orientation. (top) In the presence of extra centrosomes (three instead of two, as example), merotelic kinetochore orientation may occur: one kinetochore is bound by spindle microtubules from two centrosomes (right) instead of just one (left). (bottom) As cells move to mitosis and cluster extra centrosomes in a bipolar spindle, many attachment errors persist into anaphase, leading to lagging chromosomes.

3. Tetraploidy, centrosome amplification and spontaneous chromosomal instability in glioma

A relationship between extra centrosomes and the formation of multipolar spindles in cancer cells has been proposed by different authors (Basto et al., 2008; Cimini et al., 2004; Saunders, 2005; Sluder & Nordberg, 2004). Multipolarity in cancer cells is considered an essential transient stage prior to clustering extra centrosomes in a bipolar fashion (Brinkley, 2001). Multiple centrosomes have been detected in many types of cancer cells including glioma (Figure 4) and strongly linked to aneuploidy in a variety of studies (D'Assoro et al., 2002; Ganem et al., 2009; Ghadimi et al., 2000; Katsetos et al., 2006; Lingle et al., 2002; Magnani et al., 2009; Pihan et al., 1998).

A positive linear correlation between the percentage of cells with supernumerary centrosomes and the extent of aneuploidy within a panel of glioblastoma cell lines is shown in Figure 5.

In tumour development, aneuploidy is frequently preceded by tetraploidy, often with prolonged tetraploid precancerous status, a feature that makes it of central importance to cancer research (Margolis et al., 2003). It has been proposed that failure of cytokinesis is a key step in the formation of tetraploid karyotypes and in tumour initiation (Fujiwara et al., 2005). A tetraploid cell inherits twice the normal complement of centrosomes, a condition assessed to generate chromosomes mis-segregation in subsequent cell divisions (Ganem et al., 2007). However, tetraploid cells are observed in some normal tissues including liver and heart, indicating that cytokinesis is physiologically regulated. The possible fate of a tetraploid progeny is shown in Figure 6.

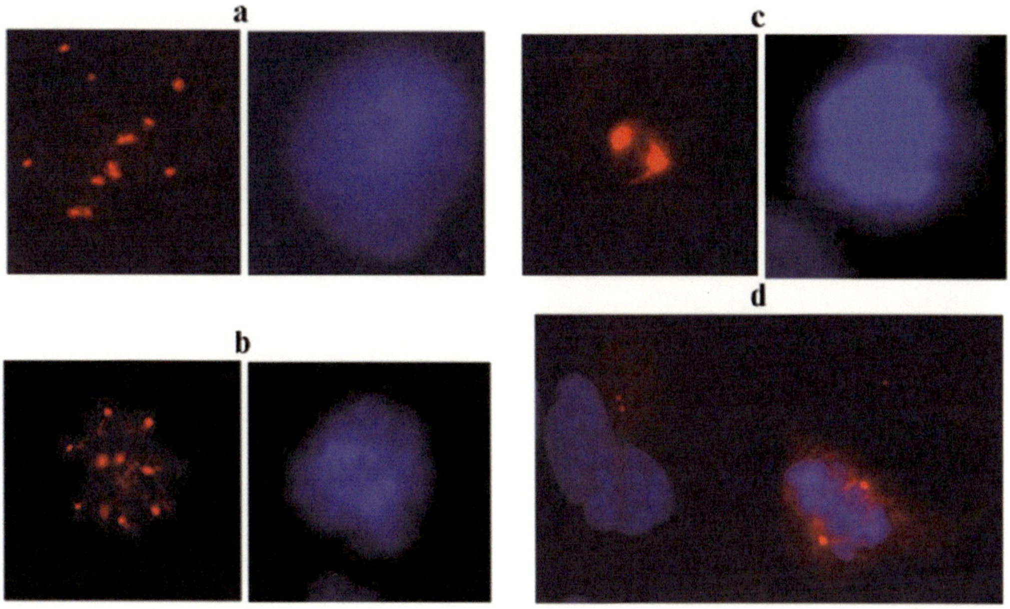

Fig. 4. Immunofluorescence with anti-γtubulin antibody (red) of representative glioblastoma cell lines, showing (a) multiple centrosomes; (b) multipolar spindles; (c) a mitotic bipolar spindle in which centrosomes are larger than the normal one (likely extra centrosomes clustered into two spindle poles), a condition that favours mitotic stability and neoplastic growth; (d) normal centrosomes and a mitotic bipolar spindle configuration. The nuclei are counterstained with DAPI (4',6-di amidino-2-phenyl indole) (blue).

Cell line	histology /grade	aneuploidies	centrosome abnormalities
MI62	OA I	0	0
G91	A II	0	15
G157	OA III	0	17
MI4	GBM IV	2	20
MI70	GBM IV	4	40
G32	GBM IV	8	40
G1	GC-GBM	7	40
MI38	GBM IV	5	50
MI60	GBM IV	4	50
MI7	GC-GBM	5	50
MI63	GBM IV	9	80
GBM	GBM IV	7	90

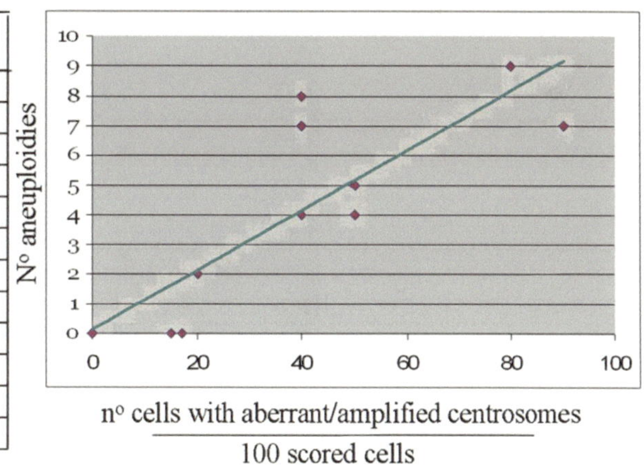

$y=0.1006x+0.1239$ $R^2=0.6805$ $r=0.82$ $P=0.001$

Fig. 5. Regression analysis between aneuploidies and centrosome aberrations in glioma cell lines, showing a statistically significant positive correlation. OA: oligoastrocytomas; A: astrocytomas; GBM: glioblastoma multiforme; GC-GBM: giant cell-GBM.

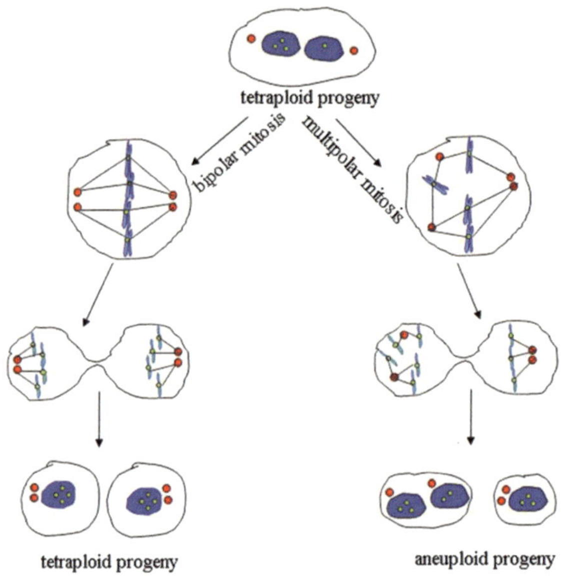

Fig. 6. Fate of a tetraploid cell: if extra centrosomes coalesce, a bipolar spindle assures the progeny maintains a tetraploid set, while lack of this *escamotage* gives rise to aneuploid progeny through a multipolar mitosis.

Binucleated tetraploid cells with multiple centrosomes are frequently observed in glioma cell lines, as illustrated by a representative image in Figure 7.

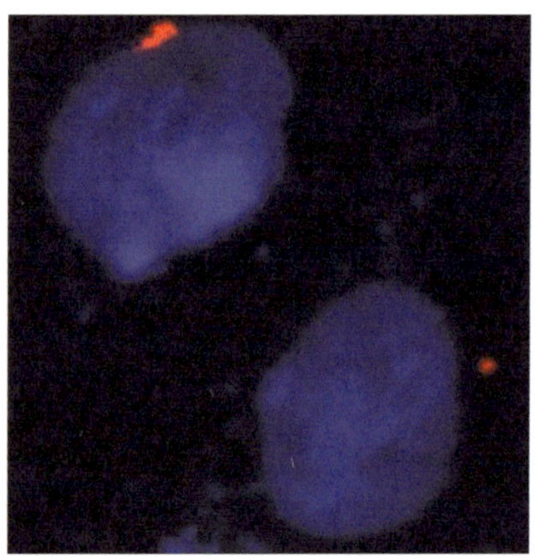

Fig. 7. Immunofluorescence with anti-γtubulin antibody (red) of a binucleated, tetraploid-derived glioblastoma cell line, showing coalesced centrosomes in one (left) of the two nuclei. Nuclei are counterstained with DAPI (blue).

To measure the occurrence of DNA damage in once-divided binucleated (BN) cells, the cytokinesis-block micronucleus cytome (CBMN Cyt) assay, an established biomarker to detect spontaneous genomic instability (Fenech, 2007), can be used. Application of CBMN Cyt to a series of glioma cell lines evidenced a high rate of micronuclei (MNi), a biomarker of chromosome breakage and/or whole chromosome loss, and chromosome aberrations such as nucleoplasmic bridges (NPBs), a biomarker of DNA misrepair and/or telomere end-fusions determining the furrow regression, and nuclear buds (NBUDSs), a biomarker of elimination of amplified DNA and/or DNA repair complexes (Figure 8a, b).

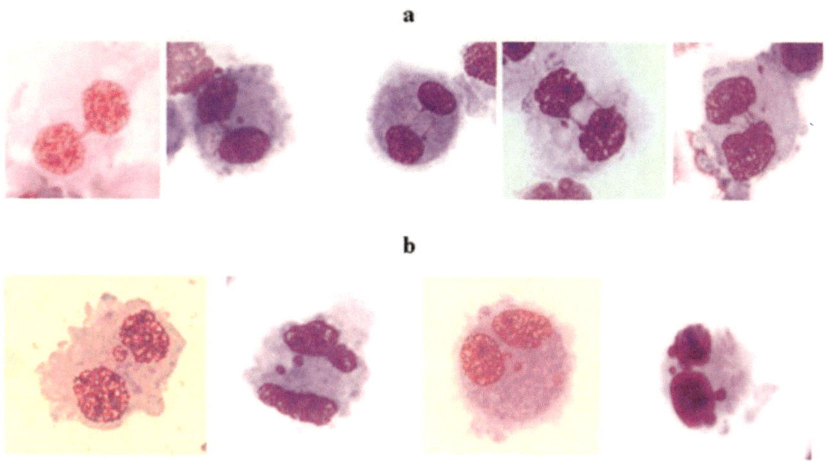

Fig. 8. Photomicrographs of glioma cell lines showing (a) typical binucleated cells with nucleoplasmic bridges and (b) binucleated cells with micronuclei and nuclear buds.

Thus, binucleated tetraploid cells may be transmitted to the progeny and enhance subsequent rounds of aberrant mitosis.

4. Cytogenomics of gliomas

Chromosomal instability can be detected by different techniques, including conventional karyotyping, fluorescence *in situ* hybridization (FISH), spectral karyotyping (SKY) and array-based comparative genomic hybridization (aCGH) analyses.
The classic assay to monitor and quantify chromosome aberrations is karyotyping (see Figure 2).
The *in situ* hybridization technique with fluorescently labelled probes targeting specific chromosomes is commonly applied on fixed glioma cells, allowing the analysis of chromosomes of interest cell by cell. Examples of FISH analysis in glioma cell lines are shown in Figure 9.
Aneuploidies are rapidly detectable by interphase FISH as well as by quantification of micronuclei formed by chromosomes that lagged behind during a previous mitosis (Figure 10).
The technique of array-CGH is considered the most powerful tool for identifying copy number changes of genetic material, since it combines high resolution and large scale genomic analysis, characteristics that are not combined by conventional approaches. Since it allows a quantification of amplifications and deletions, pointing through human genome databases directly to the affected genes, aCGH technology is more and more used in the study of tumours for the identification of potentially causative cancer genes.

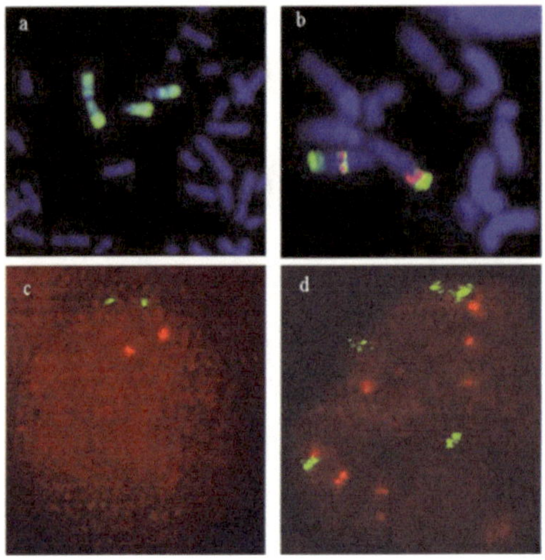

Fig. 9. Partial karyotype of MI-4 GBM cell line displaying chromosome 1 alterations by (a) whole chromosome 1 painting probe and (b) dual colour FISH of YACs 745h6, spanning the 1p36.3 breakpoint (green), and 957f12, mapping to 1p36.1 (red), showing a transposition of 1p36.1 material to der (1)(p22). DNA is counterstained with DAPI (blue). Interphase dual colour FISH of RP11-111p21, mapping to 3p21 control clone (red), and RP11-172g5, mapping to 3q26.3 (green), (c) in a normal diploid cell and (d) in MI-60 GBM cell line showing amplification of the region targeted by RP22-172g5 (green).

a

b

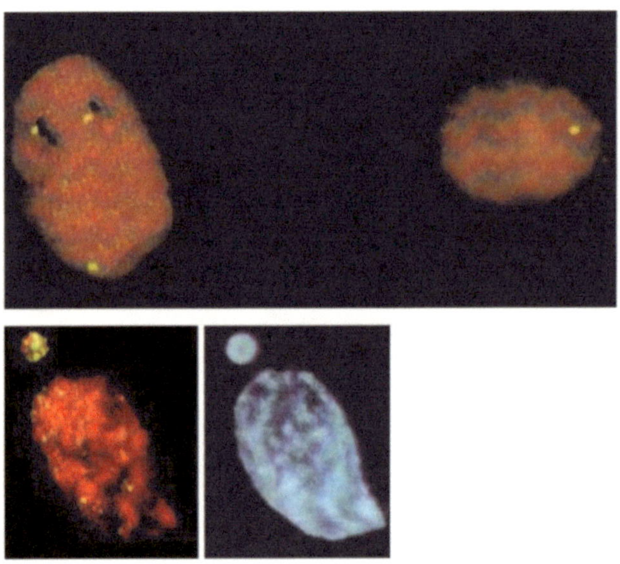

Fig. 10. (a) Interphase FISH with centromeric probes of chromosomes 7 and 10 showing trisomy of chromosome 7 and monosomy of chromosome 10 in MI-4 GBM cell line. (b) Interphase FISH with whole chromosome 19 painting probe showing a micronucleus labelled by chromosome 19 material. DNA is counterstained with DAPI (blue).

aCGH studies have been applied to gliomas and have successfully complemented previously published metaphase-CGH, SKY and LOH (loss of heterozigosity) analyses (Bredel et al, 2005; Cowell et al., 2004a, 2004b; Kitange et al., 2005; Nigro et al., 2005). Integration of the results has demonstrated an excellent correlation between the findings obtained through this genomic approach and those obtained by alternative techniques, stressing the usefulness and overall accuracy of aCGH as compared to classic previously widely employed analyses (Cowell et al., 2004a, 2004b). Comparative analysis of elaborated aCGH data led to identify copy number changes shared by various glioma grades as well as aberrations apparently related to progression to glioblastoma (GBM) (Roversi et al., 2006).

5. Non-random chromosomal aberrations in gliomas: The 19q13 abnormalities

Over the last decade, molecular approaches including mutation screening, LOH and aCGH analyses have led to identify the most frequently recurring genomic imbalances associated with each WHO glioma subtype (Kitange et al., 2005; Koschny et al., 2002; Shapiro, 2002) and hence the driver genes acting in pathways involved in glioma development, either in the initiation stages (Tp53 and Ras by PDGF-NF1) or in malignant progression (Rb-CDKN2-CDK4) (Collins, 2004; Zhu & Parada, 2002). Comprehensive genomic characterization by integrative analysis of DNA copy number, gene expression and DNA methylation aberrations in >200 glioblastomas has then refined the definition of human glioblastoma genes and core pathways (The Cancer Genome Atlas [TGCA] Research Network, 2008). Deletion of chromosome 19q is nevertheless of particular interest, as it is shared by all three glioma subtypes, occurring in approximately 75% of oligodendrogliomas, 45% of mixed oligoastrocytomas and 40% of astrocytomas (von Deimling et al., 1992, 1994), where it is associated with the transition from low-grade to anaplastic tumours (Ohgaki et al., 1995; Ritland et al., 1995; Smith et al., 1999) (Box 2).

The presence on chromosome 19 of TSGs relevant to glioma development has been inferred from LOH and cytogenetic studies

Molecular results (LOH studies)

Total loss of chromosome 19 is an unusual event in glial tumors, whereas partial genetic deletions at 19q13 are more frequently observed.

LOH on chromosome 19q13 is associated with astrocytomas, oligodendrogliomas and mixed gliomas

Cytogenetic results

Clustering of breakpoints at 19q13 is shared by all three histological types

No appreciable loss of genetic material from chromosome 19, even though microdeletions at the site of breakage cannot be ruled out

Box 2. TSGs: tumour suppressor genes.

At the cytogenetic level, chromosome 19q abnormalities are more frequently detectable in GBM than in low grade glioma, with 19q13 as the most affected region, as shown in Table1.

Case no.	Diagnosis	Partial Karyotypes
D-245	GBM	49,XY, . . . +19
D-250	GBM	47,XY, . . . +19
D-256	GBM	44,XY, . . . t(9;19)(p13;q13) ★
D-290	GBM	45,X,−X, . . . t(1;19)(q21;q13) ★
D-299	GBM	46,XY, . . . der(19)t(17,19)(q11;q13) ★
D-304	AMG	43,XY, . . . −19
D-316	GBM	46,XX, . . . der(19)t(10;19)(q11;q11)
D-340	GBM	66~77,XXYY, . . . −19,−19,der(11)t(11q19p)×2, der(11)t(11p19q),der(11)t(11;19)(cen;q13) ★
D-320	GBM	47,XX, . . . der(19)t(5;10;19)(q15–21;q11–26;q13) ★
nr	GBM	47,XX, . . . der(19)t(19; ?)(q13;?) ★
nr	GBM	79~83,Y, . . . −19,−19,der(19)t(19;?)(q13.3;?)×2 ★
37	PA	46, . . . der(19)t(19;?)(q13.1,?),der(19)t(19;?)(p13.3;?) ★
43	O	83~88,XXYY, . . . −19,der(19)t(19;?)(q13.3;?) ★
nr	GBM	39~45,der(X)t(X;?), . . . der(19)t(19;?)(p13;?)
39	GBM	43,X,−X, . . . tdic(19;22)(p13.3;q13) ★
33	GBM	43,XX, . . . +19
36	GBM	44,XY, . . . der(19)t(9;19)(q13;q13) ★
37	GBM	47~48,XY, . . . +19
40	AA	65~75,XY, . . . +19,+19
34	GBM	44,XX, . . . der(19)t(12;19)(q13;q13) ★
nr	GBM	82~90, . . . del(19)(q13.1) ★
5 MI	AA	80~86,XXXX, . . . +19
85 SJ	AA	48,XY, . . . +19
56 AW	GBM	47,XY, . . . +19
MI-4	GBM	47,XX, . . . der(1)t(1;19)(p10,q10)
MI-32	GBM	47,XX, . . . del(19)(q13.2) ★
MI-14	GBM	86~89,X,−X, . . . −19,−19
nr	O	45,XY, . . . der(1)t(1;19)(p11,q11)
T-60	GBM	45~46,XX, . . . −19,der(19)t(19;?)
3/T110	AO	44~46,XY, . . . −19
26/G227	GBM	44~45,X,−Y, . . . der(19)t(14;19)(q11.2;p13.1)
31/T35	GBM	41~45,XY, . . . der(19)t(14;19)(q13;q13.1) ★
36/T66	GBM	48~52,XY, . . . der(19)t(1;19)(q21;q13) ★
nr	PXA	46,XY, . . . t(1;11;19)(q24;q23;q13) ★
2	GBM	44,XX, . . . t(1;19)(q23;q13) ★
nr	GBM	. . . t(10;19)(q24;q13) ★

Table 1. Cytogenetic alterations of chromosome 19 in gliomas; 19q13 alterations are marked by red stars. GBM: glioblastoma multiforme; AMG: anaplastic mixed glioma; PA: pilocytic astrocytoma; O: oligodendroglioma; AA: anaplastic astrocytoma; AO: anaplastic oligodendroglioma; PXA: pleomorphic xanthoastrocytoma; nr: not reported.

Furthermore, similarly to oligodendroglioma, combined LOH of 1p and 19q was found to define a small subset of GBM patients with a significantly better survival, even if their tumours were not morphologically distinguishable from the bulk of GBMs (Schmidt et al., 2002). This finding has been translated into significant advance in the prognosis and treatment of oligodendrogliomas (van den Bent, 2004). A candidate tumour suppressor region has been assigned by LOH to 19q13.3 (Hartmann et al., 2002), but no positional or functional candidate gene in this band has yet been appointed.

Only recently an integrated analysis of human glioblastoma multiforme with the application of next generation sequencing technology disclosed a new marker associated with an increase in overall survival, represented by recurrent mutations in the active site of isocitrate dehydrogenase 1 (*IDH1*) in a large fraction of young patients with secondary GBM (Parsons et al., 2008).

6. Identification of *MARK4* gene through refined FISH mapping of 19q13 breakpoints

FISH studies of structural 19q chromosomal rearrangements in glioma (Magnani et al., 1999) and a detailed analysis of the breakpoints underlying the 19q13 alterations in the MI-4 glioblastoma cell line, led to identify a 19q13.2 intrachromosomal duplication of the MAP/microtubule affinity-regulating kinase *4 (MARK4)* gene (Beghini et al., 2003) (Figure 11). Genomic profiling by means of array-CGH interrogation of 25 primary glioma cell lines including the MI-4 GBM cell line (Roversi et al., 2006) revealed that the BAC clone encompassing *MARK4* at 19q13.2 (Figure 12) is included in a "gain" region in a few of the tested cell lines and confirmed *MARK4* duplication in the MI-4 glioblastoma cell line (Figure 13).

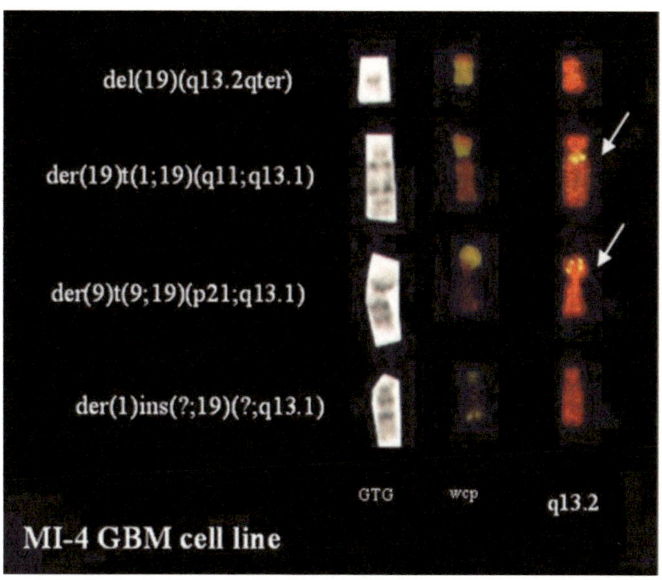

Fig. 11. 19q13.2 intrachromosomal duplication of *MARK4* in the MI-4 GBM cell line detected by G-banding and FISH analysis using a whole chromosome painting 19 probe and a *MARK4*-specific cosmid clone.

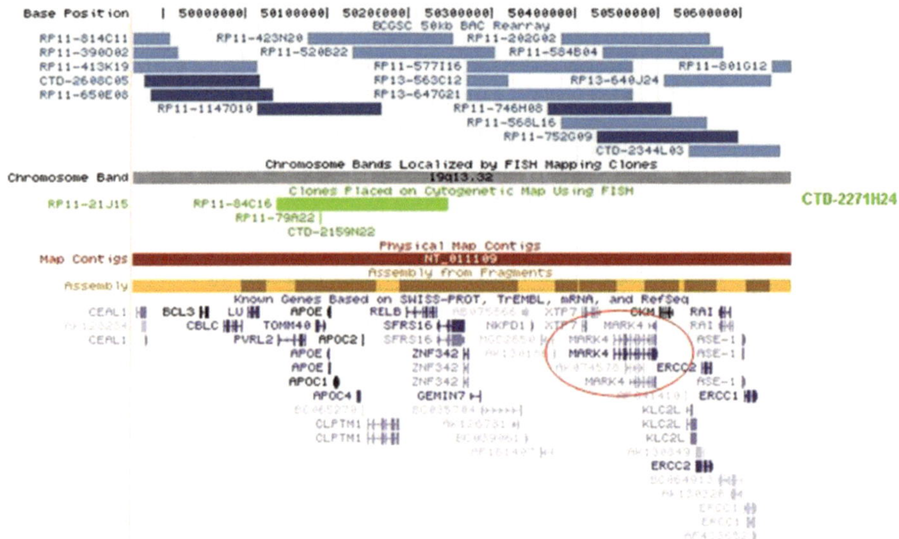

Fig. 12. *MARK4* genomic region (http://genome.ucsc.edu/). Clones of chromosome 19q full coverage (blue) overlapping *MARK4* gene are circled in red: the gene is entirely encompassed by BAC clones RP11-746H08, RP11-568L16, RP11-202G02, RP11-752G09 RP11-584B04, RP13-647G21 and partially encompassed by RP11-577I16.

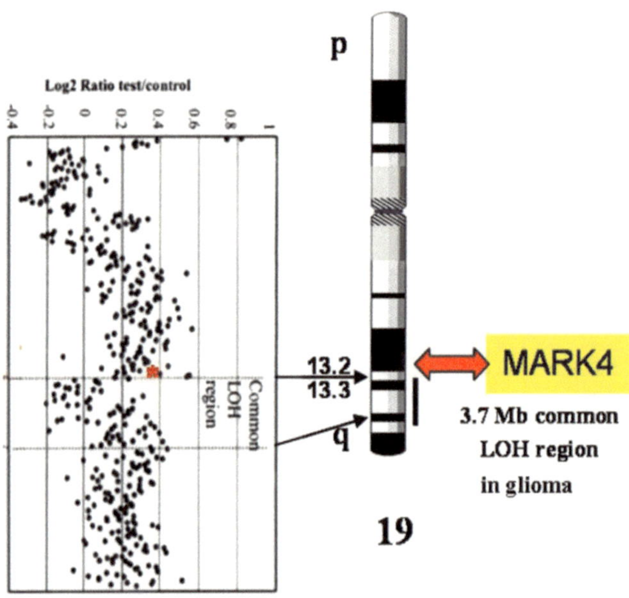

Fig. 13. (left) Chromosome 19q array-CGH of MI-4 GBM cell line, showing duplicated *MARK4* gene (red star) and the common LOH region in glioma. (right) Schematic representation of *MARK4* position on chromosome 19, at the boundary of 19q13.3 LOH region.

The combined FISH and array-CGH results provided the rationale for investigating a possible role of the serine-threonine kinase MARK4 in glioma. It's worth of note that this gene, belonging to the so called "kinome", maps at the centromeric boundary of the 19q13.3 LOH region in glioma.

7. The family of MARK kinases

MARK4 (MAP/microtubule affinity-regulating kinase 4) is a member of the MARKs family, constituted in mammals by four serine-threonine kinases (MARK1-4) which are able to phosphorylate the microtubule-associated proteins (MAPs, including Tau, MAP2, MAP4 and doublecortin) (Drewes et al., 1997). Microtubules (MTs) are cytoskeleton cylindrical structures formed by α and β tubulin dimers; dimers can quickly assemble or disassemble, causing the microtubules to grow or shorten and making them very dynamic. MAPs association stabilizes the MTs; when MARK kinases link a phosphate group to MAPs (phosphorylation), MAPs cannot associate to MTs any longer, thus microtubules become more instable and disassemble (Figure 14).

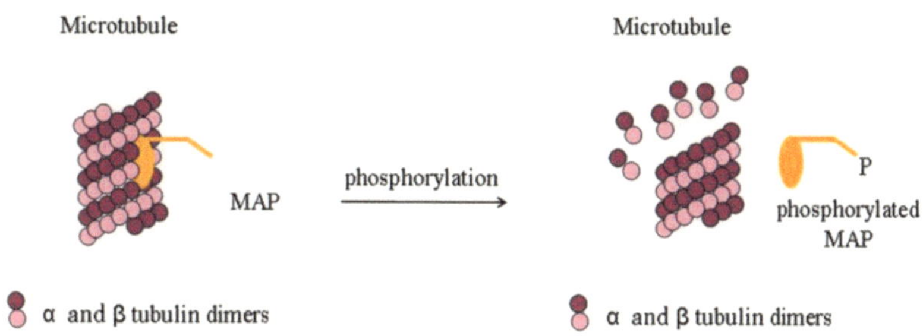

Fig. 14. Schematic representation of microtubules. Assembled α and β tubulin dimers form the microtubules, stabilized by MAP association. When MAPs are phosphorylated, they are no more able to bind microtubules, which disassemble.

7.1 MARKs protein structure

All MARK proteins have a very conserved structure, consisting of six sequence segments (Marx et al., 2010) (Figure 15):

- the N-terminal header, whose role is unknown;
- the catalytic or kinase domain, containing both the activation/inactivation loop (MARK kinases are in turn activated/inactivated by phosphorylation/dephosphorylation) and the catalytic loop, by which MARKs transfer a phosphate group to substrate proteins;
- a linker, that is a highly and negatively charged motif resembling the common docking (CD) site in MAP kinases; it may bind interactors;
- the UBA domain, a small globular domain with sequence homology to ubiquitin-associated proteins; it may exert an autoregulatory function through interaction with the catalytic domain;
- a spacer, the most variable region among MARK members; it is probably important for regulating MARK activity since it holds phosphorylation sites;
- the C-terminal tail, consisting of the kinase-associated (KA1) domain, whose function is still uncertain. It is characterized by a hydrophobic portion surrounded by positively

charged residues, which may interact with negatively charged regions of cytoskeletal proteins, MARK catalytic domain or MARK CD domain (Tochio et al., 2006) with an inhibitory effect. It has been proposed it could be involved in protein localization to the membrane, being identified as a domain that binds membrane anionic phospholipids, in particular phosphatidylserine (Moravcevic et al., 2010).

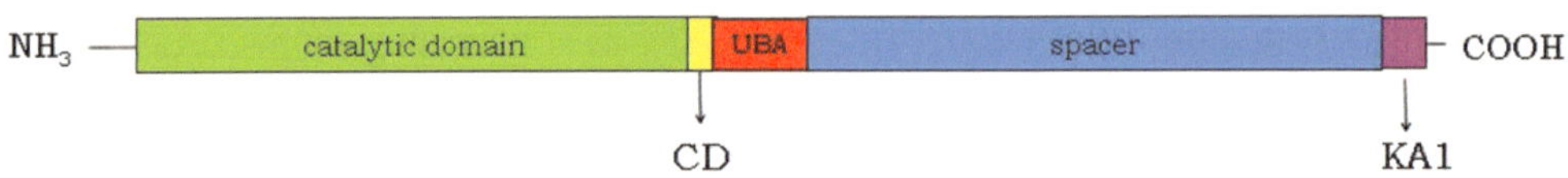

Fig. 15. Schematic representation of MARK protein structure. Boxes are not drawn to scale.

7.2 MARKs regulation

Being composed of several domains, MARK proteins are regulated by multiple mechanisms. All MARKs are activated by liver kinase B (LKB1) and MARK kinase (MARKK) by phosphorylation on the threonine residue in the activation loop (Timm et al., 2008); in addition, phosphorylation by CaMKI (calcium/calmodulin-dependent protein kinase I) activates MARK2 (Matenia & Mandelkow, 2009). On the contrary, phosphorylation by the glycogen synthase kinase 3β (GSK3β) on the serine residue in the activation loop, by aPKC (atypical protein kinase C) in the spacer region or by Pim1 kinase, down-regulates MARK activity (Matenia & Mandelkow, 2009; Timm et al., 2008). Finally, interaction between MARK catalytic domain and other proteins/MARK domains (such as 14-3-3 proteins, PAK5, MARK UBA and KA1 domains) inhibits MARK activity (Marx et al., 2010).

7.3 MARKs functions

Since MARK kinases regulate the affinity between MAPs and MTs, they are implicated in several cellular processes involving the microtubules, such as cytoskeleton dynamics, neuron motility (Schaar et al., 2004), and microtubule-dependent transport of proteins, vesicles and organelles (Mandelkow et al., 2004). Microtubules also play an important role in centrosome formation (Box 3) and in the correct distribution of the chromosomes in the two daughter cells during cell division (mitosis and cytokinesis; Box 4).

Tau is a microtubule-associated protein particularly expressed in the central nervous system. The aggregation of hyperphosphorylated *Tau* has been demonstrated to form insoluble neurofibrillary tangles (Chin et al., 2000; Gamblin et al., 2003) which are characteristic of Alzheimer's disease. MARKs role in this pathology has been evaluated in many studies, demonstrating, as an example, MARK co-localization with neurofibrillary tangles (Chin et al., 2000).

MARK2 is involved in establishing cell polarity, cooperating in the organization of the epithelial structure of liver, kidney and stomach (Cohen et al., 2004; Matenia & Mandelkow, 2009), and regulating axon formation in neuronal cells (Chen et al., 2006). Experiments in mice demonstrated that MARK2 is also implicated in many physiological functions, such as fertility, homeostasis of the immune system, memory, growth and metabolism (Bessone et al., 1999; Hurov et al., 2001; Hurov & Piwnica-Worms, 2007; Segu et al., 2008). MARK3 plays an important role in cell signaling and cell cycle control: phosphorylation of some proteins by MARK3 induces their binding to 14-3-3 proteins thus regulating many cellular pathways (Bachmann et al., 2004; Müller et al., 2001).

8. MARK4

MARK4 is the less characterized member among MARK proteins. It has been discovered by Kato and colleagues in 2001 among a few genes whose expression resulted significantly increased in hepatocarcinoma cells with elevated β-catenin levels in their nucleus (Kato et al., 2001).

MARK4 gene is located on chromosome 19q13.2, consists of 18 exons and encodes at least two isoforms, namely MARK4S and MARK4L, originated by alternative splicing (Kato et al., 2001) (Figure 16). mRNA splicing is a complex process consisting in the removal of introns, which are non-coding sequences, and in the joining of exons, the coding sequences, to generate the "edited" mRNA ready to be translated into a protein.

- MARK4S ("short") protein is the native isoform, consisting of all the 18 exons, and is 688 aminoacid-long with predicted molecular weight of 75.3 kilo Daltons (kDa);
- MARK4L protein derives from skipping of exon 16, which causes a shift of the reading frame[1] with a downstream stop codon, originating a longer protein (752 aminoacids; predicted molecular weight: 82.5 kDa).

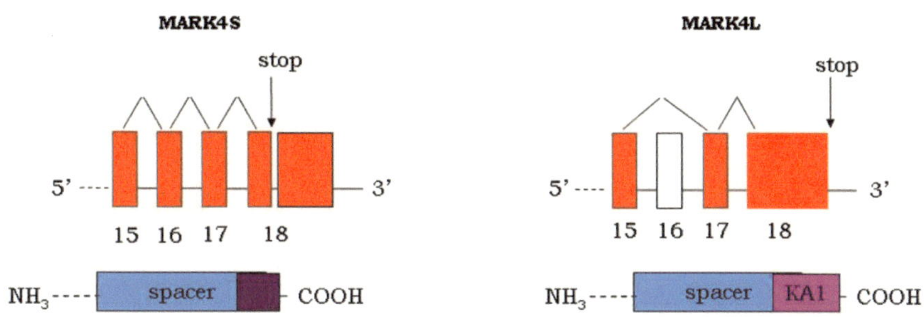

Fig. 16. Alternative splicing of exon 16 gives origin to MARK4 isoforms. When exon 16 is included in the mRNA, the stop codon is inside exon 18 and the encoded protein, MARK4S, lacks the KA1 domain at the C-terminal tail (left); when exon 16 is skipped, a shift of the reading frame occurs, changing the stop codon and generating a longer MARK4L protein, which has the classical KA1 domain (right).

Both MARK4L and S share the same protein structure of MARKs, with 90% sequence homology in the kinase domain. The two isoforms differ in the C-terminal tail, since MARK4L includes the kinase-associated 1 domain as the other MARK proteins, whereas MARK4S contains a domain with no homology to any known structure (Kato et al., 2001; Moroni et al., 2006) (Figure 16). Actually, MARK4 has less sequence homology in the C-terminus compared to the other MARKs; nevertheless MARK4L tail seems to fold in a similar shape, suggesting that the role of the C-terminal region may apply also to MARK4L (Marx et al., 2010).

[1] The mRNA sequence is "read" by an enzyme which matches a determinate "codon", made by three nucleotides, with its respective aminoacid. There are two particular codons, namely the start and the stop codon, which mark the beginning and the end of the protein.

8.1 MARK4 regulation

Phosphorylation by LKB1, in the activation loop, activates MARK4, while polyubiquitination of MARK4 inhibits the kinase activation (Al-Hakim et al., 2008). Furthermore, as MARK4 interacts with aPKC (Brajenovic et al., 2008), it could be phosphorylated and inactivated by this kinase as reported for MARK2 and MARK3.

8.2 MARK4 interactors and hypothetical functions

By tandem affinity purification and immunoprecipitation experiments, near twenty proteins have been identified as putative MARK4 interactors (Brajenovic et al., 2008). Among them, PKCλ and Cdc42 are implicated in cell polarity control and TGFβIAF (transforming growth factor β-inducing anti-apoptotic factor) is thought to be a hortologue of Miranda, a protein involved in the asymmetric division of neuroblasts in *Drosophila*. MARK4 interacts with the 14-3-3η isoform (Angrand et al., 2006; Brajenovic et al., 2008) of 14-3-3 proteins, which control multiple cellular processes by binding phosphorylated proteins and could directly regulate MARK4 or act as bridges among different pathways. Other MARK4 interactors are ARHGEF2, a cytoskeleton binding protein, and Phosphatase 2A, which is associated to microtubules and regulates *Tau* (Brajenovic et al., 2008). MARK4 protein has been also found to co-localize and co-precipitate in complex with α, β, and γ tubulin, myosin and actin (Brajenovic et al., 2008; Trinczek et al., 2004).

As the other MARK members, MARK4 phosphorylates MAPs, increasing microtubule dynamics; therefore, as also suggested by the interactions above reported, MARK4 may be involved in many processes involving microtubules, such as cytoskeleton dynamics.

9. Up-regulation of MARK4L in glioma

MARK4 gene is expressed ubiquitously in human tissues, with particularly elevated levels in brain and testis (Kato et al., 2001).

Few *MARK4* expression studies are reported in literature; they were performed with non-quantitative methods, such as northern blot (Kato et al., 2001; Schneider et al., 2004; Trinczek et al., 2004) and semi-quantitative competitive PCR (polymerase chain reaction) (Moroni et al., 2006), on different organisms (human, rat and mouse tissues) not always allowing to discern between the two MARK4 isoforms. MARK4 transcriptional variants are differentially regulated in human tissues, especially in the central nervous system: MARK4S is the predominant isoform in mouse and human brain, while MARK4L has been found highly expressed in neural progenitors and in gliomas (Beghini et al., 2003; Moroni et al., 2006).

By a semi-quantitative approach MARK4L has been found up-regulated in glioma tissue samples (fragments of glial tumours excised from patients) and glioma cell lines, of different malignancy grades, including the MI-4 GBM cell line carrying the *MARK4* duplicated gene as detected by FISH and aCGH analysis. MARK4L has been also found highly expressed in neural progenitors and down-regulated during their glial differentiation into astrocytes, suggesting that it might be necessary for proliferation, being thus highly enriched in proliferating or undifferentiated cells (Beghini et al., 2003) (Figure 17).

Protein kinase activation, often caused by gene amplification and/or mutation, is frequently associated to cancer initiation and progression, as most kinases are involved in cell proliferation. Although array-CGH analyses on glioma cell lines showed that the BAC clone encompassing *MARK4* at 19q13.2 is included in a "gain" region in a few of the tested cell lines, it did not evidence *MARK4* copy number variations, except for the MI-4 GBM cell line (Roversi et al., 2006). Only a few *MARK4* alterations are reported in the literature, namely two missense mutations (aminoacidic substitution) in exon 12 (R377Q and R418C in the spacer region), two silent mutations (no aminoacidic substitution) in exons 5 (Y137Y) and 9 (I286I) (kinase domain), while one intronic mutation (exon 8 +5 C>T; kinase domain) has been found in a few tumour samples (Greenman et al., 2007). In addition, only a splice-site mutation (exon 13 +1 G>A; spacer region) has been identified in one among 91 glioblastoma samples (TGCA Research Network, 2008). However, CpG methylation and/or promoter amplification have not yet been investigated. Based on this evidence, neither amplification nor mutations of *MARK4* gene seem to be the cause of its reported sustained expression in glioma samples.

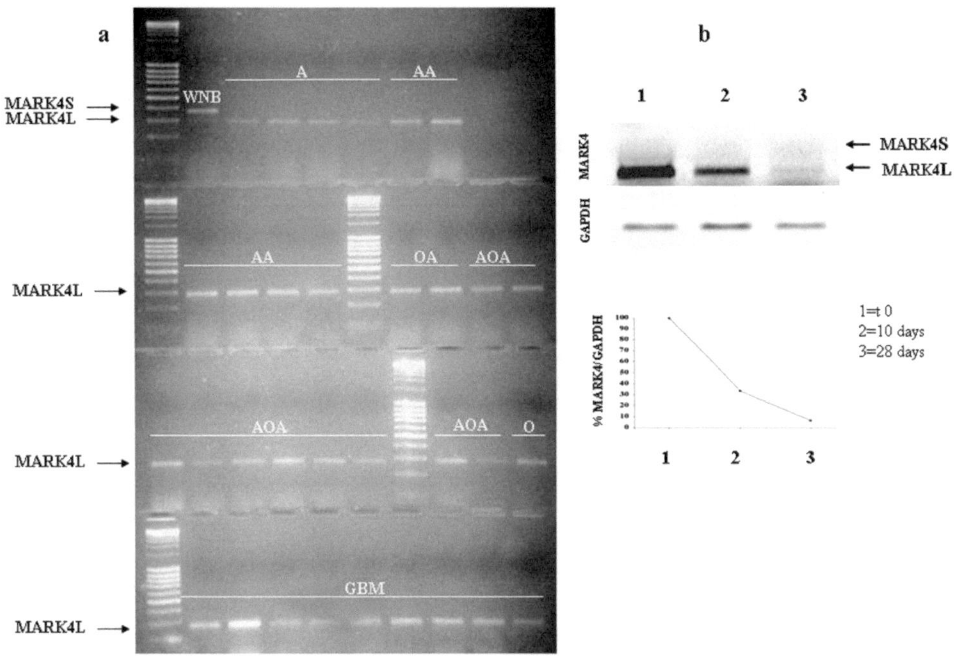

Fig. 17. (a) Semi-quantitative Reverse Transcription-PCR of MARK4S and MARK4L isoforms in whole normal brain (WNB) and in 32 glioma cell lines, subdivided according to WHO grade (A: astrocytoma; AA: anaplastic astrocytoma; OA: oligoastroctytoma; AOA: anaplastic oligoastrocytoma; O: oligodendroglioma; GBM: glioblastoma multiforme). (b) Downregulation of MARK4L expression during glial differentiation of human neural progenitors: semi-quantitative RT-PCR (top) and graph representation (bottom) of MARK4L expression in neural progenitors at times 0, 10 and 28 days of induced differentiation.

10. MARK4 sub-cellular localization in glioma cell lines

Recently, immunofluorescence analyses with a specific anti-MARK4L antibody highlighted multiple sub-cellular localizations for the endogenous MARK4L protein in glioma cell lines (Magnani et al., 2009).

10.1 Centrosome localization

It has been assessed that, under microtubule-stabilizing conditions, MARK4L localizes in the perinuclear region of glioma cell lines. By co-localization experiments with both anti-MARK4L and anti-γtubulin (the main centrosomal protein) antibodies, this perinuclear localization has been demonstrated to correspond to the centrosome (Magnani et al., 2009), as shown in Figure 18 (Box 3). This result confirms previous data referring to exogenous MARK4 protein conjugated to GFP (green fluorescent protein), which has been shown to co-localize with microtubules and centrosomes of CHO (Chinese hamster ovary) and neuroblastoma cell lines (Trinczek et al., 2004), in contrast to MARK1, MARK2 and MARK3 that exhibit uniform cytoplasmic localization. Furthermore, it has been demonstrated that the association with the centrosome is independent from microtubules, since it is not abolished when microtubules are depolimerized by nocodazole treatment (Magnani et al., 2009).

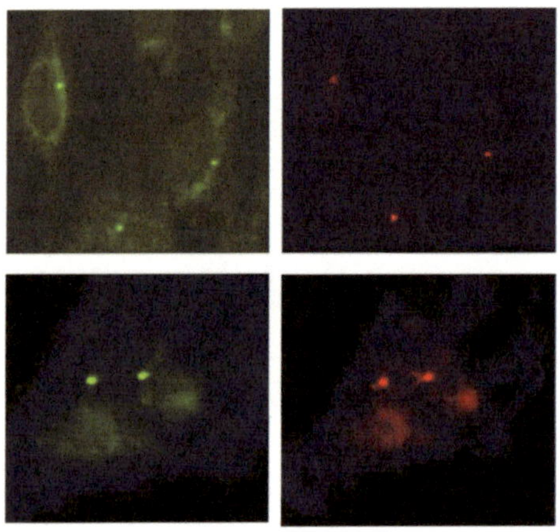

Fig. 18. Anti-MARK4L (green; left) and anti-γtubulin (red; right) antibodies showing co-localization signals in interphase (top) and mitotic (bottom) centrosomes of glioma cell lines.

The centrosome

The centrosome is a little organelle, not bound by membrane, positioned centrally in the cell near the nucleus. It is the primary MicroTubule Organizing Center (MTOC), as it can nucleate and organize microtubules. It consists of two distinct domains:

- the centriolar domain, including the centrioles, which are cylindrical organelles important for centrosome organization and replication. Each centriole consists of 9 triple microtubules;
- the pericentriolar domain, consisting of many fibers and proteins that surround the centriole. In this domain microtubules are nucleated, by associating α and β-tubulin dimers from a γ-tubulin ring (Doxsey, 2001).

The centrosome plays a key role in organizing the interphase cytoskeleton (regulating cell polarity, adhesion and motility) and the mitotic spindle (Kramer et al., 2002). It also contributes to cell cycle progression and cytokinesis (Martinez-Garay et al., 2006) and is involved in cell cycle transitions, in the cellular response to stress and signal transduction (Doxsey et al., 2005). The centrosomes duplicate only once in the cell cycle, during G1/S transition and in S phase, and form a strictly bipolar spindle during mitosis.

Box 3.

The endogenous MARK4L localizes both at normal interphase centrosomes (Figure 18) as well as at the aberrant centrosomes frequently observed in glioma cell lines (see Figure 4), suggesting a possible link between the alternatively spliced kinase and the mitotic instability frequently observed in human glioma. Two abnormal centrosome configurations are reported: a random one (multiple centrosomes randomly distributed) and a clustered one (multiple centrosomes collected in a single large aggregate) (Magnani et al., 2009), as depicted in Figure 19.

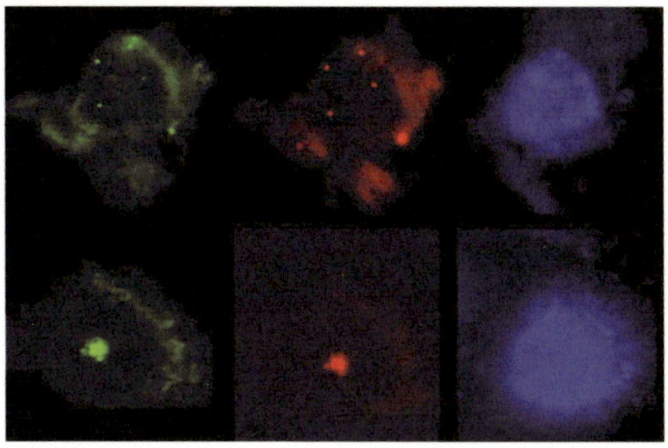

Fig. 19. Anti-MARK4L (green; left) and anti-γtubulin (red; middle) antibodies showing co-localization signals in abnormal centrosomes of glioma cell lines. Both the abnormal centrosome configurations are reported: the random one (top) and the clustered one (bottom). The nuclei are counterstained with DAPI (blue, right).

10.2 Midbody localization

The centrosome association is maintained during the entire course of mitosis, as MARK4L co-localizes with γtubulin in all the cell cycle phases. The anti-MARK4L antibody is also detected in the midbody, a microtubule structure forming at the contact point between the two daughter cells at the end of the cell division. These data demonstrate that the kinase is endogenously associated with the centrosomes during the whole cell cycle and concentrates thereafter into the midbody during cytokinesis (Magnani et al., 2009) (Figure 20) (Box 4).

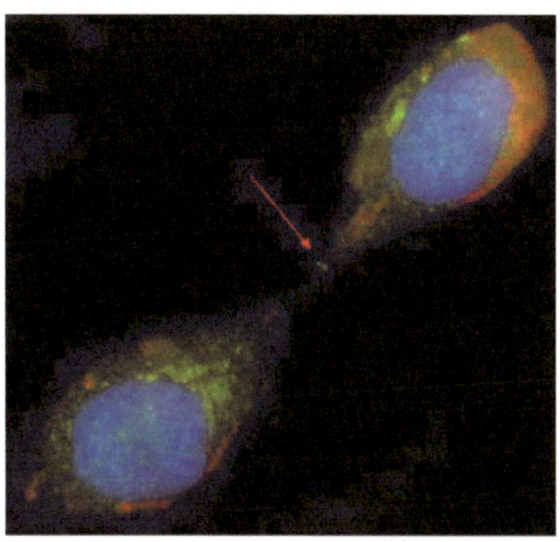

Fig. 20. Co-localization of MARK4L (green) and γtubulin (red) proteins at the midbody (arrow) during the cytokinesis of a glioma cell. The nuclei are counterstained with DAPI (blue).

Cell cycle, cytokinesis and midbody

The cell cycle corresponds to the life of a cell, beginning from its formation from a mother cell to its division into two daughter cells or to its death.
It consists of two main phases, interphase (subdivided in G1, S and G2 phases) and M phase (mitosis+cytokinesis). During interphase the cell grows and doubles its structures and DNA content; during the M phase the cell splits into two daughter cells.
In mitosis the two centrosomes move to opposite poles in the cell (asters) and organize the mitotic spindle, formed by bundles of microtubules getting off the centrosomes. The spindle binds chromosomes and segregate them toward one aster or the other, splitting the genetic material between the two poles.
During cytokinesis, the mitotic spindle locates the cleavage furrow, which will divide the cell, in a point which is equidistant from the two asters. In this furrow, a contractile ring of actin and myosin grows up and shrinks, causing the "stricture" of the cell, until the two opposing surfaces of the membrane come in contact and merge, closing and delimiting the two daughter cells (Bringmann, 2005).
Initially the two daughter cells are connected by a narrow intercellular bridge, whose core is the midbody, consisting of microtubules and a dense matrix (Mullins & McIntosh, 1982). The diameter of the intercellular bridge then decreases until it vanishes, making the two daughter cells effectively separated. The midbody is finally discarded and undergoes degradation (Mullins & Biesele, 1977).
The midbody is thought to have an important role in maintaining a bipolar spindle and in correctly separating the cytoplasm between the two daughter cells.

Box 4.

10.3 Nucleolar localization

Under standard immunofluorescence conditions, anti-MARK4L antibody is also detected in the nucleoli (Box 5).
Silver-colloid method, which allows visualizing the nucleolar organizing regions (NORs), and co-localization experiments with anti-nucleolin (a nucleolar protein) antibody allowed to assess that the nuclear structures bound by MARK4L antibody are indeed the nucleoli (Magnani et al., 2009) (Figure 21) (Box 5).

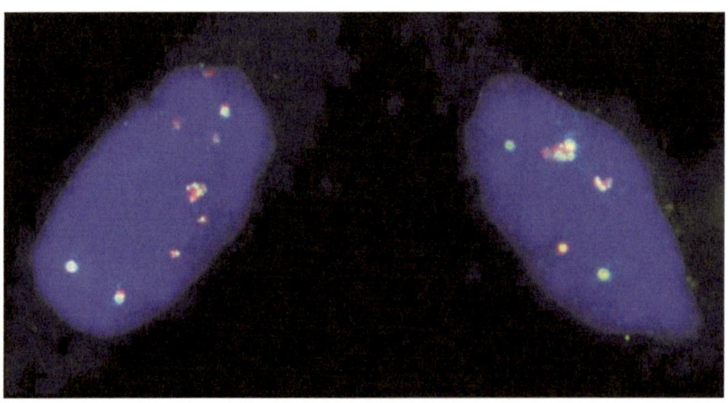

Fig. 21. Co-localization of MARK4L (green) and nucleolin (red) proteins in the nucleoli of glioma cells. The nuclei are counterstained with DAPI (blue).

The nucleolus

The nucleolus is a sub-nuclear organelle not surrounded by membranes and whose main function is ribosome biogenesis (ribosomes are involved in protein synthesis). It originates at the end of mitosis from the Nucleolus Organizing Regions (NORs), which are clusters of genes (rDNA), codifying for ribosomal RNA (rRNA), located on the acrocentric chromosomes.
The nucleolus consists of three main components, each with a different role in the formation of ribosomes, here defined starting from the inside of the nucleolus to outside:

- the fibrillar center, which is a NOR (rDNA);
- the dense fibrillar component, consisting of pre-rRNA;
- the granular component, whose granular appearance is conferred by the presence of ribosomal subunits.

The transcription of the rDNA leads to the formation of pre-rRNAs, which then undergo rearrangements and are assembled with ribosomal proteins to form the pre-ribosomes. The pre-ribosomal particles then move into the cytoplasm, passing through the nuclear pores (Carmo-Fonseca et al., 2000; Schwarzacher & Wachtler, 1983).
Besides this traditional ribosome biogenesis activity, the nucleolus is characterized by multiple functions, including the response to cellular stress, the regulation of cell cycle (Visintin & Amon, 2000) and cell growth (Zhang et al., 2010) and of post-translational modifications (phosphorylation and sumoylation) of proteins.

Box 5.

The overall immunofluorescence data on endogenous MARK4L protein confirm the previous evidence on its centrosome association and highlight two novel localization sites of MARK4L: the nucleolus and the midbody (Magnani et al., 2009).
Immunoblotting with anti-MARK4L antibody on centrosomes, midbody and nucleoli isolated by biochemical fractionation from glioblastoma cell lines confirmed the presence of MARK4L protein in each fraction, validated by antibodies specific for each cell structure: anti-γtubulin antibody for centrosomes, anti-βtubulin for the midbody (βtubulin, together with αtubulin, accounts for 30% of midbody proteins) and anti-nucleolin for the nucleolus (Magnani et al., 2009).
The localization pattern of MARK4L delineated by the above studies suggests that the kinase may take part in cell cycle progression and influence the microtubules, particularly those affecting the centrosome and midbody.
MARK4L association with the nucleolus in glial tumours is very interesting, since MARK4L could have a functional impact on this organelle, being requested for its building and maintenance like other protein kinases, as well as it could be spatially regulated by alternate translocation in and out the nucleolus. Many proteins are indeed sequestered in the nucleolus and then released according to a temporally regulated activity, since they must exert their function in certain phases of the cell cycle (Visintin & Amon, 2000). Last, the nucleolar localization of a protein may also influence its stability, protecting the protein from proteasomal degradation, since proteasomes are present in the nucleoplasm but not in nucleoli (Wojcik & DeMartino, 2003).

11. Conclusion

A few remarks can be drawn from the above synthesis on cytogenomics of human gliomas and the *MARK4* cell cycle gene as a likely "player" in gliomagenesis.

Gliomas are one of the most intractable tumours due to their "complex identity": as it has been beautifully underlined, the generation - since the earliest glioma stages - of multiple cell populations with different genotypic and phenotypic features makes unlikely to succeed therapeutic strategies targeting only clones with "dominant" or "average" characteristics of the cell population (Noble & Dietrich, 2004). The intrinsic genomic heterogeneity of human glioma has first been disclosed cytogenetically, as documented by a huge number of studies which across two decades have used the cytogenetic tools suitable to monitor the intratumour cell heterogeneity and to discern "recurrent" and potentially causative chromosomal rearrangements. A few of these rearrangements entered the diagnostic and prognostic flow chart of gliomas, others allowed to identify crucial genes which mutations or imbalance are the signature of a specific glioma type or glioma malignancy stage. In line with a research pathway that has been reiterated for several genes of relevance in cancer, focus on *MARK4* has been pinpointed by cytogenetics and deepened by multiple tools ranging from gene-targeted molecular to genomic and cytogenomic analyses. Despite its nature of serine-threonine kinase gene, *MARK4* has not be found mutated or affected by copy number alterations in glioma, while its encoded proteins represented by two different isoforms, MARK4S and MARK4L, could be featured as a potential target of dysregulation in tumours due to its dual nature. The latter isoform, produced by alternative splicing, has been found up-regulated in glioma and shown to display sub-cellular localizations, namely the centrosome, the midbody and the nucleolus, which strictly associate it with the process of cell division. Interestingly, alternative mRNA splicing has been considered a mechanism not only increasing proteomic complexity but also involved in cancer, through mechanisms of oncogenes/tumour suppressors activation/inactivation or through the generation of CIN (López-Saavedra & Herrera, 2010). CIN is a general property of aneuploid cancer cells and is generated by defects in different processes, among which the regulation of the number of centrosomes, the dynamics of microtubules attachment to the kinetochores and the overall control of cell cycle. Defects in centrosomal number and structure have been well documented in gliomas (D'Assoro et al., 2002; Katsetos et al., 2006; Magnani et al., 2009) raising the issue whether the increased MARK4L isoform, a gene involved in microtubule dynamics, may concur to errors in chromosomal segregation driving gliomagenesis.

Recent application of multidimensional technological approaches has comprehensively highlighted the scenario of glioma genes and core pathways. However, despite the impressive advances, the links between genes alteration and cellular behavior are yet hampered by the multiplicity of the genetic lesions and the interconnections among the different affected pathways. Hopefully ongoing and next years research will compose the puzzle promising to translate into the clinical set the unraveled glioma pathomechanisms.

12. Acknowledgement

We thank the *Associazione italiana per la ricerca sul cancro* (AIRC) for supporting this work (grant n 4217 to LL for 2008).

13. Methods

13.1 Cell cultures and preparation of human metaphase chromosomes

Glioma cell lines were derived from primary tumour post-surgery specimens and subsequently maintained by serial passages in RPMI 1640 medium containing 5% Fetal Calf Serum at 37°C in a 5% CO_2 atmosphere. Most of the cell lines were used within the first 30 passages.

Metaphase spreads were obtained on both fresh tumours and cultured cell lines, harvested when "peak" mitotic activity was observed; usually, a 16-hour treatment with Colcemid at a final concentration of 0.01-0.02 mg/ml is employed (Magnani et al., 1994).

13.2 Fluorescence *in situ* hybridization (FISH) analysis

Fluorescence hybridization with genomic DNA has proven to be a powerful tool for identification of chromosome rearrangements in cancer cells. Potential applications include detection of chromosome-specific aneuploidy in metaphase and interphase cells, quantification of the frequency of chromosome translocations and/or aneuploidy as a measure of genetic damage, and detection of diagnostically and prognostically relevant chromosomal lesions. Detection of translocations between human metaphase chromosomes is possible by using cocktails of chromosome-specific sequences that hybridize more or less uniformly along the chromosome. Depending on the aberration, its detection may be by visual fluorescence microscopy (see Figures 9, 10). In brief: slides carrying interphase or metaphase spreads are washed in 2x SSC (1 x SSC is 0.15 M NaCl/0.015 M sodium citrate), dehydrated in an ethanol series and denatured [70% (vol/vol) formamide/2x SSC (final concentration), pH 7, at 70°C for 2 min]. The hybridization mix consists of (final concentrations) 50% formamide, 2x SSC, 20% dextran sulfate, carrier DNA (sonicated herring sperm DNA), and biotin-labeled human genomic DNA. The mixture is applied to the slides under a glass coverslip. After overnight incubation at 37°C, the slides are washed at 45°C (50% formamide/2x SSC, pH 7), and immersed in BN buffer (0.1 M sodium bicarbonate, 0.05% Nonidet P-40, pH 8). The slides are never allowed to dry after this step. The coverslips are then removed and fluorescein-avidin DCS is applied. The coverslips are put back in their original places and the slides incubated 20 min at 37°C. They are then washed in BN buffer at 45°C. The intensity of biotin fluorescence is amplified by adding a layer of biotinylated goat anti-avidin antibody followed, after washing as above, by another layer of fluorescein-avidin DCS. After washing in BN buffer a fluorescence anti-fade solution is added. The DNA counterstain [4,6-diamidino-2-phenylindole (DAPI) or propidium iodide] is included in the anti-fade solution (Magnani et al., 1999; Pinkel et al., 1986).

13.3 Immunofluorescence

Immunofluorescence analyses enable to visualize, by fluorescence microscopy, the sub-cellular localization of a specific protein in cultured cells. The target protein is recognized by an antibody, which in turn is conjugated to a fluorochrome emitting fluorescent light. Briefly, cells are grown on glass chamber slides, then permeabilized (with solvents that extract lipids from the membranes allowing antibodies to reach a sub-cellular structure) and fixed (in order to protect the cell structure from eventual damages and to "freeze" cells in their current state). Afterwards, cells are incubated with bovine serum albumin (BSA) to block non-specific binding of antibodies. Glass slides are then incubated with a primary antibody specific to the target protein, then with a secondary antibody conjugated to the fluorochrome and finally observed under the microscope (Magnani et al., 2009).

13.4 Biochemical fractionation and immunoblotting

By biochemical fractionation we mean the whole techniques that allow to separate and isolate intact cellular components. It usually consists in carefully breaking the cell membrane with homogenizers and isotonic/hypotonic solutions, so that intact organelles can come out, and in separating cellular components by centrifugation, on the basis of differences in their mass and specific weight. Centrosome, midbody and nucleoli isolation protocols are described in Magnani et al., 2009 and based on methods respectively by Moudjou & Bornens, 1994; Chu & Sisken, 1977; Muramatsu et al., 1963. In particular, for midbody isolation cells are synchronized in mitosis by nocodazole treatment and then released from mitotic arrest in nocodazole-free medium, so that after 30 minutes near 90% of cells had formed the midbody.

After membrane breaking, all the passages are done at 4°C and with protease inhibitors, in order to prevent protein degradation, possibly exerted by released proteases. Proteins extracted from centrosome, midbody and nucleolus fractions are then analyzed by immunoblotting. Proteins are first separated, according to their molecular weight, by SDS-PAGE (Sodium Dodecyl Sulphate - PolyAcrilamide Gel Electrophoresis): this technique allows proteins to migrate, driven by electric current, in a porous gel, with speed depending exclusively on their size. Afterwards, separated proteins are transferred onto a membrane, incubated with a blocking solution (BSA or milk) to prevent non-specific binding of antibodies and then incubated with appropriate antibodies (immunoblotting). The primary antibody is specific to the target protein and is recognized by the secondary antibody conjugated to HRP (horse radish peroxidase). Antibodies are detected by covering the membrane with a peroxide/enhancer solution, which is oxidized by HRP and emits light signals.

14. References

Al-Hakim, A.K.; Zagorska, A.; Chapman, L.; Deak, M.; Peggie, M. & Alessi, D.R. (2008). Control of AMPK-related kinases by USP9X and atypical Lys^{29}/Lys^{33}-linked polyubiquitin chains. *The Biochemical Journal,* Vol.411, pp. 249-260, ISSN 0264-6021

Angrand, P.O.; Segura, I.; Völkel, P.; Ghidelli, S.; Terry, R.; Brajenovic, M.; Vintersten, K.; Klein, R.; Superti-Furga, G.; Drewes, G.; Kuster, B.; Bouwmeester, T. & Acker-Palmer, A. (2006). Transgenic mouse proteomics identifies new 14-3-3-associated proteins involved in cytoskeletal rearrangements and cell signaling. *Molecular and Cellular Proteomics,* Vol.5, No.12, pp. 2211-2227, ISSN 1535-9484

Bachmann, M.; Hennemann, H.; Xing, P.X.; Hoffmann, I. & Möröy, T. (2004). The oncogenic serine/threonine kinase Pim-1 phosphorylates and inhibits the activity of Cdc25C-associated kinase 1 (C-TAK1): a novel role for Pim-1 at the G2/M cell cycle checkpoint. *Journal of Biological Chemistry,* Vol. 279, pp. 48319-48328, ISSN 0021-9258

Basto, R.; Brunk, K.; Vinadogrova, T.; Peel, N.; Franz, A.; Khodjakov, A. & Raff, J.W. (2008). Centrosome amplification can initiate tumorigenesis in flies. *Cell*, Vol. 133, pp. 1032-1042, ISSN 0092-8674

Bayani, J.; Selvarajah, S.; Maire, G.; Vukovic, B.; Al-Romaih, K.; Zielenska, M. & Squire, J.A. (2007). Genomic mechanisms and measurement of structural and numerical instability in cancer cells. *Seminars in Cancer Biology* , Vol.17, pp. 5-18, ISSN 1044-579X

Beghini, A.; Magnani, I.; Roversi, G.; Piepoli, T.; Di Terlizzi, S.; Moroni, R.F.; Pollo, B.; Fuhrman Conti, A.M.; Cowell, J.K.; Finocchiaro, G. & Larizza, L. (2003). The neural progenitor-restricted isoform of the MARK4 gene in 19q13.2 is upregulated in human gliomas and overexpressed in a subset of glioblastoma cell lines. *Oncogene,* Vol. 22, pp. 2581-2591, ISSN 0950-9232

Bessone, S.; Vidal, F.; Le Bouc, Y.; Epelbaum, J.; Bluet-Pajot, M.T. & Darmon, M. (1999) EMK protein kinase-null mice: dwarfism and hypofertility associated with alterations in the somatotrope and prolactin pathways. *Developmental Biology,* Vol. 214, pp. 87-101, ISSN 0012-1606

Bigner, S.H.; Mark, J.; Burger, P.C.; Mahaley, M.S.Jr.; Bullard, D.E.; Muhlbaier, L.H. & Bigner, D.D. (1988). Specific chromosomal abnormalities in malignant human gliomas. *Cancer Research* , Vol.88, pp. 405-411, ISSN 0008-5472

Brajenovic, M.; Joberty, G.; Küster, B.; Bouwmeester, T. & Drewes, G. (2004). Comprehensive proteomic analysis of human Par protein complexes reveals an interconnected protein network. *The Journal of Biological Chemistry,* Vol. 279, No.13, pp. 12804-12811, ISSN 1083-351X

Bredel, M.; Bredel, C.; Juric, D.; Harsh, G.R.; Vogel, H.; Recht, L.D. & Sikic, B.I. (2005). High-resolution genome-wide mapping of genetic alterations in human glial brain tumors. *Cancer Research,* Vol. 10, pp. 4088-4096, ISSN 0008-5472

Bringmann, H. (2005). Cytokinesis and the spindle midzone. *Cell cycle,* Vol. 4, No.12, pp. 1709-1712, ISSN 1551-4005

Brinkley, B.R. (2001). Managing the centrosome numbers game: from chaos to stability in cancer cell division. *Trends in Cell Biology* , Vol.11 , pp. 18–21, ISSN 0962-8924

Carmo-Fonseca, M.; Mendes-Soares, L. & Campos, I. (2000). To be or not to be in the nucleolus. *Nature Cell Biology* , Vol. 2, No.6, pp. E107-112, ISSN 1097 -6256

Chen, Y.M.; Wang, Q.J.; Hu, H.S.; Yu, P.C.; Zhu, J., Drewes, G.; Piwnica-Worms, H. & Luo, Z.G. (2006). Microtubule affinity-regulating kinase 2 functions downstream of the PAR-3/PAR-6/atypical PKC complex in regulating hippocampal neuronal polarity. *Proceedings of the National Academy of Science of the United States of America,* Vol. 103, pp. 8534-8539, ISSN 0027-8424

Chin, J; Knowles, R.B.; Schneider, A.; Drewes, G.; Mandelkow, E.M. & Hyman, B.T. (2000). Microtubule-Affinity Regulating Kinase (MARK) is tightly associated with neurofibrillary tangles in Alzheimer brain: a fluorescence energy transfer study. *Journal of Neuropathology and Experimental Neurology,* Vol. 59, No.11, pp. 966-971, ISSN 0022-3069

Chu, L.K. & Sisken, J.E. (1977). The isolation and preliminary electrophoretic analysis of the mitotic spindle from cultured mammalian cells. *Experimental Cell Research,* Vol. 107, pp. 71-77, ISSN 0014-4827

Cimini, D.; Cameron, L.A. & Salmon, E.D. (2004). Anaphase spindle mechanics prevent mis-segregation of merotelically oriented chromosomes. *Current Biology*, Vol. 23, pp. 2149-2155, ISSN 0960-9822

Cohen, D.; Brennwald, P.J.; Rodriguez-Boulan, E. & Müsch, A. (2004). Mammalian PAR-1 determines epithelial lumen polarity by organizing the microtubule cytoskeleton. *Journal of Cell Biology*, Vol. 164, pp. 717-727, ISSN 1540-8140

Collins, V.P. (2004) . Brain tumours: classification and genes. *Journal of Neurology, Neurosurgery & Psychiatry*, Vol. 75, (Suppl 2), pp. 2-11, ISSN 0022-3050

Cowell, J. K.; Barnett, G.H. & Nowak, N.J. (2004a). Characterization of the 1p/19q chromosomal loss in oligodendrogliomas using comparative genomic hybridization arrays (CGHa). *Journal of Neuropathology & Experimental Neurology*, Vol. 63, pp. 151-158, ISSN 0022-3069

Cowell, J.K.; Matsui, S.; Wang, Y.D.; LaDuca, J.; Conroy, J.; McQuaid D. & Nowak N.J. (2004b). Application of bacterial artificial chromosome array-based comparative genomic hybridization and spectral karyotyping to the analysis of glioblastoma multiforme. *Cancer Genetics and Cytogenetics*, Vol. 151, pp.36- 51, ISSN 0165-4608

D'Assoro, A.B.; Lingle, W.L. & Salisbury, J.L. (2002). Centrosome amplification and the development of cancer. *Oncogene*, Vol. 21, pp. 6146-6153. Review, ISSN 0950-9232

Doxsey, S. (2001). Re-evaluating centrosome function. *Nature*, Vol.2, No.9, pp. 688-698, ISSN 0028-0836

Doxsey, S.; McCollum, D. & Theurkauf, W. (2005). Centrosomes in cellular regulation. *Annual Review of Cell and Developmental Biology*, Vol. 21, pp.411-434, ISSN 1081-0706

Drewes, G.; Ebneth, A.; Preuss, U.; Mandelkow, E.M. & Mandelkow, E. (1997). MARK, a novel family of protein kinases that phosphorylate microtubule-associated proteins and trigger microtubule disruption. *Cell*, Vol. 89, pp.297-308, ISSN 0092-8674

Duesberg, P.; Li, R.; Fabarius, A. & Hehlmann, R. (2006). Aneuploidy and cancer: from correlation to causation. *Contributions to Microbiology*, Vol.13, pp. 16-44, ISSN 1420-9519

Fenech, M. (2007). Cytokinesis-block micronucleus cytome assay. *Nature Protocols*, Vol.2, pp. 1084-1104, ISSN 1754-2189

Fujiwara, T.; Bandi, M.; Nitta, M.; Ivanova, E.V.; Bronson, R.T. & Pellman, D. (2005). Cytokinesis failure generating tetraploids promotes tumorigenesis in p53-null cells. *Nature*, Vol. 437, 1043-1047, ISSN 0028-0836

Gamblin, T.C.; Chen, F.; Zambrano, A.; Abraha, A.; Lagalwar, S.; Guillozet, A.L.; Lu, M.; Fu, Y.; Garcia-Sierra, F.; LaPointe, N.; Miller, R.; Berry, R.W.; Binder, L.I. & Cryns, V.L. (2003) Caspase cleavage of tau: linking amyloid and neurofibrillary tangles in Alzheimer's disease. *Proceedings of the National Academy of Sciences of the United States of America*, Vol. 100, No. 17, pp. 10032-10037, ISSN 0027-8424

Ganem, N.J.; Storchova, Z. & Pellman, D. (2007). Tetraploidy, aneuploidy and cancer. *Current Opinion in Genetics & Development*, Vol. 17, pp. 157-162, Review, ISSN 0959-437X

Ganem, N.J.; Godinho, S.A. & Pellman, D. (2009). A mechanism linking extra centrosomes to chromosomal instability. *Nature*, Vol. 460, pp.278-282 , ISSN 0028-0836

Geigl, J.B.; Obenauf, A.C.; Schwarzbraun, T. & Speicher, M.R. (2008). Defining 'chromosomal instability'. *Trends in Genetics*, Vol. 24, pp. 64-69, ISSN 0168-9525

Ghadimi, B.M.; Sackett, D.L.; Difilippantonio, M.J.; Schröck, E.; Neumann, T.; Jauho, A.; Auer, G. & Ried, T. (2000). Centrosome amplification and instability occurs exclusively in aneuploid, but not in diploid colorectal cancer cell lines, and correlates with numerical chromosomal aberrations. *Genes Chromosomes and Cancer*, Vol. 27, pp.183-190, ISSN 1045-2257

Greenman, C.; Stephens, P.; Smith, R.; Dalgliesh, G.L.; Hunter, C.; Bignell, G.; Davies, H.; Teague, J.; Butler, A.; Stevens, C.; Edkins, S.; O'Meara, S.; Vastrik, I.; Schmidt, E.E.; Avis, T.; Barthorpe, S.; Bhamra, G.; Buck, G.; Choudhury, B.; Clements, J.; Cole, J.; Dicks, E.; Forbes, S.; Gray, K.; Halliday, K.; Harrison, R.; Hills, K.; Hinton, J.; Jenkinson, A.; Jones, D.; Menzies, A.; Mironenko, T.; Perry, J.; Raine, K.; Richardson, D.; Shepherd, R.; Small, A.; Tofts, C.; Varian, J.; Webb,T.; West, S.; Widaa, S.; Yates, A.; Cahill, D.P.; Louis, D.N.; Goldstraw, P.; Nicholson, A.G.; Brasseur, F.; Looijenga, L.; Weber, B.L.; Chiew, Y.E.; De Fazio, A.; Greaves, M.F.; Green, A.R.; Campbell, P.; Birney, E.; Easton, D.F.; Chenevix-Trench, G.; Tan, M.H.; Khoo, S.K.; Teh, B.T.; Yuen, S.T.; Leung, S.Y.; Wooster, R.; Futreal, P.A. & Stratton, M.R. (2007). Patterns of somatic mutation in human cancer genomes. *Nature*, Vol. 446, pp.153-158, ISSN 0028-0836

Hartmann, C.; Johnk, L.; Kitange, G.; Wu, Y.; Ashworth, L.K.; Jenkins, R.B. & Louis, D.N. (2002). Transcript Map of the 3.7-Mb D19S112–D19S246. *Cancer Research*, Vol.62, pp. 4100-4108, ISSN 0008-5472

Hecht, B.K.; Turc-Carel, C.; Chatel, M.; Grellier, P.; Gioanni, J.; Attias, R.; Gaudray, P. & Hecht, F. (1995). Cytogenetics of malignant gliomas: I. The autosomes with reference to rearrangements. *Cancer Genetics and Cytogenetics*, Vol. 84, pp. 1-8, ISSN 0165- 4608

Hurov, J.B.; Stappenbeck, T.S.; Zmasek, C.M.; White, L.S.; Ranganath, S.H.; Russell, J.H.; Chan, A.C.; Murphy, K.M. & Piwnica-Worms, H. (2001). Immune system dysfunction and autoimmune disease in mice lacking Emk (Par-1) protein kinase. *Molecular Cell Biology*, Vol. 21, pp.3206-3219, ISSN 1098-5549

Hurov, J. & Piwnica-Worms, H. (2007). The Par-1/MARK family of protein kinases: from polarity to metabolism. *Cell cycle*, Vol.6, pp. 1966-1969, ISSN 1538-4101

Jenkins, R.B.; Kimmel, D.W.; Moertel, C.A.; Schultz, C.G.; Scheithauer, B.W.; Kelly, P.J. & Dewald, G.W. (1989). A cytogenetic study of 53 human gliomas. *Cancer Genetics and Cytogenetics*, Vol. 39, pp. 253-279, ISSN 0165- 4608

Kato, T.; Satoh, S.; Okabe, H.; Kitahara, O.; Ono, K.; Kihara, C.; Tanaka, T.; Tsunoda, T.; Yamaoka, Y.; Nakamura, Y. & Furukawa, Y. (2001). Isolation of a novel human gene, MARKL1, homologous to MARK3 and its involvement in hepatocellular carcinogenesis. *Neoplasia*, Vol. 3, No.1, pp. 4-9, ISSN 1522-8002

Katsetos, C.D.; Reddy, G.; Dráberová, E.; Smejkalová, B.; Del Valle, L.; Ashraf, Q.; Tadevosyan, A.; Yelin, K.; Maraziotis, T.; Mishra, O.P.; Mörk, S.; Legido, A.; Nissanov, J.; Baas, P.W.; de Chadarévian, J.P. & Dráber, P. (2006). Altered cellular distribution and subcellular sorting of gamma-tubulin in diffuse astrocytic gliomas and human glioblastoma cell lines. *Journal of Neuropathology and Experimental Neurology*, Vol. 65, pp. 465–477, ISSN 0022-3069

Kitange, G.; Misra, A.; Law, M.; Passe, S.; Kollmeyer, T.M.; Maurer, M.; Ballman, K.; Feuerstein, B.G. & Jenkins, R.B. (2005). Chromosomal imbalances detected by array comparative genomic hybridization in human oligodendrogliomas and mixed oligoastrocytomas. *Genes Chromosomes and Cancer*, Vol. 42, pp. 68-77, ISSN 1045-2257

Kleihues, P. & Cavenee, W.K. (2000). *Pathology and Genetics of Tumours of the Nervous System*, IARC Press, ISBN 92 83 22409 4, Lyon, France

Kleihues, P.& Ohgaki, H. (2000). Phenotype vs genotype in the evolution of astrocytic brain tumors. *Toxicologic Pathology*, Vol. 28, No.1, pp. 164-170, ISSN 0192-6233

Koschny, R.; Koschny, T.; Froster, U.G.; Krupp, W. & Zuber, M.A. (2002). Comparative genomic hybridization in glioma: a meta-analysis of 509 cases. *Cancer Genetics and Cytogenetics*, Vol. 135, pp. 147-159, ISSN 0165- 4608

Kramer, A.; Neben, K. & Ho, AD. (2002). Centrosome replication, genomic instability and cancer. *Leukemia*, Vol. 16, pp. 767-775 , ISSN 0887-6924

Lengauer, C.; Kinzler, K.W. & Vogelstein B. (1998). Genetic instabilities in human cancers. *Nature*, Vol. 396, pp. 643-649, ISSN 0028-0836

Lindstrom, E.; Salford, L.G. Heim S, Mandahl N, Stromblad S, Brun A, Mitelman F. (1991): Trisomy 7 and sex chromosome loss need not be representative of tumor parenchyma cells in malignant glioma. *Genes, Chromosomes and Cancer*, Vol. 3, pp. 474-479, ISSN 1045-2257

Lingle, W.L.; Barrett, S.L.; Negron, V.C.; D'Assoro, A.B.; Boeneman, K.; Liu, W.; Whitehead, C.M.; Reynolds, C. & Salisbury, J.L. (2002). Centrosome amplification drives chromosomal instability in breast tumor development. *Proceedings of the National Academy of Science of the United States of America*, Vol. 99, pp.1978-1983, ISSN 0027-8424

López-Saavedra, A. & Herrera, L.A. (2010). The role of alternative mRNA splicing in chromosome instability. *Mutation research*, Vol. 705, pp.246-51, ISSN 0027-5107

Louis, D.N.; Ohgaki, H.; Wiestler, O.D.; Cavenee, W.K.; Burger, P.C.; Jouvet, A.; Scheithauer, B.W. & Kleihues, P. (2007). The 2007 WHO Classification of Tumours of the Central Nervous System. *Acta Neuropathologica*, Vol. 114, No.2, pp. 97-109, ISSN 0001-6322

Magnani, I.; Guerneri, S.; Pollo, B.; Cirenei, N.; Colombo, B.M.; Broggi, G.; Galli, C.; Bugiani, O.; DiDonato, S.; Finocchiaro, G. & Fuhrman Conti, A.M. (1994). Increasing complexity of the karyotype in 50 human gliomas. *Cancer Genetics and Cytogenetics*, Vol. 75, pp. 77-89, ISSN 0165-4608

Magnani, I.; Chiariello, E.; Furhrman Conti, A.M. & Finocchiaro, G. (1999). A recurrent 19q11-12 breakpoint suggested by cytogenetic and fluorescence in situ hybridization analysis of three glioblastoma cell lines. *Cancer Genetics and Cytogenetics*, Vol. 110, pp.82-86, ISSN 0165-4608

Magnani, I.; Novielli, C.; Bellini, M.; Roversi, G.; Bello, L. & Larizza, L. (2009). Multiple localization of endogenous MARK4L protein in human glioma. *Cellular Oncology*, Vol.31, pp. 357-370, ISSN 1570-5870

Mandelkow, E.M.; Thies, E.; Trinczek, B.; Biernat, J. & Mandelkow, E. (2004). MARK/PAR1 kinase is a regulator of microtubule-dependent transport in axons. *The Journal of Cell Biology*, Vol. 167, No.1, pp. 99-110, ISSN 0021-9525

Margolis, R.L.; Lohez, O.D. & Andreassen, P.R. (2003). G1 tetraploidy checkpoint and the suppression of tumorigenesis. *Journal of Cellular Biochemistry*, Vol. 88, pp. 673-683, Review, ISSN 1097-4644

Martinez-Garay, I.; Rustom, A.; Gerdes, H.H. & Kutsche, K. (2006). The novel centrosomal associated protein CEP55 is present in the spindle midzone and the midbody. *Genomics*, Vol. 87, pp. 243–253, ISSN 0888-7543

Marx, A.; Nugoor, C.; Panneerselvam, S. & Mandelkow, E. (2010). Structure and function of polarity-inducing kinase family MARK/Par-1 within the branch of AMPK/Snf1-related kinases. *The FASEB Journal*, Vol. 24, pp. 1637-1648, ISSN 0892-6638

Matenia, D. & Mandelkow, E.M. (2009). The tau of MARK: a polarized view of the cytoskeleton. *Trends in biochemical sciences*, Vol. 34, No.7, pp. 332-342, ISSN 0968-0004

Meraldi, P.; Honda, R. & Nigg, E.A. (2002). Aurora-A overexpression reveals tetraploidization as a major route to centrosome amplification in p53-/- cells. *The EMBO Journal*, Vol. 21, pp. 483–492, ISSN 0261-4189

Moravcevic, K.; Mendrola, J.M.; Schmitz, K.R.; Wang, Y.H.; Slochower, D.; Janmey, P.A. & Lemmon, M.A. (2010). Kinase associated-1 domains drive MARK/PAR1 kinases to membrane targets by binding acidic phospholypids. *Cell*, Vol. 143, pp.966-977, ISSN 0092-8674

Moroni, R.F.; De Biasi, S.; Colapietro, P.; Larizza, L. & Beghini, A. (2006). Distinct expression pattern of microtubule-associated protein/microtubule affinity-regulating kinase 4 in differentiated neurons. *Neuroscience*, Vol. 143, pp. 83-94, ISSN 0306-4522

Moudjou, M. & Bornens, M. (1994). Method of centrosome isolation from cultured animal cells. In: *Cell biology: a laboratory handbook*, Celis J.E., pp.595-604, Academic Press, (Ed.), ISBN 0-12-164715-3, San Diego, CA

Müller, J.; Ory, S.; Copeland, T.; Piwnica-Worms, H. & Morrison, D.K. (2001). C-TAK1 regulates Ras signalling by phophorylating the MAPK scaffolds, KSR1. *Molecular Cell*, Vol. 8, pp. 983-993, ISSN 1097-2765

Mullins, J.M. & Biesele, J.J. (1977). Terminal phase of cytokinesis in D-98S cells. *The Journal of Cell Biology*, Vol. 73, pp. 672-684, ISSN 0021-9525

Mullins, J.M. & McIntosh, J.R. (1982). Isolation and initial characterization of the mammalian midbody. *The Journal of Cell Biology*, Vol. 94, pp.654-661, ISSN 0021-9525

Muramatsu, M.; Smetana, K. & Busch, H. (1963). Quantitative aspects of isolation of nucleoli of the Walker carcinosarcoma and liver of the rat. *Cancer Research*, Vol. 23, pp. 510-518, ISSN 0008-5472

Nigro, J.M.; Misra, A.; Zhang, L.; Smirnov, I.; Colman, H.; Griffin, C.; Ozburn, N.; Chen, M.; Pan, E.; Koul, D.; Yung, W.K.; Feuerstein, B.G. & Aldape, K.D. (2005). Integrated array-comparative genomic hybridization and expression array profiles identify clinically relevant molecular subtypes of glioblastoma. *Cancer Research*, Vol. 65, 1678-1686, ISSN 0008-5472

Noble, M. & Dietrich, J. (2004). The complex identity of brain tumors: emerging concerns regarding origin, diversity and plasticity. *TRENDS in Neurosciences*, Vol. 27, No.3, 148-154, ISSN 0166-2236

Ohgaki, H.; Schauble, B.; zur Hausen, A.; von Ammon, K. & Kleihues, P. (1995). Genetic alterations associated with the evolution and progression of astrocytic brain tumours. *Virchows Archive*, Vol. 427, pp. 113-118, ISSN 0945-6317

Park, H.S.; Maeda, T.; Mohapatra, G.; Waldman, F.M.; Davis, R.L. & Feuerstein, B.G. (1995). Heterogeneity, poliploidy, aneusomy and 9p deletion in human glioblastoma multiforme. *Cancer Genetics and Cytogenetics*, Vol. 83, pp. 127-135, ISSN 0165-4608

Parsons, D.W.; Jones, S.; Zhang, X.; Lin, J.C.; Leary; R.J.; Angenendt, P.; Mankoo, P.; Carter, H.; Siu, I.M.; Gallia, G.L.; Olivi, A.; McLendon, R.; Rasheed, B.A.; Keir, S.; Nikolskaya, T.; Nikolsky, Y.; Busam, D.A.; Tekleab, H.; Diaz, L.A. Jr.; Hartigan, J.; Smith, D.R.; Strausberg, R.L.; Marie, S.K.; Shinjo, S.M.; Yan, H.; Riggins, G.J.; Bigner, D.D.; Karchin, R.; Papadopoulos, N.; Parmigiani, G.; Vogelstein, B.; Velculescu, V.E. & Kinzler, K.W. (2008). An integrated genomic analysis of human glioblastoma multiforme. *Science*, Vol. 321, pp.1807-1812, ISSN 0036-8075

Pihan, G.A.; Purohit, A.; Wallace, J.; Knecht, H.; Woda, B.; Quesenberry, P. & Doxsey, S.J. (1998). Centrosome defects and genetic instability in malignant tumors. *Cancer Research*, Vol. 58, pp. 3974–3985, ISSN 0008-5472

Pinkel, D.; Straume, T. & Gray, J.W. (1986). Cytogenetic analysis using quantitative, high-sensitivity, fluorescence hybridization. *Proceedings of the National Academy of Science of the United States of America*, Vol. 83, pp. 2934-2938, ISSN 0027-8424

Ritland, S.R.; Ganju, V. & Jenkins, R.B. (1995). Region-specific loss of heterozygosity on chromosome 19 is related to the morphologic type of human glioma. *Genes, Chromosomes and Cancer*, Vol. 12, pp. 277-282, ISSN 1045-2257

Roversi, G.; Pfundt, R.; Moroni, R.F.; Magnani, I.; van Reijmersdal, S.; Pollo, B.; Straatman, H.; Larizza, L. & Schoenmakers, E.F. (2006). Identification of novel genomic markers related to progression to glioblastoma through genomic profiling of 25 primary glioma cell lines. *Oncogene*, Vol. 9, pp. 1571-1583, ISSN 0950-9232

Saunders, W. (2005). Centrosomal amplification and spindle multipolarity in cancer cells. *Seminars in Cancer Biology*, Vol. 15, pp. 25-32, Review, ISSN 1044-579X

Schaar, B.T.; Kinoshita, K. & McConnell, S.K. (2004). Doublecortin microtubule affinity is regulated by a balance of kinase and phosphatase activity at the leading edge of migrating neurons. *Neuron*, Vol. 41, pp. 203-213, ISSN 0896-6273

Schmidt, M.C.; Antweiler, S.; Urban, N.; Mueller, W.; Kuklik, A.; Meyer-Puttlitz, B; Wiestler, O.D.; Louis, D.N.; Fimmers, R. & von Deimling, A. (2002). Impact of genotype and morphology on the prognosis of glioblastoma. *Journal of Neuropathology & Experimental Neurology*, Vol.61, pp. 321-328, ISSN 0014-4886

Schneider, A.; Laage, R.; von Ahsen, O.; Fischer, A.; Rossner, M.; Scheek, S.; Grünewald, S.; Kuner, R.; Weber, D.; Krüger, C.; Klaussner, B.; Götz, B.; Hiemisch, H.; Newrzella, D.; Martin-Villalba, A.; Bach, A. & Schwaninger, M. (2004). Identification of regulated genes during permanent focal cerebral ischemia: characterization of the protein kinase 9b5/MARKL1/MARK4. *Journal of Neurochemistry*, Vol. 88, pp. 1114-1126, ISSN 1474-1644

Schwarzacher, H.G. & Wachtler, F. (1983). Nucleolus organizer regions and nucleoli. *Human genetics*, Vol. 63, pp. 89-99, ISSN 0340-6717

Segu, L.; Pascaud, A.; Costet, P.; Darmon, M. & Buhot, M.C. (2008). Impairment of spatial learning and memory in ELKL Motif Kinase 1 (EMK1/MARK2) knockout mice. *Neurobiology of aging*, Vol. 29, pp. 231-24, ISSN 0197-4580

Shapiro, J.R. (2002). Genetic alterations associated with adult diffuse astrocytic tumors. *American Journal of Medical Genetics*, Vol.115, pp. 194-201, ISSN 1552-4833

Sluder, G. & Nordberg, J.J. (2004). The good, the bad and the ugly: the practical consequences of centrosome amplification. *Current Opinion in Cell Biology*, Vol. 16, pp.49-54, Review, ISSN 09550674

Smith, J.S.; Alderete, B.; Minn, Y.; Borell, T.J.; Perry, A.; Mohapatra, G.; Hosek, S.M.; Kimmel, D.; O'Fallon, J.; Yates, A.; Feuerstein, B.G.; Burger, P.C.; Scheithauer, B.W. & Jenkins, R.B. (1999). Localization of common deletion regions on 1p and 19q in human gliomas and their association with histological subtype. *Oncogene*, Vol. 18, pp. 4144-415, ISSN 0950-9232

The Cancer Genome Atlas (TGCA) Research Network. (2008). Comprehensive genomic characterization defines human glioblastoma genes and core pathways. *Nature*, Vol. 455, No.7216, pp. 1061-1068, ISSN 0028-0836

Thiel, G.; Losanowa, T.; Kintzel, D.; Nisch, G.; Martin, H.; Vorpahl, K. & Witkowski, P. (1992). Karyotypes in 90 human gliomas. *Cancer Genetics and Cytogenetics*, Vol. 58, pp. 109-120, ISSN 0165- 4608

Timm, T.; Marx, A.; Panneerselvam, S.; Mandelkow, E. & Mandelkow, E.M. (2008). Structure and regulation of MARK, a kinase involved in abnormal phosphorylation of Tau protein. *BMC Neuroscience*, Vol. 9, Suppl 2, S9, ISSN 1471-2202

Tochio, N.; Koshiba, S.; Kobayashi, N.; Inoue, M.; Yabuki, T.; Aoki, M.; Seki, E.; Matsuda, T.; Tomo, Y.; Motoda, Y.; Kobayashi, A.; Tanaka, A.; Hayashizaki, Y.; Terada, T.; Shirouzu, M.; Kigawa, T. & Yokoyama, S. (2006). Solution structure of the kinase-associated domain 1 of mouse microtubule-associated protein/microtubule affinity-regulating kinase 3. *Protein science*, Vol. 15, 2534-2543, ISSN 1469-896X

Trinczek, B.; Brajenovic, M.; Ebneth, A. & Drewes, G. (2004). MARK4 is a novel Microtubule-associated Proteins/Microtubule Affinity-regulating Kinase that binds to the cellular microtubule network and to centrosomes. *The Journal of Biological Chemistry*, Vol. 279, No. 7, pp. 5915-5923, ISSN 0021-9258

van den Bent, M.J.(2004). Advances in the biology and treatment of oligodendrogliomas. *Current Opinion in Neurology*, Vol. 17, pp.675-680, Review, ISSN 13507540

Visintin, R. & Amon, A. (2000). The nucleolus: the magician's hat for cell cycle tricks. *Current Opinion in Cell Biology*, Vol. 12, No. 3, pp. 372-37, ISSN 09550674

von Deimling, A.; Louis, D.N.; von Ammon, K.; Petersen, I.; Wiestler, O.D. & Seizinger, B.R. (1992). Evidence for a tumor suppressor gene on chromosome 19q associated with human astrocytomas, oligodendrogliomas, and mixed gliomas. *Cancer Research*, Vol. 52, pp.4277-4279, ISSN 0008-5472

von Deimling, A.; von Ammon, K.; Schoenfeld, D.; Wiestler, O.D.; Seizinger, B.R.& Louis, D.N. (1993). Subsets of glioblastoma multiforme defined by molecular genetic analyis. *Brain Pathology*, Vol. 3, pp.19-26, ISSN 1750-3639

von Deimling, A.; Nagel, J.; Bender, B; Lenartz, D.; Schramm, J.; Louis, D.N. & Wiestler, O.D.(1994). Deletion mapping of chromosome 19 in human gliomas. *International Journal of Cancer*, Vol. 57, pp.676-680, ISSN 1097-0215

Weaver, B.A.; Silk, A.D.; Montagna, C.; Verdier-Pinard, P.& Cleveland, D.W. (2007). Aneuploidy acts both oncogenically and as a tumor suppressor. *Cancer Cell* , Vol.11, No.1, pp. 25-36 , ISSN 1535-6108

Wojcik, C. & DeMartino, G.N. (2003). Intracellular localization of proteasomes. *The International Journal of Biochemistry & Cell Biology*, Vol. 35, No.5, pp. 579-5, ISSN 1357-2725 89

Zhang, H.; Ma, X.; Shi, T.; Song, Q.; Zhao, H. & Ma, D. (2010). NSA2, a novel nucleolus protein regulates cell proliferation and cell cycle. *Biochemical and Biophysical Research Communications*, Vol. 391, No.1, p. 65, ISSN 0006-291X

Zhu, Y. & Parada, L.F. (2002). The molecular and genetic basis of neurological tumours. *Nature Reviews Cancer* , Vol. 2, pp. 616-626 , ISSN 1474-175X

8

New Insight on the Role of Transient Receptor Potential (TRP) Channels in Driven Gliomagenesis Pathways

Giorgio Santoni[1], Maria Beatrice Morelli[1,2], Consuelo Amantini[1], Matteo Santoni[1] and Massimo Nabissi[1]
[1]*School of Pharmacy, Section of Experimental Medicine, University of Camerino*
[2]*Department of Molecular Medicine, Sapienza University, Rome*
Italy

1. Role of TRP channels in glioma growth and progression

Gliomas are primary brain tumours believed to arise from glial cells or their progenitors. They account for 78% of malignant brain tumours (Shwartzbaum et al., 2006). The vast majority of gliomas is high-grade glioblastoma multiforme (GBM), and is characterized by almost unrestrained growth. Consequently, the median survival of patients with GBM was approximately 12 months (Huncharek & Muscat, 1998). While research has generated abundant information regarding the growth characteristics of these cancers, clinical care remains palliative and the prognosis dismal (Butowski et al., 2006). Gliomagenesis and progression are complex processes only partly understood. At molecular level, tumor progression and the associated heterogeneity is likely the result of multiple mutations in certain key signaling proteins (Furnari et al., 2007). Among these proteins, the Transient Receptor Potential (TRP) channel family has been identified to profoundly affect a variety of physiological and pathological processes (Kiselyov et al., 2007; Nilius et al., 2007). Members of TRP channels control cellular homeostasis by regulating calcium flux, cell proliferation, differentiation and apoptosis; moreover, in the last years an additional role for TRP ion channel family in malignant cancer growth and progression has been recognized (Xu et al., 2001; Wisnoskey et al., 2003; Xin et al., 2005; Bidaux et al., 2007; Prevarskaya et al., 2007; Gkika & Prevarskaya, 2009). Approximately thirty TRPs have been identified to date, and are classified in seven different families: TRPC (Canonical), TRPV (Vanilloid), TRPM (Melastatin), TRPML (Mucolipin), TRPP (Polycystin), and TRPA (Ankyrin transmembrane protein) and TRPN (NomPC-like) (Montell, 2003) (Fig.1).
The expression levels and activity of members of the TRPC, TRPM, and TRPV families have been correlated with malignant growth and progression (Duncan et al., 1998; Tsavaler et al., 2001; Wissenbach et al., 2001; Thebault et al., 2006; Amantini et al., 2007; Caprodossi et al., 2008; Nabissi et al., 2010). TRP channels may regulate glioma growth and progression at different levels by controlling cell proliferation, inhibiting apoptosis, stimulating angiogenesis and triggering the migration and the invasion during tumor progression (Table 1).

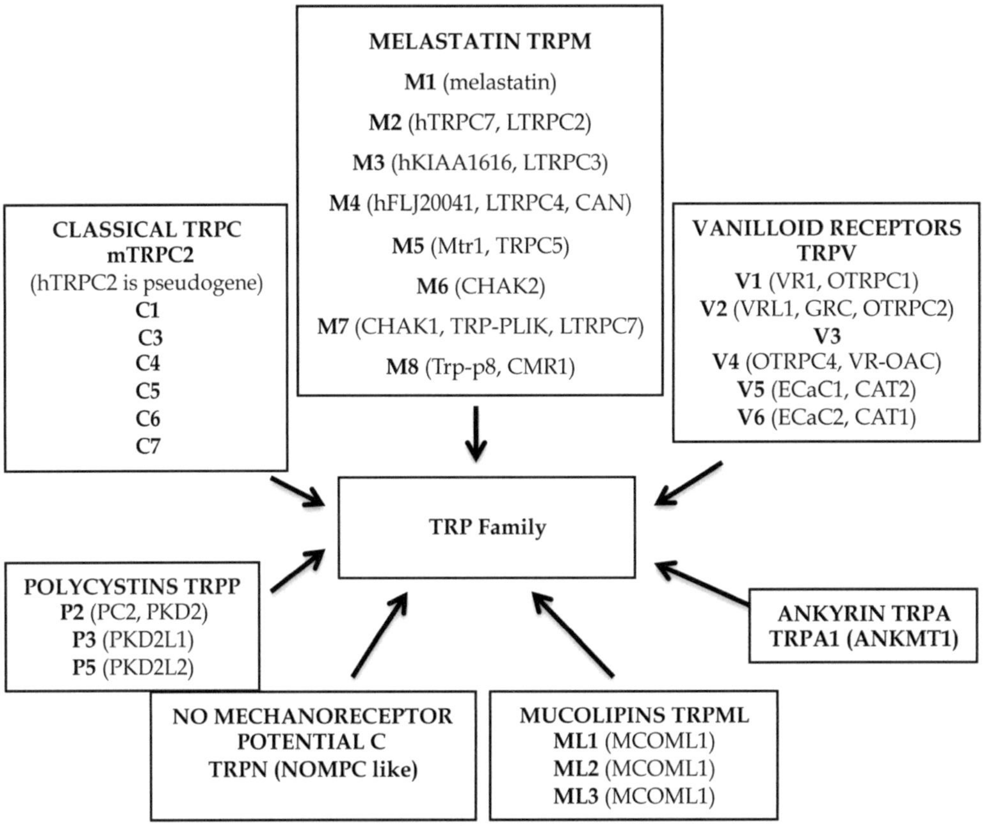

Fig. 1. TRP superfamily. TRP subgroups are represented in square, the members are indicated for each subfamily.

2. Role of TRPC and TRPV channels in cell cycle arrest and cytokinesis in malignant glioma

Growth control of cancer cell populations has been studied extensively over the past decades and research has identified a multitude of transmembrane TRP channels involved in this process (Schönherr, 2005; Santoni et al., 2011) (Fig.2). While our understanding of their exact role in the physiology of cell proliferation remains tentative, many TRP channel agonists or antagonists also stimulate or retard cell population growth, which support the notion that TRP channels are intrinsic component of the cell cycle. In particular, calcium Ca(2+) signaling plays an important role in normal and aberrant cell proliferation, and some members of the Ca(2+)-permeable TRPC family have demonstrated a role in the proliferation of many types of cancer cells (Malarkey et al., 2008). Using a combination of molecular, biochemical and biophysical approaches, it was demonstrated the expression of five TRPC channel proteins (TRPC1, TRPC3, TRPC4, TRPC5 and TRPC6) in patient biopsies and cell lines derived from glioma patients (Tables 1). Activation of TRPC channels typically occurs through the triggering of phospholipase C and this signaling cascade is the target of a number of G-protein-coupled receptors and receptor tyrosine kinases. An important form of

TRP channel	Function/s	References
TRPC1	Chemotaxis in response to EGF stimulation Calcium signaling during cytokinesis (Multinucleated-giant cells), stimulates proliferation Up-regulates hypoxia-induced VEGF expression Histamine-induced Ca(2+) entry	Sontheimer, 2010 Bomben & Sontheimer, 2018 Bomben & Sontheimer, 2010 Wang et al., 2009 Barajas et al., 2008
TRPC3	Ca(2+) influx, PAR-1-mediated astrocytic activation $[Ca(2+)]_i$ signaling	Nakao et al., 2008 Grimaldi et al., 2003
TRPC4	Histamine-induced Ca(2+) entry	Barajas et al., 2008
TRPC6	Increase intracellular Ca(2+) induced by PDGF, stimulates G2/M phase transition and clonogenic ability; increases tumor volume in a subcutaneous mouse model of xenografted human tumors and decreases mean survival in mice in an intracranial model Increases $[Ca(2+)]_i$ elevation coupled to NFAT activation; stimulates hypoxia-induced Notch1-driven growth, invasion and angiogenesis	Ding et al., 2010 Chigurupati et al., 2010
TRPV1	Ca(2+) influx, p38MAPK-dependent apoptosis	Amantini et al., 2007
TRPV2	Inhibition of cell survival and proliferation, increase sensitivity to Fas-induced apoptosis in an ERK-dependent manner	Nabissi et al., 2010
TRPM2	ROS-induced cell death	Ishii et al., 2007
TRPM8	Increases intracellular Ca(2+), BK channel activity, cell migration	Wondergem et al., 2008 Wondergem & Bartley, 2009

Table 1. Expression and function of TRP channels in human gliomas

TRPC activation has been shown downstream of the epidermal growth factor receptor (EGFR) (Odell et al.,2005) that is the major growth factor receptor activated in malignant gliomas. Indeed, mutated or amplified EGFR is often observed in malignant gliomas and has been associated with the increased cell proliferation seen in them (Bryant et al., 2004). In Cos-7 cells, EGFR activation causes phosphorylation of TRPC4 and results in channel insertion into the plasma membrane (Odell et al., 2005). Additionally, knockdown of TRPC4 in human corneal epithelial cells suppresses epidermal growth factor (EGF)-induced cell proliferation, again linking proliferation to TRPC channels (Yang et al., 2005). Among TRPC channels, TRPC6 and TRPC1 seem to play a major role in the control of cell cycle and glioma cell proliferation. Functional TRPC6 channels were overexpressed in human U251, U87, and T98G glioma cell lines. Moreover, increased TRPC6 expression was found in GBM biopsies compared with normal brain tissue, suggesting a role for TRPC6 in malignant growth of gliomas *in vitro* and *in vivo* (Ding et al., 2010). TRPC6 channels have been implicated in cell proliferation and hypertrophic gene expression through the activation of the calcineurin-nuclear factor of activated T-cell (NFAT) pathway in normal (K. Kuwahara et al., 2006; Onohara et al., 2006) and malignant cells (Bomben & Sontheimer, 2008). Because glioma cells lack the expression of voltage-gated calcium channels (Kunzelmann, 2005) and Ca(2+) signaling promotes G_1/S phase transition and cell cycle progression in a variety of cell types (Lipskaia & Lopré, 2004; M. Kuwahara et al., 2006), the TRPC6-mediated sustained elevation of $[Ca(2+)]_i$ and calcineurin-NFAT pathway activation is vital for the proliferation and malignant growth of gliomas under hypoxia. Consistently, inhibition of hypoxia-induced TRPC6 expression causes a dramatic decrease in NFAT activation (Bucholz & Ellenrieder, 2007). In glioma cells, inhibition of TRPC6 activity or expression by using a dominant-negative mutant TRPC6 (DNC6) or RNA interference, respectively, attenuated the increase in intracellular Ca(2+) induced by platelet-derived growth factor (PDGF), suppressed cell growth and clonogenic ability, induced cell cycle arrest at the G2/M phase, and enhanced the antiproliferative effect of ionizing radiation. Cyclin-dependent kinase 1 (CdK1) activation and cell division cycle 25 homolog C (Cdc25) expression regulated the DNC6-induced cell cycle arrest. Inhibition of TRPC6 activity also significantly reduced tumor volume in a subcutaneous mouse model of xenografted human tumors and increased mean survival in mice in an intracranial model (Ding et al., 2010). In addition to TRPC6 a role for TRPC3 in glioma cell proliferation has been suggested. The TRPC3 channel has been found to cause intracytoplasmic calcium oscillations in rat glial cells (Grimaldi et al., 2003). In rat cortical astrocytes, thrombin via Ca(2+) signal, induces TRPC3 upregulation and enhanced proliferation, and these effects were inhibited by TRPC3 blockers and siTRPC3 RNA (Shirakawa et al., 2010). Ca(2+) mobilization mediated by TRPC3 is associated with thrombin-induced morphological changes in human astrocytoma cells (Nakao et al., 2008). Glioblastoma multiforme proliferates extensively and cells often undergo incomplete cell divisions, resulting in multinucleated cells. Cytokinesis, which begins at the onset of anaphase, is the division of remaining cytoplasmic substances in the cell, aside from the nuclear events of mitosis (Glotzer, 2005; Eggert et al., 2006). Recent evidence (Bomben & Sontheimer, 2010) indicated that the functional loss of TRPC1 channels involved in agonist-induced calcium entry and reloading of intracellular Ca(2+) stores disrupts glioma cytokinesis leading to bizarre and greatly enlarged multinucleated glioma cells (GMGCs) showing slow growth (Palma et al., 1989). Pharmacological inhibition of TRPC1 expression using the continuously administration for up to 4 days of the chronic inhibitor of TRPC channels, SKF96365, or TRPC1 suppression using a doxycycline inducible shRNA knockdown approach, causes loss of functional channels and store-operated calcium entry in glioma cells, and a significant decrease of tumor size, respectively. This effect is associated with reduced cell proliferation and, frequently, with incomplete cell division due to arrest at the G_2/M phase of the cell cycle (Stark & Taylor, 2006). Cytokinesis is typically described with two key components being the central spindle and the contractile ring. RhoA guanosine triphosphatase GTPase is one key player in contractile ring formation, which is important for actin nucleation and myosin activation (Bement et al., 2006). Recently reports have indicated an association between TRPC1 and RhoA (Mehta et al., 2003) and independently of TRPC6 and RhoA in certain cell types (Singh et al., 2007). Finally, receptors belonging to the TRPV channel family have been found to inhibit *in vitro* glioma cell proliferation. In this regard, we have recently reported that TRPV2 mRNA was expressed in benign astrocyte tissues, and its expression progressively declined in high-grade glioma tissues as histological grade increased. TRPV2 negatively controls glioblastoma survival and proliferation. In U87 glioma cells, silencing of TRPV2 by RNA interference (siRNA) affects several genes controlling cell cycle and proliferation (Nabissi et al., 2010). Down-regulation of CD95/Fas and parallel up-regulation of CCNE1, CDK2, E2F1, Raf-1 gene expression was observed in siTRPV2-U87 glioma cells as respect to controls. Moreover, TRPV2 knock-out increased glioblastoma proliferation and survival in an ERK-dependent manner. Inhibition of ERK activation by treatment of siRNA-TRPV2 U87 glioma cells with the specific MEK-1 inhibitor PD98059, promoted Fas expression and restored Akt/PKB pathway activation leading to reduced cell survival and proliferation (Nabissi et al., 2010). Conversely, TRPV2 transfection of primary MZC glioblastoma cells also reduced glioma viability and proliferation (Nabissi et al., 2010).

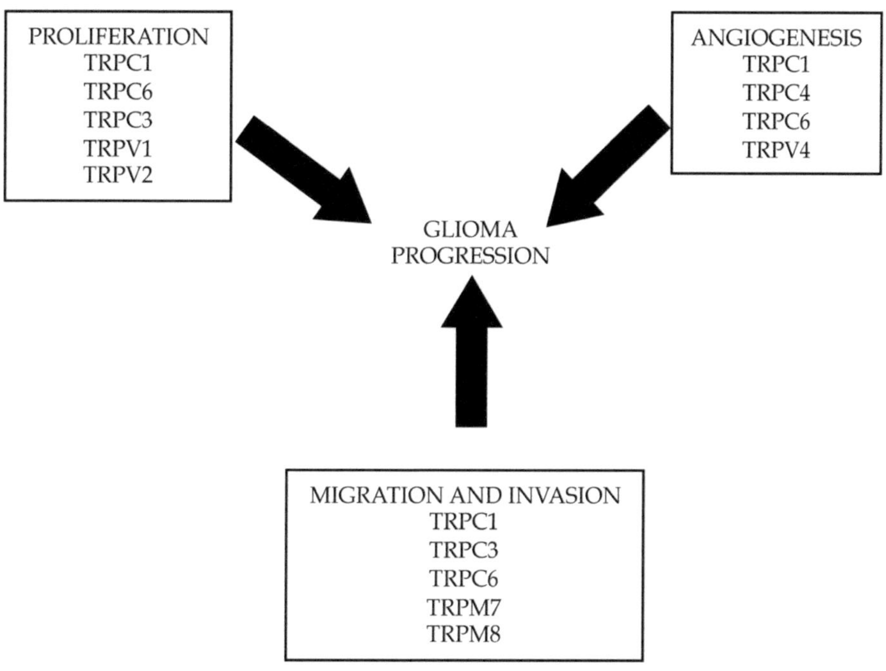

Fig. 2. TRP and glioma progression. In each square are represented the members of the TRP family, that are involved in the main processes driving glioma progression.

3. Role of TRPC and TRPV channels in hypoxia-induced angiogenesis of human gliomas: Role for VEGF and angiopoietin-1

Tumor microvessels are highly tortuous with sluggish flow and diminished gradient for oxygen delivery and increased susceptibility to thrombosis and microhemorragies. The

GBM microvasculature provides little support in oxygen/nutrient delivery, paradoxically contributing to exacerbate a metabolic mismatch between supply and demand leading to progressive hypoxia and eventually necrosis. In addition with the poor vascular architecture, endothelial cells associated with tumor vasculature fail to form tight junctions and have few associated pericytes or astrocytic foot processes leaving the integrity of the brain blood barrier compromised. This process requires that endothelial cells respond to a variety of extracellular signals that activate receptors responsible for growth and differentiation. VEGF (Vascular Endothelial Growth Factor), and Angiopoietin are key molecules in the promotion of angiogenesis via activation of the VEGFR (VEGF Receptor), and Tyrosine kinase with immunoglobulin-like and EGF-like domains 1 (TIE) expressed on vascular endothelial cells (Lutsenko et al., 2003). The Ca(2+) is another important second messenger and its entry through plasma membrane affects the angiogenesis. VEGF causes an increase in intracellular Ca(2+) concentration in cultured endothelial cells (Criscuolo et al., 1989) through both intracellular Ca(2+) release and extracellular Ca(2+) entry (Brock et al., 1991; Faehling et al., 2001; Wu et al., 1999; Cheng et al., 2006) and up-regulates vascular permeability (Criscuolo et al., 1988). Many of its physiological functions are dependent on Ca(2+) influx (Kawasaki et al., 2000; Faehling et al., 2002) through a store-independent mechanism (Pocock et al., 2000). Vascular permeability has been shown to be dependent on calcium influx, possibly through a TRPC-mediated channels. In particular, recent data indicate that TRPC6 represent an obligatory component of cation channels required for the VEGF-mediated increase in cytosolic calcium and subsequent downstream signaling that leads to processes associated with angiogenesis. The TRPC6 channel can be activated by VEGF. Overexpression of a dominant negative TRPC6 construct in human microvascular endothelial cells (HMVECs) inhibited the VEGF-mediated increase in cytosolic calcium, migration, sprouting, and proliferation. In contrast, overexpression of a wild-type TRPC6 construct increased the proliferation and migration of HMVECs (Hamdollah Zadeh et al., 2008). Inhibition of TRPC6 in HUVECs by pharmacological or genetic approaches arrested HUVECs at G2/M phase and suppressed VEGF-induced HUVEC proliferation and tube formation. Furthermore, inhibition of TRPC6 abolished VEGF-, but not FGF-induced angiogenesis in the chick embryo chorioallantoic membrane (Ge et al., 2009). Reduced oxygen availability (hypoxia) in the surrounding brain tissue is a major driving force behind GBM angiogenesis, and the low oxygen environment in the brain is positively related to GBM aggressiveness and poor prognosis (Hockel & Vaupel, 2001). The role of Hif-1α in tumor growth and invasion is well established (Semenza, 2003). Hif-1α protein was undetectable or low in glioma cells under normoxic conditions but increased markedly under hypoxia. Similarly, Notch1 activity was low in glioma cells but was elevated after the hypoxic switch. In addition to Notch1, other components of the Notch pathway were increased in glioma cells after the hypoxic switch. Specifically, the levels of Jagged-1 protein were increased under hypoxia. The molecular signals that link tissue hypoxia, Hif-1α activation to tumor angiogenesis are poorly understood. In glioma cells, the expression of TRPC6 is low or undetectable. Hypoxia by inducing Notch1 activation, increases TRPC6 expression in primary GBM and cell lines derived from GBM. Knockdown of TRPC6 expression inhibits glioma angiogenesis. Moreover, pharmacologic inhibition of Notch blocked the hypoxia-induced upregulation of TRPC6. The induction of TRPC6 expression in gliomas was TRPC subtype specific because other members of TRPC subfamily were unaffected. Although

Notch signaling is critical for TRPC6 upregulation, it remains to be determined whether the Notch pathway directly or indirectly, through cross-talk with other transcription factors (Gustafsson et al., 2005; Song et al., 2008), regulates TRPC6 transcription. TRPC6 activity is increased with EGFR activation (Odell et al., 2005), suggesting a link between growth factor response to tumor growth, and angiogenesis. Functionally, TRPC6 causes a sustained elevation of intracellular calcium that is coupled to the activation of the calcineurin-nuclear factor of activated T-cell (NFAT) pathway. Pharmacologic inhibition of the calcineurin-NFAT pathway substantially reduces hypoxia-induced glioma progression (Mosieniak et al., 1998; Chigurupati et al., 2010). The activation of TRPC6 by Galphaq induces RhoA activation and increased $[Ca(2+)]_i$ that stimulate thrombin-induced increase of actinomyosin-mediated endothelial cell contraction, cell shape change and consequently increased endothelial permeability. Inhibitor of Galphaq or phospholipase C and the Ca(2+) chelator, BAPTA-AM, abrogated thrombin-induced RhoA activation. By contrast, activation of TRPC6 by oleoyl-2-acetyl-sn-glycerol (OAG), the membrane permeable analogue of the Galphaq-phospholipase C product, diacylglycerol, induced RhoA activity. Receptor-operated Ca(2+) activation was mediated by TRPC6. Thus, TRPC6 knockdown significantly reduced Ca(2+) entry and prevented RhoA activation, myosin light chain phosphorylation, and actin stress fiber formation as well as inter-endothelial junctional gap formation in response to either OAG or thrombin (Singh et al., 2007). Lysophosphatidylcholine (lysoPC) has been also found to induce a rapid translocation of TRPC6 in endothelial cells, that triggeres calcium influx resulting in externalization of TRPC5. Activation of this novel TRPC6-TRPC5 channel cascade by lysoPC, inhibits endothelial cell migration. TRPC5 siRNA down-regulates the lysoPC-induced rise in $[Ca(2+)]_i$ and reverts the inhibition of EC migration (Chaudhuri et al., 2008), suggesting a negative role played by this channel in the regulation of EC migration. Finally, the phosphatase and tensin homologue (PTEN), has been found to serves as a scaffold for TRPC6 channel by enabling cell surface expression of the channel. Ca(2+) entry through TRPC6 induces an increase in endothelial permeability and directly promotes angiogenesis (Kini et al., 2010) (Fig 3). PTEN is a dual lipid-protein phosphatase that catalyzes the conversion of phosphoinositol 3,4,5-triphosphate to phosphoinositol 4,5-bisphosphate and thereby inhibits PI3K-Akt-dependent cell proliferation, migration, and tumor vascularization. Recently, a PTEN phosphatase-independent mechanism in regulating Ca(2+) entry through TRPC6 has been reported. PTEN tail-domain residues 394-403 permit PTEN to associate with TRPC6, and thrombin promotes this association. Deletion of PTEN residues 394-403 prevents TRPC6 cell surface expression and Ca(2+) entry (Kini et al., 2010). Other TRPC channels have been found to be involved in glioma angiogenesis. Studies in zebrafish, have demonstrated that the involvement of TRPCs channels in angiogenesis represents a reminiscent of the role of TRPC channels in axon guidance (Yu et al., 2010). Activation of TRPC1 seems to be essential for the angiogenesis *in vivo*. Knockdown of TRPC1 by antisense oligonucleotides severely disrupted angiogenic sprouting of intersegmental vessels (ISVs). *In vivo* time-lapse imaging revealed that the angiogenic defect was attributable to impairment of filopodia extension, migration, and proliferation of ISV tip cells. TRPC1 acts synergistically with VEGFA in controlling ISV growth, and appeared to be downstream to VEGFA in controlling angiogenesis (Yu et al., 2010). Recently a role for TRPC1 in hypoxia-induced VEGF expression in U87 glioma cells has been reported. TRPC1 siRNA markedly inhibits hypoxia-induced up-regulation of

VEGF mRNA and protein levels (Wang et al., 2009). TRPC1-dependent Ca(2+) influx induced by VEGF also increases endothelial permeability. Angiopoietin-1 (Ang1) that exerts a vascular endothelial barrier protective effect by blocking the action of permeability-increasing mediators such as VEGF, inhibited the VEGF-induced Ca(2+) influx and increased the endothelial permeability in a concentration-dependent manner. Ang1 interfered with downstream IP3-dependent plasmalemmal Ca(2+) entry. Anti-TRPC1 antibody (Ab) inhibited the VEGF-induced Ca(2+) entry and the increased endothelial permeability. TRPC1 overexpression in endothelial cells augmented the VEGF-induced Ca(2+) entry, and application of Ang1 opposed this effect. Consistent with the coupling hypothesis of Ca(2+) entry, Ang1 by inhibiting the association of IP3 receptor (IP3R) and TRPC1, abrogates the increase in endothelial permeability (Jho et al., 2005). Although the previously reported study has been focused on Ang1 regulation of TRPC1 activation, we cannot rule out the involvement of other relevant TRPC channels. TRPC4 acts as a functional homologue in mouse endothelia to TRPC1 in humans (Nilius et al., 2003; Tiruppathi et al., 2002). For agonist-induced Ca(2+) entry in mouse aortic endothelial cells, TRPC4 was essential as either a channel-forming subunit or a constituent required for channel activation (Freichel et al., 2001). Because TRPC1 and TRPC4 can oligomerize (Hofmann et al., 2002), it is possible that both may be needed for the VEGF-induced Ca(2+) entry. The importance of TRPC4 in regulation of endothelial permeability in mice has been reinforced by the observations that the effects of Ang1 on VEGF-induced Ca(2+) entry and permeability were mimicked by deletion of the TRPC4 gene in mice (Tiruppathi et al., 2002). Finally, VEGF-induced activation of Ca(2+) entry can also occur via TRPC6 which is activated by PLC-generated DAG (Pocock et al., 2001, 2004). TRPC4 has been also found to control thrombospondin-1 (TSP-1) secretion and angiogenesis in renal cell carcinoma (RCC) (Veliceasa et al., 2007). TRPC4 loss has been lead to impaired Ca(2+) intake, misfolding, retrograde transport and diminished secretion of antiangiogenic TSP-1, thus enabling angiogenic switch during RCC progression. TRPC4 has been recently reported to be expressed in glioma cells (Wang et al., 2009), however at present no data on the role of this channel in the inhibition of glioma angiogenesis has been provided so far. Membrane-stretch activated TRPV calcium channels have been known to mediate the orientation of endothelial cells lining blood vessels thus influencing the angiogenesis. So, TRPV4 channels expressed in the plasma membrane of capillary endothelial cells is required for mechanical-induced changes in focal adhesion assembly, cell orientation and directional migration. Recent reports indicate that activation of the mechanosensitive TRPV4 in capillary endothelial cells, stimulates phosphatidylinositol 3-kinase-dependent activation and binding of additional β1 integrin receptors, which promotes cytoskeletal remodeling and cell reorientation. Inhibition of integrin activation using blocking Abs and knock-down of TRPV4 using siRNA, suppress capillary cell reorientation. Activation of TRPV4 channels by force transfer from integrins and CD98 may enable compartmentalization of calcium signaling within focal adhesions. This early-immediate calcium signaling response required the distal region of the β1 integrin cytoplasmic tail that contains a binding site for the integrin-associated transmembrane CD98 protein, and application of external force to CD98 within focal adhesions activated the same ultra-rapid calcium signaling response (Matthews et al., 2010). Thus, mechanical forces that physically deform extracellular matrix (ECM) guide capillary cell reorientation through an "integrin-to-integrin" signaling mechanism mediated by activation of mechanically gated TRPV4 channels on the cell surface (Thodeti et al., 2009). We have recently reported the expression of TRPV4 channels in glioma cell lines (Santoni et al., 2011), however the potential role of TRPV4 in the migration of endothelial cells during glioma angionenesis is at present unknown.

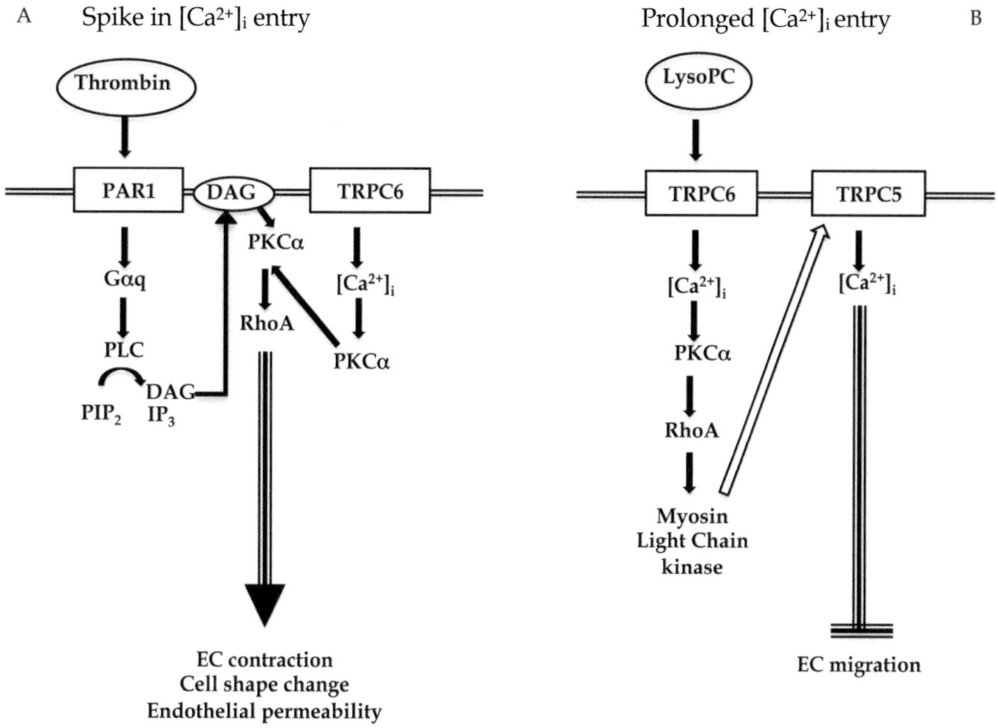

Fig. 3. Different modes of TRPC6 activation and cellular response, in glioma cells A) Spike in $[Ca^{2+}]_i$ entry induces endothelial cell (EC) contraction, cell shape and permeability; B) while prolonged $[Ca^{2+}]_i$ entry by LysoPC-induced TRPC6 activation inhibits EC migration.

4. TRPC and TRPM channels stimulate glioma cell migration and invasion

Glioblastoma multiforme is extremely invasive and consequently the clinical prognosis for patients is dismal. Invasion by glioma cells into regions of normal brain is driven by a multifactorial process involving cell interactions with ECM and with adjacent cells, as well as accompanying biochemical processes supportive of proteolytic degradation of ECM, and active cell movements (Bomben et al., 2010). These processes bear a striking resemblance to the robust inherent migration potential of glial cells during embryogenesis. Invasion and migration of glial tumors differ from other tumors where local spread is very limited and dissemination occurs hematogenously or via the lymphatic system. As they spread and form metastasis, glioma cells migrate through the narrow extracellular brain spaces often following the path of nerve fiber or blood vessels. Invading glioma cells commonly assume an elongated spindle-shaped morphology, suggesting that the cells have shrunk to fit into the narrow space into the brain (Sontheimer, 2008). Several studies have focused on the understanding of different molecular mechanisms expressed by invading tumor cells. Gliomas utilize a number of proteins and pathways to infiltrate the brain parenchyma including ion channels and calcium signaling pathways. Ion channels have recently involved in glioma invasion as a means to control cell volume or regulating Ca(2+) signaling pathways in invasive cells. Calcium signaling has been shown to play important roles in glioma cell invasion (Komuro & Kumada, 2005). Cell shrinkage by adaptation of cell size and volume to fit into narrow spaces is a prerequisite for cell movement and migration. Most immature cells that can migrate are well equipped to accumulate and release intracellular ions to shrink. How cell movement and invasion are coupled to the controlled activation of Ca(2+) channels is only partially understood (Mcferrin & Sontheimer, 2006). In glioma cells, invasion appears to involve a coordinated reduction in cell volume, which is mediated by the efflux of Cl^- and K^+ through ion channels. The Cl^- efflux is accompanied by the movement of K^+ ions. The principal pathway for K^+ efflux from glioma cells appears to be via Ca(2+)-activated bradykinin (BK) channels, which have the unique ability to couple changes in intracellular Ca(2+) to changes in membrane K^+ conductance and are expressed highly in glioma cells (Ransom & Sontheimer, 2001). In glioma cells, migration is accompanied by oscillatory changes in intracellular Ca(2+) in response to different stimuli (Grimaldi et al., 2003), which activate BK K^+ channels, and the velocity of cell migration of glioma cells correlates with oscillatory changes in intracellular Ca(2+) concentration (Bordey et al., 2000). Among ion channels contributing to Ca(2+) signaling, cytoskeleton changes, movement and migration, the TRPM and TRPC channel families seem to play an important role. Thus, triggering of TRPM8 by the specific agonist, menthol (Wondergem & Bartley, 2009), as TRPC3 and TRPC6 (Kim et al., 2009) increases glioma cell $[Ca(2+)]_i$ that in turn activates BK channels. Thus. TRP-mediated activation of Ca(2+) influx appears to be the prerequisite for cell migration and this Ca(2+) signal is instructive with regards to cell volume changes that occur down-stream. Cell shape, adhesion and migration have been regulated by actomyosin contractility. TRPM7-like transcripts current has been identified in rat microglia (Jiang et al., 2003). TRPM7 plays a role in linking receptor-mediated signals to actomyosin remodelling and cell adhesion. Activation of TRPM7 by BK, leads to a Ca(2+) and kinase-dependent interaction with the actomyosin cytoskeleton. Overexpression of TRPM7, by increasing the intracellular Ca(2+) levels resulted in cell spreading, adhesion and formation of focal adhesions (Clark et al., 2006). The effects of TRPM7 on cell morphology is directly dependent on integrin activation or is associated to increase in cytosolic Ca(2+) concentrations that affect the actomyosin cytoskeleton. The integrin activation can lead to the remodeling of the actomyosin cytoskeleton that promotes cell spreading via outside-in signaling pathways. Alternatively, Ca(2+) is an important second messenger in actin remodeling including polymerization, severing of filaments and F-actin–membrane interactions. The TRPC channels play a role in store-operated calcium entry (SOCE), and in particular TRPC1 is involved in SOCE in glioma cells (Bomben & Sontheimer, 2010). TRPC1-dependent migration and chemotaxis have been reported in different cell types such as myoblasts (Louis et al., 2008), renal epithelial (Fabian et al., 2008) and nervous cells (Wang & Poo, 2005) (Fig.2). Recently, (Bomben & Sontheimer, 2010) showed that TRPC1 channel association with lipid rafts is essential for glioma chemotaxis in response to stimuli, such as EGF, but not chemokinesis. EGF stimulation affects both TRPC trafficking (Bezzerides et al., 2004) and activation (Beech, 2005; Liu et al., 2009), and TRPC1 channel localization to the leading edge of migrating glioma cells. TRPC1 channels co-localize with the lipid raft proteins, caveolin-1. Chemotaxis toward EGF was lost when TRPC channels were pharmacologically inhibited or by shRNA knock-down of TRPC1 channels, yet without affecting unstimulated cell motility. Lipid raft integrity was required for gliomas chemotaxis; thus disruption of lipid rafts not only impaired chemotaxis but also impaired TRPC currents and decreased store-operated calcium entry. TRPC6 is markedly up-regulated under hypoxia in a manner dependent on Notch activation. The Notch-regulated transcriptional targets that are responsible for the development of the aggressive and malignant phenotypes in GBM remain poorly characterized. Notch signaling mediates hypoxia-induced tumor migration and invasion under hypoxic environment (Sahlgren et al., 2008). TRPC6 has been found to markedly inhibited glioma cell migration and invasion in response to hypoxia by regulating actin cytoskeleton assembling and disassembling which control cell shape, allowing the cell to move along the surface. The last step of invasion requires cytoskeletal rearrangements and formation of lamillipodia and fillopodia for which the family of Rho GTPases plays an important role. Most Rho proteins, cycle between GTP-bound active and GDP-bound inactive state. From the family members, Rho stimulates formation of stress fibres and focal adhesion, Rac is required for the formation of lamellipodia and Cdc42 regulates cell polarity and fillopodia formation (Teodorczyk & Martin-Villalba, 2009). A role for TRPC6 in Rho activation and actin cytoskeleton rearrangements has been suggested (Albert & Large, 2003). The TRPC6-mediated Ca(2+) entry may contribute to invasion by promoting actin-myosin interactions and the formation and disassembly of cell-substratum adhesions that are important for glioma migration (Kim & Saffen, 2005). Moreover, a role for TRPC3 activation has been also proposed. Thus, Ca(2+) entry in type I astrocytes and rat C6 glioma cells induced by OAG was InsP3-independent and inhibited by a TRPC3 antisense (Grimaldi et al., 2003). In addition, TRPC3 is functionally involved in Ca(2+) entry and thrombin stimulated morphological changes (cell rounding) induced by PAR-1 activation in 1321N1 human astrocytoma cells (Nakao et al., 2008). Finally, GBM cells express TRPM8 mRNA and protein, and its involvement in menthol and hepatocyte growth factor/scatter factor (HGF/SF) increase of $[Ca(2+)]_i$ and glioma cell migration has been reported (Wondergem et al., 2008). Menthol a TRPM8 agonist, stimulated influx of Ca(2+), membrane current, and migration of human glioblastoma DBTRG cells. The effects on Ca(2+) and migration were enhanced by pre-treatment with HGF/SF. The effects on Ca(2+) also were greater in migrating cells compared with non-migrating cells. 2-Aminoethoxydiphenyl borate inhibited all menthol stimulations. In addition, menthol, by increasing $[Ca(2+)]_i$, in human glioblastoma cells, resulted in activation of the large-conductance Ca(2+)-activated K+ membrane ion channels (BK channels). Kinetic analysis showed that menthol increased channel open probability and mean open frequency after 5 min, and this increase was abolished either by added paxilline, tetraethylammonium ion or by Ca(2+)-free external solution. In addition, inhibition of BK channels by paxillin reverses menthol-stimulated increase of $[Ca(2+)]_i$ and cell migration. Finally, menthol stimulated the rate of DBTRG cell migration into scratch wounds made in confluent cells, and this also was inhibited by paxilline or tetraethylammonium ion (Wondergem & Bartley, 2009). Invasion and metastasis are biologic hallmarks of malignant tumour. The invasion of ECM requires active degradation of ECM components. Tumour cells themselves secrete proteolytic enzymes (metalloproteinases, MMPs) or induce host cells to elaborate proteases (Pluda, 1997; Price et al., 1997; Liotta & Kohn, 1997). Glioma cells secrete MMPs to degradate the ECM surrounding invading cells (Levicar et al., 2003). In this regard, cannabidiol (CBD) has been found to impair the migration of U87 glioma cells in a cannabinoid receptor-independent manner (Vaccani et al., 2005), by increasing the tissue inhibitor of MMP1, (TIMP-1) (Ramer et al., 2010) and down-regulating the MMP-2 expression (Blazquez et al., 2008). Since CBD represents a specific ligand for TRPV2 (Qin et al., 2008), and being TRPV2 downregulated in the more invasive malignat gliomas (Nabissi et al., 2010), activation of this channel may represent an important target in anti-invasive chemotherapeutic strategy in GBM patients.

5. TRPV and TRPM channels trigger cell death in human glioma cells

Members of the TRPV and TRPM channels have been found to regulate apoptotic and necrotic cell death processes, respectively, as well as resistance to apoptotic stimuli in glioblastoma cells. In this regard, a role for TRPV1 in the apoptosis of glioma cells has been reported (Amantini et al., 2007). Thus, TRPV1 mRNA and protein expression was evidenced in normal astrocytes and glioma cells and tissues (Contassot et al., 2004; Amantini et al., 2007). TRPV1 expression inversely correlated with glioma grading, with a marked loss of TRPV1 expression in the majority of grade IV glioblastoma tissues. In addition, TRPV1 activation by the synthetic ligand, capsaicin (CPS) induced apoptosis of U373 glioma cells, and involved rise of Ca(2+) influx, p38MAPK activation, mitochondrial permeability transmembrane pore opening and transmembrane potential dissipation and caspase-3 activation (Amantini et al., 2007). Similarly, an other TRPV1 agonist, arachidonylethanolamide (AEA) induces apoptosis of human glioma cells in a TRPV1-dependent-manner (Contassot et al., 2004). Resistance of cancer cells to chemotherapeutic-induced cytotoxicity during tumor progression partially depends by a decrease sensitivity to CD95/Fas-induced apoptosis (Amantini et al., 2009). Induction of cell death by some cytotoxic drugs seems to depend to an intact Fas/FasL system. Tumour progression by exerting selective pressure alters Fas status and subsequently affects the sensitivity of cancer cells to chemotherapy (Sindhwani et al., 2001). Glioblastoma cells are resistant to Fas-induced cell death. We have recently reported that TRPV2 negatively controls glioblastoma survival as well as resistance to Fas/CD95-induced apoptosis in an ERK-dependent manner. Silencing of TRPV2 by RNA interference (siRNA) in U87 glioma cells down-regulated Fas/CD95 and procaspase-8 expression, and up-regulated Bcl-X_L mRNA expression. Moreover, TRPV2 siRNA increased glioblastoma survival to Fas/CD95-induced apoptosis in an ERK-dependent manner (Nabissi et al., 2010). Inhibition of ERK activation by treatment of the siRNA-TRPV2 U87 glioma cells with the specific MEK-1 inhibitor PD98059, reduced Bcl-X_L protein levels, promoted Fas/CD95 expression and restored Akt/PKB pathway activation leading to reduced cell survival and increased sensitivity to Fas/CD95-induced apoptosis (Nabissi et al., 2010). These events are consistent with previous evidence showing that PI3K pharmacological inhibitors inhibited calcium overload and cell death in TRPV2-transfected mouse cells (Penna et al., 2006). Consistently, TRPV2 transfection of the primary MZC glioblastoma cells also reduced glioma viability and increased spontaneous and Fas/CD95-induced apoptosis, by inducing Fas/CD95 expression (Nabissi et al., 2010). Among TRPM channels, a role for the Ca(2+) permeable TRPM2 channel in glioma cell death has been reported. Thus, insertion of TRPM2 in human A172 glioma cells enhanced cell death induced by H_2O_2 (Ishi et al., 2007).

6. TRP channels as cross-road of deregulated transcriptional activity in glioma stem like-cells

Evidence that malignant gliomas may arise from and contain a minority tumour cells with stem cell-like (GSCs) properties has been increased by the demonstration that GSCs maintain the potential for self-renewal and multi-lineage differentiation that recap the phenotype of the original glioma (Galli et al., 2004; Singh et al., 2003; Yuan et al., 2004), Since GSCs has been suggested to play an important role in glioma initiation, growth, and recurrence, it is extremely important to understand the signal pathways that contribute to their formation and maintenance, with the future aims to eliminate GSCs from the bulk tumor mass as a therapeutic strategy (Reya et al., 2001). Recent evidences adscript an emergent role of TRP channels in regulating neurogenesis (Tai et al., 2009) as well as neural differentiation (Shin et al., 2010), suggesting that deregulation of specific TRP target genes may be involved in gliomagenesis (Van Meir et al., 2010; Liu et al., 2010). In this regard, the expression of TRPV2 in normal neural stem/progenitor cells (NS/PC) from olfactory bulb and GSC lines derived from GBM patients, and a role of this TRP channel in the regulation of cellular proliferation and differentiation, have been observed (Nabissi et al., personal communication). Stem cells proliferation is maintained by a balance between proliferative and antiproliferative signals and any genetic or biochemical modifications that lead stem cells to become independent of growth signals, could induce an uncontrolled proliferation and possible tumorogenesis (Li & Neaves, 2006). GSCs divide core regulatory pathways with normal neural stem cells (NPSs), sharing developmental programs that lead NSCs to differentiate into astrocytes, oligodendrocytes and neurons (Galli et al., 2004; Singh et al., 2003), but induce in GSCs an aberrant differentiation (Cheng et al., 2010). GSCs are reported to express CD133 and nestin and to differentiate into cells expressing neuronal or glial cell markers upon growth factor depletion (Gunther et al., 2008). In addition to these NSC characteristics, glioma-derived neurospheres or CD133+ cells are tumorigenic and when transplanted into SCID mice formed secondary tumors with phenotypic and cytogenetic similarities to the patient tumor from which they were originally derived (Singh et al., 2003; Lee et al., 2006). Recent findings in GSCs demonstrated that the upregulation of classical pathways associated with neural development, as Notch, WNT, Hedgehog and TGFβ/BMT pathways (Clark et al., 2007; Silver & Steindler, 2009), induce in GSC-derived GBMs an invasive, angiogenetic, proliferative and chemoresistant phenotype (Sanai et al., 2005). So, modulation of these pathways may represent novel therapeutic approach for GBM. Notch is a family of hetero-dimeric transmembrane receptors composed of an extracellular domain responsible for ligand recognition, a transmembrane domain, and an intracellular domain involved in transcriptional regulation (Stockhausen et al., 2010). Notch proteins (and ligands)contain extracellular EGF-like repeats, which interact with the DSL domain of ligands. Activation of Notch upon ligand binding is accompanied by proteolytic processing that releases an intracellular domain of Notch (NICD) from the membrane tether. The NICD contains the RAM23 domain (RAM), which enhances interaction with the CSL protein, NLS (Nuclear Localization Signals), a CDC10/Ankyrin repeat domain ANK, which mediates interactions with CSL and other proteins, and a PEST domain rich in proline, glutamate, serine and threonine residues (Kopan, 2002). When Notch receptor is triggered by the ligands on the neighboring cells, the intracellular domain of the Notch receptor (NICD) is released from the membrane, after successive proteolytic cleavages by the γ-secretase complex. NICD then translocates into the nucleus and associates with the transcription factor RBP-J. This complex by secruiting other co-activators, stimulates the expression of downstream genes as Cyclin-D1, EGFR, and MAPK (Mitogen-Activated Protein Kinase) inducing cell proliferation, angiogenesis and chemoresistance, in GSCs (Stockhausen et al., 2010). Regarding the role of Notch signaling in GBM, gene microarray analysis have demonstrated that its expression in brain tumors correlated with good versus poor prognosis (Phillips et al., 2006). Moreover, in GBM tissue samples, high expression of Notch signal has been associated with high nestin levels, suggesting a correlation between GSCs and Notch expression (Purow et al., 2005; Lino et al.,2010; Boulay et al., 2007; Shih & Holland, 2006). Infact, Notch signaling plays a pivotal role in the maintenance of NSCs and leads to GSC-driven brain tumor development (Lino et al., 2010; Louvi & Artavanis-

Tsakonas, 2006). Recently, has been demonstrated that Notch activation is increased during hypoxia and hypoxia direct GBM to the development of an aggressive phenotype and resistance to radiation and chemotherapy (Flynn et al., 2008). Regarding the relationship between Notch signaling and TRP channels, a direct correlation has been demonstrated in human glioma cell lines where TRPC6 transcripts have been found to be increased under hypoxic condition and the involvement of Notch in hypoxia-induced TRPC6 expression in glioma has been demonstrated. Silencing of Notch1 gene inhibits TRPC6 expression suggesting that Notch1 is required for hypoxia-induced TRPC6 over-expression (Chigurupati et al., 2010). In response to hypoxia, the hypoxia inducing factors (HIF1-α and HIF-2α) are stabilized and as a consequence VEGF and TGFα are up-regulated (Birlik et al., 2006). Moreover, hypoxia-induced endothelial cell proliferation is associated with an increase of AP-1 expression, elevated store-operated calcium entry, and enhanced TRPC4 expression (Fantozzi et al., 2003), suggesting that additional TRP channels may regulate angiogenic signals (Fig.4). The interplay between GSCs and the endothelial compartement seems to be critical in gliomagenesis. Thus, GSCs closely interacting with the endothelial cells in vascular niche, promote angiogenesis through VEGF release (Bao et al., 2006a; Folkins et al., 2009). GSCs are reported to express CD133

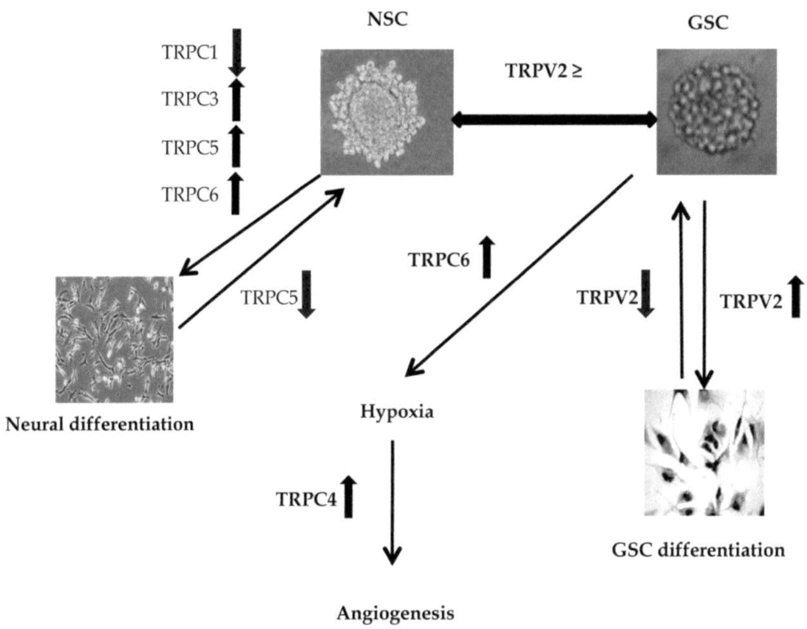

Fig. 4. The putative role of TRP channels in neural and glioma stem cell-like differentiation and angiogenesis. A schematic representation of different TRP members involved in the regulation of neuro- and glioma-genesis

and nestin (Yuan et al., 2004; Gunther et al., 2008) and have been demonstrated to have multipotent differentiative potential (Galli et al., 2004; Singh et al., 2003). Several authors have hypothesized that $CD133^+$ tumor stem cells are the source of the recurrent tumors after treatment (Chua et al., 2008; Bleau et al., 2009) and the $CD133^+$ cell population was enriched after radiation or chemotherapy and exhibited an increase in DNA repair capacity (Bao et al., 2006b). A series of pathways, including the Sonic hedgehog (Shh) and Notch, have been shown to be implicated in glioma's resistance to alkylating agents and/or the maintenance of brain tumor stem cells (Ulasov et al., 2011; Clement et al., 2007). Moreover, overexpression of *Dkk-1*, a gene encoding for a Wnt antagonist protein, has been shown to sensitize the U87 glioma cells to the cytotoxic effects of bis-chloronitrosourea (BCNU) and cisplatin (Shou et al., 2002). In this regard, an inverse correlation between TRPV2 and SHH and Notch pathways (Phillips et al., 2006; Nabissi et al., 2010) in regulating chemoresistance to the alkylating agent bis-chloronitrosourea (BCNU), can be supposed. TRPV2 expression progressively declined in high-grade glioma tissues as histological grade increased, while Notch and SHH signaling was activated in GBM. Knockdown of TRPV2 gene in gliomas increased the resistance to BCNU cytotoxicity which was associated with Ras/MEK/Erk and Akt overexpression in chemosensitive glioma cells, while TRPV2 overexpression augmented the chemosensitivity of resistant glioma cells to BCNU. In addition, down-regulation of TRPV2 reduced Fas expression and Fas-mediated apoptosis (Nabissi et al., 2010). Parallelely, upregulation of Notch 1, increased the resistance of glioma cell to apoptosis (Purow et al., 2005). Finally, forced Notch 1 overexpression in glioma cells increased the proliferation and the formation of nestin-positive, neurosphere-forming stem cells (Zhang et al., 2008). Overall, these data suggest that in gliomas, TRPV2 could be a downstream gene target of Notch signaling rescuing glioma cells to apoptosis and promoting cell proliferation.

7. Conclusions and prospectives

In this chapter, we have summarized current basic and translational changes and highlight the striking scientific advances regarding the expression and the function of the TRP channel family in glioma growth and progression, that promise to improve the clinical course of this lethal disease. These include a more comprensive view of the interplay between changes in TRP channel expression and functions (e.g., TRPC, TRPM and TRPV family) and alterations in transcriptional and growth factor pathways (e.g., Notch, PTEN, HIF-α, EGFR) driving the uncontrolled cellular proliferation, aberrant angiogenesis, intense migration and invasion, increased resistance to apoptosis. Clearly, the identification of cluster of TRP ion channels altered during glioma progression presents an opportunity for improving the understanding of this cancer. The progress and depth of understanding of the role of ion channels, including the TRP family in glioma, together with truly manipulable experimental models, now offer a real opportunities for the development of effective target therapy (Santoni & Farfariello, 2011). Despite significant gaps in our understanding, a wealth of information now exists about clinical and biological behaviour of these tumours, the genetic pathways involved in gliomagenesis and the nature and the role of their alterations. The challenge is now to integrate all of this knowledge in an interdisciplinary way to full understand this disease and how its heterogenicity contributes to the relatively poor therapeutic responses of GBM patients. In regard to stem cell issue, the fact that the glioma-like stem cells (GSCs) that play an important role in the development and recurrence of malignat glioma, not only express TRP channels, but also show functional alterations in their expression and transcriptional regulation, combined with the evidence that they displayed nearly identical Ca(2+) transients and pharmacological sensitivities to TRP channel antagonists (Nabissi et al., personal communication; Weick et al., 2009), may offer a new target for regulating GSC proliferation and developing novel therapeutic strategies. We are only at the begin of a new story; further studies on the expression and function of TRP channels in gliomas and GSCs must to be required to understand their contribute to malignant transformation and tumour progression, to delivery a specific target therapy in this devastating disease.

8. References

Albert, A.P. & Large, W.A. (2003). Synergism between inositol phosphates and diacylglycerol on native TRPC6-like channels in rabbit portal vein myocytes. *The Journal of Physiology*, Vol. 552, No. 3, pp. 789-795, ISSN 0022-3751

Amantini, C., Mosca, M., Nabissi, M., Lucciarini, R., Caprodossi, S., Arcella, A., Giangaspero, F. & Santoni, G. (2007). Capsaicin-induced apoptosis of glioma cells is mediated by TRPV1 vanilloid receptor and requires p38 MAPK activation. *Journal of Neurochemistry*, Vol. 102, No. 3, pp. 977–990, ISSN 0022-3042

Amantini, C., Ballarini, P., Caprodossi, S., Nabissi, M., Morelli, M.B., Lucciarini, R., Cardarelli, M.A., Mammana, G. & Santoni, G. (2009). Triggering of Transient Receptor Potential Vanilloid Type 1 (TRPV1) by Capsaicin induces Fas/CD95-mediated apoptosis of urothelial cancer cells in an ATM-dependent manner. *Carcinogenesis*, Vol. 30, No. 8, pp. 1320-1329, ISSN 0143-3334

Bao, S., Wu, Q., McLendon, R.E., Hao, Y., Shi, Q., Hjelmeland, A.B., Dewhirst, M.W., Bigner, D.D. & Rich, J.N. (2006b). Glioma stem cells promote radioresistance by preferential activation of the DNA damage response. *Nature*, Vol. 444, No. 7120, pp. 756-760, ISSN 0028-0836

Bao, S., Wu, Q., Sathornsumetee, S., Hao, Y., Li, Z., Hjelmeland, A.B., Shi, Q., McLendon, R.E., Bigner, D.D. & Rich, J.N. (2006a). Stem cell-like glioma cells promote tumor angiogenesis through vascular endothelial growth factor. *Cancer Research*, Vol. 66, No. 16, pp. 7843-7848, ISSN 0008-5472

Barajas, M., Andrade, A., Hernandez-Hernandez, O., Felix, R. & Arias-Montaño, J.A. (2008). Histamine-induced Ca2+ entry in human astrocytoma U373 MG cells: evidence for involvement of store-operated channels. *Journal of Neuroscience Research*, Vol. 86, No. 15, pp. 3456-3468, ISSN 0360-4012

Beech, D.J. (2005). TRPC1: store-operated channel and more. *Pflügers Archiv*, Vol. 451, No. 1, pp. 53-60, ISSN 0031-6768

Bement, W.M., Miller, A.L. & von Dassow, G. (2006). Rho GTPase activity zones and transient contractile arrays. *Bioessays*, Vol. 28, No. 10, pp.983-993, ISSN 0265-9247

Bezzerides, V.J., Ramsey, I.S., Kotecha, S., Greka, A. & Clapham, D.E. (2004). Rapid vesicular translocation and insertion of TRP channels. *Nature Cell Biology*, Vol. 6, No. 8, pp. 709-720, ISSN 1465-7392

Bidaux, G., Flourakis, M., Thebault, S., Zholos, A., Beck, B., Gkika, D., Roudbaraki, M., Bonnal, J.L., Mauroy, B., Shuba, Y., Skryma, R. & Prevarskaya, N. (2007). Prostate cell differentiation status determines transient receptor potential melastatin member 8 channel subcellular localization and function. *Journal of Clinical Investigation*, Vol. 117, No. 6, pp. 1647–1657, ISSN 0021-9738

Birlik, B., Canda, S. & Ozer, E. (2006). Tumour vascularity is of prognostic significance in adult, but not paediatric astrocytomas. *Neuropathology and Applied Neurobiology*, Vol. 32, No. 5, pp. 532-538, ISSN 0305-1846

Blázquez, C., Carracedo, A., Salazar, M., Lorente, M., Egia, A., González-Feria, L., Haro, A., Velasco, G. & Guzmán, M. (2008). Down-regulation of tissue inhibitor of metalloproteinases-1 in gliomas: a new marker of cannabinoid antitumoral activity? *Neuropharmacology*, Vol. 54, No. 1, pp. 235-243, ISSN 0952-2638

Bleau, A.M., Hambardzumyan, D., Ozawa, T., Fomchenko, E.I., Huse, J.T., Brennan, C.W. & Holland, E.C. (2009). PTEN/PI3K/Akt pathway regulates the side population phenotype and ABCG2 activity in glioma tumor stem-like cells. *Cell Stem Cell*, Vol. 4, No. 3, pp. 226-235, ISSN 1934-5909

Bomben, V.C. & Sontheimer, H. (2010). Disruption of Transient Receptor Potential Canonical Channel 1 causes incomplete cytokinesis and slows the growth of human malignant gliomas. *Glia*, Vol. 58, No. 10, pp. 1145-1156, ISSN 1098-1136

Bomben, V.C. & Sontheimer, H.W. (2008). Inhibition of transient receptor potential canonical channels impairs cytokinesis in human malignant gliomas. *Cell Proliferation*, Vol. 41, No. 1, pp. 98-121, ISSN 0960-7722

Bomben, V.C., Turner, K.L., Barclay, T.C. & Sontheimer, H. (2010). Transient Receptor Potential Canonical Channels are Essential for Chemotactic Migration of Human Malignant Gliomas. *Journal of Cellular Physiology* [Epub ahead of print], ISSN 1097-4652

Bordey, A., Sontheimer, H. & Trouslard, J. (2000). Muscarinic activation of BK channels induces membrane oscillations in glioma cells and leads to inhibition of cell migration. *Journal of Membrane Biology*, Vol. 176, No. 1, pp. 31-40, ISSN 0022-2631

Boulay, J.L., Miserez, A.R., Zweifel, C., Sivasankaran, B., Kana, V., Ghaffari, A., Luyken, C., Sabel, M., Zerrouqi, A., Wasner, M., Van Meir, E., Tolnay, M., Reifenberger, G. & Merlo, A. (2007). Loss of NOTCH2 positively predicts survival in subgroups of human glial brain tumors. *PLoS One*, Vol. 2, No. 6, pp. e576, ISSN 1932-6203

Brock, T.A., Dvorak, H.F. & Senger, D.R. (1991). Tumor-secreted vascular permeability factor increases cytosolic Ca^{2+} and von Willebrand factor release in human endothelial cells. *American Journal of Pathology*, Vol. 138, No. 1, pp. 213–221, ISSN 0002-9440

Bryant, J.A., Finn, R.S., Slamon, D.J., Cloughesy, T.F. & Charles, A.C. (2004). EGF activates intracellular and intercellular calcium signaling by distinct pathways in tumor cells. *Cancer Biology & Therapy*, Vol. 3, No. 12, pp. 1243-1249, ISSN 1538-4047

Buchholz,M. & Ellenrieder, V. (2007). An emerging role for Ca2+/calcineurin/NFAT siognaling in cancerogenesis. *Cell Cycle*, Vol. 6, No. 1, pp.16-19; ISSN 1551-4005

Butowiski, N.A., Sneed, P.K. & Chang, S.M. (2006). Diagnosis and treatment of recurrent high-grade astrocytoma. *Journal of Clinical Oncology*, Vol. 24, No. 8, pp. 1273-1280, ISSN 0732-183

Caprodossi, S., Lucciarini, R., Amantini, C., Nabissi, M., Canesin, G., Ballarini, P., Di Spilimbergo, A., Cardarelli, M.A., Servi, L., Mammana, G. & Santoni, G. (2008). Transient receptor potential vanilloid type 2 (TRPV2) expression in normal urothelium and in urothelial carcinoma of human bladder: correlation with the pathologic stage. *European Urology*, Vol. 54, No. 3, pp. 612–620, ISSN 0302-2838

Chaudhuri, P., Colles, S.M., Bhat, M., Van Wagoner, D.R., Birnbaumer, L. & Graham, L.M. (2008). Elucidation of a TRPC6-TRPC5 channel cascade that restricts endothelial cell movement. *Molecular Biology of the Cell*, Vol. 19, No. 8, pp. 3203-3211, ISSN 1059-1524

Cheng, H.W., James, A.F., Foster, R.R., Hancox, J.C. & Bates, D.O. (2006). VEGF activates receptor-operated cation channels in human microvascular endothelial cells.

Arteriosclerosis, Thrombosis, and Vascular Biology , Vol. 26, No. 8, pp. 1768–1776, ISSN 10795642

Cheng, L., Bao, S. & Rich, J.N. (2010). Potential therapeutic implications of cancer stem cells in glioblastoma. *Biochemical Pharmacology,* Vol. 80, No. 5, pp. 654-665, ISSN 0006-2952

Chigurupati, S., Venkataraman, R., Barrera, D., Naganathan, A., Madan, M., Paul, L., Pattisapu, J.V., Kyriazis, G.A., Sugaya, K., Bushnev, S., Lathia, J.D., Rich, J.N. & Chan, S.L. (2010). Receptor Channel TRPC6 Is a Key Mediator of Notch-Driven Glioblastoma Growth and Invasiveness. *Cancer Research,* Vol. 70, No. 1, pp. 418-427, ISSN 0008-5472

Chua, C., Zaiden, N., Chong, K.H., See, S.J., Wong, M.C., Ang, B.T. & Tang, C. (2008). Characterization of a side population of astrocytoma cells in response to temozolomide. *Journal of Neurosurgery,* Vol. 109, No. 5, pp. 856-866, ISSN 0022-3085

Clark, K., Langeslag, M., van Leeuwen, B., Ran, L., Ryazanov, A.G., Figdor, C.G., Moolenaar, W.H., Jalink, K. & van Leeuwen, F.N. (2006). TRPM7, a novel regulator of actomyosin contractility and cell adhesion. *The EMBO Journal,* Vol. 25, No. 2, pp. 290-301, ISSN 1469-221X

Clark, P.A., Treisman, D.M., Ebben, J. & Kuo, J.S. (2007). Developmental signaling pathways in brain tumor-derived stem-like cells. *Developmental Dynamics,* Vol. 236, No. 12, pp. 3297-3308, ISSN 1097-0177

Clement, V., Sanchez, P., de Tribolet, N., Radovanovic, I. & Ruiz i Altaba, A. (2007). HEDGEHOG-GLI1 signaling regulates human glioma growth, cancer stem cell self-renewal, and tumorigenicity. *Current Biology,* Vol. 17, No. 2, pp. 165-172, ISSN 0960-9822

Contassot, E., Wilmotte, R., Tenan, M., Belkouch, M.C., Schnüriger, V., de Tribolet, N., Burkhardt, K. & Dietrich, P.Y. (2004). Arachidonylethanolamide induces apoptosis of human glioma cells through vanilloid receptor-1. *Journal of Neuropathology & Experimental Neurology,* Vol. 63, No. 9, pp. 956–963, ISSN 0022-3069

Criscuolo, G.R., Lelkes, P.I., Rotrosen, D. & Oldfield, E.H. (1989). Cytosolic calcium changes in endothelial cells induced by a protein product of human gliomas containing vascular permeability factor activity. *Journal of Neurosurgery,* Vol. 71, No. 6, pp. 884-891, ISSN 0022-3050

Criscuolo, G.R., Merrill, M.J. & Oldfield, E.H. (1988). Further characterization of malignant glioma-derived vascular permeability factor. *Journal of Neurosurgery,* Vol. 69, No. 2, pp. 254-262, ISSN 0022-3050

Ding, X., He, Z., Zhou, K., Cheng, J., Yao, H., Lu, D., Cai, R., Jin, Y., Dong, B., Xu, Y. & Wang, Y. (2010). Essential role of TRPC6 channels in G2/M phase transition and development of human glioma. *Journal of the National Cancer Institute,* Vol. 102, No. 14, pp. 1052-1068, ISSN 0027-8874

Duncan, L.M., Deeds, J., Hunter, J., Shao, J., Holmgren, L.M., Woolf, E.A., Tepper, R.I. & Shyjan, A.W. (1998). Down-regulation of the novel gene melastatin correlates with potential for melanoma metastasis. *Cancer Research,* Vol. 58, No. 7, pp. 1515–1520, ISSN 0008-5472

Eggert, U.S., Mitchinson, T.J. & Field, C.M. (2006). Animal cytokinesis: from parts list to mechanism. *Annual Review of Biochemistry,* Vol. 75, pp. 543-566, ISSN 0066-4154

Fabian, A., Fortmann, T., Dieterich, P., Riethmuller, C., Schon, P., Mally, S., Nilius, B. & Schwab, A. (2008). TRPC1 channels regulate directionality of migrating cells. *Pflügers Archives,* Vol. 457, No. 2, pp. 475-484, ISSN 0031-6768

Faehling, M., Koch, E.D., Raithel, J., Trischler G. & Waltenberger, J. (2001). Vascular endothelial growth factor-A activates Ca^{2+}-activated K^+ channels in human endothelial cells in culture. *The International Journal of Biochemistry & Cell Biology*, Vol. 33, No. 4, pp. 337–346, ISSN 1357-2725

Faehling, M., Kroll, J., Fohr, K.J., Fellbrich, G., Mayr, U., Trischler, G. & Waltenberger, J. (2002). Essential role of calcium in vascular endothelial growth factor A-induced signaling: mechanism of the antiangiogenic effect of carboxyamidotriazole. *The FASEB Journal*, Vol. 16, No. 13, pp. 1805–1807, ISSN 0892-6638

Fantozzi, I., Zhang, S., Platoshyn, O., Remillard, C.V., Cowling, R.T. & Yuan, J.X. (2003). Hypoxia increases AP-1 binding activity by enhancing capacitative Ca2+ entry in human pulmonary artery endothelial cells. *American Journal of Physiology Lung Cellular and Molecular Physiology*, Vol. 285, No. 6, pp. L1233-1245, ISSN 1522-1504

Flynn, J.R., Wang, L., Gillespie, D.L., Stoddard, G.J., Reid, J.K., Owens, J., Ellsworth, G.B., Salzman, K.L., Kinney, A.Y. & Jensen, R.L. (2008). Hypoxia-regulated protein expression, patient characteristics, and preoperative imaging as predictors of survival in adults with glioblastoma multiforme. *Cancer*, Vol. 113, No. 5, pp. 1032-1042, ISSN 1097-0142

Folkins, C., Shaked, Y., Man, S., Tang, T., Lee, C.R., Zhu, Z., Hoffman, R.M. & Kerbel, R.S. (2009). Glioma tumor stem-like cells promote tumor angiogenesis and vasculogenesis via vascular endothelial growth factor and stromal-derived factor 1. *Cancer Research*, Vol. 69, No. 18, pp. 7243-7251, ISSN 0008-5472

Freichel, M., Suh, S.H., Pfeifer, A., Schweig, U., Trost, C., Weissgerber, P., Biel, M., Philipp, S., Freise, D., Droogmans, G., Hofmann, F., Flockerzi, V. & Nilius, B. (2001). Lack of an endothelial store-operated Ca2+ current impairs agonist-dependent vasorelaxation in TRP4–/– mice. *Nature Cell Biology*, Vol. 3, No. 2, pp. 121–127, ISSN 1465-7392

Furnari, F.B., Fenton, T., Bachoo, R.M., Mukasa, A., Stommel, J.M., Stegh, A., Hahn, W.C., Ligon, K.L., Louis, D.N., Brennan, C., Chin, L., DePinho, R.A. & Cavenee, W.K. (2007). Malignant astrocytic glioma: genetics, biology, and paths to treatment. *Genes & Devevelopment*, Vol. 21, No. 21, pp. 2683-2710, ISSN 0890-9369

Galli, R., Binda, E., Orfanelli, U., Cipelletti, B., Gritti, A., De Vitis, S., Fiocco, R., Foroni, C., Dimeco, F. & Vescovi, A. (2004). Isolation and characterization of tumorigenic, stem-like neural precursors from human glioblastoma. *Cancer Research*, Vol. 64, No. 19, pp. 7011-21, ISSN 0008-5472

Ge, R., Tai, Y., Sun, Y., Zhou, K., Yang, S., Cheng, T., Zou, Q., Shen, F. & Wang, Y. (2009). Critical role of TRPC6 channels in VEGF-mediated angiogenesis. *Cancer Letters*, Vol. 283:, No. 1, pp. 43–51, ISSN 0304-3835

Gkika, D. & Prevarskaya, N. (2009). Molecular mechanisms of TRP regulation in tumor growth and metastasis. *Biochimica et Biophysica Acta*, Vol. 1793, No. 6, pp. 953–958, ISSN 0304-4165

Glotzer, M. (2005). The molecular requirements for cytokinesis. *Science*, Vol. 307, No. 5716, pp.1735-1739, ISSN 0036-8075

Grimaldi, M., Maratos, M. & Verma, A. (2003). Transient receptor potential channel activation causes a novel form of [Ca 2+]I oscillations and is not involved in capacitative Ca 2+ entry in glial cells. *Journal of Neuroscience*, Vol. 23, No. 11, pp. 4737-4745, ISSN 0270-6474

Gunther, H.S., Schmidt, N.O., Phillips, H.S., Kemming, D., Kharbanda, S., Soriano, R., Modrusan, Z., Meissner, H., Westphal, M. & Lamszus, K. (2008). Glioblastoma-derived stem cell-enriched cultures form distinct subgroups according to molecular and phenotypic criteria. *Oncogene,* Vol. 27, No. 20, pp. 2897-2909, ISSN 0950-9232

Gustafsson, M.V., Zheng, X., Pereira, T., Gradin, K., Jin, S., Lundkvist, J., Ruas, J.L., Poellinger, L., Lendahl, U. & Bondesson, M. (2005). Hypoxia requires notch signaling to maintain the undifferentiated cell state. *Developmental Cell,* Vol. 9, No. 5, pp. 617–628, ISSN 1534-5807

Hamdollah Zadeh, M.A., Glass, C.A., Magnussen, A., Hancox, J.C. & Bates, D.O. (2008). VEGF-mediated elevated intracellular calcium and angiogenesis in human microvascular endothelial cells in vitro are inhibited by dominant negative TRPC6. *Microcirculation,* Vol. 15, No. 7, pp. 605–614, ISSN 1549-8719

Höckel, M. & Vaupel, P. (2001). Biological consequences of tumor hypoxia. *Seminars in Oncology,* Vol.28, No.2 Suppl8, pp. 36–41, ISSN 0093-7754

Hofmann, T., Schaefer, M., Shultz, G. & Gudermann, T. (2002). Subunit composition of mammalian transient receptor potential channels in living cells. *Proceedings of the National Academy of Sciences of the United States of America,* Vol. 99, No. 11, pp. 7461–7466, ISSN 0027-8424

Huncharek, M. & Muscat, J. (1998). Treatmentbof recurrent high grade astrocytoma; results of a systematic review of 1,415 patients. *Anticancer Research,* Vol. 18, No. 2B, pp.1303-1311, ISSN 0250-7005

Ishii, M., Oyama, A., Hagiwara, T., Miyazaki, A., Mori, Y., Kiuchi, Y. & Shimizu, S. (2007). Facilitation of H2O2-induced A172 human glioblastoma cell death by insertion of oxidative stress-sensitive TRPM2 channels. *Anticancer Research,* Vol. 27, No. 6B, pp. 3987-3992, ISSN 0250-7005

Jho, D., Mehta, D., Ahmmed, G., Gao, X.P., Tiruppathi, C., Broman, M. & Malik, A.B. (2005). Angiopoietin-1 opposes VEGF-induced increase in endothelial permeability by inhibiting TRPC1-dependent Ca_2 influx. *Circulation Research,* Vol. 96, No. 12, pp. 1282–1290, ISSN 0009-7330

Jiang, X., Newel, E.W. & Schlichter, L.C. (2003). Regulation of a TRPM7-like current in rat brain microglia. *Journal of Biological Chemistry,* Vol. 278, No. 44, pp. 42867-42876, ISSN 0021-9258

Kanamori, M., Kawaguchi, T., Nigro, J.M., Feuerstein, B.G., Berger, M.S., Miele, L. & Pieper, R.O. (2007). Contribution of Notch signaling activation to human glioblastoma multiforme. *Journal of Neurosurgery,* Vol. 106, No. 3, pp. 417–427, ISSN 0022-3085

Kawasaki, J., Hirano, K., Hirano, M., Nishimura, J., Nakatsuka, A., Fujishima, M. & Kanaide, H. (2000). Dissociation between the $Ca^{(2+)}$ signal and tube formation induced by vascular endothelial growth factor in bovine aortic endothelial cells. *European Journal of Pharmacology,* Vol. 398, No. 1, pp. 19–29, ISSN 0014- 2999

Kim, J.Y. & Saffen, D. (2005). Activation of M1 muscarinic acetylcholine receptors stimulates the formation of a multiprotein complex centered on TRPC6 channels. *Journal of Biological Chemistry,* Vol. 280, No. 36, (September 2005), pp. 32035-47, ISSN 0021-9258

Kim, E.Y., Alvarez-Baron, C.P. & Dryer, S.E. (2009). Canonical transient receptor potential channel (TRPC)3 and TRPC6 associate with large-conductance Ca2+-activated K+ (BKCa) channels: role in BKCa trafficking to the surface of cultured podocytes. *Molecular Pharmacology,* Vol. 75, No. 3, pp. 466-477, ISSN 0026-895X

Kini, V., Chavez, A. & Mehta, D. (2010). A new role for PTEN in regulating transient receptor potential canonical channel 6-mediated Ca2+ entry, endothelial permeability, and angiogenesis. *Journal of Biological Chemistry*, Vol. 285, No. 43, pp. 33082-33091, ISSN 0021-9258

Kiselyov, K., Soyombo, A. & Muallem, S. (2007). TRPpathies. *The Journal of Physiology*, Vol. 578, No. 3, pp. 641–653, ISSN 0022-3751

Komuro, H. & Kumada, T. (2005). Ca2+ transients control CNS neuronal migration. *Cell Calcium*, Vol. 37, No. 5, pp. 387-393, ISSN 0143-4160

Kopan, R. (2002). Notch: a membrane-bound transcription factor. *Journal of Cell Science*, Vol. 115, No. 6, pp. 1095-1097, ISSN 0021-9533

Kunzelmann, K. (2005). Ion channels and cancer. *Journal of Membrane Biology*, Vol. 205, No. 3, pp. 159-173, ISSN 0022-2631

Kuwahara, K., Wang, Y., McAnally, J., Richardson, J.A., Bassel-Duby, R., Hill, J.A. & Olson, E.N. (2006). TRPC6 fulfills a calcineurin signaling circuit during pathologic cardiac remodeling. *Journal of Clinical Investigation*, Vol. 116, No. 12, pp. 3114-3126, ISSN 0021-9738

Kuwahara, M. & Kuwahara, M. (2006). Store-mediated calcium entry in pleural mesothelial cells. *European Journal of Pharmacology*, Vol. 542, No. 1-3, pp. 16-21, ISSN 0014- 2999

Lee, J., Kotliarova, S., Kotliarov, Y., Li, A., Su, Q., Donin, N.M., Pastorino, S., Purow, B.W., Christopher, N., Zhang, W., Park, J.K. & Fine, H.A. (2006). Tumor stem cells derived from glioblastomas cultured in bFGF and EGF more closely mirror the phenotype and genotype of primary tumors than do serum-cultured cell lines. *Cancer Cell*, Vol. 9, No. 5, pp. 391-403, ISSN 1535-6108

Levicar, N., Nuttall, R.K. & Lah, T.T. (2003). Proteases in brain tumour progression. *Acta Neurochirurgica*, Vol. 145, No. 9, pp. 825-838, ISSN 0001-6268

Li, L. & Neaves, W.B. (2006). Normal stem cells and cancer stem cells: the niche matters. *Cancer Research*, Vol. 66, No. 9, pp. 4553-4557, ISSN 0008-5472

Lino, M.M., Merlo, A. & Boulay, J.L. (2010). Notch signaling in glioblastoma: a developmental drug target? *BMC Medicine*, Vol. 8, pp. 72, ISSN 1741-7015

Liotta, L.A. & Kohn, E.C. (1997). Invasion and metastasis. In: *Cancer Medicine 4th ed.*, Holland, J.F., Bast, R.C.J., Morton, D.L., Frei, III E., Kufe, D.W. & Weichselbaum, R.R. (Ed.), pp. 165-180, Williams & Wilkins, ISBN 0-683-04095-2, Baltimore

Lipskaia, L. & Lompré, A.M. (2004). Alteration in temporal kinetics of Ca2+ signaling and control of growth and proliferation. *Biology of the Cell*, Vol. 96, No. 1, pp. 55-68, ISSN 0248-4900

Liu, D., Yang, D., He, H., Chen, X., Cao, T., Feng, X., Ma, L., Luo, Z., Wang, L., Yan, Z., Zhu, Z. & Tepel, M. (2009). Increased transient receptor potential canonical type 3 channels in vasculature from hypertensive rats. *Hypertension*, Vol. 53, No. 1, pp. 70-76, ISSN 0263-6352

Liu, Y., Shete, S., Hosking, F., Robertson, L., Houlston, R. & Bondy, M. (2010). Genetic advances in glioma: susceptibility genes and networks. *Current Opinion in Genetics & Development*, Vol. 20, No. 3, pp. 239-44, ISSN 0959-437X

Louis, M., Zanou, N., Van Schoor, M. & Gailly, P. (2008). TRPC1 regulates skeletal myoblast migration and differentiation. *Journal of Cell Science*, Vol. 121, pp. 23-29, ISSN 0021-9533

Louvi, A. & Artavanis-Tsakonas, S. (2006). Notch signalling in vertebrate neural development. *Nature Reviews Neuroscience*, Vol. 7, No. 2, pp. 93-102, ISSN 1471-0048

Lutsenko, S.V., Kiselev, S.M. & Severin, S.E. (2003). Molecular mechanisms of tumor angiogenesis. *Biochemistry (Moscow)*, Vol. 68, No. 3, pp. 286-300, ISSN: 0006-2979

Malarkey, E.B., Ni, Y. & Parpura, V. (2008). Ca2+ entry through TRPC1 channels contributes to intracellular Ca2+ dynamics and consequent glutamate release from rat astrocytes. *Glia*, Vol. 56, No. 8, pp- 821-835, ISSN 1098-1136

Matthews, B.D., Thodeti, C.K., Tytell, J.D., Mammoto, A., Overby, D.R. & Ingber, D.E. (2010). Ultra-rapid activation of TRPV4 ion channels by mechanical forces applied to cell surface beta1 integrins. *Integrative Biology*, Vol. 2, No. 9, pp. 435-42, ISSN 0973-8363

Mcferrin, M.B. & Sontheimer, H. (2006). A role for ion channels in glioma cell invasion. *Neuron Glia Biology*, Vol. 2, No. 1, pp. 39-49, ISSN 1740-925X

Mehta, D., Ahmmed, G.U., Paria, B., Holinstat, M., Voyno-Yasenetskaya, T., Tiruppathi, C., Minshall, R.D. & Malik, A.B. (2003). RhoA interaction with inositol 1,4,5-trisphosphate receptor and transient receptor potential channel-1 regulates Ca2+ entry. Role in signaling increased endothelial permeability. *Journal of Biological Chemistry*, Vol. 278, No. 35, pp. 33492–33500, ISSN 0021-9258

Montell, C. (2003). Thermosensation: hot findings make TRPNs very cool. *Current Biology*, Vol. 13, No. 12, pp. R476–R478, ISSN 0960-9822

Mosieniak, G., Pyrzynska, B. & Kaminska, B. (1998). Nuclear factor of activated T cells (NFAT) as a new component of the signal transduction pathway in glioma cells. *Journal of Neurochemistry*, Vol. 71, No. 1, pp. 134-141, ISSN 0022-3042

Nabissi, M., Morelli, M.B., Amantini, C., Farfariello, V., Ricci-Vitiani, L., Caprodossi, S., Arcella, A., Santoni, M., Giangaspero, F., De Maria, R. & Santoni, G. (2010). TRPV2 channel negatively controls glioma cell proliferation and resistance to Fas-induced apoptosis in ERK-dependent manner. *Carcinogenesis*, Vol. 31, No. 5, pp. 794-803, ISSN 0143-3334

Nakao, K., Shirakawa, H., Sugishita, A., Matsutani, I., Niidome, T., Nakagawa, T. & Kaneko, S. (2008). Ca2+ mobilization mediated by transient receptor potential canonical 3 is associated with thrombin-induced morphological changes in 1321N1 human astrocytoma cells. *Journal of Neuroscience Research*, Vol. 86, No. 12, pp. 2722-2732, ISSN 0360-4012

Nilius, B., Droogmans, G. & Wondergem, R. (2003). Transient receptor potential channels in endothelium: solving the calcium entry puzzle? *Endothelium*, Vol. 10, No. 1, pp. 5–15, ISSN 1029-2373

Nilius, B., Owsianik, G., Voets, T. & Peters, J.A. (2007). Transient receptor potential cation channels in disease. *Physiological Reviews*, Vol. 87, No. 1, pp. 165–217, ISSN 0031-9333

Odell, A.F., Scott, J.L. & Van Helden D.F. (2005). Epidermal growth factor induces tyrosine phosphorylation, membrane insertion, and activation of transient receptor potential channel 4. *Journal of Biological Chemistry*, Vol. 280, No. 45, pp. 37974-37987, ISSN 0021-9258

Onohara, N., Nishida, M., Inoue, R., Kobayashi, H., Sumimoto, H., Sato, Y., Mori, Y., Nagao, T. & Kurose, H. (2006). TRPC3 and TRPC6 are essential for angiotensin II-induced cardiac hypertrophy. *EMBO Journal*, Vol. 25, No. 22, pp. 5305-5316, ISSN 1469-221X

Palma, L., Celli, P., Maleci, A., Di Lorenzo, N. & Cantore, G. (1989). Malignant monstrocellular brain tumours. A study of 42 surgically treated cases. *Acta Neurochirurgica*, Vol. 97, No. 1-2, pp. 17-25, ISSN 0001- 6268

Penna, A., Juvin, V., Chemin, J., Compan, V., Monet, M. & Rassendren, F.A. (2006). PI3-kinase promotes TRPV2 activity independently of channel translocation to the plasma membrane. *Cell Calcium*, Vol. 39, No. 6, pp. 495-507, ISSN 0143-4160

Phillips, H.S., Kharbanda, S., Chen, R., Forrest, W.F., Soriano, R.H., Wu, T.D., Misra, A., Nigro, J.M., Colman, H., Soroceanu, L., Williams, P.M., Modrusan, Z., Feuerstein, B.G. & Aldape, K. (2006). Molecular subclasses of high-grade glioma predict prognosis, delineate a pattern of disease progression, and resemble stages in neurogenesis. *Cancer Cell,* Vol. 9, No. 3, pp. 157-173, ISSN 1535-6108

Pluda, J.M. (1997). Tumor-associated angiogenesis: mechanisms, clinical implications, and therapeutic strategies. *Seminars in Oncology,* Vol. 24, No. 2, pp. 203-218, ISSN 0093-7754

Pocock, T.M., Williams, B., Curry, F.E. & Bates, D.O. (2000). VEGF and ATP act by different mechanisms to increase microvascular permeability and endothelial [Ca(2+)](i). *American Journal of Physiology Heart and Circulatory Physiology,* Vol. 279, No. 4, pp. H1625-1634, ISSN 0363-6135

Pocock, T.M. & Bates, D.O. (2001). In vivo mechanisms of vascular endothelial growth factor-mediated increased hydraulic conductivity of Rana capillaries. *The Journal of Physiology,* Vol. 534, No. 2, pp. 479–488, ISSN 0022-3751

Pocock, T.M., Foster, R.R. & Bates, D.O. (2004). Evidence of a role for TRPC channels in VEGF-mediated increased vascular permeability in vivo. *American Journal of Physiology Heart and Circulatory Physiology,* Vol. 286, No. 3, pp. H1015–H1026, ISSN 0363-6135

Prevarskaya, N., Zhang, L. & Barritt, G. (2007). TRP channels in cancer. *Biochimica and Biophysica,* Vol. 1772, No. 8, pp. 937–946, ISSN 0006-3002

Price, J.T., Bonovich, M.T. & Kohn, E.C. (1997). The biochemistry of cancer dissemination. *Critical Reviews in Biochemistry and Molecular Biology,* Vol. 32, No. 3, pp. 175–253, ISSN 1040-9238

Purow, B.W., Haque, R.M., Noel, M.W., Su, Q., Burdick, M.J., Lee, J., Sundaresan, T., Pastorino, S., Park, J.K., Mikolaenko, I., Maric, D., Eberhart, C.G. & Fine, H.A. (2005). Expression of Notch-1 and its ligands, Delta-like-1 and Jagged-1, is critical for glioma cell survival and proliferation. *Cancer Research,* Vol. 65, No. 6, pp. 2353-2363, ISSN 0008-5472

Qin, N., Neeper, M.P., Liu, Y., Hutchinson, T.L., Lubin, M.L. & Flores, C.M. (2008). TRPV2 is activated by cannabidiol and mediates CGRP release in cultured rat dorsal root ganglion neurons. *Journal of Neuroscience,* Vol. 28, No. 24, pp. 6231-6238, ISSN 0270-6474

Ramer, R., Merkord, J., Rohde, H. & Hinz, B. (2010). Cannabidiol inhibits cancer cell invasion via upregulation of tissue inhibitor of matrix metalloproteinases-1. *Biochemical Pharmacology,* Vol. 79, No. 7, pp. 955-966, ISSN 0006-2952

Ransom, C.B. & Sontheimer, H. (2001). BK channels in human glioma cells. *Journal of Neurophysiology,* Vol. 85, No. 2, pp. 790-803, ISSN 0022-3077

Reya, T., Morrison, S.J., Clarke, M.F. & Weissman, I.L. (2001). Stem cells, cancer, and cancer stem cells. *Nature,* Vol. 414, No. 6859, pp. 105-111, ISSN 0028-0836

Sahlgren, C., Gustafsson, M.V., Jin, S., Poellinger, L. & Lendahl, U. (2008). Notch signaling mediates hypoxia-induced tumor cell migration and invasion. *Proceedings of the National Academy of Sciences of the United States of America,* Vol. 105, No. 17, pp. 6392–6397, ISSN 0027-8424

Sanai, N., Alvarez-Buylla, A. & Berger, M.S. (2005). Neural stem cells and the origin of gliomas. *The New England Journal of Medicine,* Vol. 353, No. 8, pp. 811-822, ISSN 0028-4793

Santoni, G., Farfariello, V. & Amantini, C. (2011). TRPV Channels in Tumor Growth and Progression. *Advances in Experimental Medicine and Biology*, Vol. 704, pp. 947-967, ISSN 0065-2598

Santoni, G. & Farfariello, V. (2011). TRP Channels and Cancer: New Targets for Diagnosis and Chemotherapy. *Endocrine, Metabolic & Immune Disorders- Drug Targets*, Vol. 11, No. 1, pp. 54-57, ISSN 1871-5303

Schönherr, R. (2005). Clinical relevance of ion channels for diagnosis and therapy of cancer. *Journal of Membrane Biology*, Vol. 205, No. 3, pp. 175-184, ISSN 0022-2631

Schwartzbaum, J.A., Fischer, J.L., Aldape, K.D. & Wrensch,M. (2006). Epiodemiology and molecular pathology of glioma. *Nature Clinical Practice Neurology*, Vol. 2, No. 9, pp. 494-503, ISSN 1745-8358

Semenza, G.L. (2003). Targeting HIF-1 for cancer therapy. *Nature Reviews Cancer*, Vol. 3, No. 10, pp. 721–732, ISSN 1474-175X

Shih, A.H. & Holland, E.C. (2006). Notch signaling enhances nestin expression in gliomas. *Neoplasia*, Vol. 8, No. 12, pp. 1072-1082, ISSN 1522-8002

Shin, H.Y., Hong, Y.H., Jang, S.S., Chae, H.G., Paek, S.L., Moon, H.E., Kim, D.G., Kim, J., Paek, S.H. & Kim, S.J. (2010). A role of canonical transient receptor potential 5 channel in neuronal differentiation from A2B5 neural progenitor cells. *PLoS One*, Vol. 5, No. 5, pp. e10359, ISSN 1932-6203

Shirakawa, H., Nakagawa, T. & Kaneko, S. (2010). Pathophysiological roles of transient receptor potential channels in glial cells. *Yakugaku Zasshi*, Vol. 130, No. 3, pp. 281-287, ISSN 0031-6903

Shou, J., Ali-Osman, F., Multani, A.S., Pathak, S., Fedi, P. & Srivenugopal, K.S. (2002). Human Dkk-1, a gene encoding a Wnt antagonist, responds to DNA damage and its overexpression sensitizes brain tumor cells to apoptosis following alkylation damage of DNA. *Oncogene*, Vol. 21, No. 6, pp. 878-889, ISSN 0950-9232

Silver, D.J. & Steindler, D.A. (2009). Common astrocytic programs during brain development, injury and cancer. *Trends in Neurosciences*, Vol. 32, No. 6, pp. 303-311, ISSN 0166-2236

Sindhwaani, P., Hampton, J.A., Baig, M.M., Keck, R. & Selman, S.H. (2001). Curcumin prevents intravesical tumor implantation of the MBT-2 tumor cell line in C3H mice. *Journal of Urology*, Vol. 166, No. 4, pp. 1498-501, ISSN 0022-5347

Singh, I., Knezevic, N., Ahmmed, G.U., Kini, V., Malik, A.B. & Mehta, D. (2007). $G\alpha_q$-TRPC6-mediated Ca^{2+} Entry Induces RhoA Activation and Resultant Endothelial Cell Shape Change in Response to Thrombin. *The Journal of Biological Chemistry*, Vol. 282, No. 11, pp. 7833-7843, ISSN 0021-9258

Singh, S.K., Clarke, I.D., Terasaki, M., Bonn, V.E., Hawkins, C., Squire, J. & Dirks, P.B. (2003). Identification of a cancer stem cell in human brain tumors. *Cancer Research*, Vol. 63, No. 18, pp. 5821-5828, ISSN 0008-5472

Song, L.L., Peng, Y., Yun, J., Rizzo, P., Chaturvedi, V., Weijzen, S., Kast, W.M., Stone, P.J., Santos, L., Loredo, A., Lendahl, U., Sonenshein, G., Osborne, B., Qin, J.Z., Pannuti, A., Nickoloff, B.J. & Miele, L. (2008). Notch-1 associates with IKKα and regulates IKK activity in cervical cancer cells. *Oncogene*, Vol. 27, No. 44, pp. 5833–5844, ISSN 0950-9232

Sontheimer, H. (2008). An Unexpected Role for Ion Channels in Brain Tumor Metastasis. *Experimental Biology and Medicine (Maywood)*, Vol. 233, pp. 779-791, ISSN 1573-8221

Sontheimer, H. (2010). An unexpected role for ion channels in brain tumor metastasis. *Experimental Biology and Medicine*, Vol. 233, No. 7, pp. 779-791, ISSN 1535-3702

Stark, G.R. & Taylor, W.R. (2006). Control of the G2/M transition. *Molecular Biotechnology*, Vol. 32, No. 3, pp. 227-248, ISSN 1073-6085

Stockhausen, M.T., Kristoffersen, K. & Poulsen, H.S. (2010). The functional role of Notch signaling in human gliomas. *Neuro-Oncology*, Vol. 12, No. 2, pp. 199-211, ISSN 0167 -594X

Tai, Y., Feng, S., Du, W. & Wang, Y. (2009). Functional roles of TRPC channels in the developing brain. *Pflügers Archiv*, Vol. 458, No. 2, pp. 283-289, ISSN 0031-6768

Teodorczyk, M. & Martin-Villalba, A. (2009). Sensing Invasion: Cell Surface Receptors Driving Spreading of Glioblastoma. *Journal of Cellular Physiology*, Vol. 222, No. 1, pp. 1-10, ISSN 1097-4652

Thebault, S., Flourakis, M., Vanoverberghe, K., Vandermoere, F., Roudbaraki, M., Lehen'kyi, V., Slomianny, C., Beck, B., Mariot, P., Bonnal, J.L., Mauroy, B., Shuba, Y., Capiod, T., Skryma, R. & Prevarskaya, N. (2006). Differential role of transient receptor potential channels in Ca2+ entry and proliferation of prostate cancer epithelial cells. *Cancer Research*, Vol. 66, No. 4, pp. 2038–2047, ISSN 0008-5472

Thodeti, C.K., Matthews, B., Ravi, A., Mammoto, A., Ghosh, K., Bracha, A.L. & Ingber, D.E. (2009). TRPV4 channels mediate cyclic strain-induced endothelial cell reorientation through integrin-to-integrin signaling. *Circulation Research*, Vol. 104, No. 9, pp. 1123-30, ISSN 0009-7330

Tiruppathi, C., Freichel, M., Vogel, S.M., Paria, B.C., Mehta, D., Flockerzi, V. & Malik, A.B. (2002). Impairment of store-operated Ca2+ entry in TRPC4–/– mice interferes with increases in lung microvascular permeability. *Circulation Research*, Vol. 91, No. 1, pp. 70–76, ISSN 0009-7300

Tsavaler, L., Shapero, M.H., Morkowski, S. & Laus, R. (2001). Trp-p8, a novel prostate-specific gene, is up-regulated in prostate cancer and other malignancies and shares high homology with transient receptor potential calcium channel proteins. *Cancer Research*, Vol. 61, No. 9, pp. 3760–3769, ISSN 0008-5472

Ulasov, I.V., Nandi, S., Dey, M., Sonabend, A.M. & Lesniak, M.S. (2011). Inhibition of Sonic hedgehog and Notch pathways enhances sensitivity of CD133(+) glioma stem cells to temozolomide therapy. *Molecular Medicine*, Vol. 17, No. 1-2, pp. 103-112, ISSN 1076-1551

Vaccani, A., Massi, P., Colombo, A., Rubino, T. & Parolaro, D. (2005). Cannabidiol inhibits human glioma cell migration through a cannabinoid receptor-independent mechanism. *British Journal of Pharmacology*, Vol. 144, No. 8, pp. 1032-1036, ISSN 1476- 5381

Van Meir, E.G., Hadjipanayis, C.G., Norden, A.D., Shu, H.K., Wen, P.Y. & Olson, J.J. (2010). Exciting new advances in neuro-oncology: the avenue to a cure for malignant glioma. *CA Cancer Journal for Clinicians*, Vol. 60, No. 3, pp. 166-193, ISSN 0007-9235

Veliceasa, D., Ivanovic, M., Hoepfner, F.T., Thumbikat, P. Volpert, O.V. & Smith, N.D. (2007). Transient potential receptor channel 4 controls thrombospondin-1 secretion and angiogenesis in renal cell carcinoma. *FEBS Journal*, Vol. 274, No. 24, pp. 6365-6377, ISSN 1742-464X

Wang, G.X. & Poo, M.M. (2005). Requirement of TRPC channels in netrin-1-induced chemotropic turning of nerve growth cones. *Nature*, Vol. 434, No. 7035, pp. 898-904, ISSN 0028-0836

Wang, B., Li, W., Meng, X. & Zou, F. (2009). Hypoxia up-regulates vascular endothelial growth factor in U-87 MG cells: involvement of TRPC1. Neuroscience Letters ISSN 0304-3940

Weick, J.P., Austin Johnson, M. & Zhang, S.C. (2009). Developmental regulation of human embryonic stem cell-derived neurons by calcium entry via transient receptor potential channels. *Stem Cells*, Vol. 27, No. 12, pp. 2906-2916, ISSN 1549-4918

Wisnoskey, B.J., Sinkins, W.G. & Schilling, W.P. (2003). Activation of vanilloid receptor type 1 in the endoplasmic reticulum fails to activate store-operated Ca2+ entry. *Biochemical Journal*, Vol. 372, No. 2, pp. 517–528, ISSN 0264-6021

Wissenbach, U., Niemeyer, B.A., Fixemer, T., Schneidewind, A., Trost, C., Cavalie, A., Reus, K., Meese, E., Bonkhoff, H. & Flockerzi, V. (2001). Expression of CaT-like, a novel calcium-selective channel, correlates with the malignancy of prostate cancer. *Journal of Biological Chemistry*, Vol. 276, No. 22, pp. 19461–19468, ISSN 0021-9258

Wondergem, R. & Bartley, J.W. (2009). Menthol increases human glioblastoma intracellular Ca2+, BK channel activity and cell migration. *Journal of Biomedical Science*, Vol. 16, No. 1, pp. 90, ISSN 1021- 7770

Wondergem, R., Ecay, T.W., Mahieu, F., Owsianik, G. & Nilius, B. (2008). HGF/SF and menthol increase human glioblastoma cell calcium and migration. *Biochemical and Biophysical Research Communications*, Vol. 372, No. 1, pp. 210-215, ISSN 0006-291X

Wu, H.M., Yuan, Y., Zawieja, D.C., Tinsley, J. & Granger, H.J. (1999). Role of phospholipase C, protein kinase C, and calcium in VEGF-induced venular hyperpermeability. *American Journal of Physiology*, Vol. 276, No. 2, pp. H535–H542, ISSN 0363-6135

Xin, H., Tanaka, H., Yamaguchi, M., Takemori, S., Nakamura, A. & Kohama, K. (2005). Vanilloid receptor expressed in the sarcoplasmic reticulum of rat skeletal muscle. *Biochemical and Biophysical Research Communications*, Vol 332, No. 3, pp. 756–762, ISSN 0006-291X

Xu, X.Z., Moebius, F., Gill, D.L. & Montell, C. (2001). Regulation of melastatin, a TRP-related protein, through interaction with a cytoplasmic isoform. *Proceedings of the National Academy of Sciences of the United States of America*, Vol. 98, No. 19, pp. 10692–10697, ISSN 0027-8424

Yang, H., Mergler, S., Sun, X., Wang, Z., Lu, L., Bonanno, J.A., Pleyer, U. & Reinach, P.S. (2005). TRPC4 knockdown suppresses epidermal growth factor-induced store-operated channel activation and growth in human corneal epithelial cells. *Journal of Biological Chemistry* Vol. 280, No. 37, pp. 32230-32237, ISSN 0021-9258

Yu, P.C., Gu, S.Y., Bu, J.W. & Du, J.L. (2010). TRPC1 is essential for in vivo angiogenesis in zebrafish. *Circulation Research*, Vol. 106, No. 7, pp. 1221-1232, ISSN 0009-7330

Zhang, X.P., Zheng, G., Zou, L., Liu, H.L., Hou, L.H., Zhou, P., Yin, D.D., Zheng, Q.J., Liang, L., Zhang, S.Z., Feng, L., Yao, L.B., Yang, A.G., Han, H. & Chen, J.Y. (2008). Notch activation promotes cell proliferation and the formation of neural stem cell-like colonies in human glioma cells. *Molecular and Cellular Biochemistry*, Vol. 307, No. 1-2, pp. 101-108, ISSN 0300-8177

9

The Role of Stem Cells in the Glioma Growth

Sergio Garcia, Vinicius Kannen and Luciano Neder
Faculty of Medicine of Ribeirao Preto
University of Sao Paulo
Brazil

1. Introduction

Malignant glioma is the most common type of primary brain tumor and represents one of the most lethal cancers. In contrast to the long-standing and well-defined histopathology, the underlying molecular and genetic bases for gliomas are less known. (Collins, 2004; Dai & Holland, 2001).

As some other human cancers, particularly central nervous tumors are highly heterogeneous. Primarily because of its diffuse nature, relatively little is known about the processes by which they develop (Hulleman & Helin, 2005). Thus, the traditional evolution concept of tumors arising from a single mutated cell has limitations in explaining the heterogeneity observed in a single tumor nest.

Recent decades have seen only limited progress in treatment trials and basic research on human glioma, the most common central nervous malignancy (Huang et al., 2008). Unfortunately, for such gliomas, tumor recurrence after treatment is the rule due to the infiltrative nature of these tumors and the presence of cellular populations with ability to escape therapies and drive tumor recurrence and progression. At least in some cases, these resistant cells exhibit stem cell properties (Frosina, 2011). For these reasons the comprehension of the current knowledge of cancer stem cells (CSC) in relation to gliomas origin, growth and treatment is crucial. As the stem cells (for glioma, neuronal stem cells) are more susceptible to mutation, they become altered easily for their genetic composition and therefore act as the source of cancer/glioma cells. They are not actually a separate cell type and in most cases they are misinterpreted as cancer stem cells (in brain, they are glioma stem cells).

2. Glioma and the concept of cancer stem cells

For a long time it has been known that there are subpopulations of cells within solid tumors that contain different biological behaviors. Among these subpopulations, accumulating evidence supports the existence of the so-called cancer stem cells (CSCs), because these tumor cells possess stem cell properties, possibly being responsible for the initiation, growth and recurrence of tumors. Apparent similarities with non-transformed stem cells, including high self-renewal capacity and the ability to generate differentiated progeny of several cellular lineages, have led to the proposal that stem cell-like cancer cells may either originate from adult undifferentiated stem and progenitor cells or that these properties are being expressed as an effect of the genetic alterations which drive tumorigenicity (Reya et al., 2001; Gilbertson, 2006; Das et al., 2008). Basically, the CSCs, which have also been described as tumor initiating cells or tumor propagating cells, are tumor cells that self-renew and propagate tumors phenotypically similar to the parental tumor (Li et al., 2009). Furthermore, recent studies have suggested that CSC cause tumor recurrence based on their resistance to radiotherapy and chemotherapy (Inoue et al, 2010).

Although considerable controversy still surrounds the existence, behaviors and even the nomenclature of CSCs, there is no doubt that populations of cells with stem-like properties do exist inside several solid and non-solid tumors, including brain cancers. So, despite the fact that CSCs in solid tumors have not yet been precisely identified, the "CSC hypothesis" opens a new paradigm in understanding the biology of cancers. For this reason, the search for the tumor stem cells that may originate and perpetuate the tumor growth has been receiving great attention in the literature (Sanchez-Martin, 2008), but the available knowledge on this issue with regards to the gliomas is scant. Particularly, the exact identity and cell(s) of origin of the so-called glioma stem cell remains elusive (Park & Rich, 2009). Vescovi (2006) offered a functional definition of brain tumor stem cells, namely: brain tumor cells should qualify as stem cells if they show cancer-initiating ability upon orthotopic implantation, extensive self-renewal ability demonstrated either ex vivo or in vivo, karyotypic or genetic alterations, aberrant differentiation properties, capacity to generate non-tumorigenic end cells, and multilineage differentiation capacity. Furthermore, parallels between normal neurogenesis and brain tumorigenesis have been proposed (Singh et al., 2004). It has been more recently confirmed that cancer stem cells from glioblastomas share some characteristics with normal neural stem cells including the expression of neural stem cell markers, the capacity for self-renewal and long term proliferation, the formation of neurospheres, and the ability to differentiate into multiple nervous system lineages (astrocytic, oligodendrocytic and/or neuronal differentiation) (Li et al., 2009).

Among the so far evaluated stem cell markers, the transmembrane protein CD133 has been widely used to isolate putative CSC populations in several cancer types. In fact, CD133 is currently one of the best markers to characterize CSCs (Singh et al., 2004). In both human glioblastomas (GBMs) and medulloblastomas, the expression of the neural stem cell marker CD133 (also known as prominin 1) has been associated with both tumor initiation capacity and radioresistance (Pérez Castillo et al., 2008). Extensive computational comparisons with a compendium of published gene expression profiles revealed that the CD133 gene signature transcriptionally resembles human embryonic stem cells and in vitro cultured GBMs stem cells (GSC), and this signature successfully distinguishes GBMs from lower-grade gliomas. Moreover, the CD133 gene signature identifies an aggressive subtype of GBMs seen in younger patients with a shorter survival (Yan et al., 2011), confirming previous observations that Glioma stem cells are more aggressive in recurrent tumors (Huang et al., 2008). Nevertheless, it must be pointed out that the use of CD133 as a unique glioma stem cell marker is probably not sufficient to tag the whole self-renewing tumor cell reservoir (Clément et al., 2009).

Holmberg et al (2011) have recently characterized human gliomas in various malignancy grades according to the expression of stem cell regulatory proteins. These authors have shown that cells in high grade glioma co-express an array of markers defining neural stem cells (NSCs) and that these proteins can fulfill similar functions in tumor cells as in NSCs. In contrast to NSCs, the glioma cells co-express neural proteins together with pluripotent stem cell markers, including the transcription factors as Oct4, Sox2, Nanog and Klf4. In line with these findings, in high grade gliomas, mesodermal- and endodermal-specific transcription factors were detected together with neural proteins, a combination of lineage markers not normally present in the central nervous system. These findings demonstrate a general deregulated expression of neural and pluripotent stem cell traits in malignant human gliomas.

3. Stem cells and the origin of gliomas

Primarily because of the diffuse nature of gliomas, relatively little is known about the processes by which they develop (Hulleman & Helin, 2005). The concept of stem cells originating gliomas is gaining increased recognition in neuro-oncology (Richj & Eyler, 2008). Until recently, the paradigm of a tumor-initiating stem cell was confined to hematopoietic malignancies where the hierarchical lineages of stem progenitor cells are well established. Nevertheless, the demonstration of persistent stem cells and cycling progenitors in the adult brain is coupled with the expansion of the cancer stem cell concept to solid tumors, leading to the exploration of "stemness" within gliomas. Emerging data are highly suggestive of the subsistence of transformed multipotential cells within a glioma, with a subfraction of cells exhibiting increased efficiency at tumor initiation stage. However, data in support of the true glioma stem cells are inconclusive to date, particularly in respect to the functional characterization of these cells. (Panagiotakos & Tabar, 2007).

Thus, it may be considered that currently it is conceivable thought that malignant gliomas may arise from neural stem cells and appear to contain tumor stem cells. It is thought that normal stem cells live in protected pockets of the body called *niches*, where they divide infrequently to avoid accumulating damaging mutations. Upon injury or in response to normal stimuli, stem cells are mobilized to divide (Gilbertson, 2006). Hence, parallel to the role that normal stem cells play in organogenesis, stem cells are thought to be crucial for tumorigenesis.

The normal adult neural stem cells (NSCs) arise from radial glia (RG) within the central nervous system (Weiner, 2008). The RG progeny includes all the main lineages of the CNS: neurons, astrocytes, oligodendrocytes, ependymocytes and adult neural stem cells (Malatesta et al. 2003). By comparing the gene expression profiles of ependymomas with those of cells in the normal developing nervous system, it was possible to identify the RG as candidate stem cells of this brain tumor (Gilbertson, 2006). Furthermore, RG cells produce neurons in addition to glia during central nervous system development in all vertebrates and are also involved in reparative process (Weiner, 2008).

Until recently, it was thought that ependymomas originated from neuroepithelial cells, glioblastomas from abnormal astrocytes, and medulloblastomas from primitive cells in the external granular layer, but there is now evidence that all tumors can originate from a special type of stem cell called "radial glial cell" (RGC). It is interesting to note that in the human brain, most of stem cells are located in the subventricular zones (SVZ). Both supra- and infratentorially and when stimulated with carcinogens, cells in the SVZ become tumorigenic faster than those located elsewhere. In the SVZ, stem cells exist in the form of RGCs, which remain quiescent until they receive transformational signals. It is not clear whether RGCs, after receiving transformation signals, return to their initial stem cell configuration and then become tumorigenic or they transform to tumor progenitor cells

directly. In the cerebellum, depending upon the signals received, RGCs and stem cells may give origin to either ependymoma or medulloblastoma.
Tumours with the highest incidence in humans– medulloblastomas and glioblastomas – both originate from abnormal brain stem cells. . Not surprising, both of these tumors are CD133-positive, containing great neuronal differentiation, which makes them prone to be diffuse and resistant to treatment (Castilo, 2010).

4. Gliomas and the field cancerization concept

It is universally accepted that tumors growth as a clonal evolution from a single cell (Nowell, 1976). The "field cancerization theory" was introduced more than fifty years ago by Slaugher et al (1953), when studying the presence of histologically abnormal tissue surrounding carcinomas. In a classic report on oral cancer, Slaughter called "field cancerization" - a process of repeated exposure of a region's entire tissue area to carcinogenic insult (e.g., tobacco and alcohol), which increases the tissue's risk for developing multiple independent premalignant and malignant foci. The field cancerization hypothesis states that multiple cells form independent tumors on one given tissue, since carcinogenic exposure affects multiple cells in the field (Slaughter *et al.*, 1953), and predicts that second primary or synchronous tumours arise from independent genetic events (Garcia et al., 1999). The field cancerization theory may be explained by the concept that a given stem cell that acquires genetic alterations may form a "patch", a clonal unit of altered daughter cells. The proliferation of these patch cells forms expanding fields which gradually displace the normal tissue and, by clonal divergence, ultimately leads to the development of one or more tumors within a contiguous field of preneoplastic cells (Garcia et al., 1999). An important clinical implication is that fields often remain after surgery of the primary tumor and may lead to new cancers, designated presently by clinicians as "a second primary tumor" or "local recurrence," depending on the exact site and time interval (Braakhuis et al., 2003; Ryan, 2007). We had previously discussed how mutated clones from mutated stem cells may spread on tissues and that the field cancerization theory implies that the mutated genotype and molecular changes occur before the appearance of histopathological evidence of malignant cells (Garcia et al., 1999). Therefore, this "anomaly" might be due to changes that occur in a "premalignant" neoplastic condition that was histologically identified as "normal". In the clinical aspect, the field cancerization may have an etiologic role in a substantial number of recurrences. For example, a surgical resection margin that includes a genetically altered field can explain the occurrence of scar recurrence. This explanation suggests that molecular profiling of surgical margins will help reduce scar recurrences. Since multiple independent patches of cancer fields may be present in the same organ exposed to the same insults, clean molecular margins may not necessarily prevent recurrences in the residual organ (Dakubo et al., 2007). Similarly to gliomas, tumor recurrence is a major clinical concern for patients with urothelial carcinoma of the urinary bladder. Traditional morphological analysis is of limited utility for identifying cases in which recurrence will occur. However, recent studies have suggested that urothelial carcinogenesis occurs as a 'field effect' that can involve any number of sites in the bladder mucosa. Accumulating evidence supports the notion that resident urothelial stem cells in the affected field are transformed into cancer stem cells by acquiring genetic alterations that lead to tumor formation through clonal expansion (Cheng et al., 2009).

The available information in regards to the existence of a field phenomenon in gliomas is scant. In malignant gliomas, the high recurrence rates, the characteristically heterogeneous features and frequent diffuse spread within the brain have raised the question of whether malignant gliomas arise monoclonally from a single precursor cell or polyclonally from multiple transformed cells forming confluent clones (Inoue et al., 2008). To address this issue, Kattar et al (1997) have evaluated the clonality of low-grade and malignant gliomas by using polymerase chain reaction (PCR)-based assay for nonrandom X chromosome inactivation using surgical and autopsy material. The same pattern of nonrandom X chromosome inactivation was present in all areas of fifteen of 19 tumors, which were considered as monoclonal, suggesting that low-grade and malignant gliomas are, at least, usually monoclonal tumors, and extensively infiltrating tumors must result from migration of tumor cells.

Gliomatosis cerebri may shed some light in this issue. It is a rare condition in which the brain is infiltrated by an exceptionally diffusely growing of malignant glial cell population involving at least 2 lobes, though often more extensive, sometimes even affecting infratentorial regions. Kross et al (2002) have evaluated the existence of field cancerization in this affection, since *gliomatosis cerebri* may initiate as an oligoclonal process or result from collision of different gliomas. It was hypothesized that the presence of an identical set of genetic aberrations throughout the lesion would point to monoclonality of the process. In contrast, the finding of non-identical genetic changes in widely separated regions within the neoplasm would support the concept of collision of different mutated clones. For such, the authors used one autopsy case of *gliomatosis cerebri*, from which tissue samples were randomly taken from 24 locations throughout the brain and used for genetic investigation. With this aim, genome-wide screening for chromosomal aberrations was accomplished by comparative genomic hybridization (CGH). The authors found a wide distribution of particular sets of genetic aberrations, supporting the concept of monoclonal tumor proliferation (Kross et al., 2002). Nevertheless, it has been observed and well documented in one clinical case that on the long term, after initial treatment for *gliomatosis cerebri*, one glioblastoma multiforme has developed, and in a location separate from the initial lesion, suggesting that different clonal origin may had occurred (Inoue et al., 2008). More recently, Chen et al (2010) showed that the capacities for self-renewal and tumour initiation in GBM need not be restricted to a uniform population of stemlike cells.

5. The contribution of studies in animal models: Unifying the cancer stem cells and field cancerization concepts

Many genetic alterations have been identified in human gliomas, however, establishing unequivocal correlation between these genetic alterations and gliomagenesis requires accurate animal models for these cancers (Dai & Holland, 2001). Indeed, it is useful and necessary to have animal models for CNS tumors studies allowing to be carried out in different stages of tumor growth, especially in early stages, rare to be detected and observed in clinical practice (Bulnes-Sesma, 2006).

Experimental models of gliomagenesis most commonly used alkylating agents such as N-ethyl N-nitrosourea (ENU), which has been considered as a suitable model to study malignant changes. These changes were reported to appear firstly as early neoplastic proliferation (ENP) center, which continues in following stages subsequently progressing to "microtumors" until a tumor in itself. (Koestner et al., 1971; Naito et al., 1984).

By using the experimental model of gliomagenesis induced by the N-ethyl N-nitrosourea, we were able to detect putative tumor stem cells in early oncogenesis, yielding to analyze a field cancerization process and observe a close morphological relationship between metallothionein (MT) positive cells and blood vessels. With this aim, we have developed an experimental model to track putative mutated stem cells, using the ENU experimental model and metallothioneins (MT) immunostaining. MTs are metal binding proteins that take part in the homeostasis of the ions of the metals which are necessary for the proper metabolism of the organism (zinc, copper), disintoxication of metals and protect the tissues from the effects of free radicals, radiation and from mutagens (Thirumoorthy et al., 2007). MT expression is present in a significant portion of especially malignant brain tumors. In astrocytic tumors an acquired enhanced ability to produce MT has been observed as the malignant potential of a tumor increases (Hiura et al., 1998), and MT might be involved in poor response to antineoplastic drugs (Maier et al., 1997). In the murine colonic mucosa, the crypt restricted immunopositivity for MT has been shown to be reliable marker of stem cell mutation that may be induced early after mutagen treatment and that can be assayed in paraffin-fixed tissue sections (Cook et al., 2000). We have observed that 30 days after the treatment of rats with ENU, the main location of the MT positive cells have striking similarity to that of the RG cells and that the frequency of these cells (a) is strongly correlated with the increased appearing of ENP centers and new blood vessels, (b) is augmented at higher levels in long-term observation, i.e., 180 days after the carcinogen administration, (c) is related to a high staining intensity in both nucleus and cytoplasm, and (d) is very similar to the pattern of immunostaining that was observed in the nervous tissue surrounding gliomas, which were originated at an average of 321 days after the ENU administration (Fernandes-da-Silva et al., 2009). The mechanisms and reasons why MT is expressed in the preneoplastic and neoplastic lesions remain to be fully elucidated. It has been hypothesized that mutation-induced MT overexpression may interfere with the function of zinc finger DNA binding transcription factors (Zeng et al., 1991), which have been implicated in transcriptional control of various genes, including TP53, involved in cell proliferation and apoptosis. These MT-mediated effects on gene transcription are thought to confer a selective growth or survival advantage (or both) on the mutated cells (Bruewer, 2002).

6. Glioma, stem cells niche and angiogenesis

Recently in a review article, Gilbertson & Rich JN (2007) address a number of key questions which remain to be answered: do all cancer stem cells require the support of aberrant niches? Are cancer stem cell niches the primary drivers of tumor development, or are they recruited by pre-formed cancer stem cells? How do cancer stem cells and their niches subvert the tight regulatory conditions that characterize normal stem cell niches?

The stem cells of glioblastoma seem to be dependent on signals from aberrant vascular niches that mimic the normal neural stem cell niche (Gilbertson & Rich, 2007). Stem cells of various tissues are tightly regulated by the immediate microenvironment or stem cell niche (Moore & Lemischka, 2006), which is provided by capillaries in specific locations (Riquelme et al., 2008). This organization places the stem cells in close proximity to endothelial and other vascular cells, facilitating cross-talking among these cell types and affecting stem cell fate choices (Gilbertson, 2006). It is well-known that stem cells and their microenvironments may influence each other (Scadden, 2006). In fact, Cues within the niche, from cell–cell interactions to diffusible factors, are spatially and temporally coordinated to regulate proliferation and neurogenesis, ultimately (Riquelme et al., 2008).

In ENU treated rats, we have observed the existence of a close morphological relationship between MT positive cells and blood vessels. What is the relationship between them? It is known that MT is involved in the regulation of the functions of endothelial cells as well as in their protection against cytotoxic agents (Kaji et al., 1993). MT knock-out (MT-KO) mice presented dramatically decreased IL-6-induced angiogenesis caused by cortical freeze injury, suggesting that the MT have major regulatory functions in the angiogenesis process (Penkowa et al., 2000). In fact, human CD133+ Glioma CSCs are capable of producing vascular endothelial growth factor (VEGF) and thus may play an important role in glioma angiogenesis (Yao et al.,2008).

7. The concept of stemness, modulation of csc and glioma treatment

Understanding the characteristics and function of CSCs has shed light on their roles in glioma progression, including the implications for prognosis and treatment resistance. The original use of the term stemness was derived from a number of articles aimed to look for genes that could be expressed in general stem cell populations. The *stemness hypothesis* states that all stem cells use common mechanisms to regulate self-renewal and multi-lineage potential. This hypothesis has been debated and so far no conclusive evidence for a set of genes expressed in all stem cells. Certainly, identifying genes regulating stem cell properties will greatly improve our understanding of the molecular mechanisms regulating stem cell functions, our ability to manipulate stem cell fate, and the roles of stem cells in cancer (Koeva et al., 2011). Interestingly, overexpression of the transcription factor NANOG in gliomas and its close relationship with the undifferentiated state of glioma cells in vivo and in vitro indicated that NANOG may contribute to the existence of brains CSCs and may be related to tumorigenesis of the cerebrum by maintaining the undifferentiated state of glioma cells (Niu et al., 2011).

The new concept stemness is closely related to the observation that there are tissue environment factors that are able to influence or modulate CSCs. The main one is hypoxia, which activates the Hypoxia Induced Factor alpha number 1 (HIFα-1) alpha to enhance the self-renewal activity of CD133-positive cells and to inhibit their differentiation (Soeda et al., 2009). This and other signaling systems drive the transformation of normal stem cells, and perhaps of the bulk of tumor cells to cancer stem cells or to maintain the CSC phenotype (Katoh, 2011). For instance, the oxygen level of 7% has been observed to enhance the stem cell–like phenotype of $CD133^{+}$ in GBM cells (McCord et al., 2009). Furthermore, it has been observed that human glioblastoma cells from tumor biopsies, which were engrafted intracerebrally into nude rats, that CD133 negative glioma cells were tumorgenic in nude rats, and that CD133 positive cells can be obtained from these tumors. Upon the passing of the cell tumors in vivo, CD133 expression is upregulated, coinciding with the onset of angiogenesis and a shorter patient survival (Wang et al., 2008). Furthermore, the bone morphogenic protein BMP4 effectively reduces proliferation of CD133 positive cells in vitro and the tumor growth in vivo. BMP4 may act as a key inhibitory regulator of cancer initiation and therefore may be used in combined stem cell-based therapy as a non-cytotoxic therapeutic agent (Altaner, 2008).

If one accepts that there is a subpopulation of cancer cells with stem cell properties, which is responsible for tumor maintenance and progression, and may contribute to the resistance to anticancer treatments, it is very reasonable to deduce that compounds that target cancer stem-like cells could be effective to impair or even to destroy a neoplasm and nas important therapeutic implications. Various compounds have been investigated as putative influencers of stemness and malignancies in glioma stem-like cells, leading the proposal that stem cell regulatory factors may provide significant targets for therapeutic strategies (Holmberg et al., 2011). Ongoing work aims the identification of unique pathways governing self-renewal of these putative stem cells and their validation as ultimate therapeutic targets (Panagiotakos & Tabar, 2007). Additionally, it is possible to conceive that epigenetic-based drugs that modulate gene expression in CSC possibly constitute a promising alternative resource for target therapy in the treatment of these, thus far, incurable malignancy.

8. References

Altaner, C. 2008. Glioblastoma and stem cells. *Neoplasma,* Vol.55, No.5, pp.369-374.

Braakhuis BJM, Tabor MP, Kummer JA, Leemans CR, Brakenhoff RH. 2003. A genetic explanation of Slaughter's concept of field cancerization: evidence and clinical implications. *Cancer Res*, Vol.63, No.8, pp.1727-1730.

Bruewer, M.; Schmid, K.W.; Krieglstein, C.F.; Senninger, N.; Schuermann, G. 2002. Metallothionein: early marker in the carcinogenesis of ulcerative colitis-associated colorectal carcinoma. *World Journal of Surgery*, 26,6,726-731.

Bulnes-Sesma S, Ullibarri-Ortiz de Zárate N, Lafuente-Sánchez JV. 2006. Tumour induction by ethylnitrosourea in the central nervous system. *Rev Neurol*, Vol.43, No12, pp.733-738.

Castillo, M. 2010. Stem cells, radial glial cells, and a unified origin of brain tumors. *American Journal Neuroradiology*, No.3, Mar, pp.389-390.

Chen, R.; Nishimura, M.C.; Bumbaca, S.M.; Kharbanda, S.; Forrest, W.F.; Kasman, I.M.; Greve, J.M.; Soriano, R.H.; Gilmour, L.L.; Rivers, C.S.; Modrusan, Z.; Nacu, S.; Guerrero, S.; Edgar, K.A.; Wallin, J.J.; Lamszus, K.; Westphal, M.; Heim, S.; James, C.D.; VandenBerg, S.R.; Costello, J.F.; Moorefield, S.; Cowdrey, C.J.; Prados, M.; Phillips, H.S. 2010. A hierarchy of self-renewing tumor-initiating cell types in glioblastoma. *Cancer Cell,* Vol.17, No.4, April, pp.362-375.

Cheng L, Zhang S, Davidson DD, MacLennan GT, Koch MO, Montironi R, Lopez-Beltran A. 2009. Molecular determinants of tumor recurrence in the urinary bladder. *Future Oncology*, Vol.5, No.6, pp. 843-857.

Clément, V.; Dutoit, V.; Marino, D.; Dietrich, P.Y.; Radovanovic, I. 2009. Limits of CD133 as a marker of glioma self-renewing cells. *Int J Cancer*. Jul 1;125(1):244-8.

Collins, V.P. Brain tumours: classification and genes. 2004. *J Neurol Neurosurg Psychiatry*, Vol.75 Suppl 2, pp.2-11.

Cook, A.H.; Williams, D.; Thomas, A.G. 2000. Crypt-restricted metallothionein immunopositivity in murine colon: validation of a model for studies of somatic stem cell mutation. *J Pathology*, Vol.191, No.3, pp.306-312.

Dakubo, G.D.; Jakupciak, J.P.; Birch-Machin, M.A.; Parr, R.L.; 2007. Clinical implications and utility of field cancerization., *Cancer Cell International, Vol.*7, pp.2. ???

Dai, C. & Holland, E.C. 2001. Glioma models. *Biochim Biophys Acta*, Vol.1551, No.1, pp.M19-27.

Das, S.; Srikanth, M.; Kessler, J.A. 2008. Cancer stem cells and glioma. *Nat Clin Pract Neurology*, Vol.4, pp.427–435.

Fernandes da Silva, J.C.; Kanen, V.C.; Turatti, A.; Ribeiro-Silva, A.; Herrero, C.F.S.; Garcia, S.B. 2009. Overexpression of metallothioneins, stem cell niches and field cancerization in experimental gliomagenesis. *COLUNA/COLUMNA*, Vol.8, No.4, pp.428-433.

Frosina, G. 2011. Frontiers in targeting glioma stem cells. *Eur J Cancer*, Vol.47, No.4, Mar, pp.496-507.

Garcia SB, Park HS, Novelli M, Wright NA. 199. Field cancerization, clonality, and epithelial stem cells: the spread of mutated clones in epithelial sheets. *J Pathol*, Vol.187, pp.61-81.

Gilbertson, R.J. 2006. Brain tumors provide new clues to the source of cancer stem cells: does oncology recapitulate ontogeny? *Cell Cycle*, Vol.5, pp.135–137.

Gilbertson, R.J. & Rich, J.N. 2007. Making a tumour's bed: glioblastoma stem cells and the vascular niche. *Nat Rev Cancer*, Vol.7, No.10, pp.733-736.

Hiura, T.; Khalid, H.; Yamashita, H.; Tokunaga, Y.; Yasunaga, A.; Shibata, S. 1998. Immunohistochemical analysis of metallothionein in astrocytic tumors in relation to tumor grade, proliferative potential, and survival. *Cancer*, Vol.83, No.11, pp.2361-2369.

Holmberg J, He X, Peredo I, Orrego A, Hesselager G, Ericsson C, Hovatta O, Oba-Shinjo SM, Marie SK, Nistér M, Muhr J. 2011. Activation of neural and pluripotent stem cell signatures correlates with increased malignancy in human glioma. *PLoS One*, Vol.6, No.3, pp.e18454.

Huang, Q.; Zhang, Q.B.; Dong, J.; Wu, Y.Y.; Shen, Y.T.; Zhao, Y.D.; Zhu, Y.D.; Diao, Y.; Wang, A.D.; Lan, Q. 2008. Glioma stem cells are more aggressive in recurrent tumors with malignant progression than in the primary tumor, and both can be maintained long-term in vitro, *BMC Cancer*, Vol.8, Oct, pp.304.

Hulleman, E. & Helin, K. Molecular mechanisms in gliomagenesis. 2005. *Adv Cancer Research*, Vol.94, pp.1-27.

Inoue, A.; Takahashi, H.; Harada, H.; Kohno, S.; Ohue, S.; Kobayashi, K.; Yano, H.; Tanaka, Ohnishi, T. 2010. Cancer stem-like cells of glioblastoma characteristically express MMP-13 and display highly invasive activity. *Int Journal of Oncology*, Vol.37, No.5, Nov, pp.1121-1131.

Inoue, T.; Kanamori, M.; Sonoda, Y.; Watanabe, M.; Sasajima, T.; Kamisato, N.; Kumabe, T.; Tominaga, T. 2008. Glioblastoma multiforme developing separately from the initial lesion 9 years after successful treatment for gliomatosis cerebri: a case report. *No Shinkei Geka*, Vol.36, No.8, Aug, pp.709-715.

Kaji, T.; Yamamoto, C.; Tsubaki, S.; Sakamoto, M.; Sato, M.; Kozuka, H. 1993. Metallothionein induction by cadmium, cytokines, thrombin and endothelin-1 in cultured vascular endothelial cells. *Life Sci*, Vol.53, No.15, pp.1185-1191.

Katoh, M. 2011. Network of WNT and other regulatory signaling cascades in pluripotent stem cells and cancer stem cells. *Curr Pharm Biotechnol.* Vol.12, No.2, pp.160-170.

Kattar, M.M.; Kupsky, W.J.; Shimoyama, R.K.; Vo, T.D.; Olson, M.W.; Bargar, G.R.; Sarkar, F.H. 1997. Clonal analysis of gliomas. *Human Pathology*, Vol.28, No.10, Oct, pp.1166-1179.

Koestner, A.; Swenberg, J.A.; Wechsler, W. 1971. Transplacental production with ethylnitrosourea of neoplasms of the nervous system in Sprague-Dawley rats. Am J Pathology, Vol.63, No.1, Apr, pp.37-56. (PMID:4323476)

Koeva, M.; Forsberg, E.C.; Stuart, J.M. 2011 . Computational integration of homolog and pathway gene module expression reveals general stemness signatures. *PLoS One.* Vol.6, No.4, pp.e18968.

Kros, J.M.; Zheng, P.; Dinjens, W.N.; Alers, M; Janeke, C. 2002. Genetic Aberrations in Gliomatosis Cerebri Support Monoclonal Tumorigenesis. *Journal of Neuropathology & Experimental Neurology*, Vol.61, No.9, pp.806–814.

Li, Z.; Bao, S.; Wu, Q.; Wang, H.; Eyler, C.; Sathornsumetee, S.; Shi, Q.; Cao, Y.; Lathia, J.; McLendon, R.E.; Hjelmeland, A.B.; Rich, J.N. 2009. Hypoxia-inducible factors regulate tumorigenic capacity of glioma stem cells. *Cancer Cell*, Vol.15, No.6, Jun, pp.501-513.

Li, Z. & Rich JN. 2010. Hypoxia and hypoxia inducible factors in cancer stem cell maintenance. *Curr Top Microbiol Immunol*, Vol.345, pp.21-30.

Maier, H.; Jones, C.; Jasani, B.; Ofner, D.; Zelger, B.; Schmid, K.W.; Budka, H. 1997. Metallothionein overexpression in human brain tumours. *Acta Neuropathol*, Vol.94, No.6, pp.599-604.

Malatesta, P.; Hack, M.A.; Hartfuss, E.; Kettenmann, H.; Klinkert, W.; Kirchhoff, F.; Götz, M. 2003. Neuronal or glial progeny: regional differences in radial glia fate. *Neuron*, Vol.37, No.5, pp.751-764.

McCord, A.M.; Jamal, M.; Shankavaram, U.T.; Lang, F.F.; Camphausen, K.; Tofilon, P.J. 2009. Physiologic oxygen concentration enhances the stem-like properties of CD133+ human glioblastoma cells in vitro. *Mol Cancer Res*, Vol.7, No.4, Apr, pp.489-497.

Moore, K. A. & Lemischka, I. R. 2006. Stem cells and their niches. *Science*, Vol.311, pp.1880–1885.

Naito, M.; Naito, Y.; Ito, A.; Watanabe, H.; Kawashima, K. 1984. Spinal cord tumors induced by N-ethyl-N-nitrosourea in rats: presence of spinal subpial target cells. *J Natl Cancer Institute*, Vol.2, No.3, pp.715-724.

Niu, C.S.; Li, D.X.; Liu, Y.H.; Fu, X.M.; Tang, S.F.; Li, J. Expression of NANOG in human gliomas and its relationship with undifferentiated glioma cells. 2011. *Oncol Report*, May 13, doi: 10.3892/or.2011.1308. [Epub ahead of print]

Nowell, P.C. 1976. The clonal evolution of tumor cell populations. *Science*; Vol.194, pp. 23–28.

Panagiotakos, G. & Tabar, V. 2007. Brain tumor stem cells. *Current Neurology and Neuroscience Reports*, Vol.7, No.3, pp.215-220.

Park, D.M.; Rich, J.N. 2009. Biology of glioma cancer stem cells. *Mol Cells*, Vol.28, No.1, Jul, pp.7-12.

Penkowa, M.; Carrasco, J.; Giralt, M.; Molinero, A.; Hernández, J.; Campbell, I.L. 2000. Altered central nervous system cytokine-growth factor expression profiles and angiogenesis in metallothionein-I+II deficient mice. *J Cereb Blood Flow Metab.* Vol.20, No.8; pp.1174-1189.

Pérez Castillo, A.; Aguilar-Morante, D.; Morales-García, J.A.; Dorado, J. 2008. Cancer stem cells and brain tumors. *Clin Transl Oncol*, Vol.10, No.5, May, pp.262-267.

Reya, T.; Morrison, S.J.; Clarke, M.F.; Weissman, I.L. 2001. Stem cells, cancer, and cancer stem cells. *Nature.*;414:105–11.

Rich, J.N. & Eyler, C.E. 2008. Cancer stem cells in brain tumor biology. *Cold Spring Harb Symp Quant Biol*, Vol.73, pp.411-420.

Riquelme, P.A.; Drapeau, E.; Doetsch F. 2008. Brain micro-ecologies: neural stem cell niches in the adult mammalian brain. Philos Trans R Soc Lond B Biol Science, Vol.363, No.1489, pp.123-137.

Ryan, L.P. 2007. Clinical implications and utility of field cancerization. *Cancer Cell International*, 7:2.

Sanchez-Martin, M. 2008. Brain tumor stem cells: implications for cancer therapy and regenerative medicine. *Curr Stem Cell Res Ther*, Vol.3, No.3, pp.197-207.

Scadden, D. T. 2006. The stem-cell niche as an entity of action. *Nature*, Vol.441, pp.1075–1079.

Singh, S.K.; Clarke, I.D.; Hide, T.; Dirks PB. 2004. Cancer stem cells in nervous system tumors. *Oncogene*, Vol.23, No.43, Sep., pp.7267-7273.

Slaughter, D.P.; Southwick, H.W.; Smejkal, W. 1953. Field cancerization in oral stratified squamous epithelium; clinical implications of multicentric origin. *Cancer.* Vol.6, No.5, Sep., pp.963-968. (PMID:13094644)

Soeda, A.; Park, M.; Lee, D.; Mintz, A, Androutsellis-Theotokis A, McKay RD, Engh J, Iwama T, Kunisada T, Kassam AB, Pollack IF, Park DM. 2009. Hypoxia promotes expansion of the CD133-positive glioma stem cells through activation of HIF-1alpha. *Oncogene*, Vol.28, No.45, pp.3949-3959.

Thirumoorthy, N.M.; Kumar, K.T.; Shyam, S.A.; Panayappan, L.; Chatterjee, M. 2007. Metallothionein: an overview. *World J Gastroenterology*, Vol.13, No.7, pp.993-996.

Vescovi, A.L.; Galli, R.; Reynolds, B.A. 2006. Brain tumor stem cells. *Nat Rev Cancer*, Vol.6, pp.425–436

Wang, J.; Sakariassen, P.O.; Tsinkalovsky, O.; Immervoll, H.; Bøe, S.O.; Svendsen, A.; Prestegarden, L.; Røsland, G.; Thorsen, F.; Stuhr, L.; Molven, A.; Bjerkvig, R.; Enger, P.Ø. 2008. CD133 negative glioma cells form tumors in nude rats and give rise to CD133 positive cells. *Int J Cancer*, Vol.122, No.4, Feb, pp.761-768.

Weiner, L.P. 2008. Definitions and criteria for stem cells. *Methods Mol Biol.* Vol. 438, pp.3-8.

Yan, X.; Ma, L.; Yi, D.; Yoon, J.G.; Diercks, A.; Foltz, G.; Price, N.D.; Hood, L.E.; Tian, Q. 2011. A CD133-related gene expression signature identifies an aggressive glioblastoma subtype with excessive mutations. *Proc Natl Acad Science*, Vol.108, No.4, Jan, pp.1591-1596.

Yao, X.H.; Ping, Y.F.; Chen, J.H.; Xu, C.P.; Chen, D.L.; Zhang, R.; Wang, J.M.; Bian, X.W. 2008. Glioblastoma stem cells produce vascular endothelial growth factor by activation of a G-protein coupled formylpeptide receptor FPR. *J Pathology*, Vol.215, No.4, Aug, pp.369-376.

Zeng, J.; Heuchel, R.; Schaffner, W.; Kägi, J.H. 1991. Thionein (apometallothionein) can modulate DNA binding and transcription activation by zinc finger containing factor Sp1. *FEBS Lett*, Vol.279, No.2, pp.310-312.

10

Bone Marrow-Derived Cells Support Malignant Transformation of Low-Grade Glioma

Jeffrey P. Greenfield et al.*
Weill Cornell Medical College
USA

1. Introduction

Gliomas, the most common primary brain tumors, exist as a continuum between low-grade and high-grade states. Low grade gliomas are generally found in children and young adults. These tumors are characterized by well-differentiated cellularity which is mildly pleomorphic. These tumors lack mitotic figures and neovascularization and do not enhance on MRI. The average survival of patients after diagnosis is 7-10 years; the morbidity associated with these lesions is largely dependent on progression of these lesions to a higher grade state. High-grade gliomas, conversely, which exist on the other end of the glial neoplasm spectrum, are extremely malignant with poorly differentiated cells that are highly pleomorphic and display numerous mitotic figures. These tumors contain significant vascular proliferation, hemorrhage and necrosis. High grade gliomas enhance brightly on contrast MRI and often exhibit widespread invasion throughout the brain. Prognosis is poor for high grade gliomas, with a median survival of 18 months even with aggressive therapies. One of the key events in the transition from the low-grade to high-grade state has been referred to as the angiogenic switch. This is defined as the period during which the tumor undergoes a transition to an environment capable of rapid blood vessel formation supporting subsequent exponential tumor growth. It is theorized that in the low-grade state, tumor growth may be limited, at least in part, by a lack of blood supply limiting the tumor to linear growth. Once the tumor acquires the ability to recruit or form new blood vessels through this angiogenic switch, exponential growth may occur, which results in rapid clinical progression. It has been well-described in the literature that bone marrow-derived cells (BMDC) participate in the progression of cancer. BMDCs in the local tumor microenvironment have been proposed to be capable of breaking down normal structures thereby promoting vasculogenesis and invasiveness. This, in turn, provides an environment capable of sustaining and promoting tumor growth. The role of BMDC in metastatic disease has been well-documented and recent data suggests that BMDC participate in the growth and progression of brain tumors as well. This chapter will explore the role of BMDC in the transition from low-grade to high-grade gliomas particularly with respect to the angiogenic

---

* William S. Cobb, Caitlin E. Hoffman, Xueying Chen, Prajwal Rajappa,
Chioma Ihunnah, Yujie Huang and David Lyden
Weill Cornell Medical College
USA

switch. The possibility of this pathway as a potential therapeutic target will also be reviewed.

2. Low-grade glioma transformation in adults

Low-grade gliomas (LGG) are a heterogeneously diverse group of tumors with a generally benign histology and an associated variable outcome. This unpredictable course relies, in part, on the potential for malignant transformation to a higher grade. These tumors present a unique therapeutic challenge as they are typically associated with minimal symptoms and benign radiographic appearance. Initially, the majority of LGGs run an indolent clinical course but often ultimately progress into aggressive tumors with a poor prognosis. As a result, significant controversy exists as to appropriate treatment protocols for this disease. The natural history of LGG, and the risk factors for progression, have been one focus of glioma research due to the potential impact on treatment strategy. Many recent studies have helped clarify treatment recommendations including extent of resection, timing and efficacy of radiation therapy, and response to chemotherapy. Significant debate remains, however, regarding standardization of treatment for low-grade glioma given the tremendous diversity in tumor histology, biology, and outcome. While observation of low-grade gliomas was previously considered a valid treatment option to avoid the morbidity of surgery, chemotherapy, and radiation, early intervention has gradually become standard of care as the impact and incidence of malignant progression has become fully realized. Subjecting patients to the morbidity of aggressive treatment in an unpredictable tumor with variable outcome remains controversial, however. Currently, significant effort is focused on identification of risk factors and tumor characteristics that lead to progression. Better appreciation for the molecular and cellular mechanisms of malignant transformation carries the potential to create novel treatment regimens with less morbidity, thereby alleviating the use of radiation and chemotherapy which present significant toxicity to both children and adults. A review of the characteristics of low-grade gliomas, current treatment strategies, their transformation potential, and current efforts to define novel pathways involved in malignant transformation follows.

The term LGG includes World Health Organization Grade I and Grade II tumors, which are typically associated with indolent tumor growth and significantly better prognosis compared to high grade gliomas. Grade I gliomas include pilocytic astrocytoma, desmoplastic neuroectodermal tumors, subependymoma, ganglioglioma, myxopapillary ependymoma, and desmoplastic infantile tumors, which represent a spectrum of typically benign lesions. Within this class, pilocytic histology is the most common (Stieber, 2001). These pilocytic tumors are well-circumscribed, non-infiltrative, and do not generally transform to more malignant, higher grade lesions. While malignant transformation has been reported in WHOI tumors, the primary risk for malignant degeneration exists in Grade II tumors including low-grade or fibrillary astrocytoma, oligodendroglioma, or mixed oligo-astrocytoma. Ependymoma, ganglioglioma, pleomorphic xanthoastrocytoma, and choroid gliomas of the third ventricle are also considered grade II. Fibrillary astrocytomas, which comprise the majority of grade II lesions (Stieber, 2001), have garnered significant attention due to the significant morbidity and mortality of patients with this diagnosis.

While WHO I gliomas are typically well-circumscribed tumors with benign histology, WHO II gliomas are diffuse, infiltrative and have malignant potential (Stieber, 2001). Both classes, however, are associated with slow tumor growth. The incidence of LGG is reported to be between 2,700 and 4,700 cases per year, comprising approximately 30% of all malignant gliomas (Schiff et al., 2007, Wessels et al., 2003). These tumors are most common in Caucasian males, and typically present in the second to fourth decades (Schomas et al., 2009, Wessels et al., 2003). Patients greater than 60 years of age carry a poorer prognosis with generally lower Karnofsky scores and larger tumor burden at diagnosis. In adults, the most common presenting symptom is seizure followed by incidental findings on imaging. Less common presentations include trauma trauma, sinus pathology, and pituitary disorder (Wessels et al., 2003). Thirty percent of patients present with neurological deficit, and only 10% present with symptoms of raised intracranial pressure ICP. Speech and language deficits have been reported in 10% of patients (Prabhu et al., 2010), however, focal deficits are less common (Schomas et al., 2009, Wessels et al., 2003).

In adults, LGGs are generally hemispheric, supratentorial, and typically occur in the frontal and temporal lobes. They may involve eloquent cortex, which limits the capacity for gross total resection due to significant risk of morbidity (Prabhu et al., 2010, Stieber, 2001). LGG are hypointense on T1 weighted magnetic resonance imaging (MRI), hyperintense on FLAIR and T2 sequences, and enhance in 30% of cases. There is often associated vasogenic edema (Prabhu et al., 2010, Wessels et al., 2003).

LGG are typically sporadic tumors, although they can occur in association with Li Fraumeni syndrome and Neurofibromatosis Types 1 and 2 (Prabhu et al., 2010, Wessels et al., 2003). Additional risk factors include previous irradiation and exposure to industrial chemicals (Prabhu et al., 2010, Wessels et al., 2003). Allergy has been reported to lower the risk for LGG, suggesting a possible role for immune surveillance in tumor pathogenesis (Prabhu et al., 2010). Survival is highly variable for LGG as median overall survival (OS) is reported to range from 3 to 40 years. Median progression free survival (PFS) is only 50% at 5 years and 17% at 15 years (Bauman et al., 1999, Berger et al., 1994, Jaeckle et al., Stieber, 2001). Median time to progression is 7.2 years (Schomas et al., 2009). In adults, the overall malignant transformation rate ranges from 35-89% with 74% in primary astrocytoma, 70% with mixed tumors, and 45% with primarily oligodendroglial histology (Jaeckle et al., 2010). Importantly, 50% of low risk adults, defined as patients less than 40 years of age with gross total resection (GTR), underwent transformation within 5 years (Jaeckle et al., 2010, Schiff et al., 2007).

Multiple studies have found that age greater than 40 years, extent of resection, tumor diameter greater than 6cm, tumor crossing midline, neurological deficit at diagnosis, and astrocytic histology are risk factors for poor prognosis in LGG (Bauman et al., 1999, E. G. Shaw et al., 2008, Stieber, 2001, Jaeckle et al., 2010, Schiff et al., 2007, E. G. Shaw & Wisoff, 2003). The NCCTG found that astrocytomas carry a worse prognosis than oligodendroglioma. Other retrospective reports corroborate these finding and further specify gemistocytic astrocytoma as carrying a worse prognosis (Jaeckle et al., 2010, Schomas et al., 2009, Stieber, 2001, Wessels et al., 2003, E. G. Shaw et al., 2008). Contrast enhancement, Karnofsky score, mitotic activity, and genetics have also been identified as risk factors for progression (Schiff et al., 2007, Schomas et al., 2009, E. G. Shaw & Wisoff, 2003, Stieber, 2001). Additionally, a Ki67-MIB1 index greater than 4% is associated with a more rapid rate of transformation.

3. Malignant transformation of pediatric low-grade glioma

The presentation and prognosis of LGG in children differs significantly from that in adults. Overall survival and rate of malignant transformation is significantly different in the pediatric population, leading to the hypothesis that tumor biology in children is inherently different from that in adults. For LGG in children, the overall rate of malignant transformation ranges from 4.3%-38%, which is much lower than in adults (Armstrong et al., 2011, Pollack et al., 1995). This difference may be accounted for in part by the higher rate of pilocytic astrocytomas that comprise the vast majority of pediatric LGG, a histological subset that rarely transforms (Tihan et al., 1999). While no prospective studies have been performed to identify reliable risk factors for transformation in children, radiation therapy is reported to be a possible causative agent (Dirks et al., 1994). Mean time to transformation is relatively short at approximately 6.4 years (Dirks et al., 1994). While the overall rate of progression is certainly lower in children, the risk of transformation in this population is still significant and warrants active and expectant observation.

Despite this risk for malignant degeneration, overall prognosis for children with LGG is significantly better than that for adults. Overall survival in children with LGG 65-90%, however, OS is 51% when pilocytic pathology is excluded (Armstrong et al., 2011, Fisher et al., 2008, Pollack et al., 1995). Following gross total resection, survival is 90-100% with 0% progression, in comparison to the adult transformation rate of 50% even in low risk, young patients with complete resection (Pollack et al., 1995). Progression free survival is between approximately 50% at 10 years, and 53% at 15 years (Armstrong et al., 2011). Gross total resection has been the only factor currently identified to have an impact on progression free survival in children with 0% progression with GTR and 17% progression with near total resection (Pollack et al., 1995). Due to the infiltrative nature of non-pilocytic grade II astrocytomas, this histology in children is more comparable to the adult population and is associated with poorer prognosis (Pollack et al., 1995).

4. Effect of resection and adjuvant therapy on malignant transformation

Currently, initial treatment consists of pharmacologic seizure control if patients present with seizures and steroids for vasogenic edema (Prabhu et al., 2010, Stieber, 2001). For patients with lesions amenable to surgery, the goal is gross total resection as many studies have found overall survival to correlate with extent of initial resection irrespective of adjuvant therapy. At 5 years, OS was 63% with GTR versus 27% OS with STR (Prabhu et al., 2010). Recurrence is also higher with STR (Prabhu et al., 2010). Berger et al. (1994) reported no recurrences within 54 months with GTR, 14.8% recurrence with residual tumor less than $10cm^3$, and 46.2% recurrence with residual greater than $10cm^3$ (Berger et al., 1994, Stieber, 2001). In some cases, tumor location within or near eloquent cortex limits the extent of resection, therefore, newer methods including functional MRI, fiber tracking with diffuser tensor imaging (DTI), intra-operative stimulation and mapping, or intra-operative MRI have helped reduce morbidity and allow more aggressive surgery. As survival decreases with lower Karnofsky score, while the surgical goal remains complete resection, equally important is the avoidance of new neurological deficit (Gil-Robles & Duffau, 2010, Schomas et al., 2009).

The role of adjuvant therapy following surgical resection remains controversial. Although LGG are fairly slow growing tumors with low or absent mitotic activity, their infiltrative behavior and high rate of recurrence and malignant transformation has caused most centers to institute adjuvant therapy regardless of the extent of resection. Recent prospective trials have addressed the role of radiation therapy (E. Shaw et al., 2002). RT was found to improve PFS but not OS (Stieber, 2001). As a result, early RT is administered to patients at high risk for malignant transformation (defined as age > 40yrs, astrocytic histology, crossing midline, diameter > 6cm, or intractable seizures) or for control of disease at the time of progression (Prabhu et al., 2010). The study also recommended RT to all patients greater than 40 years of age irrespective of resection, as age was the most consistent prognostic factor for malignant transformation (Stieber, 2001). For patients aged 18 to 40, RT was recommended only for patients with incomplete resection. Regardless of these data, treatment protocols vary widely and are often practitioner dependant.

Chemotherapy has also been used as an initial treatment in LGG, most commonly in the setting of unresectable disease, or in patients less than 3 years of age in which RT should be deferred (Prabhu et al., 2010). The response rates to available agents are highly variable, with favorable responses reported between 10 and 60%. Poor response is often associated with low grade tumors as they tend to have lower sensitivity to chemotherapeutic agents due their inherently slow growth and minimal mitosis (Prabhu et al., 2010). The Southwest Oncology Group (SWOG) investigated the use of CCNU in addition to RT following GTR and found no added benefit of CCNU (E. G. Shaw & Wisoff, 2003). The NCCTG found a favorable response using PCV in the treatment of primary disease. Currently, the RTOG is investigating the safety and efficacy of PCV in unfavorable patients following resection and RT. Temozolamide is also under investigation for use in LGG patients at high risk for transformation (Schomas et al., 2009). Clearly, the use of adjuvant therapy requires more investigation before formal recommendations can be defined. Until then, adjuvant therapies will remain controversial and site dependant.

Treatment of pediatric gliomas is subject to a different set of considerations and standards as toxicity of therapy has a greater impact on the developing nervous and skeletal system. Surgery with GTR is the primary mode of therapy as this has been shown to be the most effective method for cure (Fisher et al., 2008, Unal et al., 2008). While rare, malignant transformation does occur so observation is not recommended with lesions that are amenable to surgery. As an exception, optic and hypothalamic gliomas are treated initially with observation and chemotherapy. Due to their slow growth and associated morbidity with surgery or radiotherapy in these locations, conservative management is standard. Ultimately, these tumors are associated with a worse prognosis due to their location and difficulty of surgical intervention in the event of progression. Similarly, first line of therapy for brainstem lesions is observation and potential biopsy only for progression of symptoms or radiographic appearance (Fisher et al., 2008). Based on the 0% progression in the setting of GTR, RT has no role following complete resection in children, as compared to adults (Pollack et al., 1995).

Although standard dose RT (50.4-54 Gy) has been shown to be effective in the pediatric population, RT is deferred in children irrespective of residual tumor burden, recurrence or progression due to the risk of toxicity including endocrine dysfunction, cognitive impairment with decreased memory, lower IQ, attention deficit, cerebrovascular disease, and secondary neoplasms (Fisher et al., 2008, Pollack et al., 1995). Standard dose RT is associated with 34% cognitive dysfunction compared to 8.6% without RT, and 17% endocrine dysfunction compared to 2.9% without RT (Pollack et al., 1995). Overall, the rate of endocrine dysfunction was 10% and cognitive dysfunction was 21%. These findings support the use of repeat surgery and chemotherapy prior to the use of RT for recurrence in children. Chemotherapeutic agents possess significant toxicity as well. While carboplatin and vincristine showed good response rates with 68% 3 year PFS, 40% of patients demonstrated hypersensitivity reactions. CCNU, vincristine, and dibromodulcitol have all been associated with significant hypersensitivity reactions (Fisher et al., 2008). As a result, TPCV is now being tested for efficacy and safety in a prospective pediatric trial (Fisher et al., 2008).

5. Histology of malignant transformation

As mentioned previously, low grade gliomas comprise a histologically diverse group of tumors. The current WHO classification describes four categories for astrocytomas (Kleihues et al., 1995, Louis et al., 2007). While it is theorized that the majority of grade IV glioblastomas (GBM) occur *de novo* (primary GBM), a significant number of lesions result from progression of a low-grade tumor (secondary GBM). Excluding Grade I pilocytic astrocytomas as they rarely progress, low grade (II) and high grade (III and IV) astrocytomas can be viewed to exist along a continuum based on the histological analysis of tumor tissue. Grade II lesions are defined by low or absent mitotic activity and, unlike Grade I gliomas, are infiltrative and invasive and should not be considered benign. Cellular density is low to moderate, and well-differentiated, mildly pleomorphic tumor cells are present. One important feature of low grade astrocytomas is the absence of neovascularization.

This is in distinct comparison to high grade gliomas, grade III anaplastic tumors and grade IV GBMs, which are poorly differentiated, widely infiltrative and display prominent mitotic activity and neovascularization. Both confer a poor prognosis. High-grade lesions display increased cellularity, marked pleomorphism and nuclear atypia and may include multinucleated giant cells. Necrosis is the defining feature of GBM and these areas are typically surrounded by pseudopalisading cells. Most importantly, extensive irregular vascular proliferation is present in GBM as these tumors have adopted the capability of undergoing the angiogenic switch to produce their own vasculature, allowing for exponential tumor growth.

While morbidity is associated with low-grade astrocytomas themselves, it is hypothesized that the majority of morbidity is caused by progression to high-grade tumor. One of the key factors in this progression is the angiogenic switch whereby the tumor adopts the ability to acquire its own vascular supply. This enables explosive growth and precipitates rapid clinical deterioration. While an increased understanding of LGG biology and behavior has led to a more aggressive approach to these tumors, clinical outcome measures still remain poor. This is due mostly in part to our inability to prevent or detect malignant degeneration. A significant amount of research is now focused on understanding the factors involved in the angiogenic switch, which is likely to lead to additional treatment targets and potentially better outcomes. This will be further discussed in the sections to follow.

6. Molecular biology of malignant transformation

While histological characteristics currently determine tumor grade in astrocytoma, important molecular differences also exist between low grade and high-grade gliomas (Table 1) (Godard et al., 2003). These molecular differences are likely to be an important factor in initiating or promoting the angiogenic switch (Wen & Kesari, 2008). Both primary and secondary GBM exhibit elevated VEGF expression and loss of heterozygosity at 10q. The majority of primary GBM show overexpression of EGFR and PTEN mutations. In particular, glioblastomas that express the EGFRvIII genetic variant have a worse prognosis and show resistance to current therapeutic regimens (Furnari et al., 2007, Hatanpaa et al., Johns et al., 2007, Pelloski et al., 2007). While PTEN mutations occur more frequently in primary glioblastoma in adults, PTEN mutations exist in high frequency in pediatric gliomas that have undergone malignant transformation (Broniscer et al., 2007).

Genetic Mutation	Incidence in Grade II Astrocytoma and Secondary GBM	Incidence in Primary GBM
p53 (TP53)	↑↑↑	↑
EGFR	↑	↑↑↑
PTEN	↑↑	↑↑↑
IDH 1&2	↑↑↑	↑↑
PDGF	↑↑↑	↑↑
BRAF	↑	--

Table 1. Various genetic mutations associated with gliomas. EGFR - epidermal growth factor receptor, PTEN - phosphatase and tensin homolog, IDH - isocitrate deyhdrogenase, PDGFR - platelet derived growth factor receptor.

In contrast, secondary GBMs often have p53 mutations and overexpress PDGF. Mutations of p53 frequently are associated with low-grade gliomas occurring in 53% of astrocytoma, 44% of oligoastrocytoma, and 13% of oligodendroglioma (Okamoto et al., 2004). Therefore, p53 may be an important molecular event involved in the malignant progression of low-grade gliomas (Louis et al., 2007). Interestingly, in children, the rate of p53 mutations is reported as only 10% in progressive pediatric LGG. While this alteration may seem to possibly explain the improved survival in pediatric gliomas, the 1p19q deletion, an indicator of a favorable response to specific chemotherapies in adults, is not found in pediatric gliomas (Fisher et al., 2008).

Other molecular changes have also been identified (Ichimura et al., 2009, Watanabe et al., 2009). IDH1 abnormalities exist in 59-88% of diffuse astrocytomas, 68-82% of oligodendrogliomas, 50-78% of anaplastic astrocytomas, 49-75% of anaplastic oligodendrogliomas, and 50-88% of secondary glioblastomas and often co-exist with p53 mutated lesions or 1p19q co-deleted tumors (Hartmann et al., 2009, Ichimura et al., 2009, Parsons et al., 2008, Sanson et al., 2009, Watanabe et al., 2009, Yan et al., 2009). While the presence of IDH mutations in low-grade tumors and secondary GBMs suggests a role for IDH in malignant progression , the literature suggests that the presence of IDH1 or IDH2 mutations correlates with better outcomes in patients (De Carli et al., 2009, Yan et al., 2009). PDGFR and the p16ink4a /RB1 pathway have also been implicated in gliomagenesis as hypermethylation of the RB1 gene may result in uncontrolled cell cycle progression, which may then drive tumor formation (Sathornsumetee et al., 2007). Both primary and secondary GBMs express PDGF, but increased RB1 gene promoter methylation appears to occur more frequently in secondary GBMs (43%) than primary GBMs (14%) (Nakamura et al., 2001).

The expression of MGMT, a DNA repair enzyme, has also been implicated in glioblastoma and low-grade gliomas (Bourne & Schiff, 2010). Of particular interest is the methylation status of MGMT as it may correlate to resistance to alkylating therapy in some patients (Hegi et al., 2005).

Finally, chromosomal e 7 (7q34) gene BRAF mutations and overexpression of B-raf, which stimulates the mitogen-activated protein kinase (MAPK) pathway, is a major factor in tumorigenesis of pilocytic astrocytomas (Pfister et al., 2008). This mutation is also present in 23-38% of adult grade II astrocytomas. The role of BRAF mutation in progression to high-grade tumors, however, has yet to be elucidated.

Defining molecular differences amongst glioma subpopulations offers an exciting new dynamic in understanding the behaviors of this highly diverse tumor although much work is required before the variability observed is completely delineated. Already, studies are underway to target tumors at the molecular level in hopes of providing better treatment options (Johns et al., 2007). As it is apparent that the angiogenic switch is important in the progression of low-grade to high-grade glioma, defining the molecular changes that promote this event may offer additional treatment benefits. Animal studies have already shown that preventing the angiogenic switch in other solid tumors reduces tumor growth (Lyden et al., 2001). Therefore, further understanding of how specific molecular changes in tumor cells promote angiogenesis may offer promising new treatment options in gliomas.

7. Advancing imaging of low-grade gliomas

MRI is the initial imaging modality of choice in brain tumors. Low-grade gliomas usually appear as well defined lesions with little mass effect. They have low-signal on T1- and high-signal on T2-weighted imaging - particularly on fluid attenuated inversion recovery (FLAIR) sequences where low-grade gliomas are very hyperintense (Kates et al., 1996). Currently, the absence of gadolinium enhancement is used to differentiate low grade versus high grade glioma (Fig. 2) (Castillo, 1994), however, a significant portion of the low-grade gliomas defined by MRI were found to be high-grade after biopsy (Kondziolka et al., 1993). As a result, MRI is not sensitive enough to definitively diagnose low-grade gliomas as there are frequently small areas within the tumor that have already undergone malignant progression. Therefore, advanced imaging technologies, such as perfusion imaging, diffusion-weighted and diffusion tensor imaging, MR spectroscopy, and position emission tomography (PET), are currently being employed to more accurately identify low-grade versus high-grade gliomas. These modalities provide exciting insight into tumor vascularity, cellularity, metabolism, and proliferation and may prove more effective in differentiating low-grade from high-grade glioma particularly in regions within a given tumor.

Since the degree of vascularity correlates with tumor grade in gliomas, (Daumas-Duport et al., 1997) perfusion MRI and MRI with gradient echo differentiates low-grade versus high-grade gliomas based on relative cerebral blood volume (rCBV) (Boxerman et al., 2006, Law et al., 2003, Law et al., 2004, Shin et al., 2002, Sugahara et al., 1998, Sugahara et al., 2001). While promising, it has been difficult to establish a reliable threshold based on rCBV for low- versus high-grade state. Diffusion-weighted MRI has also been utilized based on the apparent diffusion coefficient, which inversely correlates with tumor cellularity (Gauvain et al., 2001, Kono et al., 2001, Sugahara et al., 1999). Again, it has been difficult to reliably predict tumor grade using diffusion MRI (Bulakbasi et al., 2003, Stieber, 2001). Diffusion tensor imaging (DTI) is a modification of diffusion-weighted imaging and measures fractional anisotropy (FA), which correlated with tumor cellularity and vascularity (Price, 2010). DTI is a promising new modality as one study reports the ability to distinguish between low- and high-grade gliomas using a threshold FA value of 0.188 (Inoue et al., 2005).

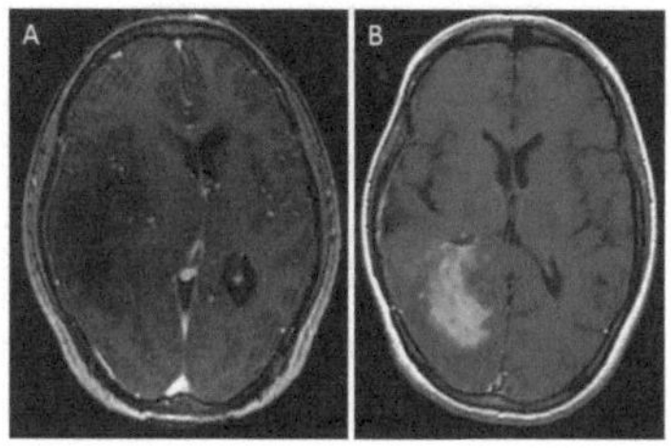

Fig. 1. Serial imaging of malignant progression of glioma. A, T1-weighted MRI with contrast. Patient presented with headache. MRI revealed hypointense lesion in right hemisphere. Note edema and mass effect but lack of contrast enhancement. Pt underwent gross total surgical resection and pathology revealed grade II astrocytoma. B, T1-weighted MRI with contrast. Subsequent imaging revealed recurrent tumor seen as a contrast enhancing lesion in the previous resection cavity. Pathology revealed progression to grade IV astrocytoma (GBM).

MR spectroscopy (MRS) also can potentially differentiate low-grade versus high-grade gliomas in the brain. All gliomas have an increased choline peak and a reduced N-acetyl aspartate peak (NAA) which are markers of membrane turnover and neuronal cell death respectively. Levels of lipid and lactate are markers of necrosis and hypoxia respectively and are decidedly elevated in high-grade compared to low-grade gliomas (McBride et al., 1995, Nafe et al., 2003, Negendank et al., 1996). Creatine (Cr), which serves as a marker of energy metabolism, is decreased in brain tumors (Meyerand et al., 1999, Moller-Hartmann et al., 2002), however, this reduction does not appear to correlate with tumor grade by itself (Moller-Hartmann et al., 2002). Using the choline/Cr ratio may be more effective, however, as low-grade gliomas tend to have a lower ratio of choline/Cr (McBride et al., 1995, Murphy et al., 2002, Sijens & Oudkerk, 2002), as well as an increase in NAA/Cr ratio (Law et al., 2003, McKnight et al., 2002, Murphy et al., 2002, Nafe et al., 2003, Negendank et al., 1996). MRS is a promising technique in differentiating low- from high-grade gliomas with sensitivity between 73% and 92% and specificity between 63% and 100% (Astrakas et al., 2004, Fayed & Modrego, 2005, Law et al., 2003, Nafe et al., 2003, Setzer et al., 2007). MRS may also be capable of identifying regions that have undergone malignant transformation within a given tumor that may not be identifiable by other imaging techniques although one such study attempting to detect malignant transformation within low-grade glioma yielded a specificity of only 57.1% (Alimenti et al., 2007).
Positron emission tomography (PET) imaging has been employed to examine gliomas in the brain by measuring the metabolic activity of tissue. Fluorinated glucose analogue 2-[18F]-fluoro-2-deoxy-D-glucose (FDG), which is administered to patients intravascularly, has high sensitivity for identifying areas of increased tumor metabolism and has been used as an index to predict tumor aggressiveness. While low-grade gliomas tend to have the same or even lower uptake of FDG than normal brain matter, high-grade gliomas demonstrate increased uptake of FDG on PET imaging (Derlon et al., 1997, Tamura et al., 1998), Studies have shown that it is possible to differentiate low- from high-grade gliomas with a sensitivity of 94% and specificity of 77% using a tumor-to-white-matter ratio of greater than 1.5 and tumor-to-grey-matter ratio of greater than 0.6 (Delbeke et al., 1995).

In addition to FDG, other tracers have been utilized in attempts to further characterize these tumors such as carbon 11 and fluorine 18 (18F)-labeled amino acid (Isselbacher, 1972). Methionine PET appears to have a higher sensitivity than FDG PET in detecting low-grade versus high-grade gliomas (Derlon et al., 1997, Giammarile et al., 2004, Ogawa et al., 1993). In particular, methionine PET exhibits a heightened sensitivity in detecting radiation necrosis from recurrent tumors, as inflammatory cells in radiation necrosis have little uptake of methionine (Thiel et al., 2000). Perhaps the most promising technique for diagnosing low-grade gliomas is 18F-FDOPA PET imaging. 18F-FDOPA PET is more accurate that FDG PET and has been shown to be highly predictive in determining tumor grade on initial diagnosis and may help differentiate tumor necrosis from recurrence (Chen et al., 2006, Fueger et al., Tripathi et al., 2009).

While there currently is no one imaging modality capable of definitively determining low-grade from high-grade tumors on its own, advanced imaging technology continues to develop and complement standard MRI. As we come to understand the behavior and variability of these tumors, advance imaging techniques provide exciting new possibilities for more precise treatments. Given the variability within a given tumor, advanced imaging techniques may allow for more precise targets for biopsy, vigilant monitoring of malignant transformation, and improved prognostic power in the management of low- and high-grade gliomas.

8. The Role of bone-marrow derived cells in malignant transformation

The vast majority of brain tumor research, molecular profiling, histological characteristics, diagnostic imaging modalities and treatment targets have focused on the actual tumor cells themselves. As mentioned earlier, one of the key events in the transition from the low-grade to the high-grade state is the angiogenic switch. It is theorized that in the low-grade state, tumor growth may be limited, at least in part, by a lack of blood supply. In this state, the tumor is only capable of a steady-state or linear growth (Mandonnet et al., 2003). Once the tumor acquires the ability to recruit or form new blood vessels, exponential growth occurs (Rees et al., 2009) resulting in rapid clinical decline. While there is considerable evidence that tumor cells undergo continued molecular changes that increase their malignant potential, these changes also allow these cells to initiate the angiogenic switch. It must also be noted that while recent evidence suggests that tumor cells may be capable of directly forming new blood vessels (Ricci-Vitiani et al., Wang et al.), a considerable body of evidence suggests that tumor cells do not do this completely on their own. While the exact details of this process still remain to be fully elucidated, tumor cells acquire the ability to transition the local tumor niche to an environment capable of rapid blood vessel formation. A variety of growth factors, signaling pathways, and indigenous populations of cells is hypothesized to participate in this process. If this theory proves to be correct, this population of cells forms an additional therapeutic target that may be as important as the tumor cells themselves. As current therapies directed at neoplastic cells are limited in part to their toxicity, elucidating other potential treatment pathways may further benefit patient outcome.

Neovascularization is a normal process in tissues and the brain during ischemia. In low oxygen states, cells release signals such as VEGF, PDGF, PlGF and HIF-1 that recruit from local existing vessels within the tissue itself (angiogenesis.) In addition, this can activate distant processes that facilitate neovascularization and may even form *de novo* blood vessels (vasculogenesis). These factors mobilize bone marrow precursor cells which then travel to the site of ischemia via the bloodstream. It is theorized that these cells facilitate vasculogenesis by breaking down existing structures and creating an environment that promotes new blood vessel growth.

Tumors are capable of adopting this machinery to increase growth and invasiveness by activating the angiogenic switch (Bergers & Benjamin, 2003, Rafii & Lyden, 2008). During early tumor development, neoplastic cells rely on existing blood flow and grow in a slow linear fashion (Mandonnet et al., 2003). Once the switch is initiated and neovascularization brings more oxygen and nutrients, tumor cells grow at a much faster rate and tumor size increases significantly (Rees et al., 2009). This initial process is thought to occur mostly by angiogenesis (Kioi, 2010). The release of proteases and proangiogenic factors causes pericytes to detach from existing vessels creating a defect in the extracellular matrix in the environment surrounding the vessel wall (Bergers & Benjamin, 2003). Endothelial cells proliferate locally and sprout outward into the tumor bed creating newly formed blood vessels feeding the tumor. While angiogenesis is an important factor in the angiogenic switch, vasculogenesis and the contribution of BMDC play a critical role as well. For example, when recruitment of BMDC is impaired in an animal model of lymphoma and lung carcinoma, tumor angiogenesis and growth is significantly decreased (Lyden et al., 2001) suggesting that BMDCs contribute significantly to neovascularization and growth in solid tumors.

In metastatic disease, the contribution of BMDC has been well described (Wels et al., 2008). Endothelial (EPCs) and hematopoietic precursor cells (HPC), mesenchymal stem cells (MSC), myeloid-derived suppressor cells (MDSCs), Tie-2 expressing monocytes (TEM) and tumor associated macrophages (TAM) all are mobilized from the bone marrow to future metastatic sites prior to tumor formation. It should be noted that these primitive cells are prominent during embryology and that a significant population of these cells is not present under normal conditions. While the exact role of each cell type has yet to be fully elucidated, their basic function is to break down normal structures and promote vasculogenesis and tumor invasiveness. The net result is a tumor friendly environment capable of sustaining tumor growth. This has been demonstrated experimentally in a murine model of metastatic disease by implanting m-cherry labeled melanoma cells into the flank of mice with GFP-labeled bone marrow and examining the lungs of these animals over time (Kaplan et al., 2005). It was observed that the first cells to arrive in future metastases were not tumor cells, but actual BMDC. This suggested, at least in metastatic disease, that the environment in future metastatic sites is primed by cells from the bone marrow before tumors can begin to grow in these distant areas (Rafii & Lyden, 2008). This also supports the hypothesis by Stephen Paget over 100 years ago that the tumor microenvironment may play as important a role as the tumor cells themselves.

In the brain, the role of BMDC has only recently garnered attention. One of the basic histological differences between low-grade and high-grade gliomas is a lack of neovascularization. Thus, activation of the angiogenic switch is a key element in the transformation of low-grade to high-grade glioma. Two elements are likely to contribute to this process. Genetic changes in tumor cells that occur during progression of disease activate pro-angiogenic factors. This has been observed in human tumor samples whereby genes involved in angiogenesis are upregulated in glioblastoma as compared to low grade astrocytoma (Godard et al., 2003). Kioi et al. also showed in their animal model that release of soluble factors by tumor cells or cells within the tumor microenvironment including

VEGF, FGF and EGF stimulates local angiogenesis (Kioi, 2010). Secondly, hypoxia is an additional critical event in triggering the switch (Kioi, 2010). As tumor size grows and metabolic demand exceeds local perfusion, hypoxic conditions occur. Release of hypoxia inducible factor-1 (HIF-1α) by tumor cells or cells within the hypoxic tumor environment, combined with stromal cell-derived factor-1 (SDF-1) and CXCR-4 receptor activation, mobilizes BMDCs to the tumor site and promotes vasculogenesis in gliomas (Du et al., 2008, Greenfield et al., 2010, Kioi, 2010).

In an attempt to further understand these processes in gliomas, Du et al. utilized an orthotopic model of GBM in mice to demonstrate recruitment of BMDC in gliomas (Du et al., 2008). Based on their results they theorize that hypoxia and the subsequent release of HIF-1α is the key event in tumor progression. Elevation of VEGF, and subsequent SDF-1 release and CXCR-4 receptor activation, mobilizes BMDC and recruits EPC and myeloid cells to the tumor. The net effect tips the balance to a pro-angiogenic state and neovascularization within the tumor bed. Kioi et al also further theorized that radiation treatment may exacerbate the vasculogenesis process and boost eventual tumor recurrence observed in current treatment regimens (Greenfield et al., 2010, Kioi, 2010). The endothelial-mesenchymal transition and MSC have also been described in metastatic disease (Singh & Settleman). MSC exist within the brain and mobilize to the tumor site as well (Hata et al., Kang et al.). The exact roles of these particular BMDC remain elusive and require more study before they are fully delineated.

In our laboratory, we have begun to investigate the correlation of BMDC mobilization and tumor grade in gliomas (unpublished data.) We used a PDGF-driven mouse model of GBM within which tumors develop slowly from low-grade to high-grade. Low-grade tumors have a clear absence of neovascularization and BMDC are not present within these lesions. In high-grade tumors, however, we have observed a profound increase in larger, irregularly shaped, hemorrhagic vessels and a significant population of BMDC exists that is not observed in low grade tumors. In addition, these cells are located near newly forming blood vessels in the perivascular niche. We have also observed that BMDC are mobilized in the bone marrow and are elevated in the peripheral blood of tumor bearing animals versus controls. In addition, a significant difference in this population of cells in the blood exists between low-grade and high-grade animals. While much work is yet to be done before this process is fully elucidated, it appears that the presence of BMDC correlates with tumor grade and the process of neovascularization. Thus, BMDC have a potential role in the angiogenic switch as tumors progress from low-grade to high-grade tumors.

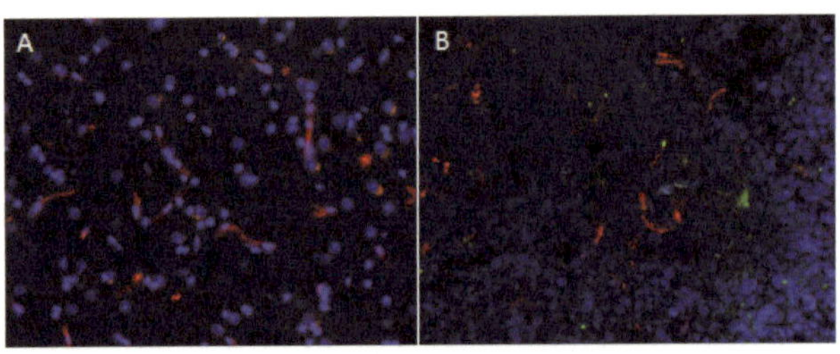

Fig. 2. Bone marrow-derived cells in human glioma. A, Immunofluorescence in grade II astrocytoma shows normal blood vessels (red, VE Cadherin) and a paucity of CD11b+ myeloid suppressor cells (Green). B, GBM shows abnormal vessel formation and an influx of CD11b+ cells (unpublished data.)

Mobilization of BMDC in peripheral blood samples has similarly been observed in patients with astrocytomas. Circulating CD133+ and VEGFR2+ EPC were measured in patients with different grade gliomas. This population of cells was significantly elevated in brain tumor patients versus controls, correlated with tumor grade, and predicted survival. In one patient, this population also predicted recurrence prior to detection by serial radiographic study. Currently, patients are followed with serial imaging in order to diagnose recurrence or malignant progression. While advances in imaging technology show promise in earlier more accurate diagnosis, the critical event has already occurred and prognosis worsens considerably. Therefore, the identification of a potential surrogate biomarker that measures tumor angiogenicity and aggressiveness may potentially serve as an index for ongoing treatment effectiveness or recurrence.

As histological and molecular differences between low-grade and high-grade gliomas are further defined and it becomes apparent that tumors cannot be loosely classified, specific treatments based on the particular characteristics of each individual tumor can potentially be designed. In addition, the presence of particular populations of BMDC in these tumors may also provide additional information on tumor behavior and serve as an additional treatment target along with tumor cells themselves. It has already been shown that the presence of BMDC in the blood correlates with tumor grade and initial animal studies suggest that BMDC are present in high-grade tumors only (Greenfield et al., 2009). In addition, TAM have been associated with poorer prognosis in metastatic lesions and other solid tumors (Wels et al., 2008). Thus histological stains aimed at identifying this population of cells may provide more accurate diagnosis and prognosis. Likewise, the molecular markers of this particular population of cells may offer an even more specific therapeutic target. Based on data collected in glioma patients, EPC can be identified by cell surface markers including CD133 and VEGFR2. Knocking down this population with specifically designed drug therapies has the potential for preventing recurrence by decreasing migration of these cells and reducing vasculogenesis within the tumor bed. Finally, one can also envision a role for advanced imaging technologies for improved diagnosis and treatment. For instance, PET has been used to specifically measure VEGF that has been labeled with copper in an orthotropic mouse model of GBM (Cai et al., 2006). If one could identify and label molecular targets that are specific to individual tumors subtypes and sensitive to new imaging techniques, this provides exciting non-invasive possibilities for tumor specific identification and treatment for each individual patient.

9. Conclusions

In summary, one of the primary factors predicting outcome in patients with low-grade glioma is malignant progression to high-grade tumor and it is evident that the angiogenic switch is an important event in this process. Initial management often entails surgical resection while adjuvant therapy for low-grade gliomas remains a controversial topic. Tumor grade is determined by histological analysis of tumor specimens, but the molecular fingerprint of these tumors is now being analyzed more thoroughly and holds promise for more exciting targeted treatment options. In addition, distinct, but as yet undefined, populations of cells are recruited to the tumor site and participate in neovascularization and promote tumor growth and invasiveness. Therefore, this population may represent an important therapeutic target in combating these tumors. Since survival is directly correlated with tumor grade, preventing tumor progression is imperative. While BMDC certainly are not the only factor in progression of disease and neovascularization, blocking recruitment of these cells to tumors has been shown to reduce growth in animal models of other tumor types. Therefore, a greater understanding of this process may define a role for targeting this population of cells. In addition, BMDC exist in the periphery, and make for an easier therapeutic target than tumor cells within the blood brain barrier. Lastly, current management of tumor recurrence relies on serial imaging studies. Therefore, an effective and accurate biomarker capable of predicting progression of disease may allow for earlier detection and better treatment outcomes. This makes the case for monitoring BMDC in the periphery in addition to therapy aimed at this population of cells as potential adjuvant therapy in glioma.

10. References

Alimenti, A., Delavelle, J., Lazeyras, F., Yilmaz, H., Dietrich, P. Y., de Tribolet, N. & Lovblad, K. O. (2007). Monovoxel 1H magnetic resonance spectroscopy in the progression of gliomas. *Eur Neurol*, Vol. 58, No. 4, pp. (198-209)

Armstrong, G. T., Conklin, H. M., Huang, S., Srivastava, D., Sanford, R., Ellison, D. W., Merchant, T. E., Hudson, M. M., Hoehn, M. E., Robison, L. L., Gajjar, A. & Morris, E. B. (2011). Survival and long-term health and cognitive outcomes after low-grade glioma. *Neuro Oncol*, Vol. 13, No. 2, pp. (223-34)

Astrakas, L. G., Zurakowski, D., Tzika, A. A., Zarifi, M. K., Anthony, D. C., De Girolami, U., Tarbell, N. J. & Black, P. M. (2004). Noninvasive magnetic resonance spectroscopic imaging biomarkers to predict the clinical grade of pediatric brain tumors. *Clin Cancer Res*, Vol. 10, No. 24, pp. (8220-8)

Bauman, G., Lote, K., Larson, D., Stalpers, L., Leighton, C., Fisher, B., Wara, W., MacDonald, D., Stitt, L. & Cairncross, J. G. (1999). Pretreatment factors predict overall survival for patients with low-grade glioma: a recursive partitioning analysis. *Int J Radiat Oncol Biol Phys*, Vol. 45, No. 4, pp. (923-9)

Berger, M. S., Deliganis, A. V., Dobbins, J. & Keles, G. E. (1994). The effect of extent of resection on recurrence in patients with low grade cerebral hemisphere gliomas. *Cancer*, Vol. 74, No. 6, pp. (1784-91)

Bergers, G. & Benjamin, L. E. (2003). Tumorigenesis and the angiogenic switch. *Nat Rev Cancer*, Vol. 3, No. 6, pp. (401-10)

Bourne, T. D. & Schiff, D. (2010). Update on molecular findings, management and outcome in low-grade gliomas. *Nat Rev Neurol*, Vol. 6, No. 12, pp. (695-701)

Boxerman, J. L., Schmainda, K. M. & Weisskoff, R. M. (2006). Relative cerebral blood volume maps corrected for contrast agent extravasation significantly correlate with glioma tumor grade, whereas uncorrected maps do not. *AJNR Am J Neuroradiol*, Vol. 27, No. 4, pp. (859-67)

Broniscer, A., Baker, S. J., West, A. N., Fraser, M. M., Proko, E., Kocak, M., Dalton, J., Zambetti, G. P., Ellison, D. W., Kun, L. E., Gajjar, A., Gilbertson, R. J. & Fuller, C. E. (2007). Clinical and molecular characteristics of malignant transformation of low-grade glioma in children. *J Clin Oncol*, Vol. 25, No. 6, pp. (682-9)

Bulakbasi, N., Kocaoglu, M., Ors, F., Tayfun, C. & Ucoz, T. (2003). Combination of single-voxel proton MR spectroscopy and apparent diffusion coefficient calculation in the evaluation of common brain tumors. *AJNR Am J Neuroradiol*, Vol. 24, No. 2, pp. (225-33)

Cai, W., Chen, K., Mohamedali, K. A., Cao, Q., Gambhir, S. S., Rosenblum, M. G. & Chen, X. (2006). PET of vascular endothelial growth factor receptor expression. *J Nucl Med*, Vol. 47, No. 12, pp. (2048-56)

Castillo, M. (1994). Contrast enhancement in primary tumors of the brain and spinal cord. *Neuroimaging Clin N Am*, Vol. 4, No. 1, pp. (63-80)

Chen, W., Silverman, D. H., Delaloye, S., Czernin, J., Kamdar, N., Pope, W., Satyamurthy, N., Schiepers, C. & Cloughesy, T. (2006). 18F-FDOPA PET imaging of brain tumors: comparison study with 18F-FDG PET and evaluation of diagnostic accuracy. *J Nucl Med*, Vol. 47, No. 6, pp. (904-11)

Daumas-Duport, C., Tucker, M. L., Kolles, H., Cervera, P., Beuvon, F., Varlet, P., Udo, N., Koziak, M. & Chodkiewicz, J. P. (1997). Oligodendrogliomas. Part II: A new grading system based on morphological and imaging criteria. *J Neurooncol*, Vol. 34, No. 1, pp. (61-78)

De Carli, E., Wang, X. & Puget, S. (2009). IDH1 and IDH2 mutations in gliomas. *N Engl J Med*, Vol. 360, No. 21, pp. (2248; author reply 2249)

Delbeke, D., Meyerowitz, C., Lapidus, R. L., Maciunas, R. J., Jennings, M. T., Moots, P. L. & Kessler, R. M. (1995). Optimal cutoff levels of F-18 fluorodeoxyglucose uptake in the differentiation of low-grade from high-grade brain tumors with PET. *Radiology*, Vol. 195, No. 1, pp. (47-52)

Derlon, J. M., Petit-Taboue, M. C., Chapon, F., Beaudouin, V., Noel, M. H., Creveuil, C., Courtheoux, P. & Houtteville, J. P. (1997). The in vivo metabolic pattern of low-grade brain gliomas: a positron emission tomographic study using 18F-fluorodeoxyglucose and 11C-L-methylmethionine. *Neurosurgery*, Vol. 40, No. 2, pp. (276-87; discussion 287-8)

Dirks, P. B., Jay, V., Becker, L. E., Drake, J. M., Humphreys, R. P., Hoffman, H. J. & Rutka, J. T. (1994). Development of anaplastic changes in low-grade astrocytomas of childhood. *Neurosurgery*, Vol. 34, No. 1, pp. (68-78)

Du, R., Lu, K. V., Petritsch, C., Liu, P., Ganss, R., Passegue, E., Song, H., Vandenberg, S., Johnson, R. S., Werb, Z. & Bergers, G. (2008). HIF1alpha induces the recruitment of bone marrow-derived vascular modulatory cells to regulate tumor angiogenesis and invasion. *Cancer Cell*, Vol. 13, No. 3, pp. (206-20)

Fayed, N. & Modrego, P. J. (2005). The contribution of magnetic resonance spectroscopy and echoplanar perfusion-weighted MRI in the initial assessment of brain tumours. *J Neurooncol*, Vol. 72, No. 3, pp. (261-5)

Fisher, P. G., Tihan, T., Goldthwaite, P. T., Wharam, M. D., Carson, B. S., Weingart, J. D., Repka, M. X., Cohen, K. J. & Burger, P. C. (2008). Outcome analysis of childhood low-grade astrocytomas. *Pediatr Blood Cancer*, Vol. 51, No. 2, pp. (245-50)

Fueger, B. J., Czernin, J., Cloughesy, T., Silverman, D. H., Geist, C. L., Walter, M. A., Schiepers, C., Nghiemphu, P., Lai, A., Phelps, M. E. & Chen, W. Correlation of 6-18F-fluoro-L-dopa PET uptake with proliferation and tumor grade in newly diagnosed and recurrent gliomas. *J Nucl Med*, Vol. 51, No. 10, pp. (1532-8)

Furnari, F. B., Fenton, T., Bachoo, R. M., Mukasa, A., Stommel, J. M., Stegh, A., Hahn, W. C., Ligon, K. L., Louis, D. N., Brennan, C., Chin, L., DePinho, R. A. & Cavenee, W. K.

(2007). Malignant astrocytic glioma: genetics, biology, and paths to treatment. *Genes Dev*, Vol. 21, No. 21, pp. (2683-710)

Gauvain, K. M., McKinstry, R. C., Mukherjee, P., Perry, A., Neil, J. J., Kaufman, B. A. & Hayashi, R. J. (2001). Evaluating pediatric brain tumor cellularity with diffusion-tensor imaging. *AJR Am J Roentgenol*, Vol. 177, No. 2, pp. (449-54)

Giammarile, F., Cinotti, L. E., Jouvet, A., Ramackers, J. M., Saint Pierre, G., Thiesse, P., Jouanneau, E., Guyotat, J., Pelissou-Guyotat, I., Setiey, A., Honnorat, J., Le Bars, D. & Frappaz, D. (2004). High and low grade oligodendrogliomas (ODG): correlation of amino-acid and glucose uptakes using PET and histological classifications. *J Neurooncol*, Vol. 68, No. 3, pp. (263-74)

Gil-Robles, S. & Duffau, H. (2010). Surgical management of World Health Organization Grade II gliomas in eloquent areas: the necessity of preserving a margin around functional structures. *Neurosurg Focus*, Vol. 28, No. 2, pp. (E8)

Godard, S., Getz, G., Delorenzi, M., Farmer, P., Kobayashi, H., Desbaillets, I., Nozaki, M., Diserens, A. C., Hamou, M. F., Dietrich, P. Y., Regli, L., Janzer, R. C., Bucher, P., Stupp, R., de Tribolet, N., Domany, E. & Hegi, M. E. (2003). Classification of human astrocytic gliomas on the basis of gene expression: a correlated group of genes with angiogenic activity emerges as a strong predictor of subtypes. *Cancer Res*, Vol. 63, No. 20, pp. (6613-25)

Greenfield, J. P., Jin, D. K., Young, L. M., Christos, P. J., Abrey, L., Rafii, S. & Gutin, P. H. (2009). Surrogate markers predict angiogenic potential and survival in patients with glioblastoma multiforme. *Neurosurgery*, Vol. 64, No. 5, pp. (819-26; discussion 826-7)

Greenfield, J. P., Cobb, W. S. & Lyden, D. (2010). Resisting arrest: a switch from angiogenesis to vasculogenesis in recurrent malignant gliomas. *J Clin Invest*, Vol. 120, No. 3, pp. (663-7)

Hartmann, C., Meyer, J., Balss, J., Capper, D., Mueller, W., Christians, A., Felsberg, J., Wolter, M., Mawrin, C., Wick, W., Weller, M., Herold-Mende, C., Unterberg, A., Jeuken, J. W., Wesseling, P., Reifenberger, G. & von Deimling, A. (2009). Type and frequency of IDH1 and IDH2 mutations are related to astrocytic and oligodendroglial differentiation and age: a study of 1,010 diffuse gliomas. *Acta Neuropathol*, Vol. 118, No. 4, pp. (469-74)

Hata, N., Shinojima, N., Gumin, J., Yong, R., Marini, F., Andreeff, M. & Lang, F. F. Platelet-derived growth factor BB mediates the tropism of human mesenchymal stem cells for malignant gliomas. *Neurosurgery*, Vol. 66, No. 1, pp. (144-56; discussion 156-7)

Hatanpaa, K. J., Burma, S., Zhao, D. & Habib, A. A. Epidermal growth factor receptor in glioma: signal transduction, neuropathology, imaging, and radioresistance. *Neoplasia*, Vol. 12, No. 9, pp. (675-84)

Hegi, M. E., Diserens, A. C., Gorlia, T., Hamou, M. F., de Tribolet, N., Weller, M., Kros, J. M., Hainfellner, J. A., Mason, W., Mariani, L., Bromberg, J. E., Hau, P., Mirimanoff, R. O., Cairncross, J. G., Janzer, R. C. & Stupp, R. (2005). MGMT gene silencing and benefit from temozolomide in glioblastoma. *N Engl J Med*, Vol. 352, No. 10, pp. (997-1003)

Ichimura, K., Pearson, D. M., Kocialkowski, S., Backlund, L. M., Chan, R., Jones, D. T. & Collins, V. P. (2009). IDH1 mutations are present in the majority of common adult gliomas but rare in primary glioblastomas. *Neuro Oncol*, Vol. 11, No. 4, pp. (341-7)

Inoue, T., Ogasawara, K., Beppu, T., Ogawa, A. & Kabasawa, H. (2005). Diffusion tensor imaging for preoperative evaluation of tumor grade in gliomas. *Clin Neurol Neurosurg*, Vol. 107, No. 3, pp. (174-80)

Isselbacher, K. J. (1972). Sugar and amino acid transport by cells in culture--differences between normal and malignant cells. *N Engl J Med*, Vol. 286, No. 17, pp. (929-33)

Jaeckle, K. A., Decker, P. A., Ballman, K. V., Flynn, P. J., Giannini, C., Scheithauer, B. W., Jenkins, R. B. & Buckner, J. C. (2010). Transformation of low grade glioma and correlation with outcome: an NCCTG database analysis. *J Neurooncol*, Vol. No. pp.

Johns, T. G., Perera, R. M., Vernes, S. C., Vitali, A. A., Cao, D. X., Cavenee, W. K., Scott, A. M. & Furnari, F. B. (2007). The efficacy of epidermal growth factor receptor-specific antibodies against glioma xenografts is influenced by receptor levels, activation status, and heterodimerization. *Clin Cancer Res*, Vol. 13, No. 6, pp. (1911-25)

Kang, S. G., Shinojima, N., Hossain, A., Gumin, J., Yong, R. L., Colman, H., Marini, F., Andreeff, M. & Lang, F. F. Isolation and perivascular localization of mesenchymal stem cells from mouse brain. *Neurosurgery*, Vol. 67, No. 3, pp. (711-20)

Kaplan, R. N., Riba, R. D., Zacharoulis, S., Bramley, A. H., Vincent, L., Costa, C., MacDonald, D. D., Jin, D. K., Shido, K., Kerns, S. A., Zhu, Z., Hicklin, D., Wu, Y., Port, J. L., Altorki, N., Port, E. R., Ruggero, D., Shmelkov, S. V., Jensen, K. K., Rafii, S. & Lyden, D. (2005). VEGFR1-positive haematopoietic bone marrow progenitors initiate the pre-metastatic niche. *Nature*, Vol. 438, No. 7069, pp. (820-7)

Kates, R., Atkinson, D. & Brant-Zawadzki, M. (1996). Fluid-attenuated inversion recovery (FLAIR): clinical prospectus of current and future applications. *Top Magn Reson Imaging*, Vol. 8, No. 6, pp. (389-96)

Kioi, M., et al. (2010). Inhibition of vasculogenesis, but not angiogenesis, prevents the recurrencec of glioblastoma following irradiation in mice. *J Clin Invest*, Vol. 120, No. pp. (XXX-YYY)

Kleihues, P., Soylemezoglu, F., Schauble, B., Scheithauer, B. W. & Burger, P. C. (1995). Histopathology, classification, and grading of gliomas. *Glia*, Vol. 15, No. 3, pp. (211-21)

Kondziolka, D., Lunsford, L. D. & Martinez, A. J. (1993). Unreliability of contemporary neurodiagnostic imaging in evaluating suspected adult supratentorial (low-grade) astrocytoma. *J Neurosurg*, Vol. 79, No. 4, pp. (533-6)

Kono, K., Inoue, Y., Nakayama, K., Shakudo, M., Morino, M., Ohata, K., Wakasa, K. & Yamada, R. (2001). The role of diffusion-weighted imaging in patients with brain tumors. *AJNR Am J Neuroradiol*, Vol. 22, No. 6, pp. (1081-8)

Law, M., Yang, S., Wang, H., Babb, J. S., Johnson, G., Cha, S., Knopp, E. A. & Zagzag, D. (2003). Glioma grading: sensitivity, specificity, and predictive values of perfusion MR imaging and proton MR spectroscopic imaging compared with conventional MR imaging. *AJNR Am J Neuroradiol*, Vol. 24, No. 10, pp. (1989-98)

Law, M., Yang, S., Babb, J. S., Knopp, E. A., Golfinos, J. G., Zagzag, D. & Johnson, G. (2004). Comparison of cerebral blood volume and vascular permeability from dynamic susceptibility contrast-enhanced perfusion MR imaging with glioma grade. *AJNR Am J Neuroradiol*, Vol. 25, No. 5, pp. (746-55)

Louis, D. N., Ohgaki, H., Wiestler, O. D., Cavenee, W. K., Burger, P. C., Jouvet, A., Scheithauer, B. W. & Kleihues, P. (2007). The 2007 WHO classification of tumours of the central nervous system. *Acta Neuropathol*, Vol. 114, No. 2, pp. (97-109)

Lyden, D., Hattori, K., Dias, S., Costa, C., Blaikie, P., Butros, L., Chadburn, A., Heissig, B., Marks, W., Witte, L., Wu, Y., Hicklin, D., Zhu, Z., Hackett, N. R., Crystal, R. G., Moore, M. A., Hajjar, K. A., Manova, K., Benezra, R. & Rafii, S. (2001). Impaired recruitment of bone-marrow-derived endothelial and hematopoietic precursor cells blocks tumor angiogenesis and growth. *Nat Med*, Vol. 7, No. 11, pp. (1194-201)

Mandonnet, E., Delattre, J. Y., Tanguy, M. L., Swanson, K. R., Carpentier, A. F., Duffau, H., Cornu, P., Van Effenterre, R., Alvord, E. C., Jr. & Capelle, L. (2003). Continuous growth of mean tumor diameter in a subset of grade II gliomas. *Ann Neurol*, Vol. 53, No. 4, pp. (524-8)

McBride, D. Q., Miller, B. L., Nikas, D. L., Buchthal, S., Chang, L., Chiang, F. & Booth, R. A. (1995). Analysis of brain tumors using 1H magnetic resonance spectroscopy. *Surg Neurol*, Vol. 44, No. 2, pp. (137-44)

McKnight, T. R., von dem Bussche, M. H., Vigneron, D. B., Lu, Y., Berger, M. S., McDermott, M. W., Dillon, W. P., Graves, E. E., Pirzkall, A. & Nelson, S. J. (2002). Histopathological validation of a three-dimensional magnetic resonance spectroscopy index as a predictor of tumor presence. *J Neurosurg*, Vol. 97, No. 4, pp. (794-802)

Meyerand, M. E., Pipas, J. M., Mamourian, A., Tosteson, T. D. & Dunn, J. F. (1999). Classification of biopsy-confirmed brain tumors using single-voxel MR spectroscopy. *AJNR Am J Neuroradiol*, Vol. 20, No. 1, pp. (117-23)

Moller-Hartmann, W., Herminghaus, S., Krings, T., Marquardt, G., Lanfermann, H., Pilatus, U. & Zanella, F. E. (2002). Clinical application of proton magnetic resonance spectroscopy in the diagnosis of intracranial mass lesions. *Neuroradiology*, Vol. 44, No. 5, pp. (371-81)

Murphy, M., Loosemore, A., Clifton, A. G., Howe, F. A., Tate, A. R., Cudlip, S. A., Wilkins, P. R., Griffiths, J. R. & Bell, B. A. (2002). The contribution of proton magnetic resonance spectroscopy (1HMRS) to clinical brain tumour diagnosis. *Br J Neurosurg*, Vol. 16, No. 4, pp. (329-34)

Nafe, R., Herminghaus, S., Raab, P., Wagner, S., Pilatus, U., Schneider, B., Schlote, W., Zanella, F. & Lanfermann, H. (2003). Preoperative proton-MR spectroscopy of gliomas--correlation with quantitative nuclear morphology in surgical specimen. *J Neurooncol*, Vol. 63, No. 3, pp. (233-45)

Nakamura, M., Yonekawa, Y., Kleihues, P. & Ohgaki, H. (2001). Promoter hypermethylation of the RB1 gene in glioblastomas. *Lab Invest*, Vol. 81, No. 1, pp. (77-82)

Negendank, W. G., Sauter, R., Brown, T. R., Evelhoch, J. L., Falini, A., Gotsis, E. D., Heerschap, A., Kamada, K., Lee, B. C., Mengeot, M. M., Moser, E., Padavic-Shaller, K. A., Sanders, J. A., Spraggins, T. A., Stillman, A. E., Terwey, B., Vogl, T. J., Wicklow, K. & Zimmerman, R. A. (1996). Proton magnetic resonance spectroscopy in patients with glial tumors: a multicenter study. *J Neurosurg*, Vol. 84, No. 3, pp. (449-58)

Ogawa, T., Shishido, F., Kanno, I., Inugami, A., Fujita, H., Murakami, M., Shimosegawa, E., Ito, H., Hatazawa, J., Okudera, T. & et al. (1993). Cerebral glioma: evaluation with methionine PET. *Radiology*, Vol. 186, No. 1, pp. (45-53)

Okamoto, Y., Di Patre, P. L., Burkhard, C., Horstmann, S., Jourde, B., Fahey, M., Schuler, D., Probst-Hensch, N. M., Yasargil, M. G., Yonekawa, Y., Lutolf, U. M., Kleihues, P. & Ohgaki, H. (2004). Population-based study on incidence, survival rates, and genetic alterations of low-grade diffuse astrocytomas and oligodendrogliomas. *Acta Neuropathol*, Vol. 108, No. 1, pp. (49-56)

Parsons, D. W., Jones, S., Zhang, X., Lin, J. C., Leary, R. J., Angenendt, P., Mankoo, P., Carter, H., Siu, I. M., Gallia, G. L., Olivi, A., McLendon, R., Rasheed, B. A., Keir, S., Nikolskaya, T., Nikolsky, Y., Busam, D. A., Tekleab, H., Diaz, L. A., Jr., Hartigan, J., Smith, D. R., Strausberg, R. L., Marie, S. K., Shinjo, S. M., Yan, H., Riggins, G. J., Bigner, D. D., Karchin, R., Papadopoulos, N., Parmigiani, G., Vogelstein, B., Velculescu, V. E. & Kinzler, K. W. (2008). An integrated genomic analysis of human glioblastoma multiforme. *Science*, Vol. 321, No. 5897, pp. (1807-12)

Pelloski, C. E., Ballman, K. V., Furth, A. F., Zhang, L., Lin, E., Sulman, E. P., Bhat, K., McDonald, J. M., Yung, W. K., Colman, H., Woo, S. Y., Heimberger, A. B., Suki, D., Prados, M. D., Chang, S. M., Barker, F. G., 2nd, Buckner, J. C., James, C. D. & Aldape, K. (2007). Epidermal growth factor receptor variant III status defines clinically distinct subtypes of glioblastoma. *J Clin Oncol*, Vol. 25, No. 16, pp. (2288-94)

Pfister, S., Janzarik, W. G., Remke, M., Ernst, A., Werft, W., Becker, N., Toedt, G., Wittmann, A., Kratz, C., Olbrich, H., Ahmadi, R., Thieme, B., Joos, S., Radlwimmer, B., Kulozik, A., Pietsch, T., Herold-Mende, C., Gnekow, A., Reifenberger, G., Korshunov, A., Scheurlen, W., Omran, H. & Lichter, P. (2008). BRAF gene duplication constitutes a mechanism of MAPK pathway activation in low-grade astrocytomas. *J Clin Invest*, Vol. 118, No. 5, pp. (1739-49)

Pollack, I. F., Claassen, D., al-Shboul, Q., Janosky, J. E. & Deutsch, M. (1995). Low-grade gliomas of the cerebral hemispheres in children: an analysis of 71 cases. *J Neurosurg*, Vol. 82, No. 4, pp. (536-47)

Prabhu, V. C., Khaldi, A., Barton, K. P., Melian, E., Schneck, M. J., Primeau, M. J. & Lee, J. M. (2010). Management of diffuse low-grade cerebral gliomas. *Neurol Clin*, Vol. 28, No. 4, pp. (1037-59)

Price, S. J. (2010). Advances in imaging low-grade gliomas. *Adv Tech Stand Neurosurg*, Vol. 35, No. pp. (1-34)

Rafii, S. & Lyden, D. (2008). Cancer. A few to flip the angiogenic switch. *Science*, Vol. 319, No. 5860, pp. (163-4)

Rees, J., Watt, H., Jager, H. R., Benton, C., Tozer, D., Tofts, P. & Waldman, A. (2009). Volumes and growth rates of untreated adult low-grade gliomas indicate risk of early malignant transformation. *Eur J Radiol*, Vol. 72, No. 1, pp. (54-64)

Ricci-Vitiani, L., Pallini, R., Biffoni, M., Todaro, M., Invernici, G., Cenci, T., Maira, G., Parati, E. A., Stassi, G., Larocca, L. M. & De Maria, R. Tumour vascularization via endothelial differentiation of glioblastoma stem-like cells. *Nature*, Vol. 468, No. 7325, pp. (824-8)

Sanson, M., Marie, Y., Paris, S., Idbaih, A., Laffaire, J., Ducray, F., El Hallani, S., Boisselier, B., Mokhtari, K., Hoang-Xuan, K. & Delattre, J. Y. (2009). Isocitrate dehydrogenase 1 codon 132 mutation is an important prognostic biomarker in gliomas. *J Clin Oncol,* Vol. 27, No. 25, pp. (4150-4)

Sathornsumetee, S., Reardon, D. A., Desjardins, A., Quinn, J. A., Vredenburgh, J. J. & Rich, J. N. (2007). Molecularly targeted therapy for malignant glioma. *Cancer,* Vol. 110, No. 1, pp. (13-24)

Schiff, D., Brown, P. D. & Giannini, C. (2007). Outcome in adult low-grade glioma: the impact of prognostic factors and treatment. *Neurology,* Vol. 69, No. 13, pp. (1366-73)

Schomas, D. A., Laack, N. N., Rao, R. D., Meyer, F. B., Shaw, E. G., O'Neill, B. P., Giannini, C. & Brown, P. D. (2009). Intracranial low-grade gliomas in adults: 30-year experience with long-term follow-up at Mayo Clinic. *Neuro Oncol,* Vol. 11, No. 4, pp. (437-45)

Setzer, M., Herminghaus, S., Marquardt, G., Tews, D. S., Pilatus, U., Seifert, V., Zanella, F. & Lanfermann, H. (2007). Diagnostic impact of proton MR-spectroscopy versus image-guided stereotactic biopsy. *Acta Neurochir (Wien),* Vol. 149, No. 4, pp. (379-86)

Shaw, E., Arusell, R., Scheithauer, B., O'Fallon, J., O'Neill, B., Dinapoli, R., Nelson, D., Earle, J., Jones, C., Cascino, T., Nichols, D., Ivnik, R., Hellman, R., Curran, W. & Abrams, R. (2002). Prospective randomized trial of low- versus high-dose radiation therapy in adults with supratentorial low-grade glioma: initial report of a North Central Cancer Treatment Group/Radiation Therapy Oncology Group/Eastern Cooperative Oncology Group study. *J Clin Oncol,* Vol. 20, No. 9, pp. (2267-76)

Shaw, E. G. & Wisoff, J. H. (2003). Prospective clinical trials of intracranial low-grade glioma in adults and children. *Neuro Oncol,* Vol. 5, No. 3, pp. (153-60)

Shaw, E. G., Berkey, B., Coons, S. W., Bullard, D., Brachman, D., Buckner, J. C., Stelzer, K. J., Barger, G. R., Brown, P. D., Gilbert, M. R. & Mehta, M. (2008). Recurrence following neurosurgeon-determined gross-total resection of adult supratentorial low-grade glioma: results of a prospective clinical trial. *J Neurosurg,* Vol. 109, No. 5, pp. (835-41)

Shin, J. H., Lee, H. K., Kwun, B. D., Kim, J. S., Kang, W., Choi, C. G. & Suh, D. C. (2002). Using relative cerebral blood flow and volume to evaluate the histopathologic grade of cerebral gliomas: preliminary results. *AJR Am J Roentgenol,* Vol. 179, No. 3, pp. (783-9)

Sijens, P. E. & Oudkerk, M. (2002). 1H chemical shift imaging characterization of human brain tumor and edema. *Eur Radiol,* Vol. 12, No. 8, pp. (2056-61)

Singh, A. & Settleman, J. EMT, cancer stem cells and drug resistance: an emerging axis of evil in the war on cancer. *Oncogene,* Vol. 29, No. 34, pp. (4741-51)

Stieber, V. W. (2001). Low-grade gliomas. *Curr Treat Options Oncol,* Vol. 2, No. 6, pp. (495-506)

Sugahara, T., Korogi, Y., Kochi, M., Ikushima, I., Hirai, T., Okuda, T., Shigematsu, Y., Liang, L., Ge, Y., Ushio, Y. & Takahashi, M. (1998). Correlation of MR imaging-determined cerebral blood volume maps with histologic and angiographic determination of vascularity of gliomas. *AJR Am J Roentgenol*, Vol. 171, No. 6, pp. (1479-86)

Sugahara, T., Korogi, Y., Kochi, M., Ikushima, I., Shigematu, Y., Hirai, T., Okuda, T., Liang, L., Ge, Y., Komohara, Y., Ushio, Y. & Takahashi, M. (1999). Usefulness of diffusion-weighted MRI with echo-planar technique in the evaluation of cellularity in gliomas. *J Magn Reson Imaging*, Vol. 9, No. 1, pp. (53-60)

Sugahara, T., Korogi, Y., Kochi, M., Ushio, Y. & Takahashi, M. (2001). Perfusion-sensitive MR imaging of gliomas: comparison between gradient-echo and spin-echo echo-planar imaging techniques. *AJNR Am J Neuroradiol*, Vol. 22, No. 7, pp. (1306-15)

Tamura, M., Shibasaki, T., Zama, A., Kurihara, H., Horikoshi, S., Ono, N., Oriuchi, N. & Hirano, T. (1998). Assessment of malignancy of glioma by positron emission tomography with 18F-fluorodeoxyglucose and single photon emission computed tomography with thallium-201 chloride. *Neuroradiology*, Vol. 40, No. 4, pp. (210-5)

Thiel, A., Pietrzyk, U., Sturm, V., Herholz, K., Hovels, M. & Schroder, R. (2000). Enhanced accuracy in differential diagnosis of radiation necrosis by positron emission tomography-magnetic resonance imaging coregistration: technical case report. *Neurosurgery*, Vol. 46, No. 1, pp. (232-4)

Tihan, T., Fisher, P. G., Kepner, J. L., Godfraind, C., McComb, R. D., Goldthwaite, P. T. & Burger, P. C. (1999). Pediatric astrocytomas with monomorphous pilomyxoid features and a less favorable outcome. *J Neuropathol Exp Neurol*, Vol. 58, No. 10, pp. (1061-8)

Tripathi, M., Sharma, R., D'Souza, M., Jaimini, A., Panwar, P., Varshney, R., Datta, A., Kumar, N., Garg, G., Singh, D., Grover, R. K., Mishra, A. K. & Mondal, A. (2009). Comparative evaluation of F-18 FDOPA, F-18 FDG, and F-18 FLT-PET/CT for metabolic imaging of low grade gliomas. *Clin Nucl Med*, Vol. 34, No. 12, pp. (878-83)

Unal, E., Koksal, Y., Cimen, O., Paksoy, Y. & Tavli, L. (2008). Malignant glioblastomatous transformation of a low-grade glioma in a child. *Childs Nerv Syst*, Vol. 24, No. 12, pp. (1385-9)

Wang, R., Chadalavada, K., Wilshire, J., Kowalik, U., Hovinga, K. E., Geber, A., Fligelman, B., Leversha, M., Brennan, C. & Tabar, V. Glioblastoma stem-like cells give rise to tumour endothelium. *Nature*, Vol. 468, No. 7325, pp. (829-33)

Watanabe, T., Nobusawa, S., Kleihues, P. & Ohgaki, H. (2009). IDH1 mutations are early events in the development of astrocytomas and oligodendrogliomas. *Am J Pathol*, Vol. 174, No. 4, pp. (1149-53)

Wels, J., Kaplan, R. N., Rafii, S. & Lyden, D. (2008). Migratory neighbors and distant invaders: tumor-associated niche cells. *Genes Dev*, Vol. 22, No. 5, pp. (559-74)

Wen, P. Y. & Kesari, S. (2008). Malignant gliomas in adults. *N Engl J Med*, Vol. 359, No. 5, pp. (492-507)

Wessels, P. H., Weber, W. E., Raven, G., Ramaekers, F. C., Hopman, A. H. & Twijnstra, A. (2003). Supratentorial grade II astrocytoma: biological features and clinical course. *Lancet Neurol*, Vol. 2, No. 7, pp. (395-403)

Yan, H., Parsons, D. W., Jin, G., McLendon, R., Rasheed, B. A., Yuan, W., Kos, I., Batinic-Haberle, I., Jones, S., Riggins, G. J., Friedman, H., Friedman, A., Reardon, D.,

Herndon, J., Kinzler, K. W., Velculescu, V. E., Vogelstein, B. & Bigner, D. D. (2009). IDH1 and IDH2 mutations in gliomas. *N Engl J Med*, Vol. 360, No. 8, pp. (765-73)

Part 3

Glioma Progression

11

Migration and Invasion of Brain Tumors

Richard A. Able, Jr.*, Veronica Dudu* and Maribel Vazquez
Department of Biomedical Engineering
The City College of The City University of New York (CCNY)
U.S.A.

1. Introduction

Recent advances in molecular biology have led to new insights in the development, growth and infiltrative behaviors of primary brain tumors (Demuth and Berens, 2004; Huse and Holland, 2010; Johnson et al., 2009; Kanu et al., 2009). These tumors are derived from various brain cell lineages and have been historically classified on the basis of morphological and, more recently, immunohistochemical features with less emphasis on their underlying molecular pathogenesis (Huse and Holland, 2010). The detailed molecular characterization of brain tumors has laid the groundwork for augmentation of standard treatment with patient-specific designed targeted therapies (Johnson et al., 2009; Kanu et al., 2009). Nevertheless, these tumors are extremely aggressive in their infiltration of brain tissue (Altman et al., 2007; Hensel et al., 1998; Yamahara et al., 2010), as well as in their metastasis outside of brain (Algra et al., 1992). Further, it now appears that the physiological conditions of the normal brain itself constitute a biological environment conducive to the uncontrolled dissemination of primary tumors (Bellail et al., 2004; Sontheimer, 2004). This review surveys the latest research on the invasive behavior of two major types of primary brain tumors: gliomas and medulloblastomas - the most common tumors diagnosed within adult and pediatric brain, respectively (Rickert and Paulus, 2001). The material has been divided into five sections: i) Characteristics of malignant brain tumors; ii) Mechanisms of tumor cell migration; iii) Models for the study of brain tumor invasion *in vivo* and *ex vivo*; iv) Models for the study of brain tumor invasion *in vitro*; and v) Future prospects of anti-invasive brain tumor therapy.

2. Characteristics of malignant brain tumors

Gliomas, commonly found in the anterior cerebral hemisphere, are a group of tumors derived from glial cells - the most abundant cells in the brain (Larjavaara et al., 2007; Lim et al., 2007; Louis et al., 2007). They are classified based on well-characterized histological features (Louis, 2006; Scheithauer, 2009; Trembath et al., 2008). The World Health Organization (WHO) defines gliomas by cell type, location and grade, and categorizes them into four classes (Lassman, 2004): i) Grade I tumors, or pilocytic astrocytomas; ii) Grade II tumors, also called low-grade astrocytomas; iii) Grade III tumors, or anaplastic astrocytomas; and iv) Grade IV tumors, also known as glioblastoma multiforme (GBM).

---

* Contributed equally

Grade I tumors typically do not invade surrounding brain and are often curable with surgery, while tumors of grades II to IV are diffuse and invade normal brain, with grade III and IV tumors being most aggressive. Grade III and IV tumors are called "high-grade" or "malignant" tumors although they almost never metastasize to other tissues of the body (Lassman, 2004).

The etiological events causing glioma formation have not been clearly defined, but are thought to involve genetic alterations (Figure 1A). Such alterations disrupt cell cycle arrest pathways (Zhou et al., 2005; Zhou et al., 2010), and cause aberrant receptor tyrosine kinase activity in the brain cells (Dai et al., 2001). For instance, activation of receptors such as Hepatocyte Growth Factor Receptor (HGF) c-Met (Gentile et al., 2008), Platelet-Derived Growth Factor Receptor (PDGFR) (Cattaneo et al., 2006; Natarajan et al., 2006), and Epidermal Growth Factor Receptor (EGFR) (Chicoine and Silbergeld, 1997) is now well-known to stimulate glioma motility. Additionally, marker specific glial progenitor populations, neural stem cells and cancer stem cells are being investigated for their roles as possible initiators of gliomagenesis (Briancon-Marjollet et al., 2010).

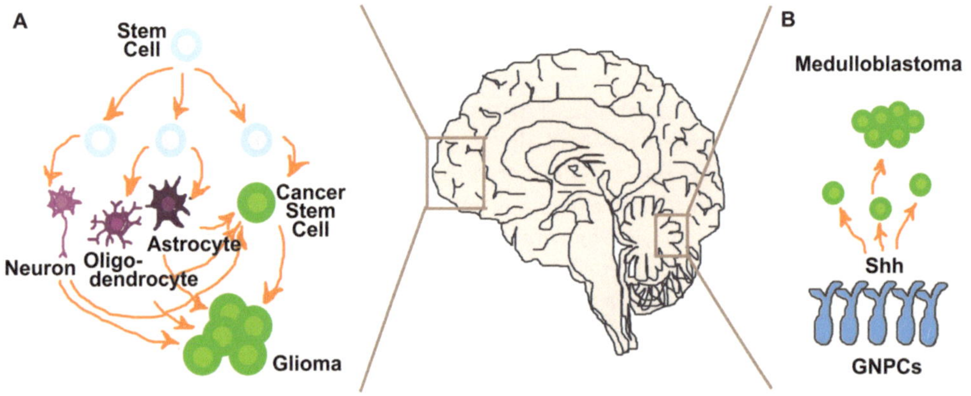

Fig. 1. Origin of brain tumors: development gone wrong. (A) During normal brain development, neural stem cells give rise to three main adult cell types: neurons, oligodendrocytes and astrocytes. Genetic alterations occur within these differentiated cells that can lead to the rise of malignant tumors. Alternatively, immature stem cells may serve as cancer stem cells that confer both radio- and chemoresistance phenotypes to gliomas. (B) Medulloblastomas originate in the cerebellum, from granule neuron precursor cells (GNPCs), upon un-controlled activation of Sonic Hedgehog (Shh) signaling pathway.

The current standard of care for gliomas is surgical removal of the tumor followed by post-operative radio- and chemotherapy (Stupp and Weber, 2005). However, due to their diffusely invasive properties, gliomas are one of the most difficult tumors to isolate or treat (Burger et al., 1985). Furthermore, while cell migration is fundamental to normal brain development and homeostasis, unconstrained migration of pathological and diseased cells makes the complete resection of tumor lesions, often performed for other types of tumors, an ineffective clinical treatment in brain. Prior to the advance of high-throughput genetic screening techniques clinicians depended primarily on glioma recurrence for prognosis of patient survival. Later, the generation of models that combined gene expression and molecular markers made it possible to subcategorize gliomas, enabling the increase in grade-specific predictability (Zhou et al., 2010). Recent findings suggest the possibility that the recurrent growth of glioma is derived from chemo- and radio-resistant cancer stem cell renewal and/or growth of diffusively invasive cells (Hadjipanayis and Van Meir, 2009). Evidence emerging over the past decade has suggested the existence of stem-like cells within brain tumors, which are currently examined as potential sources of tumor resistance and recurrence (Galli et al., 2004; Lenkiewicz et al., 2009; Singh and Dirks, 2007). The inability to remove high-grade gliomas in their entirety, or to prohibit their migration to other parts of the brain has led to low survival rates among brain cancer patients (Demuth and Berens, 2004). Patients with GBM have a median survival of about 1 year, while patients with anaplastic gliomas can survive 2-3 years, and those with grade II gliomas often survive 10-15 years (Louis et al., 2007).

Medulloblastomas (MBs) encompass a collection of clinically and molecularly diverse tumor subtypes, and are characterized by high tumor invasiveness to extraneural tissues and reoccurrence in the cerebellum after total resection (Dhall, 2009). Four different MB subtypes have been included in the current WHO classification (Louis et al., 2007): i) Classic MB; ii) Demoplastic/nodular MB; iii) MB with extensive nodularity; and iv) Anaplastic or large cell MB. Two other variants, medullomyoblastoma and melanotic MB, are much more rare. MBs are overwhelmingly found in pediatric patients, but can rarely occur within adult brain, where the tumor characteristics become very atypical. Adult MB is arguably a biologically distinct challenge in that it exhibits a higher proportion of desmoplastic histological characteristics, shows more proclivity toward cerebellar hemispheric origin, possesses different proliferative and apoptotic indices, and demonstrates a notorious tendency for late relapse with respect to the pediatric variants (Chan et al., 2000; Sarkar et al., 2002).

MBs are thought to arise within the cerebellum, with approximately 25% originating from granule neuron precursor cells (GNPCs) (Gibson et al., 2010) after aberrant activation of the Sonic Hedgehog (Shh) pathway (Figure 1B). A number of genetic alterations have been associated with MB (Biegel et al., 1997; Bigner et al., 1997; Herms et al., 2000; Yin et al., 2002). Studies of the receptors and intracellular signaling pathways that support proliferation and survival of GNPCs have shown a dysregulation of the Shh pathway, the canonical Wnt pathway, or the ERB-B pathway in both familiar and sporadic MBs (Gilbertson, 2004). A recent study showed that Wnt-subtype tumors infiltrate the dorsal brainstem, whereas Shh-subtype tumors are located within the cerebellar hemispheres (Gibson et al., 2010). These results have profound implications for future research and treatment of this childhood cancer, because to date, few data link such genetic alterations to metastasis in MB.

The treatment of patients with standard risk tumors, i.e. those who had tumors completely resected and with no evidence of dissemination to any other part of the body (Nishikawa, 2010), has been partially successful with survival rates of up to 40% for gliomas over the last five years (Van Meir et al., 2010) and 78% for MBs (Gajjar et al., 2006). In contrast, the cure of metastatic disease has been limited until recently to single cases (Fruhwald and Plass, 2002). Even though promising, the current treatment options for high-risk brain tumors are associated with neural and neuroendocrine side effects, with a tremendous decline in quality of life among survivors (Edelstein et al., 2011; Palmer et al., 2001), as well as growth reoccurrence and aggressive brain infiltration (Farin et al., 2006).

In the cases of both gliomas and MBs, the migration of cells from primary tumors to other locations, within brain or otherwise, has been one of the most clinically challenging and poorly understood processes that contributes to the poor life prognosis of patients. The following sections will discuss the fundamental mechanisms of cellular migration, the common *in vivo* models used to examine tumor cell migration within brain, and current *in vitro* technologies used to characterize and better understand the migration of cells derived from gliomas and MBs.

3. Mechanisms of tumor cell migration

The migration of brain cancer cells is highly complex, involving interactions with extracellular matrix (ECM), and chemoattractants that either diffuse from blood vessels and/or are produced by neighboring cells (Condeelis and Segall, 2003; Sahai, 2005). As a consequence of such complexity, the molecular mechanisms of primary brain tumor migration and metastasis are poorly understood. Over the last several years, a group of critical growth factors has been the topic of research for their role as regulators of tumor biology and chemotaxis (Hamel and Westphal, 2000). It is believed that over time secreted cytokines diffuse and generate concentration gradients that are sensed by glioma and MB-derived cells, leading to the detachment and migration of these cells away from the primary tumor (Chicoine and Silbergeld, 1997; Piperi et al., 2005). Therefore, brain tumor invasion is believed to be induced by soluble cytokines that stimulate directional and/or random tumor cell motility (Brockmann et al., 2003). Alternatively, cancer cells may communicate with specific distant targets through secreted microvesicles that contain growth factors and receptors, functional mRNAs, and miRNAs (Cocucci et al., 2009; Skog et al., 2008; Valadi et al., 2007). Such microvesicles are shed by most cell types, including cancer cells, and have been found in sera from numerous cancer patients (Cocucci et al., 2009; Skog et al., 2008).

While the effects of mitogens on the *in vitro* motility and invasion of glioma cells have been well documented using conventional assays, such as transwell chambers and spheroid models (discussed later in this chapter), the ability of soluble cytokines to drive various cellular functions (i.e. migration and/or proliferative growth) has been shown to depend upon several determinant factors. Some of these factors have been addressed in the literature, such as dosage-dependence (Gonzalez-Perez and Quinones-Hinojosa, 2010; Shih et al., 2004), contact inhibition (Weidner et al., 1990), as well as autocrine and paracrine signaling-driven tumor growth via extensive proliferation and aggressive recruitment of surrounding cells to the tumor (Betsholtz et al., 1984; Fomchenko and Holland, 2005; Hermansson et al., 1988; Rood et al., 2004). The diligent study of Central Nervous System tumor cell (CNSTC) invasion has identified four commonly overexpressed receptor tyrosine kinases as targets for anti-invasive therapies (EGFR, c-MET, PDGFR, and Vascular Epidermal Growth Factor Receptor (VEGFR)) (Abounader, 2009; Arora and Scholar, 2005; Huang et al., 2009; Zwick et al., 2001).

Cancer cell locomotion is highly sensitive to stimuli from the ECM as well as from the surrounding media. Receptors on the plasma membrane can activate cellular signaling pathways that alter the mechanotransduction of a cell via reorganization of motility-related organelles and cellular compartments. As an example, tumor-derived cells are known to increase cell motility in response to protease inhibitors and adhesion inhibitors (Sahai, 2005). The modes of cancer cell migration vary according to whether the cells undergo single cell chain, or collective migration. Tumor-derived cells disseminate from the bulk tumor mass individually via mesenchymal or amoeboid movement. However, in many tumors both single cell and collective cell migration may be present depending on the molecular cues dictating migration (Friedl and Wolf, 2003).

During the mesenchymal-type migration often observed in gliomas, cells exhibit a highly polarized and fibroblastic morphology. Cells undergo the classical, overlapping processes generally exhibited during mammalian cell migration: cell polarization, protrusion of leading edge, traction at the trailing edge, and detachment (Lauffenburger and Horwitz, 1996). First, cells become highly fibroblast-like, with bipolar opposites. Second, a growing number of actin filaments begin to push the cell membrane outwards on the leading edge via the formation of lamellipodia or filopodia. Actin polymerization then initiates signal transduction pathways along the leading edge. Next, cell integrins come into contact with ECM ligands and cluster to recruit intracellular signaling proteins that induce phosphorylation signaling, or so-called "outside in" signaling (Hynes, 2002; Miyamoto et al., 1995) via focal adhesion kinases. Afterwards, surface proteases act to cleave ECM molecules via production of soluble matrix metalloproteases (MMPs) in order to degrade surrounding ECM. Finally, cell contraction occurs via myosin that leads to focal contact disassembly at the trailing edge and actin cleavage and filament turnover (Wear et al., 2000).

Contrarily, during amoeboid movement, cells utilize a "fast gliding" mechanism driven by weak interactions with the substrate. As such, cells like neutrophils and lymphocytes exhibit a shape-driven migration with appreciable lack of focal adhesions that allows them to circumnavigate rather than degrade surrounding ECM during migration (Friedl et al., 2001). The result is an increased cell motility, as well as cell ability to undergo early detachment and metastatic spread from primary tumors. Cancer cells may undergo conversion from mesenchymal to amoeboid type migration in order to alter integrin distribution and actin cytoskeleton organization for increased dissemination (Wolf et al., 2003).

Collective migration is a well-studied phenomenon that is characteristic of embryological development, such as during the migration of cell clusters or sheets in the ectoderm following closure of the neural tube (Davidson and Keller, 1999). *In vitro* studies (Friedl et al., 1995; Nabeshima et al., 1995) showed that cells can migrate as a functional unit, and that in contrast to single motile cells, cell-cell adhesion can lead to a particular form of cortical actin filament present along cell junctions. This enables formation of a larger, multicellular contractile body. Here, a select group of highly motile cells are designated as so-called "path-generating" cells that create migratory traction via pseudopod activity (Friedl et al., 1995; Hegerfeldt et al., 2002; Nabeshima et al., 1995). It is then believed that cells located in the inner and trailing regions are passively dragged behind during dissemination. In tumors, collective migration has been observed as protruding sheets that maintain contact with the primary site, or as cell clusters that detach from their origin and extend along paths of least resistance (Byers et al., 1995; Hashizume et al., 1996; Madhavan et al., 2001). Collective migration offers the advantage of protection from immunological response. Further, heterogeneous sets of cells that move as one functional unit can work together to promote the invasion of less motile, but potentially apoptosis-resistant, sub-populations that increase tumor survival. To complicate matters, cells may transition between collective and individual cell migration with dedifferentiated cells to increase dissemination and metastatic spread (Friedl and Wolf, 2003).

4. Models for the study of brain tumor invasion *in vivo* and *ex vivo*

Glioma and MB models have been largely developed by studying altered oncogene expression through retroviral transfection of murine neural tissue of genetically engineered mouse models (GEMMs) (Fisher et al., 1999; Hatton et al., 2008; Heyer et al., 2010; Huse and

Holland, 2010; Pazzaglia et al., 2002; Pazzaglia et al., 2006; Romer and Curran, 2004). Via this powerful methodology, diverse tumor types with distinct histological features have been generated dependent upon the specific genetic background of the cell of tumor origin and the disease location of interest (Furnari et al., 2007). In particular, the histological features of GEMM and implanted xenograph derived tumors have been shown to be similar to human brain tumors presented in identical CNS locations, and have shed light on the diverse nature of human gliomas found clinically (Candolfi et al., 2007).

Historically, it has been suggested that glioma cell infiltration throughout the brain primarily utilizes mechanisms of migration innately patterned by neural progenitors during normal brain development (Cayre et al., 2009; Kakita and Goldman, 1999; Scherer, 1940). Confirmation of this similarity has been accomplished *in vivo* via implanted xenographs that result in spontaneous intracranial GBMs in six different animal model variations that show reproducible invasion of tumor cells into non-neoplastic brain regions (Figure 2) (Candolfi et al., 2007). More recently, several labs began utilizing GEMMs to specifically examine glial progenitor recruitment *in vivo* (Assanah et al., 2006; Masui et al., 2010). For instance, Assanah and colleagues have demonstrated via histological analysis of cortical sections from GEMMs that overexpression of tumor inducing proteins like PDGF can induce malignant glioma cells to invade across the corpus callosum into the contralateral hemisphere and overlying cortex (Assanah et al., 2006; Assanah et al., 2009).

The diffusive invasion and increased recurrence of gliomas post-operatively have been attributed to the same therapies used to treat the disease. Narayana and colleagues reported clinical results of 61 high-grade GBM patients treated with an anti-angiogenesis drug, bevacizumab. Their results showed that 82% of the patients treated with bevacizumab suffer from tumor regrowth and 70% died from the disease within 19 months (Narayana et al., 2009). Pàez-Ribes and colleagues reported similar results showing that although the use of angiogenesis inhibitors, such as Sunitinib and SU10944, extend that survival time of treated mice to an additional 7 weeks versus non-treated mice, the kinase inhibitors tend to also evoke an increase in glioma cell invasion as well as to promote tumor progression (Pàez-Ribes et al., 2009). A closer examination using xenographs of human tumor spheroid implanted into rat brains, and further treated with the bevacizumab, led to a reduction in contrast enhancement in magnetic resonance imaging (MRI) analysis while enhancing glioma cell diffusion by 68% versus non-treated rats (Figure 3) (Keunen et al., 2011).

Characterization of MB migration *in vivo* has yet to be analyzed at large, as most of the reports to-date focused on tumor growth and not its dissemination. Nevertheless, a select number of *in vivo* studies examined tumor cell migration and invasion. Hatton and colleagues illustrated in a GEMM for MB that 94% of the mice developed MB by 2 months of age, and that these tumors frequently exhibited leptomeningeal spread, a common feature of the human disease (Hatton et al., 2008). MacDonald and colleagues implanted human MB cells in the brain of nude mice, and thereafter followed them *in vivo* at single-cell level via fluorescence microscopy (MacDonald et al., 1998). These MB cells were shown to invade the brain and to form distant micro-metastases. In another study, MB cells were engineered to overexpress HGF and were implanted subcutaneously and intra-cranially (Li et al., 2005). The study reported activated c-Met that strongly increased MB xenograft growth and invasive characteristics with finger-like protrusions, metastatic growth, and leptomeningeal spread. Such findings illustrate that the HGF/c-Met pathway is one of the mediators of MB malignancy.

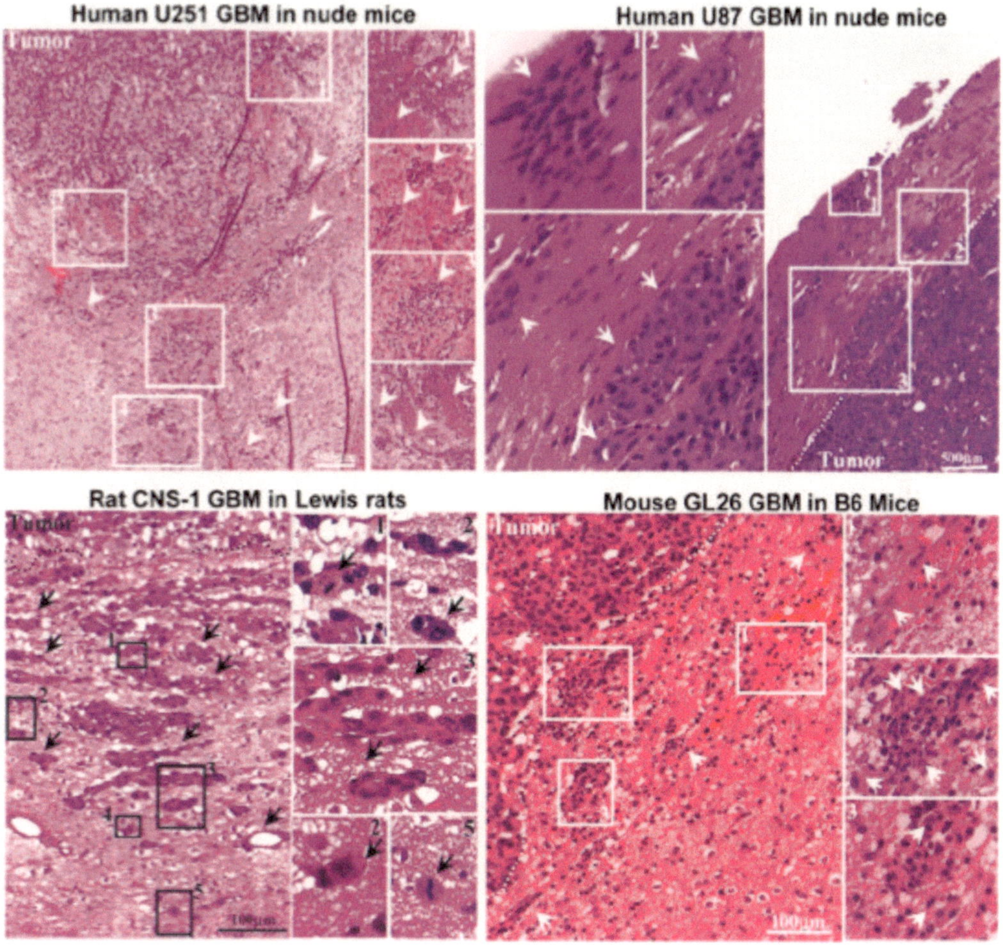

Fig. 2. Neoplastic cellular infiltration into surrounding non-neoplastic brain tissue in syngeneic rat (CNS-1) and mouse (GL26) GBM models and human glioma xenografts in nude mice (U251 and U87). Paraffin sections (5 μm) from GBM were stained with hematoxylin and eosin for evaluating neoplastic invasion. The numbers in low-magnification microphotographs depict areas magnified in the microphotographs on the right. *Arrows* indicate malignant cells, clusters of GBM cells, and tumoral blood vessels infiltrating surrounding brain parenchyma. The indistinct tumor borders and the malignant cells clearly entering the non-neoplastic brain tissue suggest an invasive phenotype. (Courtesy of Candolfi et al., 2007)

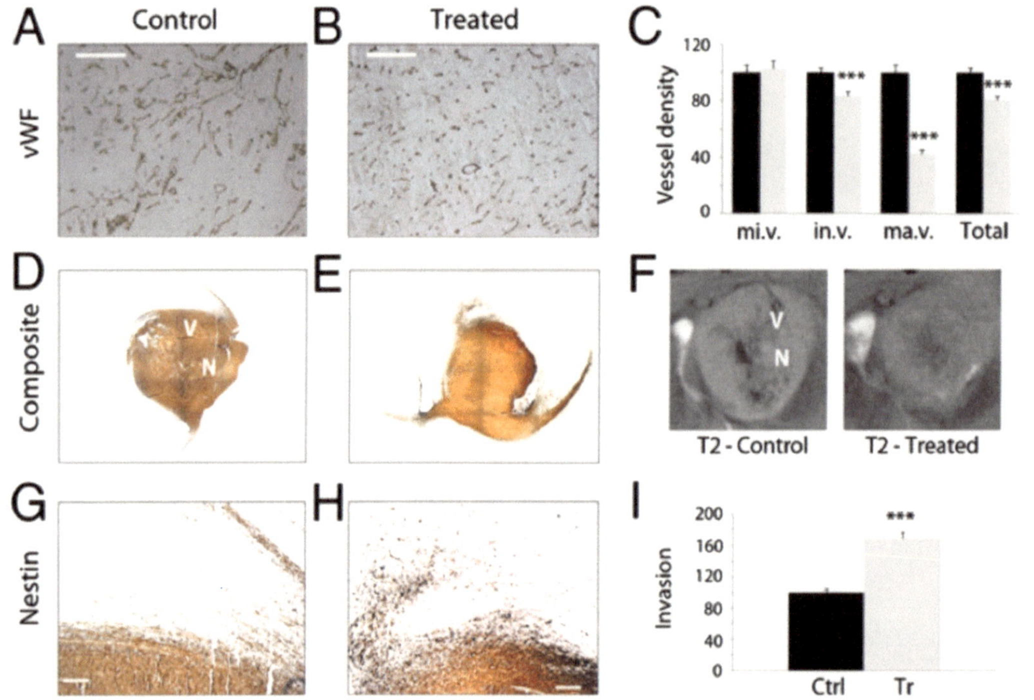

Fig. 3. Changes in blood vessel morphology and tumor cell invasion after bev treatment. Immunostaining for von Willebrand factor (vWF) (A and B) and quantification thereof (C), indicating a significant reduction in the density of medium and large blood vessels and in total vessel number after bev treatment. (Scale bar: 200 µm.) Nestin-stained composite images (D and E) reveal a more homogeneous appearance of the treated compared with untreated tumors, also reflected in corresponding T2-weighted MRI images (F). Large vessels ("V") appear as dark tortuous lines in nestin and T2- weighted images and necrotic areas ("N") as brighter spots. Quantification of the nestin-positive cells outside the tumor core (G and H) shows a 68% increase in cell invasion after treatment (I). mi.v: microvessels; in.v: intermediate-sized vessels; ma.v: macrovessels; Ctrl: controls; Tr: treated. (Scale bars: ± SE.) ***$P < 0.001$. (Courtesy of Keunen et al., 2011)

The ability to visualize brain tumor invasion in direct response to specific genetic aberrations and alterations made to the immediate environment has been critical in understanding the characteristics of this process. An advance made in this direction was accomplished via the detection of specific biomarkers involved in the progression or migration of CNSTCs, such as Receptor Tyrosine Kinases (RTKs), using conjugated antibodies that enabled *in vivo* monitoring via MRI (Towner et al., 2008). Alternatively, to *in vivo* imaging procedures, *ex vivo* brain tumor invasion assays that enable the study of tissue outside of the living system have had a tremendous impact in the field. Brain slices from mice and rats have been used to quantify the invasion of human gliomas (Nakada et al., 2004), and have demonstrated suppressed invasion on 2D surfaces, suggesting that the brain environment alone is capable of regulating protein function and, consequentially, the pattern and directionality of glioma migration (Beadle et al., 2008). Additionally, not only have *ex vivo* cell cultures been used to study the invasive properties of CNS tumors, but also to characterize the expression molecular markers (Riffkin et al., 2001), and to evaluate the therapeutic potential of co-cultured T-cells for anti-tumor activity (Ahmed et al., 2007).

By reducing the incidence of recurrent growth, clinicians envision the possibility of detecting and directly tracking migratory tumor cells *in vivo*, and therefore enabling operative procedures limited to a single total resection surgery. In order to accomplish this goal, there is a stringent need for development of enhanced imaging tools to allow visualization of migrating tumor cells. Meanwhile, the most successful quantitative assessment of CNSTCs migration has been accomplished outside of the brain itself, in engineered systems redesigned to mimic specific *in vivo* conditions. We will discuss these *in vitro* assays further, which have been utilized to evaluate a variety of cellular functions, from growth patterns and rates, to invasive motility of cells derived from highly malignant brain tumors.

5. Models for the study of brain tumor invasion *in vitro*

Tumor cells of the brain have been characterized as having a highly infiltrative phenotype for spreading into the healthy surrounding parenchyma. This malignant property is arguably the principle reason for tumor recurrence and high mortality rates (Lim et al., 2007). The interaction of integrins, membrane anchored heterodimeric proteins, with various ECM proteins has been explored extensively, as it is one of the key events that occurs during the invasion of tumor cells within their local microenvironments (Teodorczyk and Martin-Villalba, 2010). Another key process of tumor invasion is the cellular secretion/production of proteases that degrade ECM proteins in order to create pores through which the cells may migrate; such proteases include serine proteases, various MMPs, and cathepsins (Rao, 2003). In addition to stimulating tumor invasion via degradation of ECM protein components, it is assumed that MMPs are capable of enhancing tumor growth by indirectly triggering the release of growth factors trapped within the basement membrane itself (Mott and Werb, 2004). Lastly, another key aspect of tumor dissemination is played by the activation of RTK signaling pathways. During the destruction of the basement membrane by MMPs, soluble growth factors are sequestered from the ECM and bind to their cognate cellular receptors to trigger a cascade of events that enhance cellular migration (Zucker et al., 2000).

In vitro invasion assays are important tools for investigating the tumor-matrix interactions and the effects of extracellular macromolecules on these interactions. While not entirely identical to *in vivo* behavior, the study of tumor cell migration *in vitro* is advantageous due to the tightly-controlled experimental conditions, higher experimental throughput, and lower costs. The following section discusses the most commonly used *in vitro* assays, in the order of increased complexity.

5.1 Culture dish assays

Culture dish assays have the advantage of design simplicity and execution, while providing insightful information pertaining to cell-to-cell and cell-to-environment interactions. Coated culture dishes have been widely used to examine the roles played by specific ECM proteins, integrins, MMPs, and RTKs in stimulating the migration of brain tumor-derived cells, as detailed here.

Integrins are membrane heterodimeric proteins that mediate cell-environment attachment (Hynes, 1987; Tucker, 2006). In addition to anchoring cells to their environment, integrins have been shown to serve as signal mediators for ECM proteins that were found to stimulate tumor migration *in vitro* (Ohnishi et al., 1997; Tysnes et al., 1996). The most abundant ECM proteins found to interact with integrins in the brain are fibronectin, laminin, fibrinogen, tenascin-C, thrombodpondin, neuron-glia cell adhesion molecules (Ng-CAMs), and collagens IV and V (Rutka et al., 1988). Giese and colleagues evaluated astrocytoma migration as a function of integrin adhesiveness on various ECM proteins (collagen IV, fibronectin, laminin and vitronectin) (Giese et al., 1994). Based on the examination of eight different astrocytoma cell lines, the group concluded that the migration of glioma cells was subject to alteration depending on tumor expressed integrins and the availability of complementary matrix proteins. Furthermore, even though laminin frequently enabled tumor cells to adhere and migrate with increased adhesion, overall it was stated that there was no specific ECM protein that would always result in increased astrocytoma binding (Giese et al., 1994).

Friedlander and colleagues examined the migration trends of twenty-four excised human astrocytomas, ten GBM cell lines, and three MB cell lines on nine different ECM protein coated culture dishes (Friedlander et al., 1996). The comparative migration of astrocytomas (grades I, II and III), GBMs and MBs demonstrated that most tumor cells, regardless of their grade, were capable of migrating on fibronectin and laminin at rates exceeding 30 µm over a 16 hour period. A closer comparison between low-grade and high-grade tumor migration on all tested substrates revealed that, on average, high-grade tumors migrated approximately 14 µm more than low-grade tumor cells under similar conditions. Specifically, type IV collagen substrates induced a 4-fold increase in distances traveled by high-grade tumor cells over low-grade cells. Collagen IV coated substrates also stimulated approximately 100 µm migration over 16 hours of thirteen excised GBMs and eight well studied GBMs cell lines, with cell lines being more motile than the excised tumors (Friedlander et al., 1996). Finally, monoclonal antibodies specific for the α_v and β_1 integrins were used to reduce the migration of four GBMs cell lines (U-373 MG, U-118 MG, U-251 MG and U-87 MG) on several migration enhancing ECM substrates, including collagen IV (Friedlander et al., 1996). These results illustrate that brain tumor-derived cells can migrate remarkably large distances within the brain, often to varied regions of the brain. However, tumor cell populations are very diverse, and such studies have not identified the lineage of motile cells, or whether certain sub-populations of cells could migrate farther than others within brain.

MB samples revealed type I collagen present in the leptomeninges, and in the ECM surrounding blood vessels and tumor cells (Liang et al., 2008). Expression of both type I collagen and β_1 integrin, a subunit of a known type I collagen receptor, localized to the same area of MB. The same study showed that the adherence of MB cells to type I collagen matrix *in vitro* depends on the presence of β_1 integrin (Liang et al., 2008).

A study by Corcoran and Del Maestro revealed that MB cell lines do not defer cell proliferation for migration across an uncoated surface or invasion of a type I collagen matrix, contrary to the "Go or Grow" hypothesis (Corcoran and Del Maestro, 2003). The "Go or Grow" hypothesis proposes that cell division and cell migration are temporally exclusive events, and that tumor cells defer cell division to migrate (Giese et al., 1996). Migrating and invading MBs continued to proliferate and migrate/invade, irrespective of the number of divisions that took place (Corcoran and Del Maestro, 2003). These findings emphasize the need to evaluate the effect of future therapies on both biological events and, if possible, to identify intracellular signaling proteins that negatively regulate MB migration/invasion and proliferation.

Matrix-degrading proteases are involved in the hydrolytic breakdown of ECM proteins and have been shown to regulate tumor cell progression and invasion (Levicar et al., 2003; Rao, 2003; Rooprai and McCormick, 1997). Additionally, proteases have been well-studied and shown to display differential expression and activation patterns, correlated to their invasion-associated effects, i.e. angiogenesis (Forsyth et al., 1999; Thorns et al., 2003). These proteases are either located in the membrane of the cell or secreted into its surroundings, respectively denoted as MT-MMP and MMP. Diffusely invasive glioma cells express MMPs that enable them to catabolize ECM proteins that have been shown to prohibit the migration of other cells that lack these MMPs. For instance, specific membrane proteins expressed by CNS myelin have been shown to have anti-spreading functionality on neurite outgrowth, astrocytes and fibroblasts (Schwab and Caroni, 1988; Spillmann et al., 1998).

The migration of glioma-, MB- and meningioma- cell lines on CNS myelin was found to be tumor grade-dependent and to involve active unspecified MMPs (Amberger et al., 1998). Culture dishes were coated with 15 μg/dish rat spinal cord myelin, a concentration shown to reduce by 80% the fibroblast migration, followed by the seeding with various cell lines and the recording of cell ability to adhere and spread (Amberger et al., 1998). The results conclude that high grade GBMs, like U-251 MG, were able to strongly attach and spread, while low grade gliomas and MBs exhibited poor attachment and inhibited spreading (Amberger et al., 1998). Additionally, spreading of GBM and anaplastic astrocytomas cells on CNS myelin was strongly blocked when cells were treated with the MMP blocker O-phenanthroline (Felber et al., 1962), and temporarily inhibited with carbobenzoxy-Phe-Ala-Phe-Tyr-amide (Amberger et al., 1997) confirming the role played by MMPs in ECM modification as a precursory for migration.

Belien and colleagues studied the role of MT1-MMP in enhanced spreading and migration of gliomas (Belien et al., 1999). As a substrate, they utilized myelin-coated culture dishes, since it was previously shown that invasion of gliomas predominantly occurs along the white matter of the CNS (Giese et al., 1996; Pedersen et al., 1995), which is heavily composed of myelin (Baumann and Pham-Dinh, 2001; McLaurin and Yong, 1995), to seed both gliomas and MT1-MMP-transfected fibroblasts. In this case, MT1-MMP was shown to be responsible for altering the cellular environment to enable migration of both gliomas and the transfected fibroblasts (Belien et al., 1999).

When the invasiveness of five MB cell lines within a 3D *in vitro* collagen I or IV-based model was studied, the data showed that within hours of implantation, individual cells readily detached from the surface of the cell aggregates and invaded the collagen matrix, to distances of up to 1,200 μm and at rates of up to 300 μm per day (Ranger et al., 2010). Furthermore, MB invasiveness within this 3D model appears to depend upon a combination of metalloproteinase (MMP-1 and -2, TIMP-1 and -2) and cysteine protease activity (Ranger et al., 2010).

The RTKs, like integrins, function as signal mediators of extracellular proteins yet in a different way. Integrins, as mentioned above, interact primarily with static, structural ECM proteins that are the composite materials of the cellular environment (Tucker, 2006). Meanwhile, RTKs interact with soluble macromolecules present in the environment, e.g. growth factors, that trigger a cascade of events in the cells, spanning from the extracellular surface of the plasma membrane to the nucleus, to elicit various cellular responses (Konopka and Bonni, 2003; Mueller et al., 2003; Teodorczyk and Martin-Villalba, 2010). Additionally,

genetically modified and overexpressed RTKs are capable of eliciting cellular signals in the absence of ligand binding, thus bypassing the need for an extracellular trigger (Akbasak and Sunar-Akbasak, 1992; Dong et al., 2011; Strommer et al., 1990; Torp et al., 2007). Ding and colleagues employed U-87 MG cells grown on coated cultured dishes to demonstrate a strong adhesion to vitronectin, as opposed to collagen or laminin, which was mediated through the $\alpha_v\beta_3$ and $\alpha_v\beta_5$ integrins (Ding et al., 2003). Additionally, the group was able a to link the specific cooperative interaction between the RTK PDGFRβ and the $\alpha_v\beta_3$ integrin to induce migration of U-87 MG cells into the wounded area in a scratch-wound assay after stimulation of the culture with PDGF (Ding et al., 2003). Therefore, these results suggest the direct correlation between the ability of RTKs to transmit extracellular signals into the cell and to convert these signals into direct and measurable cellular response.
As an improvement upon the simple use of cell culture dishes for study of tumor cell migration, micropipette turning assays have been used to create gradients within culture dishes that enable changes in cell migration with micropipette position. Gradients, defined as fields where biochemical concentrations are varied along a specific distance, are generated via simple diffusion of biological molecules from the micropipette into the culture medium. Gradient formation and stability are functions of the molecular properties of the stimulant being used (i.e. diffusivity constant and molecular weight), as well as pipette mechanics (i.e. dimensions and flow rates) (Lohof et al., 1992), and for these reasons make gradient measurement difficult. Wyckoff and colleagues used the micropipette method to collect subpopulations of motile mammary carcinoma and macrophage cells into microneedles filled with Matrigel™ and a range of EGF concentrations from confluent culture dishes (Wyckoff et al., 2000). The Matrigel™ matrix is a solubilized basement membrane preparation extracted from Engelbreth-Holm-Swarm mouse sarcoma (Ohashi et al., 2006; Reed et al., 2009), commonly used in cell-matrix interaction studies. The contents of the microneedles were then emptied into new culture dishes and allowed to grow for at least 6 days before quantifying cell populations. A bell-shaped curve of normalized cell numbers was reported and had the maximal number of collected cells for 25 nM EGF, 8-fold greater than controls (Wyckoff et al., 2000). Such results illustrate that growth factor concentration gradients, or differences in concentrations along given distances, stimulate brain tumor cell migration.

5.2 Spheroids

A key question regarding cancer cell migration and invasion is based on determining the reason why tumor cells detach from the bulk tumor mass. Some studies have suggested that lack of contact-inhibition may be responsible for cell migration away from the bulk (Pedersen et al., 1995). While normal cells go into a quiescent state that allows apoptosis during nutrient depleted states, cancer cells do not rely on contact-dependent growth and therefore can detach and venture out to diffusely invade the parenchyma. The Spheroid Model utilizes the natural tendency of cancer cells to form colonies and to grow into localized spheres (Santini and Rainaldi, 1999; Zhang et al., 2005). This model mimics the 3D characteristics of cell migration, while culture dish experiments described in the previous subsection provide important data on 2D cell migration. As a result, the spheroid model has been used to study the directional migration of tumor cells from the bulk spheroid mass in response to specific motogens and chemotherapeutic agents, as well as to measure the penetration of various molecules into the tumor (Carlsson and Nederman, 1983; Nederman et al., 1983).

Spheroids grown from several different GBM cell lines were placed on uncoated 24-well dishes and treated with EGF, which triggered a strong stimulation of cellular invasion and increased growth (Lund-Johansen et al., 1990). Similarly, spheroids grown from several human glioma cell lines exhibited enhanced growth and directional migration when cultured in 10 ng/ml EGF or 10 ng/ml bFGF concentrations, compared to control and other growth factors, such as PDGFBB (Engebraaten et al., 1993). When MB cultures were induced to generate spheroids, gene expression of CD133 (a hallmark of the brain cancer stem cells and radioresistant tumors), MT1-MMP, and MMP-9 were induced and correlated with increased invasiveness of the spheroid cells (Annabi et al., 2008). Additionally, Corcoran and Del Maestro revealed that MB cells from an established cell line, UW228-13, could exhibit elevated levels of invasion into a 3D matrix of type 1 collagen compared to biopsied DAOY cells (Figure 4) (Corcoran and Del Maestro, 2003).

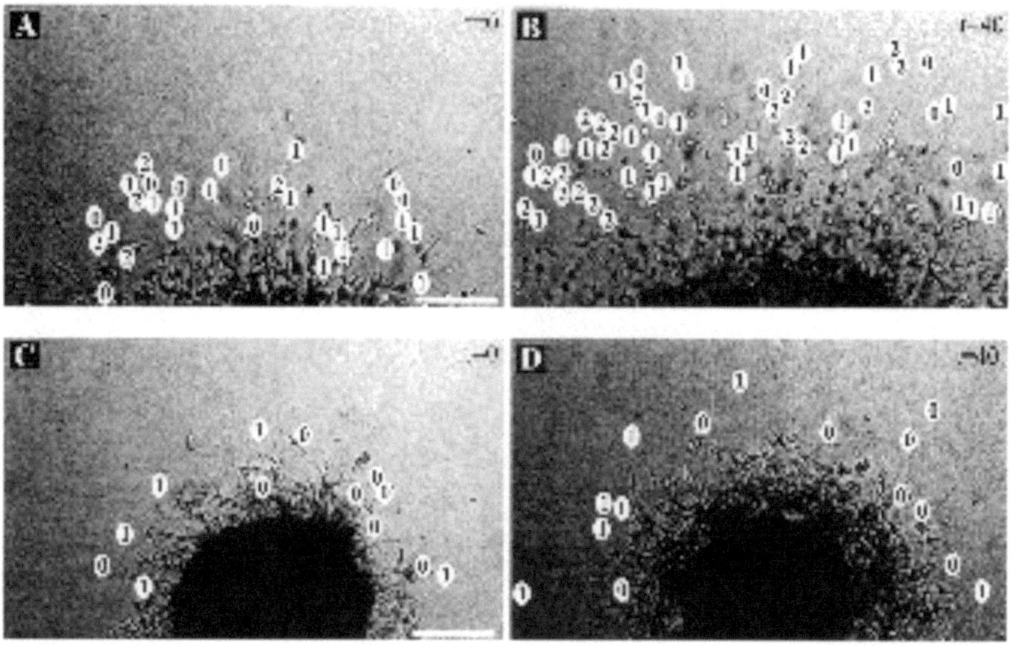

Fig. 4. First and last images extracted from time-lapse videos of DAOY (A and B) and UW228-3 (C and D) spheroids invading Type I collagen matrices. Spheroids were recorded 48 hours after implantation. The numbers identify cells that divided zero, one, or two times in 40 hours; parent cells are labeled in A and C and daughter cells in B and D. The number of hours elapsed from the start time of the videos (t) are indicated at the top right corner of images. Scale bars, 250 µm. (Courtesy of Corcoran and DelMaestro, 2003)

Wild-Bode and colleagues grew glioma spheroids on agar base-coated culture flasks until they were ~200 µm in diameter, followed by their transfer to 96-well plates. In order to examine the cause of glioma relapse in close proximity to the excised lesion, they measured the radial distance of migration as function of irradiation at 3 Gy. Irradiation led to increased migration of all cell lines, compared to non-irradiated cells, a phenomenon which was linked to increased expression and activation of MMP-2, MMP-9 and MT1-MMP (Wild-Bode et al., 2001).

Just as the spheroid model employs a 3D environment in order to better mimic *in vivo* conditions, other *in vitro* technologies were developed to imitate the biochemical environment of the brain. In particular, transwell assays were developed in order to expose tumor-derived cells to different concentration gradients of cytokines present within brain.

5.3 Transwell migration assays

The transwell migration assay is a commonly-used test to study the migratory response of cells to inducers or inhibitors. This assay is also known as the Boyden or modified Boyden chamber assay, and was originally used to evaluate leukocyte chemotaxis (Boyden, 1962). In this assay, a chamber that is separated into two compartments by a polyethylene terephthalate filter (Figure 5A) and the cells placed into the upper compartment are allowed to settle, while the solution being tested for chemotactic activity is placed in the lower compartment. The membrane contains randomly distributed pores through which the cells migrate (Figure 5B), in response to the chemoattractant from the bottom compartment. Invasive cells migrated to the underside of the filter can be stained and quantified (Figure 5C).

Different ECM components can be used to coat the filter in order to mimic the basement membrane that cells must penetrate while invading *in vivo,* while exposing the cells to various chemicals for different time lengths. The main advantage of this assay is its detection sensitivity. Migration through the permeable membrane can be caused by very low levels of chemoattractants (Kreutzer et al., 1978). Prolonged studies are difficult, due to the fact that the chemoattractant concentration will quickly equalize between the compartment below the membrane and the compartment above the membrane. Another disadvantage is the relative difficulty in setting up the transwells. Despite these disadvantages, transwell assays are commonly the test of choice for migration and invasion studies *in vitro.*

Over the last 50-years, several modifications have been implemented to this technology by various research groups in order to circumvent difficulties encountered with its use. For instance, upon crossing the membrane and reaching the lower surface of the chamber, cells may detach from the filter, thus resulting in an underestimate of transmigrated cells (Li and Zhu, 1999). Albini and colleagues were among the first researchers to use filters coated with ECM. They used radiolabeled proteins to demonstrate an 8-10 hour gradient stabilization period within the Boyden chamber, and showed that cell invasion time was very much dependent on the volume of the coated matrix barrier (Albini et al., 1987). Li and Zhu pioneered the use of different cell populations to attract other cells, by growing a monolayer of bovine aortic endothelial cells on filters, and investigating the transendothelial migration of six cell lines of different human tumors (Li and Zhu, 1999).

Chemotactic migration of GMB cells in response to several growth factors, predominately PDGF, EGF, and HGF, has been extensively studied (Hoelzinger et al., 2007). These studies have demonstrated dosage-dependent motogenic responses to various concentrations and combinations of these cytokines (Brockmann et al., 2003). For example, Moriyama and colleagues demonstrated, through a checkerboard analysis of various HGF concentrations, that a dose-dependent response to HGF induces both chemotaxis and chemokinesis of U-251 MG cells (Moriyama et al., 1996). In this study the concept of an "optimal concentration" was introduced, and the authors reported a decline in the chemotactic activity of U-251 MG cells at concentrations exceeding the reported optimal concentration of 50 ng/ml (Moriyama et al., 1996). Similarly, Koochekpour and colleagues used transwell assays to show dose-dependent migration and invasion of five different human glioma cell lines toward various concentrations of HGF, in addition to reducing basal migration of these cells using an anti-HGF neutralizing antibody (Koochekpour et al., 1997). Brockmann and colleagues reported increases in U-87 MG migration, as high as 33-fold greater than controls, in the presence of 100 pM HGF concentrations. In the same study, 1 nM TGFα and 50 nM FGF1 stimulated U-87 MG migration 17- and 4-fold, respectively (Brockmann et al., 2003). Transwell assays were used to demonstrate the chemotaxis of metastatic breast adenocarcinomas toward bone and brain extracts, rather than extracts from liver or lung (Hujanen and Terranova, 1985). Interestingly, it was found that C6-GFP rat glioma cells could extend their leading cytoplasmic processes through membrane pores, as a function of actin dynamics alone, but they required myosin IIA/B to generate additional cytoplasmic contractile forces to push the nucleus through pores having a smaller diameter (Beadle et al., 2008).

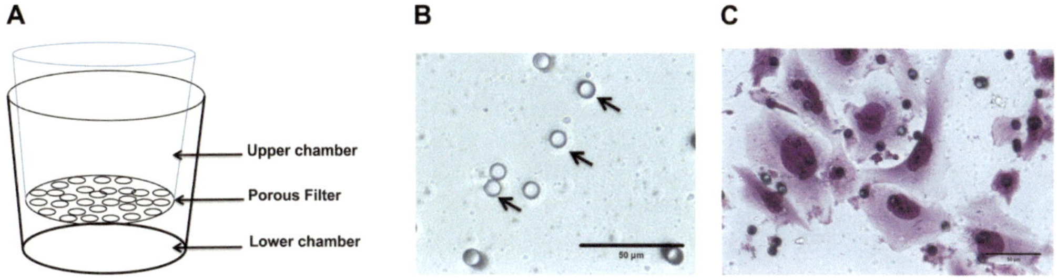

Fig. 5. Boyden chamber assay. (A) Transwell migration assays are composed of a well insert with a porous filter bottom that temporarily separates the cell solution from the test solution. (B) The filter has randomly distributed microscale diameter pores as shown by arrows. (C) Invasive Daoy cells on the underside of the filter stained and imaged for migration analysis. Scale bar = 50 μm.

A study that looked at the inhibitory effect of dietary-derived flavonols on the HGF receptor c-Met activity suggests that such an effect may contribute to the chemopreventive properties of these molecules (Labbe et al., 2009). The authors showed that the flavonols quercetin, kaempferol, and myricetin inhibited HGF/c-Met signaling in MB, preventing the formation of actin-rich membrane ruffles and resulting in the inhibition of c-Met-induced cell migration in Boyden chambers (Labbe et al., 2009). Furthermore, quercetin and kaempferol also strongly diminished HGF-mediated Akt activation (Labbe et al., 2009).

While investigating the effect of ionizing irradiation on the invasiveness of glioma cells via transwell assays, Park and colleagues reported increased Matrigel™ invasion of PTEN null gliomas, U-251 MG and U-373 MG, as a result of elevated levels irradiation treatment, which the group suggested correlates with increases in MMP-2 secretion (Park et al., 2006). Similarly, Wild-Bode and colleagues found that the sublethal irradiation doses of 1, 3, and 6 Gy increased the chemotactic migration and invasion of three different human glioma cell lines with increasing dosage (Wild-Bode et al., 2001). Similarly to glioma, radiation enhanced invasion and migration of 7 Gy irradiated MB compared to non-irradiated MB cells, as assessed via Boyden chamber assays (Nalla et al., 2010). Increased expression of urokinase-type plasminogen activator (uPA) and its receptor (uPAR), focal adhesion kinase (FAK), N-cadherin and integrin subunits (e.g., α_3, α_5 and β_1) was detected in irradiated cells.

Conversely, down-regulation of uPAR reduced the radiation-induced adhesion, migration and invasion of the irradiated cells, primarily by inhibiting phosphorylation of FAK, Paxillin and Rac-1/Cdc42 (Nalla et al., 2010).
Transwell assays were also used to study the activated RTK-dependent MB migration. These studies have shown that MB migration is dependent on estrogen-receptor (Belcher et al., 2009), c-Met (Guessous et al., 2010), and PDGFR-β activation (Yuan et al., 2010). Via a combination of wound-healing assays and modified Boyden chamber assays, two groups showed that PDGF-induced overexpression of Rac1, a Rho GTPase, is involved in MB cell migration and invasion, whereas knockdown of Rac1 expression dramatically inhibited migration and invasion of MBs (Chen et al., 2011; Yuan et al., 2010). These findings may promote the evaluation of Rac1 as a novel therapeutic agent impairing medulloblastoma PDGF-induced migration/invasion. Additional work has demonstrated that PDGFR-β activity may guide the migration of MB by transactivating EGFR (Abouantoun and MacDonald, 2009). These results are of particular interest, since EGFR is known to be expressed in GNPCs of the human cerebellum, participating in its normal development and function (Seroogy et al., 1995). Recently, the multifunctional signaling protein neurotrophin receptor $p75^{NTR}$ was shown to be a central regulator for GBM (Johnston et al., 2007) and MB spinal invasion while γ-secretase inhibitor, which blocks $p75^{NTR}$ proteolytic processing, significantly abrogates $p75^{NTR}$ induced MB migration and invasion *in vitro* and *in vivo* (Wang et al., 2010).
The transwell assays, even though used commonly for cell migration experiments, often yield inconsistent results across research groups due to the experimental individual assay modifications made by each group. For example, the ECM component used for filter coating can serve as a chemoattractant via integrin signaling (triggered by the interaction with laminin contained in the matrix), or via the release of growth factors embedded in the matrix itself. Although a reduced-growth factor form of Matrigel™ is generally used (i.e. reduced amounts of the above mentioned molecules are present in the matrix), there are a plethora of ECM proteins and growth factors, reconstituted along with Matrigel™, whose concentrations may vary with each batch purchased, and cause variations in the results. Yet, perhaps the largest shortcoming of transwell assays with respect to quantifying migration is that the cytokine microenvironments they create are very complex to model mathematically. Diffusion gradients of molecules across the membrane pores are difficult to measure or predict analytically, with or without matrix coating. Among *in vitro* approaches, microfluidics has proven to be a powerful technology to study cell migration over the past few years, due to the ability to generate a precise cell microenvironment that can be both predicted by analytical models and validated experimentally (Kong et al., 2010), as summarized further on.

5.4 Microdevices

Advances in microfabrication have made microfluidics systems easier to design and manufacture. Currently, the majority of devices are constructed of polydimethylsiloxane (PDMS) via soft lithography pioneered by the Whitesides group (McDonald and Whitesides, 2002). The polymer allows the construction of systems with high transparency and low thickness that are highly-compatible with biological microscopy. As dissemination of glioma or MB cells can often follow the path of white matter tracks or other heterogeneous structures, mechanical properties of the microenvironment play significant roles in tumor cell locomotion (Guck et al., 2010). PDMS microsystems pre-define the cell migratory path within microsized channels that mimic *in vivo* conditions. As such, cell motility and directionality can be examined and measured via conventional time-lapse imaging. Pioneering applications of microdevices for cancer cell study utilized microchannels coated and filled with various extracellular matrixes in 2D and 3D (Schoen et al., 2010; Sung et al., 2009) to illustrate the selectivity of cancer cell migration on distinct ECM, as well as to measure traction forces and leading edge protrusions of a variety of cancer cell types (Li et al., 2009). More recently, biomedical engineers have begun to develop systems that generate linear and non-linear cytokine gradients in order to more accurately investigate the chemotactic behavior of cells derived from primary tumors.

Establishment of steady-state gradient profiles has been examined using flow-based gradient generators, diffusion-based gradient generators, as well as hybrid generators (mixture of convection and diffusion). One of the original microdesigns for migration study was developed by Li Jeon and colleagues, in a gradient mixer design initially used for neutrophil chemotaxis (Li Jeon et al., 2002). This device contains multiple inlets that enable the loading of different ligand solutions that are then mixed in channels perpendicular to the flow direction (Figure 6A). Subsequently, a variety of system designs have been developed to generate alterative gradient shapes for further chemotaxis study (Kim et al., 2010). In such flow-based designs, two concentrations of biomolecules flow separately into a network of microchannels, where mixers are patterned to combine adjacent streams via convection in order to generate a chemical gradient. While flow-based devices are able to finely control the spatiotemporal resolution of the gradient, they require constant flow rates of reagents that remove molecules secreted from cells that are critical to regulation of tumor cell migration (Huang et al., 2011).

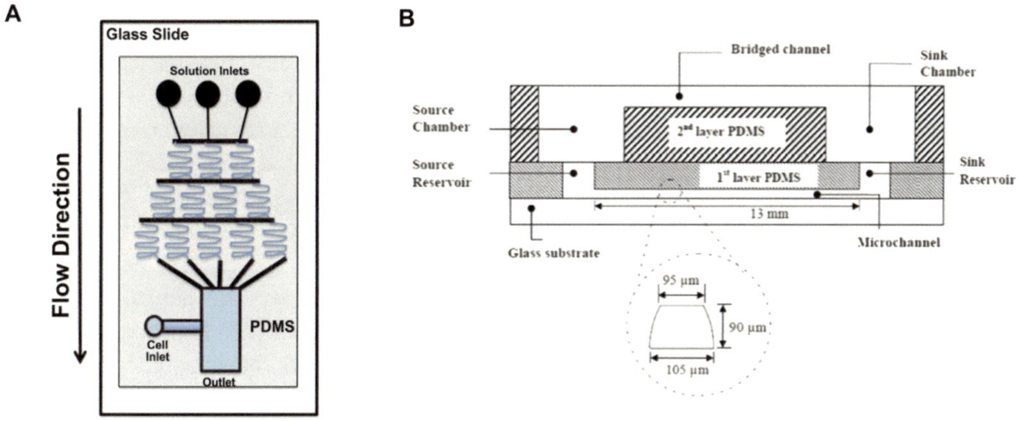

Fig. 6. Schematics of microdevices currently used to generate concentration gradients (not to scale). The flow mixer device was first proposed by Li Jeon and colleagues to create highly controllable concentrations along specific distances via continuous convective flow. (A) Schematic representation of a premixing gradient generating device pioneered by Li Jeon and colleagues. (B) A hybrid microlane system uses interconnected reservoirs to create concentration gradients via both convection and diffusion. The microchannel approximately measures 13 mm in length, 90 µm in depth and 100 µm in width (averaged with the upper side of 95 µm and the lower side of 105 µm), as its semi-hemispherical cross-section shown in inset. (Courtesy of Kong et al., 2010)

Subsequent microdevice designs now often generate soluble gradients by using passive diffusion. These systems can eliminate fluid flow near the surroundings of cells by using 3D hydrogels or high resistance channels so that transport occurs predominantly via diffusion (Beebe et al., 2002). In this configuration, two reservoirs are typically used to maintain given chemical concentration in a specified sink and source. Diffusion along adjoining microchannels then facilitates the formation of a concentration gradient between the reservoirs that enables cells to migrate along the defined gradient (Paguirigan and Beebe, 2008). While these systems eliminate the flow stresses imposed upon cells in flow-based devices, they require several hours to generate desired gradients, and rapid adjustment to the gradient profile is often difficult if not impractical. As a result, hybrid microsystems have been developed to enable the use diffusion with a minute level of convection to bolster formation of a desired gradient. For example, our group was able to generate steady-state gradients that were stable for 2-3 days using a bridge design and by exploiting the ultra-low bulk velocities generated by density differences between the reagents used (Figure 6B) (Kong et al., 2010).

The development of microfluidic platforms that incorporate real-time control of cell imaging and measurement of chemotactic concentration gradients is highly needed for understanding the dynamics of brain tumor interactions, an area which remains relatively unexplored when the majority of microfluidic studies focus on measurement of end-point cellular responses.

6. Future prospects of anti-invasive brain tumor therapy

The impetus for the development of anti-migratory therapeutic agents for brain tumors has been the desire to ease the manageability of the disease, by arresting tumor cells to their primary local environment. Such strategies can reduce the need to utilize the so-called "Search and Destroy" approach that is the currently suggested clinical necessity. Elucidation of possible mechanisms used by diffusely infiltrative glioma and MB cells will enable a better understanding of how to render these cells static, while providing targets for the development of pharmacological products capable of such a task.

More recently it has been suggested that enhancing the recruitment of endogenous progenitors toward tumor masses will aid in restoring the brain regions that have been resected or lost via necrosis (Cayre et al., 2009). Neural stem cells (NSCs) have aroused attention in the field of neurooncology as delivery vehicles of therapeutic genes. In addition to their multipotential capabilities that allow them to differentiate into neurons, astrocytes and oligodendrocytes, NSCs are also characterized by their remarkable capability to migrate through the brain (Gage, 2000; Yandava et al., 1999). The ability of implanted NSCs to distribute themselves throughout the tumors and follow invasive glioma cells has raised the idea of their therapeutic potential in targeting invasive glioma cells *in vivo* (Aboody et al., 2000; Staflin et al., 2009). Shimato and colleagues demonstrated *in vitro* that human NSCs exhibited extensive tropism for MB cells (Shimato et al., 2007). Using leptomeningeal dissemination mouse models, they confirmed *in vivo* that NSCs were able to distribute diffusely to MB cells that had spread throughout the entire spinal cord after implantation in the cisterna magna, and that genetically transformed NSCs functioned effectively in killing MB cells (Shimato et al., 2007). Similarly, genetically-modified NSCs were delivered intra-cranially and shown to target MBs (Kim et al., 2006). Recently, it was shown that human umbilical cord blood-derived stem cells can integrate into human MB after local delivery, and that MMP-2 expression by the tumor cells mediates this response through the SDF1/CXCR4 pathway (Bhoopathi et al., 2011). These results offer a new promising therapeutic modality that uses human stem cells for targeting intra-cranial as well as leptomeningeal dissemination of MBs.

Although significant results are being generated from the stem cell community, brain tumor researchers have only recently begun to reflect on the specifics of glial progenitor recruitment as a form of treatment for the disease. Glial progenitor cells have shown increased healing potential after supplementing the cultures with exogenous concentrations of VEGF D when compared to controls (Kranich et al., 2009). Using transwell assays, a dose dependent invasive response of murine neural stem cells towards human glioma conditioned media (Heese et al., 2005) and bi-potential O-2A progenitors toward PDGF (Gallo et al., 1996) has been displayed.

Ideally, as has been the case in previous years, the focus should be to target cytokines and their cognate receptors involved in glioma and MB chemotaxis signaling events. Moving forward, the community is in great need of technologies and strategies that can both approximate the chemical microenvironment present in the *in vivo* brain, and replicate these environments *in vitro*. In so doing, migration strategies can be developed that examine how combinations of cytokine and/or pharmacological cocktails can be used to limit the diffusive migration of tumor-derived cells into healthy brain.

7. Conclusion

The migration of glioma and medulloblastoma tumor cells into healthy brain tissue is a critical, yet poorly-understood, component of the tumor invasion and metastasis that contributes to poor patient prognosis. Extensive *in vivo* studies of brain tumors have generated invaluable data to elucidate the molecular alterations and genetic backgrounds present in diseased cells, the signaling mechanisms cells use to communicate with their surrounding microenvironment, and the characteristic patterns of dissemination used by specific tumor cell types. Additionally, *in vitro* studies of brain tumor-derived cells have established the chemotactic potential of various cytokines and extracellular matrixes, evaluated the effectiveness of pharmaceutical cocktails on tumor growth, as well as enabled fundamental measurement of motility and directionality in tumor cell samples. While the majority of research efforts to date have focused on the origin and nature of tumorigenesis in glioma and medulloblastoma, the community is now beginning to examine the integrated role of cell migration in tumor growth and dissemination. Future research is needed to examine the existence and characteristics of tumor cell populations with highly motile phenotypes in order to establish cell migration as a viable therapeutic target, and start designing treatment regimens based on cell migratory behaviors.

8. References

Aboody, K.S., Brown, A., Rainov, N.G., Bower, K.A., Liu, S., Yang, W., Small, J.E., Herrlinger, U., Ourednik, V., Black, P.M., Breakefield, X.O., Snyder, E.Y., 2000. Neural stem cells display extensive tropism for pathology in adult brain: evidence from intracranial gliomas. Proceedings of the National Academy of Sciences of the United States of America. 97, 12846-51.

Abouantoun, T.J., MacDonald, T.J., 2009. Imatinib blocks migration and invasion of medulloblastoma cells by concurrently inhibiting activation of platelet-derived growth factor receptor and transactivation of epidermal growth factor receptor. Molecular cancer therapeutics. 8, 1137-47.

Abounader, R., 2009. Interactions between PTEN and receptor tyrosine kinase pathways and their implications for glioma therapy. Expert review of anticancer therapy. 9, 235-45.

Ahmed, N., Ratnayake, M., Savoldo, B., Perlaky, L., Dotti, G., Wels, W.S., Bhattacharjee, M.B., Gilbertson, R.J., Shine, H.D., Weiss, H.L., Rooney, C.M., Heslop, H.E., Gottschalk, S., 2007. Regression of experimental medulloblastoma following transfer of HER2-specific T cells. Cancer research. 67, 5957-64.

Akbasak, A., Sunar-Akbasak, B., 1992. Oncogenes: cause or consequence in the development of glial tumors. Journal of the neurological sciences. 111, 119-33.

Albini, A., Iwamoto, Y., Kleinman, H.K., Martin, G.R., Aaronson, S.A., Kozlowski, J.M., McEwan, R.N., 1987. A rapid in vitro assay for quantitating the invasive potential of tumor cells. Cancer research. 47, 3239-45.

Algra, P.R., Postma, T., Van Groeningen, C.J., Van der Valk, P., Bloem, J.L., Valk, J., 1992. MR imaging of skeletal metastases from medulloblastoma. Skeletal radiology. 21, 425-30.

Altman, D.A., Atkinson, D.S., Jr., Brat, D.J., 2007. Best cases from the AFIP: glioblastoma multiforme. Radiographics : a review publication of the Radiological Society of North America, Inc. 27, 883-8.

Amberger, V.R., Avellana-Adalid, V., Hensel, T., Baron-van Evercooren, A., Schwab, M.E., 1997. Oligodendrocyte-type 2 astrocyte progenitors use a metalloendoprotease to spread and migrate on CNS myelin. The European journal of neuroscience. 9, 151-62.

Amberger, V.R., Hensel, T., Ogata, N., Schwab, M.E., 1998. Spreading and migration of human glioma and rat C6 cells on central nervous system myelin in vitro is correlated with tumor malignancy and involves a metalloproteolytic activity. Cancer research. 58, 149-58.

Annabi, B., Rojas-Sutterlin, S., Laflamme, C., Lachambre, M.P., Rolland, Y., Sartelet, H., Beliveau, R., 2008. Tumor environment dictates medulloblastoma cancer stem cell expression and invasive phenotype. Molecular cancer research : MCR. 6, 907-16.

Arora, A., Scholar, E.M., 2005. Role of tyrosine kinase inhibitors in cancer therapy. The Journal of pharmacology and experimental therapeutics. 315, 971-9.

Assanah, M., Lochhead, R., Ogden, A., Bruce, J., Goldman, J., Canoll, P., 2006. Glial progenitors in adult white matter are driven to form malignant gliomas by platelet-derived growth factor-expressing retroviruses. The Journal of neuroscience : the official journal of the Society for Neuroscience. 26, 6781-90.

Assanah, M.C., Bruce, J.N., Suzuki, S.O., Chen, A., Goldman, J.E., Canoll, P., 2009. PDGF stimulates the massive expansion of glial progenitors in the neonatal forebrain. Glia. 57, 1835-47.

Baumann, N., Pham-Dinh, D., 2001. Biology of oligodendrocyte and myelin in the mammalian central nervous system. Physiological reviews. 81, 871-927.

Beadle, C., Assanah, M.C., Monzo, P., Vallee, R., Rosenfeld, S.S., Canoll, P., 2008. The role of myosin II in glioma invasion of the brain. Molecular biology of the cell. 19, 3357-68.

Beebe, D.J., Mensing, G.A., Walker, G.M., 2002. Physics and applications of microfluidics in biology. Annual review of biomedical engineering. 4, 261-86.

Belcher, S.M., Ma, X., Le, H.H., 2009. Blockade of estrogen receptor signaling inhibits growth and migration of medulloblastoma. Endocrinology. 150, 1112-21.

Belien, A.T., Paganetti, P.A., Schwab, M.E., 1999. Membrane-type 1 matrix metalloprotease (MT1-MMP) enables invasive migration of glioma cells in central nervous system white matter. The Journal of cell biology. 144, 373-84.

Bellail, A.C., Hunter, S.B., Brat, D.J., Tan, C., Van Meir, E.G., 2004. Microregional extracellular matrix heterogeneity in brain modulates glioma cell invasion. The international journal of biochemistry & cell biology. 36, 1046-69.

Betsholtz, C., Westermark, B., Ek, B., Heldin, C.H., 1984. Coexpression of a PDGF-like growth factor and PDGF receptors in a human osteosarcoma cell line: implications for autocrine receptor activation. Cell. 39, 447-57.

Bhoopathi, P., Chetty, C., Gogineni, V.R., Gujrati, M., Dinh, D.H., Rao, J.S., Lakka, S.S., 2011. MMP-2 mediates mesenchymal stem cell tropism towards medulloblastoma tumors. Gene therapy. 2011 Mar 3. [Epub ahead of print].

Biegel, J.A., Janss, A.J., Raffel, C., Sutton, L., Rorke, L.B., Harper, J.M., Phillips, P.C., 1997. Prognostic significance of chromosome 17p deletions in childhood primitive neuroectodermal tumors (medulloblastomas) of the central nervous system. Clinical cancer research : an official journal of the American Association for Cancer Research. 3, 473-8.

Bigner, S.H., McLendon, R.E., Fuchs, H., McKeever, P.E., Friedman, H.S., 1997. Chromosomal characteristics of childhood brain tumors. Cancer genetics and cytogenetics. 97, 125-34.

Boyden, S., 1962. The chemotactic effect of mixtures of antibody and antigen on polymorphonuclear leucocytes. The Journal of experimental medicine. 115, 453-66.

Briancon-Marjollet, A., Balenci, L., Fernandez, M., Esteve, F., Honnorat, J., Farion, R., Beaumont, M., Barbier, E., Remy, C., Baudier, J., 2010. NG2-expressing glial precursor cells are a new potential oligodendroglioma cell initiating population in N-ethyl-N-nitrosourea-induced gliomagenesis. Carcinogenesis. 31, 1718-25.

Brockmann, M.A., Ulbricht, U., Gruner, K., Fillbrandt, R., Westphal, M., Lamszus, K., 2003. Glioblastoma and cerebral microvascular endothelial cell migration in response to tumor-associated growth factors. Neurosurgery. 52, 1391-9; discussion 1399.

Burger, P.C., Vogel, F.S., Green, S.B., Strike, T.A., 1985. Glioblastoma multiforme and anaplastic astrocytoma. Pathologic criteria and prognostic implications. Cancer. 56, 1106-11.

Byers, S.W., Sommers, C.L., Hoxter, B., Mercurio, A.M., Tozeren, A., 1995. Role of E-cadherin in the response of tumor cell aggregates to lymphatic, venous and arterial flow: measurement of cell-cell adhesion strength. Journal of cell science. 108 (Pt 5), 2053-64.

Candolfi, M., Curtin, J.F., Nichols, W.S., Muhammad, A.G., King, G.D., Pluhar, G.E., McNiel, E.A., Ohlfest, J.R., Freese, A.B., Moore, P.F., Lerner, J., Lowenstein, P.R., Castro, M.G., 2007. Intracranial glioblastoma models in preclinical neuro-oncology: neuropathological characterization and tumor progression. Journal of neuro-oncology. 85, 133-48.

Carlsson, J., Nederman, T., 1983. A method to measure the radio and chemosensitivity of human spheroids. Advances in experimental medicine and biology. 159, 399-417.

Cattaneo, M.G., Gentilini, D., Vicentini, L.M., 2006. Deregulated human glioma cell motility: inhibitory effect of somatostatin. Molecular and cellular endocrinology. 256, 34-9.

Cayre, M., Canoll, P., Goldman, J.E., 2009. Cell migration in the normal and pathological postnatal mammalian brain. Progress in neurobiology. 88, 41-63.

Chan, A.W., Tarbell, N.J., Black, P.M., Louis, D.N., Frosch, M.P., Ancukiewicz, M., Chapman, P., Loeffler, J.S., 2000. Adult medulloblastoma: prognostic factors and patterns of relapse. Neurosurgery. 47, 623-31; discussion 631-2.

Chen, B., Gao, Y., Jiang, T., Ding, J., Zeng, Y., Xu, R., Jiang, X., 2011. Inhibition of tumor cell migration and invasion through knockdown of rac1 expression in medulloblastoma cells. Cellular and molecular neurobiology. 31, 251-7.

Chicoine, M.R., Silbergeld, D.L., 1997. Mitogens as motogens. Journal of neuro-oncology. 35, 249-57.

Cocucci, E., Racchetti, G., Meldolesi, J., 2009. Shedding microvesicles: artefacts no more. Trends in cell biology. 19, 43-51.

Condeelis, J., Segall, J.E., 2003. Intravital imaging of cell movement in tumours. Nature reviews. Cancer. 3, 921-30.

Corcoran, A., Del Maestro, R.F., 2003. Testing the "Go or Grow" hypothesis in human medulloblastoma cell lines in two and three dimensions. Neurosurgery. 53, 174-84; discussion 184-5.

Dai, C., Celestino, J.C., Okada, Y., Louis, D.N., Fuller, G.N., Holland, E.C., 2001. PDGF autocrine stimulation dedifferentiates cultured astrocytes and induces oligodendrogliomas and oligoastrocytomas from neural progenitors and astrocytes in vivo. Genes & development. 15, 1913-25.

Davidson, L.A., Keller, R.E., 1999. Neural tube closure in Xenopus laevis involves medial migration, directed protrusive activity, cell intercalation and convergent extension. Development. 126, 4547-56.

Demuth, T., Berens, M.E., 2004. Molecular mechanisms of glioma cell migration and invasion. Journal of neuro-oncology. 70, 217-28.

Dhall, G., 2009. Medulloblastoma. Journal of child neurology. 24, 1418-30.

Ding, Q., Stewart, J., Jr., Olman, M.A., Klobe, M.R., Gladson, C.L., 2003. The pattern of enhancement of Src kinase activity on platelet-derived growth factor stimulation of glioblastoma cells is affected by the integrin engaged. The Journal of biological chemistry. 278, 39882-91.

Dong, Y., Jia, L., Wang, X., Tan, X., Xu, J., Deng, Z., Jiang, T., Rainov, N.G., Li, B., Ren, H., 2011. Selective inhibition of PDGFR by imatinib elicits the sustained activation of ERK and downstream receptor signaling in malignant glioma cells. International journal of oncology. 38, 555-69.

Edelstein, K., Spiegler, B.J., Fung, S., Panzarella, T., Mabbott, D.J., Jewitt, N., D'Agostino, N.M., Mason, W.P., Bouffet, E., Tabori, U., Laperriere, N., Hodgson, D.C., 2011. Early aging in adult survivors of childhood medulloblastoma: Long-term neurocognitive, functional, and physical outcomes. Neuro-oncology. 13, 536-45.

Engebraaten, O., Bjerkvig, R., Pedersen, P.H., Laerum, O.D., 1993. Effects of EGF, bFGF, NGF and PDGF(bb) on cell proliferative, migratory and invasive capacities of human brain-tumour biopsies in vitro. International journal of cancer. Journal international du cancer. 53, 209-14.

Farin, A., Suzuki, S.O., Weiker, M., Goldman, J.E., Bruce, J.N., Canoll, P., 2006. Transplanted glioma cells migrate and proliferate on host brain vasculature: a dynamic analysis. Glia. 53, 799-808.

Felber, J.P., Coombs, T.L., Vallee, B.L., 1962. The mechanism of inhibition of carboxypeptidase A by 1,10-phenanthroline. Biochemistry. 1, 231-8.

Fisher, G.H., Orsulic, S., Holland, E., Hively, W.P., Li, Y., Lewis, B.C., Williams, B.O., Varmus, H.E., 1999. Development of a flexible and specific gene delivery system for production of murine tumor models. Oncogene. 18, 5253-60.

Fomchenko, E.I., Holland, E.C., 2005. Stem cells and brain cancer. Experimental cell research. 306, 323-9.

Forsyth, P.A., Wong, H., Laing, T.D., Rewcastle, N.B., Morris, D.G., Muzik, H., Leco, K.J., Johnston, R.N., Brasher, P.M., Sutherland, G., Edwards, D.R., 1999. Gelatinase-A (MMP-2), gelatinase-B (MMP-9) and membrane type matrix metalloproteinase-1 (MT1-MMP) are involved in different aspects of the pathophysiology of malignant gliomas. British journal of cancer. 79, 1828-35.

Friedl, P., Noble, P.B., Walton, P.A., Laird, D.W., Chauvin, P.J., Tabah, R.J., Black, M., Zanker, K.S., 1995. Migration of coordinated cell clusters in mesenchymal and epithelial cancer explants in vitro. Cancer research. 55, 4557-60.

Friedl, P., Borgmann, S., Brocker, E.B., 2001. Amoeboid leukocyte crawling through extracellular matrix: lessons from the Dictyostelium paradigm of cell movement. Journal of leukocyte biology. 70, 491-509.

Friedl, P., Wolf, K., 2003. Tumour-cell invasion and migration: diversity and escape mechanisms. Nature reviews. Cancer. 3, 362-74.

Friedlander, D.R., Zagzag, D., Shiff, B., Cohen, H., Allen, J.C., Kelly, P.J., Grumet, M., 1996. Migration of brain tumor cells on extracellular matrix proteins in vitro correlates with tumor type and grade and involves alphaV and beta1 integrins. Cancer research. 56, 1939-47.

Fruhwald, M.C., Plass, C., 2002. Metastatic medulloblastoma--therapeutic success through molecular target identification? The pharmacogenomics journal. 2, 7-10.

Furnari, F.B., Fenton, T., Bachoo, R.M., Mukasa, A., Stommel, J.M., Stegh, A., Hahn, W.C., Ligon, K.L., Louis, D.N., Brennan, C., Chin, L., DePinho, R.A., Cavenee, W.K., 2007. Malignant astrocytic glioma: genetics, biology, and paths to treatment. Genes & development. 21, 2683-710.

Gage, F.H., 2000. Mammalian neural stem cells. Science. 287, 1433-8.

Gajjar, A., Chintagumpala, M., Ashley, D., Kellie, S., Kun, L.E., Merchant, T.E., Woo, S., Wheeler, G., Ahern, V., Krasin, M.J., Fouladi, M., Broniscer, A., Krance, R., Hale, G.A., Stewart, C.F., Dauser, R., Sanford, R.A., Fuller, C., Lau, C., Boyett, J.M., Wallace, D., Gilbertson, R.J., 2006. Risk-adapted craniospinal radiotherapy followed by high-dose chemotherapy and stem-cell rescue in children with newly diagnosed medulloblastoma (St Jude Medulloblastoma-96): long-term results from a prospective, multicentre trial. The lancet oncology. 7, 813-20.

Galli, R., Binda, E., Orfanelli, U., Cipelletti, B., Gritti, A., De Vitis, S., Fiocco, R., Foroni, C., Dimeco, F., Vescovi, A., 2004. Isolation and characterization of tumorigenic, stem-like neural precursors from human glioblastoma. Cancer research. 64, 7011-21.

Gallo, V., Zhou, J.M., McBain, C.J., Wright, P., Knutson, P.L., Armstrong, R.C., 1996. Oligodendrocyte progenitor cell proliferation and lineage progression are regulated by glutamate receptor-mediated K+ channel block. The Journal of neuroscience : the official journal of the Society for Neuroscience. 16, 2659-70.

Gentile, A., Trusolino, L., Comoglio, P.M., 2008. The Met tyrosine kinase receptor in development and cancer. Cancer metastasis reviews. 27, 85-94.

Gibson, P., Tong, Y., Robinson, G., Thompson, M.C., Currle, D.S., Eden, C., Kranenburg, T.A., Hogg, T., Poppleton, H., Martin, J., Finkelstein, D., Pounds, S., Weiss, A., Patay, Z., Scoggins, M., Ogg, R., Pei, Y., Yang, Z.J., Brun, S., Lee, Y., Zindy, F., Lindsey, J.C., Taketo, M.M., Boop, F.A., Sanford, R.A., Gajjar, A., Clifford, S.C., Roussel, M.F., McKinnon, P.J., Gutmann, D.H., Ellison, D.W., Wechsler-Reya, R., Gilbertson, R.J., 2010. Subtypes of medulloblastoma have distinct developmental origins. Nature. 468, 1095-9.

Giese, A., Rief, M.D., Loo, M.A., Berens, M.E., 1994. Determinants of human astrocytoma migration. Cancer research. 54, 3897-904.

Giese, A., Loo, M.A., Tran, N., Haskett, D., Coons, S.W., Berens, M.E., 1996. Dichotomy of astrocytoma migration and proliferation. International journal of cancer. Journal international du cancer. 67, 275-82.

Gilbertson, R.J., 2004. Medulloblastoma: signalling a change in treatment. The Lancet oncology. 5, 209-18.

Gonzalez-Perez, O., Quinones-Hinojosa, A., 2010. Dose-dependent effect of EGF on migration and differentiation of adult subventricular zone astrocytes. Glia. 58, 975-83.

Guck, J., Lautenschlager, F., Paschke, S., Beil, M., 2010. Critical review: cellular mechanobiology and amoeboid migration. Integrative biology : quantitative biosciences from nano to macro. 2, 575-83.

Guessous, F., Zhang, Y., diPierro, C., Marcinkiewicz, L., Sarkaria, J., Schiff, D., Buchanan, S., Abounader, R., 2010. An orally bioavailable c-Met kinase inhibitor potently inhibits brain tumor malignancy and growth. Anti-cancer agents in medicinal chemistry. 10, 28-35.

Hadjipanayis, C.G., Van Meir, E.G., 2009. Tumor initiating cells in malignant gliomas: biology and implications for therapy. Journal of molecular medicine. 87, 363-74.

Hamel, W., Westphal, M., 2000. Growth factors in gliomas revisited. Acta neurochirurgica. 142, 113-37; discussion 137-8.

Hashizume, R., Koizumi, H., Ihara, A., Ohta, T., Uchikoshi, T., 1996. Expression of beta-catenin in normal breast tissue and breast carcinoma: a comparative study with epithelial cadherin and alpha-catenin. Histopathology. 29, 139-46.

Hatton, B.A., Villavicencio, E.H., Tsuchiya, K.D., Pritchard, J.I., Ditzler, S., Pullar, B., Hansen, S., Knoblaugh, S.E., Lee, D., Eberhart, C.G., Hallahan, A.R., Olson, J.M., 2008. The Smo/Smo model: hedgehog-induced medulloblastoma with 90% incidence and leptomeningeal spread. Cancer research. 68, 1768-76.

Heese, O., Disko, A., Zirkel, D., Westphal, M., Lamszus, K., 2005. Neural stem cell migration toward gliomas in vitro. Neuro-oncology. 7, 476-84.

Hegerfeldt, Y., Tusch, M., Brocker, E.B., Friedl, P., 2002. Collective cell movement in primary melanoma explants: plasticity of cell-cell interaction, beta1-integrin function, and migration strategies. Cancer research. 62, 2125-30.

Hensel, T., Amberger, V.R., Schwab, M.E., 1998. A metalloprotease activity from C6 glioma cells inactivates the myelin-associated neurite growth inhibitors and can be neutralized by antibodies. British journal of cancer. 78, 1564-72.

Hermansson, M., Nister, M., Betsholtz, C., Heldin, C.H., Westermark, B., Funa, K., 1988. Endothelial cell hyperplasia in human glioblastoma: coexpression of mRNA for platelet-derived growth factor (PDGF) B chain and PDGF receptor suggests autocrine growth stimulation. Proceedings of the National Academy of Sciences of the United States of America. 85, 7748-52.

Herms, J., Neidt, I., Luscher, B., Sommer, A., Schurmann, P., Schroder, T., Bergmann, M., Wilken, B., Probst-Cousin, S., Hernaiz-Driever, P., Behnke, J., Hanefeld, F., Pietsch, T., Kretzschmar, H.A., 2000. C-MYC expression in medulloblastoma and its prognostic value. International journal of cancer. Journal international du cancer. 89, 395-402.

Heyer, J., Kwong, L.N., Lowe, S.W., Chin, L., 2010. Non-germline genetically engineered mouse models for translational cancer research. Nature reviews. Cancer. 10, 470-80.

Hoelzinger, D.B., Demuth, T., Berens, M.E., 2007. Autocrine factors that sustain glioma invasion and paracrine biology in the brain microenvironment. Journal of the National Cancer Institute. 99, 1583-93.

Huang, T.T., Sarkaria, S.M., Cloughesy, T.F., Mischel, P.S., 2009. Targeted therapy for malignant glioma patients: lessons learned and the road ahead. Neurotherapeutics : the journal of the American Society for Experimental NeuroTherapeutics. 6, 500-12.

Huang, Y., Agrawal, B., Sun, D., Kuo, J.S., Williams, J.C., 2011. Microfluidics-based devices: New tools for studying cancer and cancer stem cell migration. Biomicrofluidics. 5, 13412.

Hujanen, E.S., Terranova, V.P., 1985. Migration of tumor cells to organ-derived chemoattractants. Cancer research. 45, 3517-21.

Huse, J.T., Holland, E.C., 2010. Targeting brain cancer: advances in the molecular pathology of malignant glioma and medulloblastoma. Nature reviews. Cancer. 10, 319-31.

Hynes, R.O., 1987. Integrins: a family of cell surface receptors. Cell. 48, 549-54.

Hynes, R.O., 2002. Integrins: bidirectional, allosteric signaling machines. Cell. 110, 673-87.

Johnson, R., Wright, K.D., Gilbertson, R.J., 2009. Molecular profiling of pediatric brain tumors: insight into biology and treatment. Current oncology reports. 11, 68-72.

Johnston, A.L., Lun, X., Rahn, J.J., Liacini, A., Wang, L., Hamilton, M.G., Parney, I.F., Hempstead, B.L., Robbins, S.M., Forsyth, P.A., Senger, D.L., 2007. The p75 neurotrophin receptor is a central regulator of glioma invasion. PLoS biology. 5, e212.

Kakita, A., Goldman, J.E., 1999. Patterns and dynamics of SVZ cell migration in the postnatal forebrain: monitoring living progenitors in slice preparations. Neuron. 23, 461-72.

Kanu, O.O., Hughes, B., Di, C., Lin, N., Fu, J., Bigner, D.D., Yan, H., Adamson, C., 2009. Glioblastoma Multiforme Oncogenomics and Signaling Pathways. Clinical medicine. Oncology. 3, 39-52.

Keunen, O., Johansson, M., Oudin, A., Sanzey, M., Rahim, S.A., Fack, F., Thorsen, F., Taxt, T., Bartos, M., Jirik, R., Miletic, H., Wang, J., Stieber, D., Stuhr, L., Moen, I., Rygh, C.B., Bjerkvig, R., Niclou, S.P., 2011. Anti-VEGF treatment reduces blood supply and increases tumor cell invasion in glioblastoma. Proceedings of the National Academy of Sciences of the United States of America. 108, 3749-54.

Kim, S., Kim, H.J., Jeon, N.L., 2010. Biological applications of microfluidic gradient devices. Integrative biology : quantitative biosciences from nano to macro. 2, 584-603.

Kim, S.K., Kim, S.U., Park, I.H., Bang, J.H., Aboody, K.S., Wang, K.C., Cho, B.K., Kim, M., Menon, L.G., Black, P.M., Carroll, R.S., 2006. Human neural stem cells target experimental intracranial medulloblastoma and deliver a therapeutic gene leading to tumor regression. Clinical cancer research : an official journal of the American Association for Cancer Research. 12, 5550-6.

Kong, Q., Able, R.A., Jr., Dudu, V., Vazquez, M., 2010. A microfluidic device to establish concentration gradients using reagent density differences. Journal of biomechanical engineering. 132, 121012.

Konopka, G., Bonni, A., 2003. Signaling pathways regulating gliomagenesis. Current molecular medicine. 3, 73-84.

Koochekpour, S., Jeffers, M., Rulong, S., Taylor, G., Klineberg, E., Hudson, E.A., Resau, J.H., Vande Woude, G.F., 1997. Met and hepatocyte growth factor/scatter factor expression in human gliomas. Cancer research. 57, 5391-8.

Kranich, S., Hattermann, K., Specht, A., Lucius, R., Mentlein, R., 2009. VEGFR-3/Flt-4 mediates proliferation and chemotaxis in glial precursor cells. Neurochemistry international. 55, 747-53.

Kreutzer, D.L., O'Flaherty, J.T., Orr, W., Showell, H.J., Ward, P.A., Becker, E.L., 1978. Quantitative comparisons of various biological responses of neutrophils to different active and inactive chemotactic factors. Immunopharmacology. 1, 39-47.

Labbe, D., Provencal, M., Lamy, S., Boivin, D., Gingras, D., Beliveau, R., 2009. The flavonols quercetin, kaempferol, and myricetin inhibit hepatocyte growth factor-induced medulloblastoma cell migration. The Journal of nutrition. 139, 646-52.

Larjavaara, S., Mantyla, R., Salminen, T., Haapasalo, H., Raitanen, J., Jaaskelainen, J., Auvinen, A., 2007. Incidence of gliomas by anatomic location. Neuro-oncology. 9, 319-25.

Lassman, A.B., 2004. Molecular biology of gliomas. Current neurology and neuroscience reports. 4, 228-33.

Lauffenburger, D.A., Horwitz, A.F., 1996. Cell migration: a physically integrated molecular process. Cell. 84, 359-69.

Lenkiewicz, M., Li, N., Singh, S.K., 2009. Culture and isolation of brain tumor initiating cells. Current protocols in stem cell biology. Chapter 3, Unit3 3.

Levicar, N., Nuttall, R.K., Lah, T.T., 2003. Proteases in brain tumour progression. Acta neurochirurgica. 145, 825-38.

Li Jeon, N., Baskaran, H., Dertinger, S.K., Whitesides, G.M., Van de Water, L., Toner, M., 2002. Neutrophil chemotaxis in linear and complex gradients of interleukin-8 formed in a microfabricated device. Nature biotechnology. 20, 826-30.

Li, Y., Lal, B., Kwon, S., Fan, X., Saldanha, U., Reznik, T.E., Kuchner, E.B., Eberhart, C., Laterra, J., Abounader, R., 2005. The scatter factor/hepatocyte growth factor: c-met pathway in human embryonal central nervous system tumor malignancy. Cancer research. 65, 9355-62.

Li, Y.H., Zhu, C., 1999. A modified Boyden chamber assay for tumor cell transendothelial migration in vitro. Clinical & experimental metastasis. 17, 423-9.

Li, Z., Song, J., Mantini, G., Lu, M.Y., Fang, H., Falconi, C., Chen, L.J., Wang, Z.L., 2009. Quantifying the traction force of a single cell by aligned silicon nanowire array. Nano letters. 9, 3575-80.

Liang, Y., Diehn, M., Bollen, A.W., Israel, M.A., Gupta, N., 2008. Type I collagen is overexpressed in medulloblastoma as a component of tumor microenvironment. Journal of neuro-oncology. 86, 133-41.

Lim, D.A., Cha, S., Mayo, M.C., Chen, M.H., Keles, E., VandenBerg, S., Berger, M.S., 2007. Relationship of glioblastoma multiforme to neural stem cell regions predicts invasive and multifocal tumor phenotype. Neuro-oncology. 9, 424-9.

Lohof, A.M., Quillan, M., Dan, Y., Poo, M.M., 1992. Asymmetric modulation of cytosolic cAMP activity induces growth cone turning. The Journal of neuroscience : the official journal of the Society for Neuroscience. 12, 1253-61.

Louis, D.N., 2006. Molecular pathology of malignant gliomas. Annual review of pathology. 1, 97-117.

Louis, D.N., Ohgaki, H., Wiestler, O.D., Cavenee, W.K., Burger, P.C., Jouvet, A., Scheithauer, B.W., Kleihues, P., 2007. The 2007 WHO classification of tumours of the central nervous system. Acta neuropathologica. 114, 97-109.

Lund-Johansen, M., Bjerkvig, R., Humphrey, P.A., Bigner, S.H., Bigner, D.D., Laerum, O.D., 1990. Effect of epidermal growth factor on glioma cell growth, migration, and invasion in vitro. Cancer research. 50, 6039-44.

MacDonald, T.J., Tabrizi, P., Shimada, H., Zlokovic, B.V., Laug, W.E., 1998. Detection of brain tumor invasion and micrometastasis in vivo by expression of enhanced green fluorescent protein. Neurosurgery. 43, 1437-42; discussion 1442-3.

Madhavan, M., Srinivas, P., Abraham, E., Ahmed, I., Mathew, A., Vijayalekshmi, N.R., Balaram, P., 2001. Cadherins as predictive markers of nodal metastasis in breast cancer. Modern pathology : an official journal of the United States and Canadian Academy of Pathology, Inc. 14, 423-7.

Masui, K., Suzuki, S.O., Torisu, R., Goldman, J.E., Canoll, P., Iwaki, T., 2010. Glial progenitors in the brainstem give rise to malignant gliomas by platelet-derived growth factor stimulation. Glia. 58, 1050-65.

McDonald, J.C., Whitesides, G.M., 2002. Poly(dimethylsiloxane) as a material for fabricating microfluidic devices. Accounts of chemical research. 35, 491-9.

McLaurin, J.A., Yong, V.W., 1995. Oligodendrocytes and myelin. Neurologic clinics. 13, 23-49.

Miyamoto, S., Teramoto, H., Coso, O.A., Gutkind, J.S., Burbelo, P.D., Akiyama, S.K., Yamada, K.M., 1995. Integrin function: molecular hierarchies of cytoskeletal and signaling molecules. The Journal of cell biology. 131, 791-805.

Moriyama, T., Kataoka, H., Seguchi, K., Tsubouchi, H., Koono, M., 1996. Effects of hepatocyte growth factor (HGF) on human glioma cells in vitro: HGF acts as a motility factor in glioma cells. International journal of cancer. Journal international du cancer. 66, 678-85.

Mott, J.D., Werb, Z., 2004. Regulation of matrix biology by matrix metalloproteinases. Current opinion in cell biology. 16, 558-64.

Mueller, M.M., Werbowetski, T., Del Maestro, R.F., 2003. Soluble factors involved in glioma invasion. Acta neurochirurgica. 145, 999-1008.

Nabeshima, K., Moriyama, T., Asada, Y., Komada, N., Inoue, T., Kataoka, H., Sumiyoshi, A., Koono, M., 1995. Ultrastructural study of TPA-induced cell motility: human well-differentiated rectal adenocarcinoma cells move as coherent sheets via localized modulation of cell-cell adhesion. Clinical & experimental metastasis. 13, 499-508.

Nakada, M., Niska, J.A., Miyamori, H., McDonough, W.S., Wu, J., Sato, H., Berens, M.E., 2004. The phosphorylation of EphB2 receptor regulates migration and invasion of human glioma cells. Cancer research. 64, 3179-85.

Nalla, A.K., Asuthkar, S., Bhoopathi, P., Gujrati, M., Dinh, D.H., Rao, J.S., 2010. Suppression of uPAR retards radiation-induced invasion and migration mediated by integrin beta1/FAK signaling in medulloblastoma. PloS one. 5, e13006.

Narayana, A., Kelly, P., Golfinos, J., Parker, E., Johnson, G., Knopp, E., Zagzag, D., Fischer, I., Raza, S., Medabalmi, P., Eagan, P., Gruber, M.L., 2009. Antiangiogenic therapy using bevacizumab in recurrent high-grade glioma: impact on local control and patient survival. Journal of neurosurgery. 110, 173-80.

Natarajan, M., Stewart, J.E., Golemis, E.A., Pugacheva, E.N., Alexandropoulos, K., Cox, B.D., Wang, W., Grammer, J.R., Gladson, C.L., 2006. HEF1 is a necessary and specific downstream effector of FAK that promotes the migration of glioblastoma cells. Oncogene. 25, 1721-32.

Nederman, T., Acker, H., Carlsson, J., 1983. Penetration of substances into tumor tissue: a methodological study with microelectrodes and cellular spheroids. In vitro. 19, 479-88.

Nishikawa, R., 2010. Standard therapy for glioblastoma--a review of where we are. Neurologia medico-chirurgica. 50, 713-9.

Ohashi, K., Yokoyama, T., Nakajima, Y., Kosovsky, M., 2006. Methods for Implantation of BD MatrigelTM Matrix into Mice and Tissue Fixation. BD Biosciences Technical Bulletin #455.

Ohnishi, T., Arita, N., Hiraga, S., Taki, T., Izumoto, S., Fukushima, Y., Hayakawa, T., 1997. Fibronectin-mediated cell migration promotes glioma cell invasion through chemokinetic activity. Clinical & experimental metastasis. 15, 538-46.

Paez-Ribes, M., Allen, E., Hudock, J., Takeda, T., Okuyama, H., Vinals, F., Inoue, M., Bergers, G., Hanahan, D., Casanovas, O., 2009. Antiangiogenic therapy elicits malignant progression of tumors to increased local invasion and distant metastasis. Cancer cell. 15, 220-31.

Paguirigan, A.L., Beebe, D.J., 2008. Microfluidics meet cell biology: bridging the gap by validation and application of microscale techniques for cell biological assays. BioEssays : news and reviews in molecular, cellular and developmental biology. 30, 811-21.

Palmer, S.L., Goloubeva, O., Reddick, W.E., Glass, J.O., Gajjar, A., Kun, L., Merchant, T.E., Mulhern, R.K., 2001. Patterns of intellectual development among survivors of pediatric medulloblastoma: a longitudinal analysis. Journal of clinical oncology : official journal of the American Society of Clinical Oncology. 19, 2302-8.

Park, C.M., Park, M.J., Kwak, H.J., Lee, H.C., Kim, M.S., Lee, S.H., Park, I.C., Rhee, C.H., Hong, S.I., 2006. Ionizing radiation enhances matrix metalloproteinase-2 secretion and invasion of glioma cells through Src/epidermal growth factor receptor-mediated p38/Akt and phosphatidylinositol 3-kinase/Akt signaling pathways. Cancer research. 66, 8511-9.

Pazzaglia, S., Mancuso, M., Atkinson, M.J., Tanori, M., Rebessi, S., Majo, V.D., Covelli, V., Hahn, H., Saran, A., 2002. High incidence of medulloblastoma following X-ray-irradiation of newborn Ptc1 heterozygous mice. Oncogene. 21, 7580-4.

Pazzaglia, S., Tanori, M., Mancuso, M., Gessi, M., Pasquali, E., Leonardi, S., Oliva, M.A., Rebessi, S., Di Majo, V., Covelli, V., Giangaspero, F., Saran, A., 2006. Two-hit model for progression of medulloblastoma preneoplasia in Patched heterozygous mice. Oncogene. 25, 5575-80.

Pedersen, P.H., Edvardsen, K., Garcia-Cabrera, I., Mahesparan, R., Thorsen, J., Mathisen, B., Rosenblum, M.L., Bjerkvig, R., 1995. Migratory patterns of lac-z transfected human glioma cells in the rat brain. International journal of cancer. Journal international du cancer. 62, 767-71.

Piperi, C., Zisakis, A., Lea, R.W., Kalofoutis, A., 2005. Role of Cytokines in the Regulation of Glioma Tumour Growth and Angiogenesis. American Journal of Immunology. 1, 106-113.

Ranger, A., McDonald, W., Moore, E., Delmaestro, R., 2010. The invasiveness of five medulloblastoma cell lines in collagen gels. Journal of neuro-oncology. 96, 181-9.

Rao, J.S., 2003. Molecular mechanisms of glioma invasiveness: the role of proteases. Nature reviews. Cancer. 3, 489-501.

Reed, J., Walczak, W.J., Petzold, O.N., Gimzewski, J.K., 2009. In situ mechanical interferometry of matrigel films. Langmuir : the ACS journal of surfaces and colloids. 25, 36-9.

Rickert, C.H., Paulus, W., 2001. Epidemiology of central nervous system tumors in childhood and adolescence based on the new WHO classification. Child's nervous system : ChNS : official journal of the International Society for Pediatric Neurosurgery. 17, 503-11.

Riffkin, C.D., Gray, A.Z., Hawkins, C.J., Chow, C.W., Ashley, D.M., 2001. Ex vivo pediatric brain tumors express Fas (CD95) and FasL (CD95L) and are resistant to apoptosis induction. Neuro-oncology. 3, 229-40.

Romer, J.T., Curran, T., 2004. Medulloblastoma and retinoblastoma: oncology recapitulates ontogeny. Cell cycle. 3, 917-9.

Rood, B.R., Macdonald, T.J., Packer, R.J., 2004. Current treatment of medulloblastoma: recent advances and future challenges. Seminars in oncology. 31, 666-75.

Rooprai, H.K., McCormick, D., 1997. Proteases and their inhibitors in human brain tumours: a review. Anticancer research. 17, 4151-62.

Rutka, J.T., Apodaca, G., Stern, R., Rosenblum, M., 1988. The extracellular matrix of the central and peripheral nervous systems: structure and function. Journal of neurosurgery. 69, 155-70.

Sahai, E., 2005. Mechanisms of cancer cell invasion. Current opinion in genetics & development. 15, 87-96.

Santini, M.T., Rainaldi, G., 1999. Three-dimensional spheroid model in tumor biology. Pathobiology : journal of immunopathology, molecular and cellular biology. 67, 148-57.

Sarkar, C., Pramanik, P., Karak, A.K., Mukhopadhyay, P., Sharma, M.C., Singh, V.P., Mehta, V.S., 2002. Are childhood and adult medulloblastomas different? A comparative study of clinicopathological features, proliferation index and apoptotic index. Journal of neuro-oncology. 59, 49-61.

Scheithauer, B.W., 2009. Development of the WHO classification of tumors of the central nervous system: a historical perspective. Brain pathology. 19, 551-64.

Scherer, H.J., 1940. The forms of growth in gliomas and their practical significance. Brain. 63, 1-35.

Schoen, I., Hu, W., Klotzsch, E., Vogel, V., 2010. Probing cellular traction forces by micropillar arrays: contribution of substrate warping to pillar deflection. Nano letters. 10, 1823-30.

Schwab, M.E., Caroni, P., 1988. Oligodendrocytes and CNS myelin are nonpermissive substrates for neurite growth and fibroblast spreading in vitro. The Journal of neuroscience : the official journal of the Society for Neuroscience. 8, 2381-93.

Seroogy, K.B., Gall, C.M., Lee, D.C., Kornblum, H.I., 1995. Proliferative zones of postnatal rat brain express epidermal growth factor receptor mRNA. Brain research. 670, 157-64.

Shih, A.H., Dai, C., Hu, X., Rosenblum, M.K., Koutcher, J.A., Holland, E.C., 2004. Dose-dependent effects of platelet-derived growth factor-B on glial tumorigenesis. Cancer research. 64, 4783-9.

Shimato, S., Natsume, A., Takeuchi, H., Wakabayashi, T., Fujii, M., Ito, M., Ito, S., Park, I.H., Bang, J.H., Kim, S.U., Yoshida, J., 2007. Human neural stem cells target and deliver therapeutic gene to experimental leptomeningeal medulloblastoma. Gene therapy. 14, 1132-42.

Singh, S., Dirks, P.B., 2007. Brain tumor stem cells: identification and concepts. Neurosurgery clinics of North America. 18, 31-8, viii.

Skog, J., Wurdinger, T., van Rijn, S., Meijer, D.H., Gainche, L., Sena-Esteves, M., Curry, W.T., Jr., Carter, B.S., Krichevsky, A.M., Breakefield, X.O., 2008. Glioblastoma microvesicles transport RNA and proteins that promote tumour growth and provide diagnostic biomarkers. Nature cell biology. 10, 1470-6.

Sontheimer, H., 2004. Ion channels and amino acid transporters support the growth and invasion of primary brain tumors. Molecular neurobiology. 29, 61-71.

Spillmann, A.A., Bandtlow, C.E., Lottspeich, F., Keller, F., Schwab, M.E., 1998. Identification and characterization of a bovine neurite growth inhibitor (bNI-220). The Journal of biological chemistry. 273, 19283-93.

Staflin, K., Zuchner, T., Honeth, G., Darabi, A., Lundberg, C., 2009. Identification of proteins involved in neural progenitor cell targeting of gliomas. BMC cancer. 9, 206.

Strommer, K., Hamou, M.F., Diggelmann, H., de Tribolet, N., 1990. Cellular and tumoural heterogeneity of EGFR gene amplification in human malignant gliomas. Acta neurochirurgica. 107, 82-7.

Stupp, R., Weber, D.C., 2005. The role of radio- and chemotherapy in glioblastoma. Onkologie. 28, 315-7.

Sung, K.E., Su, G., Pehlke, C., Trier, S.M., Eliceiri, K.W., Keely, P.J., Friedl, A., Beebe, D.J., 2009. Control of 3-dimensional collagen matrix polymerization for reproducible human mammary fibroblast cell culture in microfluidic devices. Biomaterials. 30, 4833-41.

Teodorczyk, M., Martin-Villalba, A., 2010. Sensing invasion: cell surface receptors driving spreading of glioblastoma. Journal of cellular physiology. 222, 1-10.

Thorns, V., Walter, G.F., Thorns, C., 2003. Expression of MMP-2, MMP-7, MMP-9, MMP-10 and MMP-11 in human astrocytic and oligodendroglial gliomas. Anticancer research. 23, 3937-44.

Torp, S.H., Gulati, S., Johannessen, E., Dalen, A., 2007. Coexpression of c-erbB 1-4 receptor proteins in human glioblastomas. An immunohistochemical study. Journal of experimental & clinical cancer research : CR. 26, 353-9.

Towner, R.A., Smith, N., Doblas, S., Tesiram, Y., Garteiser, P., Saunders, D., Cranford, R., Silasi-Mansat, R., Herlea, O., Ivanciu, L., Wu, D., Lupu, F., 2008. In vivo detection of c-Met expression in a rat C6 glioma model. Journal of cellular and molecular medicine. 12, 174-86.

Trembath, D., Miller, C.R., Perry, A., 2008. Gray zones in brain tumor classification: evolving concepts. Advances in anatomic pathology. 15, 287-97.

Tucker, G.C., 2006. Integrins: molecular targets in cancer therapy. Current oncology reports. 8, 96-103.

Tysnes, B.B., Larsen, L.F., Ness, G.O., Mahesparan, R., Edvardsen, K., Garcia-Cabrera, I., Bjerkvig, R., 1996. Stimulation of glioma-cell migration by laminin and inhibition by anti-alpha3 and anti-beta1 integrin antibodies. International journal of cancer. Journal international du cancer. 67, 777-84.

Valadi, H., Ekstrom, K., Bossios, A., Sjostrand, M., Lee, J.J., Lotvall, J.O., 2007. Exosome-mediated transfer of mRNAs and microRNAs is a novel mechanism of genetic exchange between cells. Nature cell biology. 9, 654-9.

Van Meir, E.G., Hadjipanayis, C.G., Norden, A.D., Shu, H.K., Wen, P.Y., Olson, J.J., 2010. Exciting new advances in neuro-oncology: the avenue to a cure for malignant glioma. CA: a cancer journal for clinicians. 60, 166-93.

Wang, X., Cui, M., Wang, L., Chen, X., Xin, P., 2010. Inhibition of neurotrophin receptor p75 intramembran proteolysis by gamma-secretase inhibitor reduces medulloblastoma spinal metastasis. Biochemical and biophysical research communications. 403, 264-9.

Wear, M.A., Schafer, D.A., Cooper, J.A., 2000. Actin dynamics: assembly and disassembly of actin networks. Current biology : CB. 10, R891-5.

Weidner, K.M., Behrens, J., Vandekerckhove, J., Birchmeier, W., 1990. Scatter factor: molecular characteristics and effect on the invasiveness of epithelial cells. The Journal of cell biology. 111, 2097-108.

Wild-Bode, C., Weller, M., Rimner, A., Dichgans, J., Wick, W., 2001. Sublethal irradiation promotes migration and invasiveness of glioma cells: implications for radiotherapy of human glioblastoma. Cancer research. 61, 2744-50.

Wolf, K., Mazo, I., Leung, H., Engelke, K., von Andrian, U.H., Deryugina, E.I., Strongin, A.Y., Brocker, E.B., Friedl, P., 2003. Compensation mechanism in tumor cell migration: mesenchymal-amoeboid transition after blocking of pericellular proteolysis. The Journal of cell biology. 160, 267-77.

Wyckoff, J.B., Segall, J.E., Condeelis, J.S., 2000. The collection of the motile population of cells from a living tumor. Cancer research. 60, 5401-4.

Yamahara, T., Numa, Y., Oishi, T., Kawaguchi, T., Seno, T., Asai, A., Kawamoto, K., 2010. Morphological and flow cytometric analysis of cell infiltration in glioblastoma: a comparison of autopsy brain and neuroimaging. Brain tumor pathology. 27, 81-7.

Yandava, B.D., Billinghurst, L.L., Snyder, E.Y., 1999. "Global" cell replacement is feasible via neural stem cell transplantation: evidence from the dysmyelinated shiverer mouse brain. Proceedings of the National Academy of Sciences of the United States of America. 96, 7029-34.

Yin, X.L., Pang, J.C., Ng, H.K., 2002. Identification of a region of homozygous deletion on 8p22-23.1 in medulloblastoma. Oncogene. 21, 1461-8.

Yuan, L., Santi, M., Rushing, E.J., Cornelison, R., MacDonald, T.J., 2010. ERK activation of p21 activated kinase-1 (Pak1) is critical for medulloblastoma cell migration. Clinical & experimental metastasis. 27, 481-91.

Zhang, X., Wang, W., Yu, W., Xie, Y., Zhang, Y., Ma, X., 2005. Development of an in vitro multicellular tumor spheroid model using microencapsulation and its application in anticancer drug screening and testing. Biotechnology progress. 21, 1289-96.

Zhou, Y.H., Hess, K.R., Liu, L., Linskey, M.E., Yung, W.K., 2005. Modeling prognosis for patients with malignant astrocytic gliomas: quantifying the expression of multiple genetic markers and clinical variables. Neuro-oncology. 7, 485-94.

Zhou, Y.H., Hess, K.R., Raj, V.R., Yu, L., Liu, L., Yung, A.W., Linskey, M.E., 2010. Establishment of prognostic models for astrocytic and oligodendroglial brain tumors with standardized quantification of marker gene expression and clinical variables. Biomarker insights. 5, 153-68.

Zucker, S., Cao, J., Chen, W.T., 2000. Critical appraisal of the use of matrix metalloproteinase inhibitors in cancer treatment. Oncogene. 19, 6642-50.

Zwick, E., Bange, J., Ullrich, A., 2001. Receptor tyrosine kinase signalling as a target for cancer intervention strategies. Endocrine-related cancer. 8, 161-73.

12

Extracellular Matrix Microenvironment in Glioma Progression

Marzenna Wiranowska[1] and Mumtaz V. Rojiani[2]
[1]Department of Pathology and Cell Biology
College of Medicine, University of South Florida, Tampa, Florida
[2]Departments of Medicine and Pathology, GHSU Cancer Center Augusta, Georgia
USA

1. Introduction

Malignant gliomas are primary brain tumors, which are highly invasive but not known to metastasize outside the central nervous system (CNS). The median survival time of patients with glioma is only 6 months to 2 years depending on various patient, tumor and treatment parameters (Louis et al. 2007). The highly aggressive character of gliomas with glioblastoma multiforme (GBM) being the most aggressive subtype are characterized by their diffuse infiltration into the normal brain parenchyma and interaction with the extracellular matrix (ECM) components in the brain. Standard brain tumor therapies, which include surgery followed by chemotherapy and radiation are not effective in eradicating single glioma cells that migrated into the normal brain establishing new tumor foci. Glioma cells are locally invasive and when migrating through the ECM within several millimeters or centimeters from the main lesion they initiate recurrent tumors often distant to the primary lesion (Bolteus et al. 2001). The infiltrative path of glioma into the normal brain parenchyma involves the basement membrane of blood vessels and myelinated nerve fibers of white matter tracts (Rao 2003, Lefranc et al. 2005).

The pattern of glioma cell invasion is related to the unique composition of the cerebral ECM microenvironment, which is remodeled during invasion by activated matrix metalloproteinases (MMPs) (reviewed by Rojiani et al. 2011). In addition, new ECM molecules are secreted and receptor adhesion molecules are expressed by glioma promoting the glioma cell-ECM interaction and signaling. Some of the secreted ECM molecules such as tenascin-C are known to be associated with cell motility and angiogenesis which are both essential for tumor development. Another important microenvironment component affecting glioma development was found to be mechanical force determined by ECM rigidity. More rigid ECM promotes glioma migration and proliferation and lower rigidity of ECM (similar to that of normal brain) would have an opposite effect (Ulrich et al. 2009).

The recent sequencing data presented by the Cancer Genome Atlas Research Network (2008) revealed genomic abnormalities in GBM that relate to several signaling pathways such as Epidermal Growth Factor Receptor (EGFR) / Ras / PI3K known to be associated with ECM-related signaling (Ulrich et al. 2009). In addition, the recent integrated genomic analysis identified clinically relevant subtypes of GBM with its characteristic abnormalities in platelet derived growth factor receptor A (PDGFRA), isocitrate dehydrogenase 1 (IDH1), neurofibromin 1 (NF1), and confirmed EGFR mutations across all newly defined subtypes of GBM such as classical, proneural, neural and mesenchymal (Verhaak et al. 2010). The most recent studies by Holland (2011) in PDGF-driven mouse models of proneural GBMs with a focus on the biology, therapeutic response and the complexity of the microenvironment showed that some of the genes found in mice are predictive of the survival of patients with this proneural subtype of GBM. Interestingly, many of these genes are rather expressed in the stroma of the tumor than by the tumor cells themselves.

In this chapter, the most recent information pertaining to the glioma extracellular microenvironment and the possible biological targets within ECM for anti-glioma therapy will be reviewed.

2. Extracellular matrix molecules in the normal brain

In the central nervous system (CNS) approximately only 15-25% of the CNS volume is taken up by the extracellular space, while the majority of the CNS volume consists of cellular elements such as neurons, glia, astrocytic processes and blood vessels (Sykova 2002, Quirico-Santos et al. 2010). The components found within the extracellular space include various ions, metabolites, neurohormones, peptides and ECM molecules produced by neurons and glia. The ECM environment of the normal brain contains high levels of space-filling carbohydrate molecules unbound to proteins such as the large glycosaminoglycan (GAG) hyaluronan (HA). HA binds to specific cell surface receptors such as cluster determinant 44 (CD44) adhesion molecule and receptor for hyaluronate mediated motility (RHAMM) regulating properties of ECM and tissue, e.g., proliferation, adhesion, motility etc. Protein-bound carbohydrate molecules, which are present in the normal brain at high levels, include sulfated proteoglycans such as chondroitin sulfate proteoglycans (CSPGs) and heparan sulfate proteoglycans (HSPGs). In addition, fibrous proteins associated with the basement membranes of the brain's vasculature include collagens, fibronectin, and laminin (Wiranowska and Plaas 2008). The levels of these fibrous proteins in the normal brain are low compared to the connective tissue outside the central nervous system (Bellail et al. 2004, Quirico-Santos et al. 2010). However, the ECM microenvironment of glioma differs from the normal brain and varies depending on the grade of glioma, e.g., with the highly aggressive GBM producing collagen, fibronectin or laminin (Mahesparan et al. 2003). Several classes of ECM molecules play an important role in the normal CNS development but have altered functions in glioma are reviewed below.

The main classes of ECM components in the normal brain are GAG hyaluronan (HA), also called hyaluronic acid, and proteoglycans (PGs), which consist of a core protein attached to GAG chain. HA plays multiple roles in providing an organization of the pericellular matrix. There is a high diversity of PGs due to various core proteins, and variations in GAG side chains. Two classes of transmembrane PGs, glypicans and syndecans, which contain heparan sulphate (HS) side chains called HSPGs are found at high levels in the CNS.

An important class of PGs are chondroitin sulfate PGs (CSPGs), which are expressed at high levels in the regions of the developing fetal brain and later in mature brain in astrocytes and neurons (Rao 2003, Quirico-Santos et al. 2010). CSPGs, and especially the subclass of lecticans, are one of the major families of HA binding matrix glycoproteins in the CNS. A second family of PGs that bind HA in the CNS are HA- and proteoglycan-link proteins (HAPLNs) also called "link proteins", which bind both HA and lecticans. The PGs called lecticans contain lectin and HA-binding domains and within that group there are molecules such as aggrecan, versican, neurocan, and brain enriched hyaluronic acid binding protein/brevican (BEHAB/brevican) that act as linkers to ECM components. They bind to HA as well as to cell-surface receptors regulating many processes within the CNS during development, e.g., cell motility, axonal navigation etc. (Sim et al. 2009). Some of these molecules such as versican are known to be produced by glial cells and neural stem cells (Abaskharoun et al. 2010). Another member of CSPGs is phosphocan, an astroglial proteoglycan that binds to neural cell adhesion molecules and tenascin-C. Neuroglial protein-2 (NG2), also a CSPG proteoglycan, which is known as a characteristic marker of oligodendrocyte progenitor cells and pericytes in developing vasculature, is expressed by many gliomas. The NG2 positive cells have been suggested to be the originating cells for glioma (Stallcup and Huang 2008).

Tenascins (C and R), a family of glycoproteins exist in the ECM as assemblies of several subunits expressed in zones of proliferation, migration, and morphogenesis and are known to play an important role in the developing CNS. For example, tenascin-C was found highly expressed in the subventricular zone and essential for neural stem cell development (reviewed by Wiranowska and Plaas 2008). Galectins (Gal) , mannose- binding lectins, are glycan-binding proteins found inside and outside the cells. Gal-1 is highly represented in the CNS and takes part in the development of neural and non-neural networks and Gal-3 interacts with other neural tissue derived glycoproteins and is expressed by astrocytes and endothelial cells (Quirico-Santos et al. 2010). The role of many ECM components of the normal brain described above, are altered dramatically in glioma.

In the normal brain, the ECM complexes containing HA and PGs such as versican, brevican, neurocan, aggrecan, phosphacan and tenascin-C, tenascin-R, and link proteins form the ECM domains called perineuronal nets first described by Camillo Golgi in 1893. These perineuronal net aggregates enwrap the neuronal cell bodies and proximal dendrites of certain neurons and fill the space between neurons and glial processes. More recently, it was proposed that perineuronal nets within the brain are more heterogenous and include structures called "interstitial clefts" (Brightman 2002). As described by Brightman (Brightman 2002), interstitial clefts comprised of astrocytic walls, basal lamina and ECM molecules may vary in size , shape and content depending on the brain region. In addition, the size and the content of interstitial clefts was found to be different in the mature brain by being narrower with limited capacity for cell movement compared to that in the fetal brain. Here, in the fetal brain, the size and the content of interstitial clefts permit cell migration and outgrowth of neurites while in the mature brain cell migration in the interstitial clefts could only occur after enzymatic degradation of the ECM (Brightman 2002).

2.1 Extracellular matrix in the brain as a cytokine and growth factor depot

In the normal brain some regions are especially rich in ECM. These brain regions include subarachnoid space, supependymal packets, circumventricular organs (CVOs) supplied by fenestrated capillaries without blood-brain barrier (BBB), and perivascular space around arterioles and venules. These vessels are associated with stromal connective tissue space and lined by basal laminae containing heparan sulfate proteoglycans (HSPGs). HSPGs which are also components of ependymal, astroglial, and endothelial interfaces in the CNS (including interstitial clefts) have been suggested to serve as a storage site of growth factors and cytokines (Brightman and Kaya 2000). A large number of growth factors, for example, insulin-like growth factor (IGF), transforming growth factor-beta (TGF-beta), hepatocyte growth factor (HGF) were found to bind to HSPG (Folkman 1998). A similar observation was made for certain cytokines (reviewed by Wiranowska and Plaas 2008). It was suggested by Mercier et al. (Mercier et al. 2003) that cytokines and growth factors secreted by cells of connective tissue may accumulate in the basal lamina, interact with ECM proteins and affect biological processes including cytogenesis of stem cells in the CNS.

2.2 Extracellular matrix stem cell niche in the brain

In the CNS, the ability of normal stem cells to self-renew and to differentiate into specific cell types is controlled by the microenvironment of a CNS area in which these cells reside and which is called niche. Similarly, in other tissues and organs, stem cells are found in the protective microenvironment of niches, which are composed of ECM molecules and various differentiated cell types that release regulatory factors and provide direct contact with stem cells maintaining their quiescence. The CNS microenvironment of the neural stem cells (NSC) niche is also called vascular niche, because stem cells concentrate near blood vessels. The NSC niche consists of several ECM components, and includes the basal lamina and endothelial cells of vasculature (Doetsch 2003). These mature, differentiated vascular endothelial cells have an intimate association with stem cells and play a regulatory role in the NSC niche through secreted soluble factors. These factors were shown to promote activation of Notch, a neural precursor receptor, resulting in self-renewal of neural stem cells (Shen et al. 2004). In addition, the basement membrane (also known as basal lamina) contributes to the microenvironment and provides a substrate for stem cells' movement. The subventricular zone, a highly neurogenic area in the CNS, contains transmembrane HSPGs bound to the supependymal basal lamina located in proximity to the stem cells. As mentioned earlier (Section 2.1), HSPGs have the capacity to bind and to store a number of growth factors and cytokines thereby serving as a cytokine and growth factor depot. The growth factors and cytokines can diffuse quickly, and because of close proximity, they can reach high concentrations near the stem cells and regulate their development (Kearns et al. 2003) . For example, EGF and basic fibroblast growth factor (bFGF) stored in the ECM of the subventricular zone can have a stimulatory effect on stem cells by enhancing their proliferation. The growth factors and cytokines can be stored in the ECM throughout life.

As mentioned earlier, one of ECM molecules, tenascin-C, is highly expressed in the subventricular zone and essential for neural stem cell development (Wiranowska and Plaas 2008). Tenascin-C plays a key role in the regulation of the developmental program of oligodendrocyte precursor cells (OPCs) and therefore confirming the importance of tenascin-C as an ECM component of the niche (Scadden 2006). Other ECM molecules, such as laminin and fibronectin, stimulate motility of stem/progenitor cells while CSPGs have an inhibitory effect (Kearns et al. 2003). It was also observed that upon activation of MMPs by proinflammatory cytokines, the neural progenitor cells were stimulated to migrate to the site of injury (Ben-Hur et al. 2006). In summary, many modulatory molecules were described within the ECM of the stem cell niche and, interestingly, many of them were found in glioma, but at higher levels than in the normal brain. In addition, not only the levels but also the functions of many of these molecules differ between the normal brain and glioma such as CSPGs, which are inhibitory for stem cells migration within the niche of the normal brain but stimulatory for glioma cell migration (Kearns et al. 2003, Sim et al. 2009).

3. Extracellular matrix in glioma

3.1 Role of ECM and MMP molecules in vasculogenic mimicry in glioma: Historical perspective

It was observed previously by Maniotis et al. (Maniotis et al. 1999) that blood vessels of highly aggressive tumors such as uveal melanoma originated from tumor cells, rather than from endothelial cells as it was originally expected. This phenomenon named vasculogenic mimicry (VM) was reported later also for other tumors including glioma (Yue and Chen 2005). Although the mechanism of VM could not be explained at that time, many studies evaluated MMPs and ECM interactions in search for clues. It was suggested that several components of the tumor microenvironment may be contributing to the development of VM. For example, consideration was given to MMPs' cleavage of laminin, VE-cadherin-promoted adherence of newly formed vascular channels to tumor cells, and dedifferentiation of tumor cells (Zhang et al. 2007). Three main factors were suspected to play a role in VM: 1) plasticity of malignant tumor cells, 2) remodeling of the ECM by MMPs secreted by tumor cells to obtain space for VM, and 3) the connection of newly formed VM channels with existing blood vessels to acquire blood from the host (Zhang et al. 2007). It was proposed by Maniotis et al. (Maniotis et al. 1999) that the level of the VM channel formation was directly proportional to the level of tumor aggressiveness and influenced by interstitial fluid pressure (IFP), a microenviromental factor known to affect angiogenesis. Tumors that proliferate rapidly have high IFP and compromised blood circulation. In addition, there is a limited blood supply from the host due to decreased endothelial cell sprouting and decreased formation of endothelium-lined blood vessels. Therefore, tumor cells that form VM channels obtain a sufficient blood supply to sustain tumor growth. It was observed that the blood vessels formed as a result of VM had a different structure than normal endothelial-lined blood vessels. VM channels were found to be lined by highly aggressive and poorly differentiated tumor cells that could degrade the base membrane of blood vessels by releasing proteases and migrate into the normal tissue. Recent data (Inoue et al. 2010) support this observation by showing that GBM cancer stem cells express MMP-13 responsible for invasion and migration of these cells.

Anti-vascular and anti-angiogenic therapies that used molecules such as angiostatin or endostatin that target endothelial cells, showed no effect on tumors with VM. To overcome the lack of understanding of the molecular mechanisms underlying VM, several *in vitro* studies were initiated in search of new therapeutic approaches based on the concept of ECM involvement in VM formation. For example, laminin was targeted *in vitro* showing that an anti-laminin antibody was able to inhibit VM channel formation by tumor cells (Sanz et al. 2003). Other *in vitro* studies targeted and inhibited MMP-2 and MMP-9 involved in VM by using doxcyline (Zhang et al. 2007). Also, it was shown that the Cox-2 inhibitor, celecoxib, inhibited *in vitro* VM formation in a dose-dependent manner (Basu et al. 2005). Although, these results were only obtained *in vitro*, there may be a recent indirect *in vivo* confirmation. Interestingly, recent *in vivo* studies using a glioma mouse model, showed that non-steroidal anti-inflammatory drugs (NSAID) such as Cox-2 inhibitors suppress gliomagenesis (Fujita et al. 2011). Although the primary conclusion of this study was that gliomagenesis was suppressed due to inhibition of prostaglandin E2-dependent accumulation of myeloid derived suppressor cells in the tumor microenvironment, a secondary effect of Cox-2 inhibitors on VM may be involved as addressed in section 6.2.2.

3.2 Microenvironment of glioma stem cell vascular niche: New theory of vascular mimicry

Recently, a new concept of cancer progenitor cells, also known as cancer-initiating cells or cancer stem cells (CSCs), was proposed. These self-renewing, multipotent CSCs are highly tumorigenic and resistant to conventional therapies (Lakka and Rao 2008). Glioblastoma CSCs resemble the normal NSC and express the markers Nestin+/ CD133+ found in the neural stem cell population. Also, glioma CSCs, similar to NSCs, concentrate around blood vessels in the vascular niches with easy access to nutrients, signaling molecules, and the vasculature itself as a substrate for migration (Calabrese et al. 2007, Denysenko et al. 2010). However, CSCs differ from NSCs in their distribution in the brain and their capacity to proliferate. For example, the normal NSCs, which proliferate at a low rate are found only in specific CNS regions such as hippocampus and subventricular zone. In contrast, highly proliferative glioma CSCs can be found distributed across in all regions of cerebrum and cerebellum within the tumors. It was proposed that the main difference between the normal NSCs and glioma CSCs may be the way in which these cells are modulated by the microenvironment of the vasculature within the niche (Calabrese et al. 2007). The vascular niche in brain tumors is abnormal in such that it contributes to the propagation of CSCs thereby enhancing tumor growth. Furthermore, the endothelial cells from this abnormal vascular niche can interact with brain tumor CSCs, as shown *in vitro,* providing certain extracellular regulatory factors and maintaining the self-renewal capability and undifferentiated state of these cells (Calabrese et al. 2007). In that way the glioma vasculature establishes a microenvironment of the niche in which CSCs can transmit and receive signals from the ECM. For example, it was shown that upon stimulation of CSCs by ECM of the vascular niche, the CSCs can secrete vascular endothelial growth factor (VEGF) promoting angiogenesis and thereby enhancing tumor growth (Bao et al. 2006). In addition, the vascular niche was shown to interfere with radiation and chemotherapy by shielding the CSCs and contributing to the resistance to treatments (Denysenko et al. 2010). It was also suggested that the microenvironment of the niche may play a role in tumor initiation based on the observation that non-tumorigenic cell populations may become tumorigenic depending on a certain microenvironment (Rosen and Jordan 2009). Recent reports show that GBM stem cells have similar capabilities as the normal NSCs and undergo differentiation into endothelial cells forming the majority of new blood vessels in gliomas (El Hallani et al. 2010, Ricci-Vitiani et al. 2010, Wang et al. 2010). Blocking VEGF or silencing VEGF receptor 2 inhibits the maturation of tumor endothelial progenitors into endothelium but does not stop the differentiation of CSCs (CD133+ cells) into endothelial cells. However, silencing of Notch (neural precursor receptor as mentioned in section 2.2) blocks the transition of CSCs (CD133+ cells) into endothelial progenitors (Wang et al. 2010). Further studies of the microenvironmental components within the brain tumor vascular niche could lead to new therapeutic targets for treatments of glioma.

3.3 Extracellular matrix and mechanical rigidity in glioma

There are anatomic variations in stiffness in the normal brain parenchyma (Elkin et al. 2007) with basement membrane of blood vessels and the myelinated fiber tracts of white matter exhibiting a higher mechanical rigidity (Lefranc et al. 2005) and both serving as an infiltrative path for glioma invasion (Rao 2003, Ulrich et al. 2009, Kumar 2009). It was first observed *in vitro* that directed migration of fibroblasts occurs from soft to stiff areas of the ECM, a phenomenon named mechanotaxis (Lo et al. 2000). A similar observation was made for glioblastoma where changes in ECM rigidity can both increase and decrease cell motility and the extent of the effect was cell–type dependent (Thomas and DiMilla 2000). It was found that high ECM stiffness enhanced the expression of contractility-mediating proteins such as Rho (Paszek et al. 2005). ECM components have been found to be the main regulators of cell motility in the brain. For example, previous studies showed a stimulatory effect of ECM proteins such as fibronectin, collagen, laminin and others on glioma cell migration (Mahesparan et al. 2003). Ulrich et al. (Ulrich et al. 2009) had shown that glioma cells cultured on fibronectin-coated polymeric ECM with varied but defined mechanical rigidity exhibited altered cell morphology and cytoskeletal organization. These authors showed that glioma cells cultured on softer substrates showed a decreased spreading area, disappearing stress fibers and focal adhesions. Interestingly, all evaluated glioma cell lines cultured on the softest substrates were rounded but viable with cortical rings of F-actin and punctuate vinculin-positive focal complexes, and with no indication of apoptosis (Ulrich et al. 2009). The rigidity of the soft substrates used in that study was comparable to the ECM rigidity of normal brain parenchyma while an increased stiffness was characteristic for glioma and its surrounding stroma.

In addition, it was shown that increasing ECM rigidity resulted in increased cell spreading, motility and proliferation. It was suggested previously that glioma cells actively remodel their microenvironment changing it from normal brain ECM to rigid tumor-like ECM (Nakada et al. 2007). Therefore, it was suggested that glioma cells modify their ECM through proteolytic degradation of the normal brain matrix and secretion of new ECM components, thereby providing for a stiffer and more rigid microenvironment which in turn sends mechanobiological signals that support glioma cell invasion (Ulrich et al. 2009). This was observed previously also for invading breast cancer cells (Provenzano et al. 2008). By targeting either the signaling pathways for mechanotaxis or mechanical remodeling itself, new therapeutic approaches could be developed for the treatment of glioma which would affect glioma invasion and proliferation.

3.4 Extracellular matrix molecules in glioma

3.4.1 Glycosaminoglycan hyaluronan and CD44 adhesion molecule

Glioma cells constitutively produce HA and its production is increased during cell proliferation (Wiranowska and Naidu 1994, Wiranowska et al. 2010) promoting glioma invasion (Park et al. 2008). HA is synthesized at the plasma membrane by HA-synthases and the synthesis can be enhanced by various growth factors, e.g., epidermal growth factor (Knudson and Knudson 1993) Interestingly, the content of HA in glioma resembles that of embryonic brain cells (Delpech et al. 1993). HA binds to the HA-binding proteins called hyaladherins which include the CD44 surface receptor. CD44 is a transmembrane glycoprotein expressed by many cell types and by glioma. CD44 serves as a surface receptor for ECM molecules such as HA and CSPGs (Ranuncolo et al. 2002).

CD44 receptor is overexpressed in glioma cells *in vitro* (Wiranowska et al. 2000, Yu et al. 2010) and found *in vivo* at the leading edge of glioma at the brain-tumor interface (Wiranowska et al. 2006). The HA-CD44 interaction and CD44 shedding from the cell surface were found to be associated with glioma cell motility, migration, and infiltration into the normal brain parenchyma (Annabi et al. 2005). These authors also described that CD44 shedding was mediated by HA and accompanied by up-regulation of MT1-MMP expression.

After binding to the CD44 receptor, HA can be endocytosed, transported into lysosomes and degraded by hyaluronidases into small oligosaccharides shown to have glioma - stimulatory activity (Novak et al. 1999). It was previously reported that while small HA fragments were found in the tumor tissues, native HA of high molecular mass was found in the normal and benign tissue (Rooney et al. 1995). Both the high levels of full length polymeric HA and its low molecular weight degradation products, HA fragments, known as oligosaccharides support glioma growth (Novak et al. 1999). The HA oligosaccharides, e.g., hexamer oligoHA-6 (HA-6) or decamer oligoHA-10 (HA-10) are able to displace full length HA via competition for CD44 receptor binding. HA can be effectively displaced by HA decasaccharides, such as HA-10, but not by HA oligosaccharides that are shorter than 10-mer (Tammi et al. 1998). It was observed that full length, large size HA had an anti-angiogenic property, whereas smaller oligosaccharides after degradation (3-10 disaccharide units) were no longer anti-angiogenic (Deed et al. 1997). We found that small size oligosaccharide, decamer HA-10, exogenously added to the cell culture stimulated HA production by glioma cells (Wiranowska et al. 2010), as previously described for normal human fibroblasts (Luke and Prehm 1999). These authors found that displacement of nascent HA from the receptors by HA oligosaccharides led to stimulation of HA synthesis (Luke and Prehm 1999). Further studies of HA and the role of HA-CD44 interaction in glioma growth and invasiveness may provide new therapeutic targets for the treatment of glioma. Recent therapeutic approaches targeting HA-CD44 interaction are discussed in the Section 5.2.

3.4.2 Chondroitin sulfate proteoglycans (CSPGs)

CSPGs are expressed at elevated levels in the developing brain (as described in sections: 2 & 2.2). In the normal brain, they are known for their inhibitory effect on stem cell migration (section 2.2). In glioma however, CSPGs are upregulated and stimulate glioma cell migration (Kearns et al. 2003, Sim et al. 2009). The two members of the CSPG subclass of lecticans (described in section 2) such as versican and BEHAB/brevican are expressed at a higher level in glioma than in the normal brain tissue. In addition, it was reported that the VO/VI versican isoform expressed by migratory glioma cells interacts with surface receptors e.g., EGFR activating the ERK signaling pathway involved in tumor promotion (Ricciardelli et al. 2009). In addition, versican and brevican can form complexes with mesenchymal matrix proteins found in the ECM of glioma, but not in the ECM of the normal brain (Sim et al. 2009). Gliomas of various grades, e.g., astrocytoma and GBM secrete high levels of BEHAB/brevican. The CSPG lectican has an N-terminal HA-binding domain that interacts with fibronectin, thereby further stimulating glioma progression (Viapiano and Matthews 2006). Several other ECM molecules such as HA, CD44, tenascin and transforming growth factor beta2 (TGFbeta2) also interact with versican and promote brain tumor cell invasion. Recently, the link proteins HAPLN4 and HAPLN2 were shown to be reduced in malignant gliomas and it was suggested that this reduction may be associated with matrix remodeling by glioma. Therefore, in contrast to the normal brain tissue where CSPGs lecticans associated to HAPLNs serve as inhibitors of cell motility, in glioma this stabilizing role of link proteins may be reduced or lost resulting in proinvasive activity of CSPGs in glioma (Sim et al. 2009).

Another member of CSPGs family, neuroglial protein 2 (NG2), is also overexpressed in glioma (Schrappe et al. 1991, Wiranowska et al. 2006). NG2 was first found to be expressed by oligodendrocyte progenitor cells (section 2). NG2 expressed by glioma cells has a strong association with ECM ligands such as collagen VI and cellular ligands such as CD44. It has been implicated in the invasive behavior of glioma and found to be expressed *in vitro* and *in vivo* by highly migratory glioma cells while not found in non migratory cells (Lin et al. 1996, Galli et al. 2004, Wiranowska et al. 2006, Stallcup and Huang 2008). NG2 is not only expressed by oligodendrocyte progenitor cells and glioma cells but also by pericytes, which are associated with microvasculature and may play a role in the development of glioma vasculature (Stallcup and Huang 2008). Therefore, NG2 may be considered as one of the main CSPGs involved in glioma progression.

3.4.3 Vasculature-associated ECM molecules expressed by gliomas

The basement membrane of the cerebral vasculature contains collagens (type IV and V), fibronectin, laminin, vitronectin and HSPGs such as glypicans and syndecans. Some HSPGs, e.g., syndecan-2 were reported to be increased in brain tumors (Theocharis et al. 2010). Laminin, collagen and fibronectin were also shown to be expressed by normal brain tissue bordering with glioma cells in spheroids (Knott et al. 1998). In addition, some of these molecules are also expressed by cells of highly aggressive gliomas. For example, it was found that fibronectin was expressed by GBM *in vitro* and in gliomesenchymal junctions in tumors and their blood vessels (Rao 2003). Another molecule, vitronectin, was found to be expressed in late stage GBM while it was absent in normal brain and early stage of glioma (Yamamoto et al. 1994). Laminins, which were found in blood vessels and in the glial limitants externa in glioma, were also shown to be expressed by human glioma cells positive for glial fibrillary astrocytic protein (GFAP) (Tysnes et al. 1999). An active site on laminin which was capable of binding to CD44 was identified (Hibino et al. 2004). In addition, Ljubimova et al. (Ljubimova et al. 2004) found that highly invasive GBMs overexpressed laminin-8, a member of the subset of laminins characterized by containing the alpha4 chain. Moreover, these authors also found that laminin-8 not only facilitated tumor invasion *in vitro*, but was involved in tumor regrowth after completion of a therapy. On the contrary, a different isoform, laminin-9, was found in lower grade gliomas, astrocytomas, and at low levels in benign brain tumors and in normal brain tissue. Therefore, many of these ECM molecules originally known to be associated with vasculature and now found at various levels expressed by glioma cells could be considered as biomarkers of glioma progression.
Tenascin -C , a proteoglycan synthesized by glial and neural crest cells is highly expressed in the subventricular zone and essential for the development of neural stem cells (as described in sections 2 & 2.2). Tenascin-C, which is believed to be produced by endothelial cells, was found around blood vessels in astrocytoma and its expression correlated with angiogenesis and tumor progression from grade II to grade III (Zagzag et al. 1995, Quirico-Santos et al. 2010). Tenascin-C was found overexpressed in invasive glioma both *in vitro* and *in vivo* (Mahesparan et al. 2003) thus confirming its significance as an ECM molecule in glioma pathology. Also, galectins are upregulated in glioma and shown to be involved in glioma cell migration and angiogenesis. While high levels of Gal-1 are correlated with aggressiveness of many tumors, the expression of Gal-3 by astrocytes and endothelial cells can be used diagnostically to differentiate GBM from other, less malignant types of glioma (Quirico-Santos et al. 2010). The schematic representation of ECM glioma microenvironment and the summary of representative ECM molecules and their functional significance are shown in Figure 1 and Table1.

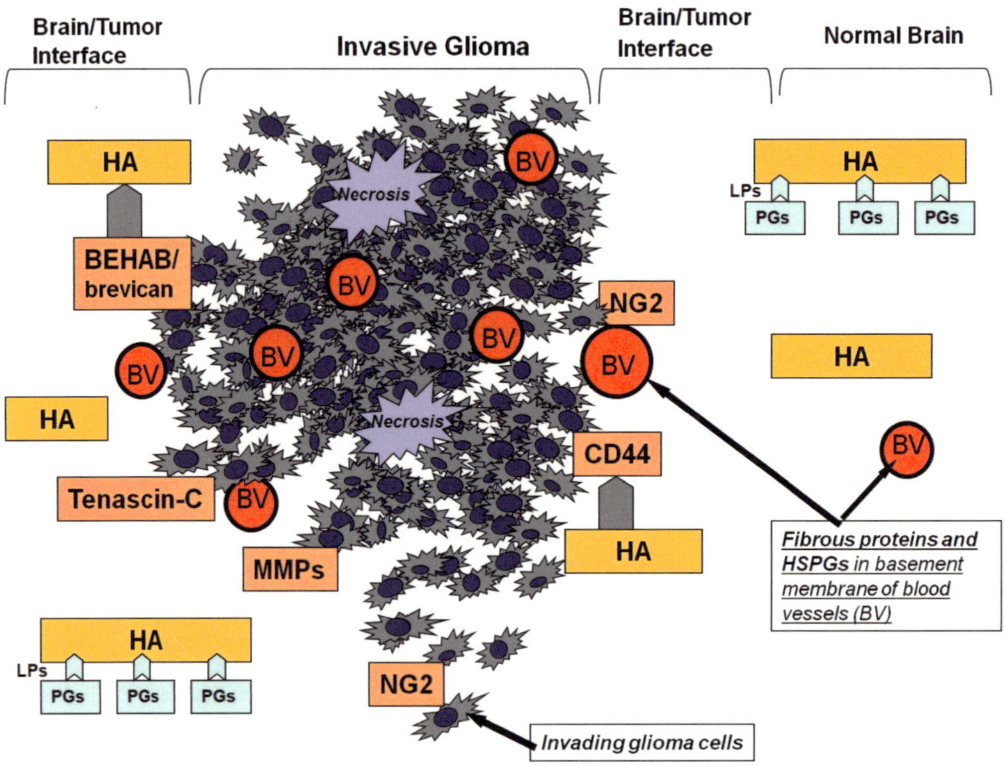

Fig. 1. Schematic representation of the extracellular matrix (ECM) microenvironment of invasive glioma with necrotic centers and associated brain parenchyma. Hyaluronic acid (HA), a long space-filling molecule composed of a carbohydrate chain is shown either unbound or bound to proteoglycans (PGs) via link proteins (LPs) or bound to CD44 receptor. Also shown are two glioma associated ECM molecules (both chondroitin sulfate proteoglycans): brain enriched hyaluronic acid binding protein/brevican (BEHAB/brevican) and neuroglial protein-2 (NG2) with the latter expressed by glioma cells and pericytes of blood vessels. In addition, glycoprotein tenascin-C, and matrix metalloproteinases (MMPs) are shown. Blood vessels (BV) shown in the glioma and the associated brain parenchyma contain fibrous proteins such as collagens, laminins etc. and heparan sulfate proteoglycans (HSPGs) associated with the BV basement membrane.

4. Proteases, Matrix Metalloproteinases (MMPs), Their Inhibitors (TIMPS) and remodeling of ECM in glioma

Matrix Metalloproteinases (MMPs) are a class of enzymes known to be involved in normal tissue remodeling, but also produced by glioma cells (Wiranowska et al. 2000) and involved in modification of glioma ECM. In the past, MMPs were considered a potential target for anti-cancer therapies. The result of ECM degradation by MMPs is the release and diffusion of cytokines and growth factors stored in the ECM with subsequent further activation of MMPs by these factors (Wiranowska and Plaas 2008). Since upregulation of MMPs was traditionally associated with inflammation and cancer progression, MMPs were considered a logical target for anti-cancer therapy. Supporting evidence was generated using transgenic mouse models overexpressing MMPs (Ha et al. 2001).

Molecules	Location		Function
	Brain	Glioma	
Glycosaminoglycans (GAGs):			
-Hyaluronan (HA)	+	+++	HA: space filling molecule, binds to cell surface receptors: CD44 and RHAMM; regulation of ECM; regulates cell proliferation, adhesion, motility.
-Proteoglycans (PG)s:			PGs: HA binding proteins
. Chondroitin sulfate PGs(CSPGs)	+	+++	CSPGs: high levels in the developing fetal brain and glioma
.. lecticans:			Lecticans: aggrecan (neurons), neurocan (neurons & glia), versican (glia), brevican (glia & neurons); bind to HA and cell surface receptors, regulate cell motility, axonal navigation; enhance migration of glioma cells; inhibit normal brain stem cell migration.
aggrecan	+	?	
neurocan	+	++	
versican	+	+++	
BEHAB/brevican	+	+++	
.. NG2	+	+++	NG2: expressed by CNS progenitor, pericytes, glioma cells; binds to collagen VI and CD44.
. Link proteins (LPs)/ HAPLNs	+	+ /-	LPs: bind to HA & lecticans; stabilize binding of core protein to HA.
. Heparan sulfate PGs (HSPGs) (glypicans, syndecans: syn.)	+	+ ++ (syn.-2)	HSPGs: bind to basal lamina of blood vessels, ependymal, astroglial, endothelial surfaces; storage site for cytokines and growth factors.
Tenascin:C & R, (glycoproteins)	+	+++	Tenascins: expressed in zones of proliferation, migration and morphogenesis; Tenascin-C is over expressed in glioma.
Galectins, (lectins)	+	+++	Galectins: (glia & endothelial cells), glycan binding proteins; neuronal and non-neuronal network development, angiogenesis.
Fibrous Proteins	In blood vessels only		Fibrous proteins: structural elements of connective tissue in blood vessels' basement membrane in normal brain and glioma; in high grade glioma also expressed by glioma cells.
• collagens		+	
• fibronectin		+	
• laminins		+	
• vitronectin		+	
Matrix metalloproteinases (MMPs), proteases	+	+++	MMPs: tissue, ECM remodeling, angiogenesis; MMP-2,-9, -13 and MT1-MMP play a role in glioma progression

Table 1. ECM molecules and their functional significance

4.1 Proteases in glioma

The local infiltration of neoplastic cells into healthy CNS parenchyma is the hallmark of gliomas. In this context it is relevant to note that the brain extracellular matrix differs in its composition from other such matrices and that glioma cells have the ability to exploit this environment for invasion. Glioma cells aggressively disseminate as single cells through this unique ECM of the central nervous system. They infiltrate along the periphery of blood vessels or along the longitudinal white matter tracts utilizing different proteolytic enzymes, to achieve their goal of both invasion and metastasis. Serine, cysteine and metalloproteinases are employed to breakdown connective tissue barriers, induce angiogenesis and penetrate normal brain tissue thereby achieving the invasive phenotype (reviewed by Rao 2003). The urokinase plasminogen activator (uPA)/plasmin system of the serine protease family have been shown to be up-regulated in gliomas (Lakka and Rao 2008) and high uPA levels are associated with poor prognosis. Cathepsin B is a lysosomal cysteine protease shown to be secreted at increased levels in gliomas, with expression being significantly higher in glioblastoma than in low-grade glioma and normal brain (Rao 2003, Lakka and Rao 2008).

The third and the most widely studied protease system implicated in gliomas are the matrix metalloproteinases (MMPs). MMPs are a diverse family of endopeptidases that utilize zinc at their active site and encompass a broad spectrum of substrates. Common structural features of MMPs include a signal peptide, a catalytic domain which harbors the conserved zinc-binding site and a hemopexin-like domain. The proteolytic activity of MMPs affects diverse cellular functions such as cell proliferation, adhesion, migration, angiogenesis, bone development, wound healing and mammary involution, among others, by virtue of cleavage of ECM constituents, pro-growth factors, growth factor receptors and cell adhesion molecules. Within the tumor microenvironment, MMPs have been well documented to play a critical role in metastasis and angiogenesis (Kessenbrock et al. 2010).
The family of Metzincin proteinases to which the MMPs belong also includes ADAM (a disintegrin and metalloproteinase) and ADAMTS (a disintegrin and metalloproteinase with thrombospondin motifs). The ADAMs are mostly cell associated, and responsible for cleavage of other proteins like amyloid precursor protein and Notch and hence are also called "sheddases". On the other hand the ADAMTS are secreted (Murphy 2008). The role of ADAMs family members in nervous system development has been documented (Yang et al. 2006).Though these two subfamilies have not been extensively studied in glioma, there is some documentation of their role in these tumors. In this context, it has been shown that ADAM 8 and 19 are overexpressed in glioma correlating with invasion. ADAMTS 4 and 5 cleave brevican, a component of the ECM in the normal brain and have been shown to be upregulated in glioma cells (Rivera et al. 2010).

4.2 MMPs and their inhibitors (TIMPs) in glioma

MMPs span a wide range of subtypes within this family of endopeptidases that utilize zinc at their active site and interact with different targets. The proteolytic activity of MMPs affects diverse cellular functions as mentioned above, particularly impacting cell proliferation, adhesion, migration and angiogenesis. Thus they are important effectors of tissue remodeling, acting at various levels. The human MMP family comprises of over 23 members and cleaves every component of the ECM. They are classified as follows:

1. The archetypal MMPs: these include the collagenases i.e. MMP-1, MMP-8 and MMP-13; Stromelysins include MMP-3, MMP-10, MMP-11; Other archetypal MMPs e.g. the metalloelastase i.e MMP-12, also includes MMP-12, MMP-19, MMP-20 and MMP-27
2. Matrilysins include MMP-7 and MMP-26
3. Gelatinases include MMP-2 and MMP-9
4. Membran-type (MT)-MMPs include MMP-14, MMP-15, MMP-16, MMP-17, MMP-24 and MMP-25 A subgroup of glycosylphosphatidylinositol (GPI) MT-MMP includes MMP-17 and MMP-25.
5. Type II transmembrane MMPs include MMP-23A and MMP-23B-identical proteins encoded by distinct genes.

The MT-MMPs are covalently linked to the cell surface, however secreted ones can also attach to the cell membrane by either binding to integrins or to CD44. MMPs are produced in cells as zymogens where cysteine from the pro-domain is bound to zinc at the catalytic site and require proteolytic cleavage for activation. Activation of MMPs often requires cleavage by other MMPs, or serine proteases outside the cell. However some, including the membrane-type MMPs, are activated intracellularly (Egeblad and Werb 2002). Besides activation of pro-enzymes, MMP activity is also regulated by gene expression, compartmentalization and inhibition of active enzymes by their specific tissue inhibitors.

Tissue inhibitors of metalloproteinases (TIMPs) are specific endogenous inhibitors of MMPs that have been correlated both positively and negatively in glioma invasion.

4.2.1 MMPs in glioma

MMP up-regulation has been implicated in several broad disease categories including inflammation, vascular pathologies, and cancer. Analysis of MMP expression in cancer patients show strong correlation between increased expression of many MMPs and tumor progression in a wide range of malignancies including gliomas. Within the tumor, MMPs are secreted by tumor cells, as well as by stromal cells of the tumor (Rojiani et al. 2010). It appears that tumor cells produce a potent factor called extracellular matrix metalloproteinase inducer (EMMPRIN) a cell surface glycoprotein of the immunoglobulin superfamily. EMMRPIN stimulates MMP expression in stromal cells and also in tumor cells (Jodele et al. 2006).

Several studies have documented overexpression of MMPs in gliomas compared to normal brain tissue. However the MMPs involved in gliomas have almost exclusively been the gelatinases MMP-2 and MMP-9 (reviewed by Rao 2003).

The glioma vasculature as well as infiltrating inflammatory cells, which form a portion of the glioma mass have been implicated in MMP expression (VanMeter et al. 2001). Strong gelatinase expression correlates with tumor grade (Forsyth et al. 1999, Wang et al. 2003). Intracranial implantation of glioblastoma cells in nude mice resulted in increased levels of MMP-9 during growth (Sawaya et al. 1998, Chintala et al. 1999). Raithatha et al. (Raithatha et al. 2000) carried out an RNA and protein localization study for gelatinases in a set of human gliomas with varied malignancy. They found that MMP-2 expression was most prominent in tumor cells whereas MMP-9 expression was seen in tumor cell but was more strongly expressed in the vasculature. Nakagawa et al. (Nakagawa et al. 1994) reported increased MMP-9 levels in blood vessels at proliferating margins. Recently Zhang et al. (Zhang et al. 2009) showed that knockdown of Akt2 resulted in decreased MMP-9 expression with concomitant decrease in glioma invasion *in vitro* and *in vivo*. It should be pointed out that EMMPRIN levels have been shown to increase in glioma and correlate with tumor grade (Sameshima et al. 2000). EMMPRIN has also been shown to increase hyaluronan and co-localizes with its receptor CD44 (Toole and Slomiany 2008). Given that Hyaluronan and CD44 are important players in the CNS and in gliomas (see section 3.4.1) EMMPRIN may play a significant role in glioma invasion.

In vitro studies also manifest a strong correlation between the expression of gelatinases and glioma cell invasion (reviewed by Bellail et al. 2004). Using matrigel assay, it was shown that the most invasive GBM cell line produced the highest level of gelatinases (Uhm et al. 1996, Abe et al. 1994). Besides the gelatinases, there are a number of studies documenting the role of MT1-MMP as well as reports of other MMPs involved in gliomas. Lampert et al. (Lampert et al. 1998) found increased levels of gelatinases as well as MT1-MMP and MT2-MMP in brain tumors. Yamamoto et al. (Yamamoto et al. 1996) found that increased MT1-MMP expression is associated with the expression of activated form of MMP-2 which in turn correlated with malignant glioma progression *in vivo*. Overexpression of MT1-MMP in glioma cell lines leads to activation of pro-MMP-2 (Nakada et al. 2001, Deryugina et al. 1997). Additionally, other studies show that MT1-MMP is increased in glioma-associated microglia and that glioma-released factors trigger this expression by microglia. The MT1-MMP then activates glioma-derived proMMP-2 and promotes glioma expansion (Markovic et al. 2009). The known classical function of MT1-MMP is activation of proMMP-2 in conjunction with TIMP-2. A complex of MT1-MMP and TIMP-2 interacts with proMMP-2 thus resulting in cleavage of the pro-domain from MMP-2 (Murphy et al. 1999). Hence, it is not surprising that many studies on glioma define activation of proMMP-2.

The gelatinases MMP-2 and MMP-9 as well as the membrane-type protease MT1-MMP have been well documented to play pivotal roles in invasion and angiogenesis (Handsley and Edwards 2005). Vascular basement membrane components are well recognized substrates of MMP-2 and MMP-9. MMP-9 is a known component of the angiogenic switch regulating the bioavailability of VEGF (Bergers et al. 2000). MMP-2 expression has been correlated with the degree of vascularization of tumor nodules (Fang et al. 2000). MT1-MMP deficient mice have provided convincing evidence for its role in angiogenesis (reviewed by Handsley and Edwards 2005). These same MMPs are found at the invasive front of the tumor. Invadopodia are actin-rich protrusions of tumor cells with proteolytic activity. The gelatinases and the MT1-MMP localize to or become activated at the invadopodia (Stylli et al. 2008).

Within the realm of glioma angiogenesis, the gelatinases remain crucial. MMP-2 and MMP-9 showed positive correlation with glioma invasion and angiogenesis (Wang et al. 2003). In a mouse model, glioma growth required host MMP-2 to support angiogenesis (Takahashi et al. 2002). Small interferring RNA (siRNA)-mediated targeting of MMP-9 inhibits glioma angiogenesis in *in vitro* and *in vivo* models (Lakka et al. 2005). Hypoxia-inducible factor-1 α (HIF1α) was shown to induce recruitment of CD45+ cells amongst other cellular components, in a murine glioblastoma model. MMP-9 activity of these bone marrow derived CD45+ cells was essential and sufficient to initiate angiogenesis by increasing VEGF bioavailability (Du et al. 2008).

With regard to other MMPs, Lettau et al. (Lettau et al. 2010) have found that MMP-19 is strongly expressed in astroglial tumors and is also responsible for the invasion of glioma cells *in vitro*. In a study using the glioma cell line U251, Deng et al. (Deng et al. 2010) found that MMP-26 promoted cell invasion *in vitro* and *in vivo*. Stojic et al. (Stojic et al. 2008) have shown enhanced expression of MMP-1, MMP-11 and MMP-19 in glioblastoma multiforme in comparison to low grade astrocytomas and normal brain. Tenascin-C is an ECM protein of the brain parenchyma and its synthesis is known to be up-regulated in glioma. MMP-12 was implicated in the invasion of glioma cell lines using tenascin-C in a three-dimensional matrix model (Sarkar et al. 2006).

Hence, it appears that MMPs play a pivotal role in glioma aggressiveness which would appear to make them potential targets for therapy. However, it should be pointed out that MMPs, by virtue of their degradation capacity also generate endogenous angiogenesis inhibitors. Proteolytic cleavage of plasminogen by several MMPs generates angiostatin and endostatin is generated from the C-terminal fragment of collagen type XVIII. MMP-9 is involved in the release of Tumstatin, another inhibitor of angiogenesis. MMPs as potential targets are further discussed below.

4.2.2 Tissue Inhibitors of Matrix Metalloproteinases (TIMPS) in glioma

As mentioned above, MMP regulation occurs at four different levels i.e. transcription, zymogen activation, compartmentalization and natural endogenous inhibition. Inhibition by α_2-macroglobulin and tissue inhibitors of metalloproteinases (TIMPs) occurs in the liquid phase and in tissues, respectively (Nagase et al. 1999, Brew et al. 2000). Although TIMPs have been known for their primary function of inhibiting MMPs, it has now been widely recognized that TIMPs exhibit additional biological activities independent of their MMP inhibitory function. There are four TIMP members: TIMP-1, TIMP-2, TIMP-3 and TIMP-4, all of which inhibit MMP activity. TIMP-1, -2 and -4 are secreted, whereas TIMP-3 is associated with the extracellular matrix. They are differentially regulated i.e. TIMP-1 expression is inducible, whereas TIMP-2 expression is constitutive (Gomez et al. 1997, Nagase et al. 1999).

The MMP-independent activity of TIMPs includes promotion of cell growth as exhibited by TIMP-1 and TIMP-2, apoptosis, angiogenesis as well as a role in cell signaling. These roles of TIMPs surfaced when overexpression of these molecules gave conflicting results. There are several earlier studies showing an inhibitory role of TIMPs in tumor growth and metastasis; however, a number of studies have also demonstrated a tumor-promoting function and serum levels of TIMP correlated with poor prognosis as well (reviewed by Rojiani et al. 2010).

This paradoxical tumor promoting and tumor inhibiting role of TIMPs extends to gliomas as well. In the normal murine brain TIMP-2, -3 and -4 are strongly expressed whereas there is very little TIMP-1 expression (reviewed by Crocker et al. 2004) . Studies demonstrating the classical role of TIMP show, for example, that adding TIMP-2 to cultured glioblastoma cells reduces their invasion (Rao et al. 1994). Likewise, use of recombinant TIMP-1 on glioma cells showed reduced glioma invasion (VanMeter et al. 2001). Also, TIMP-1 was shown to cause significant reduction in brain metastasis of implanted fibrosarcoma cells (Kruger et al. 1998) and a decrease in TIMP-2 levels in glioblastomas has been noted as well (Lampert et al. 1998). TIMP-3 overexpression suppresses glioma cell infiltration (Baker et al. 1999). Interestingly, *TIMP-3* gene is one of the most highly methylated genes found in brain tumors (Esteller et al. 2001) and has been referred to as a tumor suppressor.

Nakada et al. (Nakada et al. 2001) found that TIMP-1 but not TIMP-2 levels were significantly higher in glioblastoma multiforme compared to other glioma grades when using sandwich enzyme immunoassays. The same study developed stable transfectants of MT1-MMP and found that invasion and gelatinase activity of these transfectants could be totally inhibited by recombinant TIMP-2 but not recombinant TIMP-1. Lampert et al. (Lampert et al. 1998) have demonstrated a significant increase in TIMP-1 levels in glioblastomas compared to low grade tumors. Pagenstecher et al. (Pagenstecher et al. 2001) investigated the expression profiles of 9 MMPs and all TIMPs in different gliomas and found that TIMP-1 expression was the highest in GBMs and grade I gliomas with expression being confined to walls of neovessels. Groft et al. (Groft et al. 2001) carried out an extensive study looking at the expression and localization of all four TIMPs in normal human brains and gliomas. A detailed analysis of the expression of mRNA and protein levels showed that TIMP-2 and TIMP-3 expression pattern did not alter with tumor grade. However TIMP-1 levels correlated positively with glioma malignancy, whereas TIMP-4 correlated negatively. TIMP-1 transcript expression was localized to tumor cell and the surrounding tumor vasculature while TIMP-4 transcripts were found mainly in tumor cells with minor expression seen in vessels. These authors also showed that in an *in vitro* assay, recombinant TIMP-4 reduced invasion of U251 glioma cells through Matrigel. Thus, although TIMPs have clearly been shown to play a significant role in the invasive and growth aspects of glioma, their precise roles remain elusive. However, TIMPs deserve further consideration in the search for targeted therapies.

5. Therapeutic targeting of ECM molecules in glioma

5.1 Targeting metalloproteinases

MMPs play a crucial role in tumor growth, metastasis and angiogenesis and therefore have been the targets of antitumor therapy. Due to highly pleiotropic activities of MMPs the outcomes of the clinical studies targeting these molecules have been disappointing, resulting often in increased tumor growth (reviewed by Rojiani et al. 2011). The initial use of broad spectrum MMP inhibitors interfering with the function of many of these enzymes in clinical trials had unforeseen consequences and resulted in early termination of these studies (reviewed by Coussens et al. 2002). These disappointing results led to the realization that the experimental data had to be reevaluated. For example, in animal studies the inhibitors were administered in early or intermediate stages of cancer whereas in humans they were administered in advanced stages. Besides, it has now been well documented that a number of MMPs play a protective role and their elimination can have adverse consequences (Martin and Matrisian 2007).

However, given their significant contribution to tumor progression, MMPs still remain strong potential target candidates for therapeutic interventions. Therefore, it is not surprising that there are a number of MMP inhibitors (MMPI) in clinical trials (reviewed by Roy et al. 2009). Their effectiveness has yet to be proven. Also, the timing of delivery has been reconsidered since drugs given at earlier stages of cancer appear to be more effective than when given in advanced stages (Roy et al. 2009).

Despite the adaptation of clinical trials and because of the pleiotropic activities of MMPs, a prediction of outcome is still difficult. Therefore, attention is now also given to other ECM molecules in the glioma microenvironment. New classes of targets need to be identified, eg. ECM molecules found within the cancer stem cell niche. Examples of other ECM targets are discussed below (sections 5.2, 6.1 and 6.2).

5.2 Targeting HA and CD44 adhesion molecule

We showed previously that blocking CD44 and interfering with HA-CD44 ligand-receptor interaction resulted in inhibition of glioma cell invasion, decreased HA production and led to glioma cell apoptosis (Wiranowska et al. 1998, Wiranowska et al. 2010). In addition, recent data by Xu et al. (Xu et al. 2010) showed that CD44 attenuates activation of the Hippo signaling pathway and that knockdown of CD44 expression resulted in the inhibition of glioblastoma. It was suggested that CD44 is a prime therapeutic target for treatment of glioblastoma (Xu et al. 2010). Therefore, further studies of this promising biological target molecule in glioma are warranted. The soluble recombinant CD44-HA-binding domain (CD44-HABD) inhibited proliferation of endothelial cells *in vitro* , blocked angiogenesis *in vivo* and inhibited growth of various tumors (Pall et al. 2004) providing hope for a new therapeutic approach to glioma. In addition, HA was recently used *in vivo* as a delivery carrier for chemotherapeutic paclitaxel (HA-paclitaxel) targeting CD44 positive ovarian carcinoma (Auzenne et al. 2007). Also, recently cisplatin carrying HA nanoparticles were evaluated as potential treatment for cancer (Jeong et al. 2008).

6. Future therapies of glioma

6.1 ECM therapeutic targets: Hopes and disappointments

Current therapies like surgery, radiotherapy and chemotherapy are aimed at debulking of the brain tumor mass as well as targeting and eradicating proliferating tumor cells. However, these therapies do not address the quiescent population of the cancer stem cells. These cells, which are nourished and protected from therapeutic interventions by the microenvironment of the CSCs vascular niche can repopulate and initiate new tumor foci in the brain (Denysenko et al. 2010)

The modulation of the ECM microenvironment of the stem cell niche may be a promising approach especially in light of the finding that many of the genes and their products prognostic for the faith of proneural GBM were identified in the stroma of the brain tumor but not in the brain tumor cells themselves (as mentioned in Section 1: Holland 2011). Therapies targeting solely the brain tumors and their CSCs population may not be successful due to the high complexity and heterogeneity of brain tumors as demonstrated by the existence of various subtypes of GBMs. In addition, the genetic instability in expressing markers for undifferentiated cells within these tumors makes it difficult to assign the correct differentiation status of the tumor cells (Denysenko et al. 2010). Therefore, other therapeutic options should be pursued including therapies targeting the ECM of the CSCs vascular niches which would disrupt the microenvironment protective and supportive of the CSCs' self-renewal.

One of the stimulatory pro-angiogenic molecules released within the CSCs niche which enhances the survival of neural stem cells is VEGF (section 3.2). It has been shown that targeting VEGF and disruption of the niches by anti-VEGF treatment *in vivo* resulted in CSCs depletion and tumor growth inhibition (Calabrese et al. 2007). Some other studies however, showed that blocking VEGF *in vivo* resulted in growth of satellite tumors (Rubenstein et al. 2000). The early data obtained from clinical trials of GBM patients using VEGF-specific inhibitors such as bevacizumab combined with chemotherapeutic drug CPT-11, showed promising results (Calabrese et al. 2007). However, recent finding by Ricci-Vitiani et al. (Ricci-Vitiani et al. 2010) and Wang et al. (Wang et al. 2010) showed that newly formed blood vessels originating from the GBM stem cells that differentiated into endothelial cells were not responsive to anti-VEGF therapy (section 3.2). Most recently, it has been shown (di Tomaso et al. 2011) that patients treated with anti-VEGF therapy still contained Nestin + cells, a characteristic marker of the CSCs, despite a decreased vascularization of the brain tumors. The phase II results from anti-VEGF therapy in combination with chemotherapeutic CPT-11 failed to show prolonged survival of the GBM patients (Lai et al. 2011). Similar results were obtained from phase III clinical studies with recurrent GBM patients treated with cediranib, an inhibitor of VEGF alone or in combination with chemotherapeutic lomustine (Batchelor, 2010). In addition, it was shown recently by Takano et al. (Takano et al. 2010) that failure of bevacizumab treatment was associated with the high incidence of infiltrative tumors and MMP activity in the samples of urine. Therefore, based on the current state of knowledge, other approaches targeting ECM molecules of the vascular niche of CSCs need to be developed.

6.2 Glioma possible new prognostic factors and new targets

6.2.1 ECM prognostic factors

There is evidence that some ECM molecules could serve as prognostic markers of anti-angiogenic therapy of glioma indicative of the fate of the therapy. For example, Takano et al. (Takano et al. 2010) found that failure of bevacizumab (anti-VEGF antibody) treatment was associated with the high incidence of infiltrative tumors and levels of MMP activity in urine. Therefore, early detection and measurement of urine MMPs activity in samples from patients could be indicative of progressive disease. The detection of this biomarker could allow for earlier therapeutic intervention or alteration of a given anti-glioma therapy. Another ECM prognostic factor of potential therapeutic value could be presence of soluble collagen IV in the blood. It was shown by Sorensen et al. (Sorensen et al. 2009) that in patients treated with anti-angiogenic therapy using cediranib (pan-VEGF receptor tyrosine kinase inhibitor) increased levels of collagen IV were found. This increase in circulating collagen IV was explained as the result of "blood vessels normalization" involving thinning of the abnormally thick tumor associated basement membrane of blood vessels. Increased levels of circulating collagen IV were associated with progression-free and overall patient survival.

6.2.2 New ECM targets

Recent data by Inoue et al. (Inoue et al. 2010) showed that cancer stem-like cells of GBM express MMP-13 responsible for invasion and migration of these cells suggesting that, MMP-13 might be a potential new therapeutic target for glioblastomas. Blocking VEGF or silencing VEGF receptor 2 inhibits the maturation of tumor endothelial progenitors into endothelium but does not stop the differentiation of CSCs (CD133+ cells) into endothelial cells. However, silencing of Notch (neural precursor receptor as mentioned in section 2.2) blocks the transition of CSCs (CD133+ cells) into endothelial progenitors (Wang et al. 2010). Therefore, Notch may be another potential new target in the stem cell niche. Fujita et al. (Fujita et al. 2011) showed that non-steroidal anti-inflammatory drugs (NSAID) such as Cox-2 inhibitors suppressed gliomagenesis via inhibition of prostaglandin E2 mediated accumulation of myeloid derived suppressor cells. In addition, as mentioned earlier (section 3.1) the Cox-2 inhibitor, celecoxib, inhibited *in vitro* microvascular channel formation associated with VEGF down regulation (Basu et al. 2005). The effect was more pronounced and prostaglandin E2-independent in a highly invasive breast cancer cell line when compared to a less invasive cell line. Based on these findings, it could be hypothesized that the NSAID class may have potential application in highly invasive glioma by targeting of the inflammatory molecules and immune cells as well as VM channel formation in the ECM.

7. Summary and conclusions

Despite years of research, glioma therapy remains a challenge due to very limited therapeutic options and short survival of glioma patients (as described in section 1). Until recently the focus of research evaluating possible target molecules for treatment was mainly on the cancer cell itself and its genetic characterization. Therefore, routine anti-glioma therapies such as chemotherapy or radiation are solely focused on targeting proliferating glioma cells by interfering with their cell cycle and resulting in glioma cell death. Very little attention was given to evaluation and validation of therapeutic targets in the extracellular matrix in glioma, its vasculature and brain stroma outside the tumor. Recent clinical trials targeting glioma vasculature with anti-angiogenic molecules initially provided encouraging results but later failed to be effective in slowing glioma progression. On the contrary, some of the anti-angiogenic treatments despite achieving blood vessel "normalization" within the tumor later resulted in the development of new glioma foci in the brain parenchyma away from the main lesion. It became known recently that a population of glioma CSCs present within the tumors was capable of escaping this anti-angiogenic therapy giving rise to tumor endothelium which had no markers for anti-angiogenic therapy.

Another attempt to stop glioma cell invasion into the normal brain parenchyma involved targeting various MMPs responsible for remodeling ECM during glioma progression. Although there were high expectations, the results of these studies were disappointing again. It was found that many of the targeted MMPs had anti-tumor as well as tumorigenic activities and blocking or eliminating their activity lead to glioma regrowth. Clearly, the

ECM and the surrounding stroma play an essential role in glioma progression but more studies need to be done in order to find proper targets within the ECM to slow or inhibit glioma growth. This is supported by most recent finding by Holland (Holland 2011) that genes expressed in the microenvironment of the stroma rather than in the glioma itself may be predictive of glioma patient survival. This chapter provides a review of recent information relating to ECM targets for anti-glioma therapy. Consideration was given to various ECM molecules within the normal brain, in glioma and in the vascular niche harboring glioma stem cells. Consideration was also given to ECM rigidity and its effect on glioma progression. In addition to discussing some pertinent ECM molecules in glioma progression, also new emerging ECM targets and new prognostic markers candidates were discussed. All in all, ECM molecules are of great importance in the development of new therapeutic strategies and the information compiled in this chapter summarizing their role should be suitable to give guidance for the search and the development of new ECM anti-glioma targets.

8. References

Abaskharoun, M., Bellemare, M., Lau, E. and Margolis, R. U. (2010). "Expression of hyaluronan and the hyaluronan-binding proteoglycans neurocan, aggrecan, and versican by neural stem cells and neural cells derived from embryonic stem cells." Brain Res 1327: 6-15.

Abe, T., Mori, T., Kohno, K., Seiki, M., Hayakawa, T., Welgus, H. G., Hori, S. and Kuwano, M. (1994). "Expression of 72 kDa type IV collagenase and invasion activity of human glioma cells." Clin Exp Metastasis 12(4): 296-304.

Annabi, B., Bouzeghrane, M., Moumdjian, R., Moghrabi, A. and Beliveau, R. (2005). "Probing the infiltrating character of brain tumors: inhibition of RhoA/ROK-mediated CD44 cell surface shedding from glioma cells by the green tea catechin EGCg." J Neurochem 94(4): 906-16.

Auzenne, E., Ghosh, S. C., Khodadadian, M., Rivera, B., Farquhar, D., Price, R. E., Ravoori, M., Kundra, V., Freedman, R. S. and Klostergaard, J. (2007). "Hyaluronic acid-paclitaxel: antitumor efficacy against CD44(+) human ovarian carcinoma xenografts." Neoplasia 9(6): 479-86.

Baker, A. H., George, S. J., Zaltsman, A. B., Murphy, G. and Newby, A. C. (1999). "Inhibition of invasion and induction of apoptotic cell death of cancer cell lines by overexpression of TIMP-3." Br J Cancer 79(9-10): 1347-55.

Batchelor, T.(2010) 15th Annual Scientific Meeting of Society for Neuro-Oncology , Abstract OT-25, November, 19, 2010

Bao, S., Wu, Q., Sathornsumetee, S., Hao, Y., Li, Z., Hjelmeland, A. B., Shi, Q., McLendon, R. E., Bigner, D. D. and Rich, J. N. (2006). "Stem cell-like glioma cells promote tumor angiogenesis through vascular endothelial growth factor." Cancer Res 66(16): 7843-8.

Basu, G. D., Pathangey, L. B., Tinder, T. L., Gendler, S. J. and Mukherjee, P. (2005). "Mechanisms underlying the growth inhibitory effects of the cyclo-oxygenase-2 inhibitor celecoxib in human breast cancer cells." Breast Cancer Res 7(4): R422-35.

Bellail, A. C., Hunter, S. B., Brat, D. J., Tan, C. and Van Meir, E. G. (2004). "Microregional extracellular matrix heterogeneity in brain modulates glioma cell invasion." Int J Biochem Cell Biol 36(6): 1046-69.

Ben-Hur, T., Ben-Yosef, Y., Mizrachi-Kol, R., Ben-Menachem, O. and Miller, A. (2006). "Cytokine-mediated modulation of MMPs and TIMPs in multipotential neural precursor cells." J Neuroimmunol 175(1-2): 12-8.

Bergers, G., Brekken, R., McMahon, G., Vu, T. H., Itoh, T., Tamaki, K., Tanzawa, K., Thorpe, P., Itohara, S., Werb, Z. and Hanahan, D. (2000). "Matrix metalloproteinase-9 triggers the angiogenic switch during carcinogenesis." Nat Cell Biol 2(10): 737-44.

Bolteus, A. J., Berens, M. E. and Pilkington, G. J. (2001). "Migration and invasion in brain neoplasms." Curr Neurol Neurosci Rep 1(3): 225-32.

Brew, K., Dinakarpandian, D. and Nagase, H. (2000). "Tissue inhibitors of metalloproteinases: evolution, structure and function." Biochim Biophys Acta 1477(1-2): 267-83.

Brightman, M. W. (2002). "The brain's interstitial clefts and their glial walls." J Neurocytol 31(8-9): 595-603.

Brightman, M. W. and Kaya, M. (2000). "Permeable endothelium and the interstitial space of brain." Cell Mol Neurobiol 20(2): 111-30.

Cancer Genome Atlas Res. Network, 2008 Comprehensive genomic charachterization defines human glioblastoma genes
and core pathways, *Nature,* vol. 455, No 7216, pp.1061-1068

Calabrese, C., Poppleton, H., Kocak, M., Hogg, T. L., Fuller, C., Hamner, B., Oh, E. Y., Gaber, M. W., Finklestein, D., Allen, M., Frank, A., Bayazitov, I. T., Zakharenko, S. S., Gajjar, A., Davidoff, A. and Gilbertson, R. J. (2007). "A perivascular niche for brain tumor stem cells." Cancer Cell 11(1): 69-82.

Chintala, S. K., Kyritsis, A. P., Mohan, P. M., Mohanam, S., Sawaya, R., Gokslan, Z., Yung, W. K., Steck, P., Uhm, J. H., Aggarwal, B. B. and Rao, J. S. (1999). "Altered actin cytoskeleton and inhibition of matrix metalloproteinase expression by vanadate and phenylarsine oxide, inhibitors of phosphotyrosine phosphatases: modulation of migration and invasion of human malignant glioma cells." Mol Carcinog 26(4): 274-85.

Coussens, L. M., Fingleton, B. and Matrisian, L. M. (2002). "Matrix metalloproteinase inhibitors and cancer: trials and tribulations." Science 295(5564): 2387-92.

Crocker, S. J., Pagenstecher, A. and Campbell, I. L. (2004). "The TIMPs tango with MMPs and more in the central nervous system." J Neurosci Res 75(1): 1-11.

Deed, R., Rooney, P., Kumar, P., Norton, J. D., Smith, J., Freemont, A. J. and Kumar, S. (1997). "Early-response gene signalling is induced by angiogenic oligosaccharides of hyaluronan in endothelial cells. Inhibition by non-angiogenic, high-molecular-weight hyaluronan." Int J Cancer 71(2): 251-6.

Delpech, B., Maingonnat, C., Girard, N., Chauzy, C., Maunoury, R., Olivier, A., Tayot, J. and Creissard, P. (1993). "Hyaluronan and hyaluronectin in the extracellular matrix of human brain tumour stroma." Eur J Cancer 29A(7): 1012-7.

Deng, Y., Li, W., Li, Y., Yang, H., Xu, H., Liang, S. and Zhang, L. (2010). "Expression of Matrix Metalloproteinase-26 promotes human glioma U251 cell invasion in vitro and in vivo." Oncol Rep 23(1): 69-78.

Denysenko, T., Gennero, L., Roos, M. A., Melcarne, A., Juenemann, C., Faccani, G., Morra, I., Cavallo, G., Reguzzi, S., Pescarmona, G. and Ponzetto, A. (2010). "Glioblastoma cancer stem cells: heterogeneity, microenvironment and related therapeutic strategies." Cell Biochem Funct 28(5): 343-51.

Deryugina, E. I., Bourdon, M. A., Luo, G. X., Reisfeld, R. A. and Strongin, A. (1997). "Matrix metalloproteinase-2 activation modulates glioma cell migration." J Cell Sci 110 (Pt 19): 2473-82.

di Tomaso, E., Snuderl, M., Kamoun, W. S., Duda, D. G., Auluck, P. K., Fazlollahi, L., Andronesi, O. C., Frosch, M. P., Wen, P. Y., Plotkin, S. R., Hedley-Whyte, E. T., Sorensen, A. G., Batchelor, T. T. and Jain, R. K. (2011). "Glioblastoma recurrence after cediranib therapy in patients: lack of "rebound" revascularization as mode of escape." Cancer Res 71(1): 19-28.

Doetsch, F. (2003). "A niche for adult neural stem cells." Curr Opin Genet Dev 13(5): 543-50.

Du, R., Lu, K. V., Petritsch, C., Liu, P., Ganss, R., Passegue, E., Song, H., Vandenberg, S., Johnson, R. S., Werb, Z. and Bergers, G. (2008). "HIF1alpha induces the recruitment of bone marrow-derived vascular modulatory cells to regulate tumor angiogenesis and invasion." Cancer Cell 13(3): 206-20.

Egeblad, M. and Werb, Z. (2002). "New functions for the matrix metalloproteinases in cancer progression." Nat Rev Cancer 2(3): 161-74.

El Hallani, S., Boisselier, B., Peglion, F., Rousseau, A., Colin, C., Idbaih, A., Marie, Y., Mokhtari, K., Thomas, J. L., Eichmann, A., Delattre, J. Y., Maniotis, A. J. and Sanson, M. (2010). "A new alternative mechanism in glioblastoma vascularization: tubular vasculogenic mimicry." Brain 133(Pt 4): 973-82.

Elkin , B.S., BS., Azeloglu, EU., Costa KD., Morrison B3rd (2007). "Mechanical heterogeneity of the rat hippocampus measured by atomic force microscope indentation". J.Neurotrama, 24, 812-822.

Esteller, M., Corn, P. G., Baylin, S. B. and Herman, J. G. (2001). "A gene hypermethylation profile of human cancer." Cancer Res 61(8): 3225-9.

Fang, J., Shing, Y., Wiederschain, D., Yan, L., Butterfield, C., Jackson, G., Harper, J., Tamvakopoulos, G. and Moses, M. A. (2000). "Matrix metalloproteinase-2 is required for the switch to the angiogenic phenotype in a tumor model." Proc Natl Acad Sci U S A 97(8): 3884-9.

Folkman, J. (1998). "Antiangiogenic gene therapy." Proc Natl Acad Sci U S A 95(16): 9064-6.

Forsyth, P. A., Wong, H., Laing, T. D., Rewcastle, N. B., Morris, D. G., Muzik, H., Leco, K. J., Johnston, R. N., Brasher, P. M., Sutherland, G. and Edwards, D. R. (1999). "Gelatinase-A (MMP-2), gelatinase-B (MMP-9) and membrane type matrix metalloproteinase-1 (MT1-MMP) are involved in different aspects of the pathophysiology of malignant gliomas." Br J Cancer 79(11-12): 1828-35.

Fujita, M., Kohanbash, G., Fellows-Mayle, W., Hamilton, R. L., Komohara, Y., Decker, S. A., Ohlfest, J. R. and Okada, H. (2011). "COX-2 Blockade Suppresses Gliomagenesis by Inhibiting Myeloid-Derived Suppressor Cells." Cancer Res 71(7): 2664-74.

Galli, R., Binda, E., Orfanelli, U., Cipelletti, B., Gritti, A., De Vitis, S., Fiocco, R., Foroni, C., Dimeco, F. and Vescovi, A. (2004). "Isolation and characterization of tumorigenic, stem-like neural precursors from human glioblastoma." Cancer Res 64(19): 7011-21.

Gomez, D. E., Alonso, D. F., Yoshiji, H. and Thorgeirsson, U. P. (1997). "Tissue inhibitors of metalloproteinases: structure, regulation and biological functions." Eur J Cell Biol 74(2): 111-22.

Groft, L. L., Muzik, H., Rewcastle, N. B., Johnston, R. N., Knauper, V., Lafleur, M. A., Forsyth, P. A. and Edwards, D. R. (2001). "Differential expression and localization of TIMP-1 and TIMP-4 in human gliomas." Br J Cancer 85(1): 55-63.

Ha, H. Y., Moon, H. B., Nam, M. S., Lee, J. W., Ryoo, Z. Y., Lee, T. H., Lee, K. K., So, B. J., Sato, H., Seiki, M. and Yu, D. Y. (2001). "Overexpression of membrane-type matrix metalloproteinase-1 gene induces mammary gland abnormalities and adenocarcinoma in transgenic mice." Cancer Res 61(3): 984-90.

Handsley, M. M. and Edwards, D. R. (2005). "Metalloproteinases and their inhibitors in tumor angiogenesis." Int J Cancer 115(6): 849-60.

Hibino, S., Shibuya, M., Engbring, J. A., Mochizuki, M., Nomizu, M. and Kleinman, H. K. (2004). "Identification of an active site on the laminin alpha5 chain globular domain that binds to CD44 and inhibits malignancy." Cancer Res 64(14): 4810-6.

Holland, E C. (2011). "PDGF/Proneural GBMs: Microenvironment and Therapeutic response". Program of 102 Annual Am. Assoc for Cancer Res, April 2-6, 2011, p.190.

Inoue, A., Takahashi, H., Harada, H., Kohno, S., Ohue, S., Kobayashi, K., Yano, H., Tanaka, J. and Ohnishi, T. (2010). "Cancer stem-like cells of glioblastoma characteristically express MMP-13 and display highly invasive activity." Int J Oncol 37(5): 1121-31.

Jeong, Y. I., Kim, S. T., Jin, S. G., Ryu, H. H., Jin, Y. H., Jung, T. Y., Kim, I. Y. and Jung, S. (2008). "Cisplatin-incorporated hyaluronic acid nanoparticles based on ion-complex formation." J Pharm Sci 97(3): 1268-76.

Jodele, S., Blavier, L., Yoon, J. M. and DeClerck, Y. A. (2006). "Modifying the soil to affect the seed: role of stromal-derived matrix metalloproteinases in cancer progression." Cancer Metastasis Rev 25(1): 35-43.

Kearns, S. M., Laywell, E. D., Kukekov, V. K. and Steindler, D. A. (2003). "Extracellular matrix effects on neurosphere cell motility." Exp Neurol 182(1): 240-4.

Kessenbrock, K., Plaks, V. and Werb, Z. (2010). "Matrix metalloproteinases: regulators of the tumor microenvironment." Cell 141(1): 52-67.

Knott, J. C., Mahesparan, R., Garcia-Cabrera, I., Bolge Tysnes, B., Edvardsen, K., Ness, G. O., Mork, S., Lund-Johansen, M. and Bjerkvig, R. (1998). "Stimulation of extracellular matrix components in the normal brain by invading glioma cells." Int J Cancer 75(6): 864-72.

Knudson, C. B. and Knudson, W. (1993). "Hyaluronan-binding proteins in development, tissue homeostasis, and disease." FASEB J 7(13): 1233-41.

Kruger, A., Sanchez-Sweatman, O. H., Martin, D. C., Fata, J. E., Ho, A. T., Orr, F. W., Ruther, U. and Khokha, R. (1998). "Host TIMP-1 overexpression confers resistance to experimental brain metastasis of a fibrosarcoma cell line." Oncogene 16(18): 2419-23.

Kumar, S. (2009). "Cell-matrix mechanobiology: applications to brain tumors and design of tissue engineering scaffolds." Conf Proc IEEE Eng Med Biol Soc 2009: 3350-2.

Lai, A., Tran, A., Nghiemphu, P. L., Pope, W. B., Solis, O. E., Selch, M., Filka, E., Yong, W. H., Mischel, P. S., Liau, L. M., Phuphanich, S., Black, K., Peak, S., Green, R. M., Spier, C. E., Kolevska, T., Polikoff, J., Fehrenbacher, L., Elashoff, R. and Cloughesy, T. (2011). "Phase II study of bevacizumab plus temozolomide during and after radiation therapy for patients with newly diagnosed glioblastoma multiforme." J Clin Oncol 29(2): 142-8.

Lakka, S. S., Gondi, C. S. and Rao, J. S. (2005). "Proteases and glioma angiogenesis." Brain Pathol 15(4): 327-41.

Lakka, S. S. and Rao, J. S. (2008). "Antiangiogenic therapy in brain tumors." Expert Rev Neurother 8(10): 1457-73.

Lampert, K., Machein, U., Machein, M. R., Conca, W., Peter, H. H. and Volk, B. (1998). "Expression of matrix metalloproteinases and their tissue inhibitors in human brain tumors." Am J Pathol 153(2): 429-37.

Lefranc, F., Brotchi, J. and Kiss, R. (2005). "Possible future issues in the treatment of glioblastomas: special emphasis on cell migration and the resistance of migrating glioblastoma cells to apoptosis." J Clin Oncol 23(10): 2411-22.

Lettau, I., Hattermann, K., Held-Feindt, J., Brauer, R., Sedlacek, R. and Mentlein, R. (2010). "Matrix metalloproteinase-19 is highly expressed in astroglial tumors and promotes invasion of glioma cells." J Neuropathol Exp Neurol 69(3): 215-23.

Lin, X. H., Dahlin-Huppe, K. and Stallcup, W. B. (1996). "Interaction of the NG2 proteoglycan with the actin cytoskeleton." J Cell Biochem 63(4): 463-77.

Ljubimova, J. Y., Fugita, M., Khazenzon, N. M., Das, A., Pikul, B. B., Newman, D., Sekiguchi, K., Sorokin, L. M., Sasaki, T. and Black, K. L. (2004). "Association between laminin-8 and glial tumor grade, recurrence, and patient survival." Cancer 101(3): 604-12.

Lo, C. M., Wang, H. B., Dembo, M. and Wang, Y. L. (2000). "Cell movement is guided by the rigidity of the substrate." Biophys J 79(1): 144-52.

Louis, D. N., Ohgaki, H., Wiestler, O. D., Cavenee, W. K., Burger, P. C., Jouvet, A., Scheithauer, B. W. and Kleihues, P. (2007). "The 2007 WHO classification of tumours of the central nervous system." Acta Neuropathol 114(2): 97-109.

Luke, H. J. and Prehm, P. (1999). "Synthesis and shedding of hyaluronan from plasma membranes of human fibroblasts and metastatic and non-metastatic melanoma cells." Biochem J 343 Pt 1: 71-5.

Mahesparan, R., Read, T. A., Lund-Johansen, M., Skaftnesmo, K. O., Bjerkvig, R. and Engebraaten, O. (2003). "Expression of extracellular matrix components in a highly infiltrative in vivo glioma model." Acta Neuropathol 105(1): 49-57.

Maniotis, A. J., Folberg, R., Hess, A., Seftor, E. A., Gardner, L. M., Pe'er, J., Trent, J. M., Meltzer, P. S. and Hendrix, M. J. (1999). "Vascular channel formation by human melanoma cells in vivo and in vitro: vasculogenic mimicry." Am J Pathol 155(3): 739-52.

Markovic, D. S., Vinnakota, K., Chirasani, S., Synowitz, M., Raguet, H., Stock, K., Sliwa, M., Lehmann, S., Kalin, R., van Rooijen, N., Holmbeck, K., Heppner, F. L., Kiwit, J., Matyash, V., Lehnardt, S., Kaminska, B., Glass, R. and Kettenmann, H. (2009). "Gliomas induce and exploit microglial MT1-MMP expression for tumor expansion." Proc Natl Acad Sci U S A 106(30): 12530-5.

Martin, M. D. and Matrisian, L. M. (2007). "The other side of MMPs: protective roles in tumor progression." Cancer Metastasis Rev 26(3-4): 717-24.

Mercier, F., Kitasako, J. T. and Hatton, G. I. (2003). "Fractones and other basal laminae in the hypothalamus." J Comp Neurol 455(3): 324-40.

Murphy, G. (2008). "The ADAMs: signalling scissors in the tumour microenvironment." Nat Rev Cancer 8(12): 929-41.

Murphy, G., Stanton, H., Cowell, S., Butler, G., Knauper, V., Atkinson, S. and Gavrilovic, J. (1999). "Mechanisms for pro matrix metalloproteinase activation." APMIS 107(1): 38-44.

Nagase, H., Meng, Q., Malinovskii, V., Huang, W., Chung, L., Bode, W., Maskos, K. and Brew, K. (1999). "Engineering of selective TIMPs." Ann N Y Acad Sci 878: 1-11.

Nakada, M., Kita, D., Futami, K., Yamashita, J., Fujimoto, N., Sato, H. and Okada, Y. (2001). "Roles of membrane type 1 matrix metalloproteinase and tissue inhibitor of metalloproteinases 2 in invasion and dissemination of human malignant glioma." J Neurosurg 94(3): 464-73.

Nakada, M., Nakada, S., Demuth, T., Tran, N. L., Hoelzinger, D. B. and Berens, M. E. (2007). "Molecular targets of glioma invasion." Cell Mol Life Sci 64(4): 458-78.

Nakagawa, T., Kubota, T., Kabuto, M., Sato, K., Kawano, H., Hayakawa, T & Okada, Y. (1994). "Production of matrix metalloproteinases and tissue inhibitor of metalloproteinases-1 by human brain tumors." J Neurosurg 81 : 69-77

Novak, U., Stylli, S. S., Kaye, A. H. and Lepperdinger, G. (1999). "Hyaluronidase-2 overexpression accelerates intracerebral but not subcutaneous tumor formation of murine astrocytoma cells." Cancer Res 59(24): 6246-50.

Pagenstecher, A., Wussler, E. M., Opdenakker, G., Volk, B. and Campbell, I. L. (2001). "Distinct expression patterns and levels of enzymatic activity of matrix metalloproteinases and their inhibitors in primary brain tumors." J Neuropathol Exp Neurol 60(6): 598-612.

Pall, T., Gad, A., Kasak, L., Drews, M., Stromblad, S. and Kogerman, P. (2004). "Recombinant CD44-HABD is a novel and potent direct angiogenesis inhibitor enforcing endothelial cell-specific growth inhibition independently of hyaluronic acid binding." Oncogene 23(47): 7874-81.

Park, J. B., Kwak, H. J. and Lee, S. H. (2008). "Role of hyaluronan in glioma invasion." Cell Adh Migr 2(3): 202-7.

Paszek, M. J., Zahir, N., Johnson, K. R., Lakins, J. N., Rozenberg, G. I., Gefen, A., Reinhart-King, C. A., Margulies, S. S., Dembo, M., Boettiger, D., Hammer, D. A. and Weaver, V. M. (2005). "Tensional homeostasis and the malignant phenotype." Cancer Cell 8(3): 241-54.

Provenzano, P. P., Inman, D. R., Eliceiri, K. W., Beggs, H. E. and Keely, P. J. (2008). "Mammary epithelial-specific disruption of focal adhesion kinase retards tumor formation and metastasis in a transgenic mouse model of human breast cancer." Am J Pathol 173(5): 1551-65.

Quirico-Santos, T., Fonseca, C. O. and Lagrota-Candido, J. (2010). "Brain sweet brain: importance of sugars for the cerebral microenvironment and tumor development." Arq Neuropsiquiatr 68(5): 799-803.

Raithatha, S. A., Muzik, H., Rewcastle, N. B., Johnston, R. N., Edwards, D. R. and Forsyth, P. A. (2000). "Localization of gelatinase-A and gelatinase-B mRNA and protein in human gliomas." Neuro Oncol 2(3): 145-50.

Roijani M.V., Wiranowska, M., & Roijani A.M.. (2011). "Matrix Metalloproteinases and Their Inhibitors-Friend or Foe" in Tumor Microenvironment (ed Dietmar W. Siemann) J. Wiley and Sons, Ltd.

Ranuncolo, S. M., Ladeda, V., Specterman, S., Varela, M., Lastiri, J., Morandi, A., Matos, E., Bal de Kier Joffe, E., Puricelli, L. and Pallotta, M. G. (2002). "CD44 expression in human gliomas." J Surg Oncol 79(1): 30-5; discussion 35-6.

Rao, J. S. (2003). "Molecular mechanisms of glioma invasiveness: the role of proteases." Nat Rev Cancer 3(7): 489-501.

Rao, J. S., Steck, P. A., Tofilon, P., Boyd, D., Ali-Osman, F., Stetler-Stevenson, W. G., Liotta, L. A. and Sawaya, R. (1994). "Role of plasminogen activator and of 92-KDa type IV

collagenase in glioblastoma invasion using an in vitro matrigel model." J Neurooncol 18(2): 129-38.
Ricci-Vitiani, L., Pallini, R., Biffoni, M., Todaro, M., Invernici, G., Cenci, T., Maira, G., Parati, E. A., Stassi, G., Larocca, L. M. and De Maria, R. (2010). "Tumour vascularization via endothelial differentiation of glioblastoma stem-like cells." Nature 468(7325): 824-8.
Ricciardelli, C., Sakko, A. J., Ween, M. P., Russell, D. L. and Horsfall, D. J. (2009). "The biological role and regulation of versican levels in cancer." Cancer Metastasis Rev 28(1-2): 233-45.
Rivera, S., Khrestchatisky, M., Kaczmarek, L., Rosenberg, G. A. and Jaworski, D. M. (2010). "Metzincin proteases and their inhibitors: foes or friends in nervous system physiology?" J Neurosci 30(46): 15337-57.
Rooney, P., Kumar, S., Ponting, J. and Wang, M. (1995). "The role of hyaluronan in tumour neovascularization (review)." Int J Cancer 60(5): 632-6.
Rosen, J. M. and Jordan, C. T. (2009). "The increasing complexity of the cancer stem cell paradigm." Science 324(5935): 1670-3.
Roy, R., Yang, J. and Moses, M. A. (2009). "Matrix metalloproteinases as novel biomarkers and potential therapeutic targets in human cancer." J Clin Oncol 27(31): 5287-97.
Rubenstein, J. L., Kim, J., Ozawa, T., Zhang, M., Westphal, M., Deen, D. F. and Shuman, M. A. (2000). "Anti-VEGF antibody treatment of glioblastoma prolongs survival but results in increased vascular cooption." Neoplasia 2(4): 306-14.
Sameshima, T., Nabeshima, K., Toole, B. P., Yokogami, K., Okada, Y., Goya, T., Koono, M. and Wakisaka, S. (2000). "Expression of emmprin (CD147), a cell surface inducer of matrix metalloproteinases, in normal human brain and gliomas." Int J Cancer 88(1): 21-7.
Sanz, L., Feijoo, M., Blanco, B., Serrano, A. and Alvarez-Vallina, L. (2003). "Generation of non-permissive basement membranes by anti-laminin antibody fragments produced by matrix-embedded gene-modified cells." Cancer Immunol Immunother 52(10): 643-7.
Sarkar, S., Nuttall, R. K., Liu, S., Edwards, D. R. and Yong, V. W. (2006). "Tenascin-C stimulates glioma cell invasion through matrix metalloproteinase-12." Cancer Res 66(24): 11771-80.
Sawaya, R., Go, Y., Kyritisis, A. P., Uhm, J., Venkaiah, B., Mohanam, S., Gokaslan, Z. L. and Rao, J. S. (1998). "Elevated levels of Mr 92,000 type IV collagenase during tumor growth in vivo." Biochem Biophys Res Commun 251(2): 632-6.
Scadden, D. T. (2006). "The stem-cell niche as an entity of action." Nature 441(7097): 1075-9.
Schrappe, M., Klier, F. G., Spiro, R. C., Waltz, T. A., Reisfeld, R. A. and Gladson, C. L. (1991). "Correlation of chondroitin sulfate proteoglycan expression on proliferating brain capillary endothelial cells with the malignant phenotype of astroglial cells." Cancer Res 51(18): 4986-93.
Shen, Q., Goderie, S. K., Jin, L., Karanth, N., Sun, Y., Abramova, N., Vincent, P., Pumiglia, K. and Temple, S. (2004). "Endothelial cells stimulate self-renewal and expand neurogenesis of neural stem cells." Science 304(5675): 1338-40.
Sim, H., Hu, B. and Viapiano, M. S. (2009). "Reduced expression of the hyaluronan and proteoglycan link proteins in malignant gliomas." J Biol Chem 284(39): 26547-56.
Sorensen, A. G., Batchelor, T. T., Zhang, W. T., Chen, P. J., Yeo, P., Wang, M., Jennings, D., Wen, P. Y., Lahdenranta, J., Ancukiewicz, M., di Tomaso, E., Duda, D. G. and Jain, R. K. (2009). "A "vascular normalization index" as potential mechanistic biomarker

to predict survival after a single dose of cediranib in recurrent glioblastoma patients." Cancer Res 69(13): 5296-300.

Stallcup, W. B. and Huang, F. J. (2008). "A role for the NG2 proteoglycan in glioma progression." Cell Adh Migr 2(3): 192-201.

Stojic, J., Hagemann, C., Haas, S., Herbold, C., Kuhnel, S., Gerngras, S., Roggendorf, W., Roosen, K. and Vince, G. H. (2008). "Expression of matrix metalloproteinases MMP-1, MMP-11 and MMP-19 is correlated with the WHO-grading of human malignant gliomas." Neurosci Res 60(1): 40-9.

Stylli, S. S., Kaye, A. H. and Lock, P. (2008). "Invadopodia: at the cutting edge of tumour invasion." J Clin Neurosci 15(7): 725-37.

Sykova, E. (2002). "Plasticity of extracellular space". In The Neuronal Environment. Walz W.Ed: Humana Press Inc. pp 57-81

Takahashi, M., Fukami, S., Iwata, N., Inoue, K., Itohara, S., Itoh, H., Haraoka, J. and Saido, T. (2002). "In vivo glioma growth requires host-derived matrix metalloproteinase 2 for maintenance of angioarchitecture." Pharmacol Res 46(2): 155-63.

Takano, S., Mashiko, R., Osuka, S., Ishikawa, E., Ohneda, O. and Matsumura, A. (2010). "Detection of failure of bevacizumab treatment for malignant glioma based on urinary matrix metalloproteinase activity." Brain Tumor Pathol 27(2): 89-94.

Tammi, R., MacCallum, D., Hascall, V. C., Pienimaki, J. P., Hyttinen, M. and Tammi, M. (1998). "Hyaluronan bound to CD44 on keratinocytes is displaced by hyaluronan decasaccharides and not hexasaccharides." J Biol Chem 273(44): 28878-88.

Theocharis, A.D., Skandalis S.S., Tzanakakis, G.N., Karamanos, N.K.. (2010). "Proteoglycans in health and disease: novel roles for proteoglycans in malignancy and their pharmacological targeting". FASEB J. 277 (19):3904-23.

Thomas, T. W. and DiMilla, P. A. (2000). "Spreading and motility of human glioblastoma cells on sheets of silicone rubber depend on substratum compliance." Med Biol Eng Comput 38(3): 360-70.

Toole, B. P. and Slomiany, M. G. (2008). "Hyaluronan, CD44 and Emmprin: partners in cancer cell chemoresistance." Drug Resist Updat 11(3): 110-21.

Tysnes, B. B., Mahesparan, R., Thorsen, F., Haugland, H. K., Porwol, T., Enger, P. O., Lund-Johansen, M. and Bjerkvig, R. (1999). "Laminin expression by glial fibrillary acidic protein positive cells in human gliomas." Int J Dev Neurosci 17(5-6): 531-9.

Uhm, J. H., Dooley, N. P., Villemure, J. G. and Yong, V. W. (1996). "Glioma invasion in vitro: regulation by matrix metalloprotease-2 and protein kinase C." Clin Exp Metastasis 14(5): 421-33.

Ulrich, T. A., de Juan Pardo, E. M. and Kumar, S. (2009). "The mechanical rigidity of the extracellular matrix regulates the structure, motility, and proliferation of glioma cells." Cancer Res 69(10): 4167-74.

VanMeter, T. E., Rooprai, H. K., Kibble, M. M., Fillmore, H. L., Broaddus, W. C. and Pilkington, G. J. (2001). "The role of matrix metalloproteinase genes in glioma invasion: co-dependent and interactive proteolysis." J Neurooncol 53(2): 213-35.

Verhaak, R. G., Hoadley, K. A., Purdom, E., Wang, V., Qi, Y., Wilkerson, M. D., Miller, C. R., Ding, L., Golub, T., Mesirov, J. P., Alexe, G., Lawrence, M., O'Kelly, M., Tamayo, P., Weir, B. A., Gabriel, S., Winckler, W., Gupta, S., Jakkula, L., Feiler, H. S., Hodgson, J. G., James, C. D., Sarkaria, J. N., Brennan, C., Kahn, A., Spellman, P. T., Wilson, R. K., Speed, T. P., Gray, J. W., Meyerson, M., Getz, G., Perou, C. M. and Hayes, D. N.

(2010). "Integrated genomic analysis identifies clinically relevant subtypes of glioblastoma characterized by abnormalities in PDGFRA, IDH1, EGFR, and NF1." Cancer Cell 17(1): 98-110.

Viapiano, M. S. and Matthews, R. T. (2006). "From barriers to bridges: chondroitin sulfate proteoglycans in neuropathology." Trends Mol Med 12(10): 488-96.

Wang, M., Wang, T., Liu, S., Yoshida, D. and Teramoto, A. (2003). "The expression of matrix metalloproteinase-2 and -9 in human gliomas of different pathological grades." Brain Tumor Pathol 20(2): 65-72.

Wang, R., Chadalavada, K., Wilshire, J., Kowalik, U., Hovinga, K. E., Geber, A., Fligelman, B., Leversha, M., Brennan, C. and Tabar, V. (2010). "Glioblastoma stem-like cells give rise to tumour endothelium." Nature 468(7325): 829-33.

Wiranowska, M., Ladd, S., Moscinski, L. C., Hill, B., Haller, E., Mikecz, K. and Plaas, A. (2010). "Modulation of hyaluronan production by CD44 positive glioma cells." Int J Cancer 127(3): 532-42.

Wiranowska, M., Ladd, S., Smith, S. R. and Gottschall, P. E. (2006). "CD44 adhesion molecule and neuro-glial proteoglycan NG2 as invasive markers of glioma." Brain Cell Biol 35(2-3): 159-72.

Wiranowska, M. and Naidu, A. K. (1994). "Interferon effect on glycosaminoglycans in mouse glioma in vitro." J Neurooncol 18(1): 9-17.

Wiranowska, M. and Plaas, A . (2008). "Cytokines and Extracellular Matrix Remodeling in the Central Nervous System". In: Neuroimmune Biology (I.Berczi, and A. Szentivanyi, eds.), vol. 6, Cytokines and the Brain, Elsevier B.V. Science.

Wiranowska, M., Rojiani, A. M., Gottschall, P. E., Moscinski, L. C., Johnson, J. and Saporta, S. (2000). "CD44 expression and MMP-2 secretion by mouse glioma cells: effect of interferon and anti-CD44 antibody." Anticancer Res 20(6B): 4301-6.

Wiranowska, M., Tresser, N. and Saporta, S. (1998). "The effect of interferon and anti-CD44 antibody on mouse glioma invasiveness in vitro." Anticancer Res 18(5A): 3331-8.

Xu, Y., Stamenkovic, I. and Yu, Q. (2010). "CD44 attenuates activation of the hippo signaling pathway and is a prime therapeutic target for glioblastoma." Cancer Res 70(6): 2455-64.

Yamamoto, M., Mohanam, S., Sawaya, R., Fuller, G. N., Seiki, M., Sato, H., Gokaslan, Z. L., Liotta, L. A., Nicolson, G. L. and Rao, J. S. (1996). "Differential expression of membrane-type matrix metalloproteinase and its correlation with gelatinase A activation in human malignant brain tumors in vivo and in vitro." Cancer Res 56(2): 384-92.

Yamamoto, M., Sawaya, R., Mohanam, S., Bindal, A. K., Bruner, J. M., Oka, K., Rao, V. H., Tomonaga, M., Nicolson, G. L. and Rao, J. S. (1994). "Expression and localization of urokinase-type plasminogen activator in human astrocytomas in vivo." Cancer Res 54(14): 3656-61.

Yang, P., Baker, K. A. and Hagg, T. (2006). "The ADAMs family: coordinators of nervous system development, plasticity and repair." Prog Neurobiol 79(2): 73-94.

Yue, W. Y. and Chen, Z. P. (2005). "Does vasculogenic mimicry exist in astrocytoma?" J Histochem Cytochem 53(8): 997-1002.

Zagzag, D., Friedlander, D. R., Miller, D. C., Dosik, J., Cangiarella, J., Kostianovsky, M., Cohen, H., Grumet, M. and Greco, M. A. (1995). "Tenascin expression in astrocytomas correlates with angiogenesis." Cancer Res 55(4): 907-14.

Zhang, B., Gu, F., She, C., Guo, H., Li, W., Niu, R., Fu, L., Zhang, N. and Ma, Y. (2009). "Reduction of Akt2 inhibits migration and invasion of glioma cells." Int J Cancer 125(3): 585-95.

Zhang S., Zhang, D., & Sun, B. (2007). "Vascular mimicry: Current status and future prospects." *Cancer Letters*, vol. 254, pp157-164.

13

The Role of Chemoattractant Receptors in the Progression of Glioma

Xiao-hong Yao et al.*
[1]Third Military Medical University, Chongqing,
[2]National Cancer Institute at Frederick, Frederick, MD
[1]People's Republic of China
[2]USA

1. Introduction

Chemoattractant receptors are a superfamily of G-protein coupled seven transmembrane cell surface receptors (GPCRs), which transduce extracellular signals into intracellular effector pathways through the activation of heterotrimeric G proteins. This superfamily includes GPCRs for classical chemoattractants such as formyl peptides (fMLF) produced by Gram negative bacteria and host cell mitochondria, the complement cleavage components, leukotriene B4 (LTB4), and platelet activating factor (PAF) as well as GPCRs for chemokines (Le et al., 2002).

Chemoattractant GPCRs have the ability to mediate directional migration of cells along a gradient of a chemoattractant. Initially, these receptors were identified mainly on leukocytes, where they play an important role in the trafficking of such cells to sites of inflammation and to lymphoid organs in immune responses (Le et al., 2004). However, during the past few years, both hematopoietic and nonhematopoietic cells have been found to express various chemoattractant GPCRs and are capable of migrating in response to agonists produced in tissue microenvironment. The interaction of chemoattractant GPCRs with their agonists participates in a variety of essential pathophysiological processes including immune responses, inflammation, host defense against microbial infection, hematopoiesis as well as cancer progression and metastasis (Huang et al., 2008).

Chemoattractants and their GPCRs are widely expressed in the brain by neurons, glial and microglia cells. They are involved not only in cell migration during development and inflammation, but also act as regulators of neuronal survival, neurotransmission and cell-cell communications (Ambrosini and Aloiso, 2004), as the third major transmitter system in the brain (Adler and Rogers, 2005). In addition, chemoattractants and their GPCRs are disregulated in neurodegenerative diseases, multiple sclerosis and brain tumors (Balkwill, 2004; Ransohoff et al., 2007). A number of chemoattractant GPCRs have been detected in glioma cells including FPR1 and chemokine GPCRs (Table 1).

---

*Ying Liu, Jian Huang, Ye Zhou, Keqiang Chen, Wanghua Gong,
Mingyong Liu, Xiu-wu Bian and Ji Ming Wang
Third Military Medical University, Chongqing, China
Fudan University, Shanghai, China
National Cancer Institute at Frederick, Frederick, MD, USA

Chemoattractant GPCRs (expressing cells)	Ligand (cell sources)	Major effects on glioma	References
FPR1 (glioma cells)	fMLF (bacteria); Annexin1(necrotic glioma cells)	Growth; Invasion; Angiogenesis	Zhou et al., 2005; Huang et al., 2007, 2008, and 2010
CXCR1 (glioma cells)	CXCL8 (glioma cells)	Invasion	Raychaudhuri et al., 2011
CXCR2 (glioma cells)	CXCL8 (glioma cells)	Angiogenesis	Brat DJ et al., 2005
CXCR3 (glioma cells)	CXCL10 (glioma cells) ; CXCL9 (glioma cells)	Proliferation; Growth	Liu et al., 2010; Maru et al., 2008
CXCR4 (glioma cells)	CXCL12 (glioma cells and stromal cells)	Growth; Angiogenesis; Migration	Ping et al., 2007 and 2011
CXCR5 (glioma cells)	CXCL13 (glioma cells)	Not clear	Bajetto et al., 2006
CXCR7 (glioma cells)	CXCL12 (glioma cells and stromal cells)	Anti-apoptosis	Hattermann et al., 2010
CCR2A (glioma cells)	CCL2 (glioma cells)	Migration	Liang Y et al., 2008
CCR3 (glioma cells)	CCL3L1 (glioma cells)	Proliferation	Kouno et al., 2004
CCR4 (Treg cells)	CCL22 (glioma cells)	Treg infiltration	Jacobs et al., 2010
CCR5 (glioma cells)	CCL3L1 (glioma cells)	Proliferation	Kouno et al., 2004
CX3CR1 (glioma cells and GIMs)	CX3CL1 (glioma cells)	Tumorigenesis; Pro-or anti-invasion based on whether CX3CL1 is soluble or membrane bound.	Liu et al., 2008

GIMs: glioma infiltrating macrophages; Treg: regulatory T cells.

Table 1. The expression of chemoattractant GPCRs in glioma

Glioma is the most common tumor type in human brain. Nearly two-thirds of human gliomas are highly malignant with rapid progression, high invasiveness, vigorous angiogenesis and resistance to chemotherapy and radiation treatment (Bar, 2011). Glioblastoma (GBM), the most aggressive form of malignant glioma, is characterized by extensive infiltration into the surrounding normal brain tissues and multifocal necrosis. Despite multiple therapeutic regimens (Jahraus and Friedman, 2010), the 2-year survival rate of patients with GBM is less than 30% and has not changed over the past two decades. Because of the increasing incidence of GBM and very poor prognosis, a better understanding of GBM initiation and progression is crucial for the development of more effective therapeutic approaches. GBM cells utilize the normal physiological functions of chemoattractant GPCRs to promote their growth by sensing cognate ligands produced in the microenvironment that enhance tumor cell proliferation, invasion and the production of angiogenic factors such as vascular endothelial cell growth factor (VEGF) and the chemokine CXCL8 (IL-8) (Yao et al., 2008; Ping et al., 2007). Recently, the chemoattractant GPCRs FPR1 and CXCR4 were also found to be expressed by glioma stem-like cells (GSLCs) and to mediate GSLC chemotaxis and the production of VEGF (Ping et al., 2007; Yao et al.,

2008; Ping et al., 2011), suggesting the important role of these GPCRs in glioma initiation. In this article, we will review the contribution of chemoattractant GPCRs in glioma progression and discuss the potential for GPCRs as therapeutic targets in glioma.

2. The role of the classical chemoattractant GPCR, FPR1, in the progression of GBM

2.1 Identification of FPR1 in GBM

Human FPR1 (originally named FPR) was detected in 1976 on the surface of human neutrophils, and was cloned in 1990 from a myeloid leukemia-cell line. FPR1 binds N-formyl-methionyl-leucyl-phenylalanine (fMLF), a product of the Gram negative bacteria, as well as mitochondria formylated peptide, and elicits a cascade of signal transduction events mediated by pertussis toxin-sensitive G proteins of the Gi subtype and controlled by phospholipase C (PLC) and phosphoinositide (PI) 3 kinases (Pan et al., 2000). Human myeloid cells activated by FPR1 agonist peptides undergo rapid shape change, showing increased adhesion, chemotaxis, phagocytosis and release of bactericidal and proinflammatory mediators. These functions of FPR1 enable myeloid cells to have proinflammatory and antimicrobial activities. In fact, depletion of the human FPR1 counterpart mFPR1 from mice decreased their resistance to infection by Listeria monocytogenes. Although FPR1 has been shown to be a GPCR that mediates host defense against bacterial infection by phagocytic leukocytes, we found that FPR1 was also selectively expressed by tumor cells in more highly malignant human glioma specimens (Zhou et al., 2005). These findings prompted us to use established human glioma cell lines to investigate the relationship between FPR1 expression and the biological behavior of the tumor cells. For example, the human GBM cell line U87 expresses higher levels of FPR1 and forms more rapidly growing tumors in nude mice than glioma cell lines derived from low grade gliomas, which do not express FPR1 (Zhou et al., 2005). Therefore, observations with glioma cell lines lead us to hypothesize that FPR1 is selectively expressed by more highly malignant glioma cells and may play a role in promoting tumor growth.

2.2 Function of FPR1 in GBM cells

The function of FPR1 in GBM cells was extensively examined by using the prototype chemotactic agonist peptide, bacterial fMLF as a stimulator. In addition to inducing robust chemotaxis and calcium mobilization of GBM cells by fMLF, FPR1 exhibited several unique properties that are closely related to tumor progression. For instance, activation of FPR1 in GBM cells under suboptimal culture conditions (i.e. at low fetal calf serum (FCS) concentration) supports the survival of tumor cells in association with increased intracellular levels of the anti-apoptotic protein Bcl-2. In addition, FPR1 agonist peptide activated two important transcription factors, namely NF-κB and STAT3 in GBM cells. Increased NF-κB translocation has been observed as a consequence of FPR1 signaling pathway also in phagocytic leukocytes (Huang et al., 2001); FPR1 signaling in GBM cells stimulated the phosphorylation of STAT3 at Ser-727 and Tyr-105 residues, while only Ser-727 was phosphorylated in human monocytes. Another transcription factor hypoxia inducible factor-1α (HIF-1α), which induces the adaptation to hypoxic microenvironment by regulating the gene transcription in several processes such as cell oxygen uptake, glucose metabolism, angiogenesis, cell survival and apoptosis, was also activated by FPR1 agonists in GBM cells (Zhou et al., 2005).

Since both STAT3 and HIF-1α are implicated in the transcriptional activation of the gene coding for VEGF, we investigated the effect of activating FPR1 on the production of VEGF by tumor cells. We found that supernatants from fMLF-stimulated GBM cells induced the migration and tubule formation of human vascular endothelial cells (EC) (Zhou et al., 2005). This property of the tumor cell supernatant was abolished by a neutralizing anti-human VEGF antibody (Zhou et al., 2005), suggesting VEGF was released by FPR1 agonist-stimulated GBM cells. FPR1 in GBM cells was subsequently shown to promote the release of another angiogenic factor, the chemokine CXCL8 (IL-8) (Yao et al., 2008). The contribution of FPR1 to GBM progression was then tested in vivo in nude mice. Tumor cells containing small interference (si) RNA targeting FPR1 mRNA yielded tumors in nude mice with markedly reduced rate of growth as compared to control cells transfected with random siRNA (Zhou et al., 2005). Thus, the functional studies provide strong evidence for the involvement of FPR1 in supporting the rapid progression of GBM.

Crosstalk between GPCRs and growth factor receptors plays an important role in orchestrating the interaction of intracellular signaling molecules implicated in tumor growth, angiogenesis and metastasis (Lappano and Maggiolini, 2011). The crosstalk between GPCRs and the receptor for epidermal growth factor (EGFR) has been shown to promote the progression of colon, lung, breast, ovarian, prostate, and head and neck carcinomas (Hart et al., 2005). Like many malignant tumors of human and mouse origin, human GBM cells express high levels of EGFR and stimulation with EGF increases tumor cell chemotaxis and proliferation with rapid phosphorylation of at least 4 tyrosine residues in the C-terminal domain of EGFR (Huang et al., 2007). When GBM cells were stimulated with the FPR1 agonist fMLF, EGFR was also rapidly phosphorylated but with restriction to a single tyrosine residue Tyr992. This transactivation of EGFR by FPR1 agonist peptide accounted for approximately 40% of the biological activity of FPR1 in GBM cells and was dependent on a Src kinase pathway (Huang et al., 2007). Moreover, GBM cells depleted of either FPR1 or EGFR grew more slowly as compared with parental cells and depletion of both receptors further reduced the tumorigenicity of the GBM cells (Huang et al., 2007). Thus, FPR1 aberrantly expressed in GBM cells is capable of exploiting the function of EGFR to exacerbate the malignant behavior of the tumor cells. Since interference with both receptors additionally reduced tumor growth, FPR1 and EGFR also had non-redundant functions (Huang et al., 2008).

2.3 The involvement of FPR1 in GBM cell invasion

The ability of GBM cells to invade into surrounding brain tissue is a critical pathological event in the progression of GBM. In the human GBM cell line U87, there are FPR1+ and FPR1- subpopulations which could be isolated and cloned. FPR1+ cells showed a more "motile" phenotype in vitro as compared with cells lacking FPR1 expression (Huang et al., 2010). Moreover, although both FPR1+ and FPR- GBM cells implanted subcutaneously into nude mice developed tumors, only tumors formed by FPR1+ cells invaded the surrounding connective tissues. In addition, FPR1- cells transfected with FPR1 showed enhanced mobility in vitro and the in vivo capacity to form more rapidly growing and invasive tumors in mice. Tumor invasion depends not only on tumor cell mobility, but also on the capacity of tumor cells to secrete metal matrimetalloproteases (MMPs) that degrade extracellular matrix (ECM) and facilitate the detachment of highly motive tumor cells. Stimulation of GBM cells with FPR1 agonist peptide up-regulates the expression of MMP2 and MMP9 and increases the release of pro-MMP2. As reported in the literature, regulation of MMPs is controlled by AP1 transcription factor complex through MAP kinase pathways and PKC, which are activated by FPR1 agonist in GBM cells. Thus stimulation of FPR1 activates MMPs in GBM cells and increases proteolytic processes in the tumor microenvironment (Huang et al., 2010).

2.4 Identification of endogenous FPR1 agonist released by necrotic GBM cells

Despite extensive characterization of FPR1 function in GBM cells, whether host-derived agonists are present in the tumor microenvironment remains unknown. We tested GBM cell responses to the neutrophil granule protein cathepsin G, which is an endogenous agonist for FPR1 and induces the migration of myloid cells. We determinated that cathepsin G is capable of inducing the migration of GBM cells expressing FPR1 (Sun et al., 2004). However, cathepsin G is unlikely to be present in brain unless substantial tissue damage compromises the blood brain barrier and results in the release of this FPR1 agonist into the brain by neutrophils. We therefore examined other possible sources of potential FPR1 agonists that may act on GBM cells. Since mitochondrial peptides are also potential endogenous FPR1 agonists and GBMs frequently contain necrotic foci in the rapidly growing tumor mass that may release mitochondrial components, we examined the presence of FPR1 agonists in supernatants of necrotic tumor cells. Indeed, supernatants of necrotic GBM cells and tumors formed by GBM cells in nude mice induced potent chemotaxis of live GBM cells as well as a rat basophil leukemia-cell line transfected to express human FPR1 (ETFR cells). The chemotactic activity released by necrotic GBM cells and tumor tissues was blocked by an anti-FPR1 antibody and by a FPR-specific antagonist tBoc-MLF (Zhou et al., 2005). The robust intracellular Ca2+ mobilization induced in GBM cells by necrotic GBM cell supernatant attenuated the subsequent cell response to fMLF, suggesting that agonist contained in the supernatants of necrotic tumor cells share a receptor with fMLF (Zhou et al., 2005). Further evidence to support the release of FPR1 agonists by necrotic GBM cells was provided by the observation that the tumor cell supernatant down-regulated FPR1 expressed on the surface of human monocytes and FPR1 expressing ETFR cells. These observations confirm that FPR1 expressed on GBM cells is able to recognize agonist activity released in the tumor microenvironment in a paracrine and/or autocrine loop (Zhou et al., 2005). Our recent effort to characterize the biochemical nature of the FPR1 agonist activity released by necrotic GBM cells revealed that the glucocorticoid binding protein annexin1 (AnxA1), which has been reported to be an agonist for FPR1 and its variant receptor FPR2, can promote tumor cell invasion and angiogenesis. AnxA1 accounts for the majority of the FPR1 agonist activity released by necrotic GBM cells because depletion of AnxA1 from the necrotic tumor supernatant markedly reduced its capacity to stimulate FPR1 on viable GBM cells (Yang et al., unpublished observation). We therefore established a paradigm for the role of FPR1 in GBM progression in which FPR1 in GBM cells by responding to necrotic tumor cell-released agonist such as AnxA1 transactivates EGFR and the two receptors co-operate to promote the growth, invasion, angiogenesis and progression of GBM (Fig 1A).

3. The role of the chemokine GPCR CXCR4 in glioma progression

3.1 CXCR4 and its ligand CXCL12

CXCR4 selectively binds the CXC chemokine stromal cell-derived factor 1 (SDF-1), also known as CXCL12 (Furusato et al., 2010). CXCR4 is normally expressed in a wide variety of cells and tissues. The CXCR4 agonist CXCL12 was first cloned from a murine bone marrow stromal cell line, and was produced in high quantity by marrow stromal cells. In addition to mediating cell chemotaxis in response to CXCL12, CXCR4 also acts as a co-receptor for CD4 cell entry of T tropic HIV. In mouse models, deletion of CXCL12 or CXCR4 results in embryonic death with defects in the development of cardiac and central nervous systems as well as reduction in hematopoietic stem-cell homing (Zou et al., 1998). CXCR4 is up-regulated in more than 20 different types of malignant tumors (Kryczek et al., 2007). Further studies show that CXCR4 regulates tumor progression by mediating tumor cell proliferation and metastasis as well as angiogenesis.

3.2 The effect of CXCR4 on glioma invasion and metastasis

CXCR4 expression was detected in primary human glioma specimens and the level of CXCR4 was correlated with the degree of malignancy of the tumors. In vitro, CXCR4+ malignant glioma cells secrete its ligand CXCL12, suggesting that two molecules may exert paracrine and autocrine regulation of glioma progression (Bajetto et al., 2006). Studies performed in human GBM specimens demonstrated that tumor cells infiltrating into surrounding brain tissues express higher levels of CXCR4, suggesting CXCR4 expression may define more highly invasive tumor cells. This is corroborated by in vitro experiments showing that invasive human glioma cells overexpress CXCR4 as compared with noninvasive tumor cells (Ehtesham et al., 2006). Invasive cells isolated from rat C6 glioma cell line express both CXCR4 and CXCL12 at high levels (Ehtesham et al., 2006). Moreover, application of CXCR4 antagonist or siRNA targeting CXCR4 in vivo inhibited the invasion of tumors formed by invasive C6 glioma cells.

The invasion process of GBM requires the detachment of invading cells from tumor mass, attachment of tumor cells to ECM components, ECM degradation, and subsequent cell infiltration into surrounding brain tissues. Attachment of tumor cells to ECM components is an essential phase of invasion mediated by integrins that are overexpressed on both glioma cells and tumor vasculature. Recognition of CXCL12 by CXCR4 activates tumor-associated integrins, such as α2, α4, α5, and β1 to promote tumor dissemination (Hartman et al., 2004, and 2005). Inhibition of integrin function disrupts GBM cell migration. In vitro, interference of CXCR4 with the urokinase-receptor (uPAR) reduces the adhesion of CXCL12-mediated CXCR4+ GBM cells to collagen, the main component of ECM (Montuori et al., 2010).

ECM degradation by MMPs enhances tumor invasion. In vitro, glioma cells with lower production of MMP-9 show diminished migration and invasion and such cells no longer form tumors following intracranial injection into nude mice. MMP-2 and -9 have been identified as MMPs in high grade gliomas and their level of expression directly correlates with the grade of glioma malignancy (Stojic et al., 2008). Similar to FPR1, CXCR4 mediated glioma invasion in vivo was also associated with its capacity to activate MMPs (Kryczek et al., 2007). It has been reported that CXCR4/ERK/NF-κ B signaling pathway induces the up-regulation of MMPs in glioma cells. Activation of CXCR4 by its ligand CXCL12 also promotes tumor invasion by release of MMP-9.

3.3 CXCR4 in glioma growth and angiogenesis

3.3.1 Role of CXCR4/CXCL12 in malignant glioma growth and survival

The CXCR4 ligand CXCL12 produced by tumor and stromal cells interacting with CXCR4 on tumor cells results in the activation of several downstream pathways, including MAPK/ERK1/2, PI3k and Akt, as well as NF-κB. These pathways are known to participate in the regulation of cell proliferation and survival in normal or malignant glial cells. In vitro activation of CXCR4 promotes the proliferation of GBM cell lines based on the activation of ERK1/2 and PI3K/Akt (Bian et al., 2007). In agreement with data obtained from GBM cell lines, 80% of clinical GBM samples express high levels of phosphorylated Akt (Hambardzumyan et al., 2008). CXCL12 induces the proliferation of primary GBM cells expressing CXCR4 by significantly increasing DNA synthesis in tumor cells (do Carmo et al., 2010). CXCR4-mediated tumor cell proliferation may also be amplified by EGFR signaling, since stimulation of CXCR4 has been reported to transactivate EGFR in many tumors of the epithelial lineage (Dolce et al., 2011). In fact, as discussed earlier, EGFR in GBM cells is transactivated by another chemoattractant GPCR FPR1, and the two receptors co-operate to promote the growth of GBM (Huang et al., 2007). The role of CXCR4 in promoting glioma growth was further supported by the use of a small molecule CXCR4 antagonist, AMD3100, which significantly inhibited tumor cell proliferation in vitro and tumorigenicity in nude mice (do Carmo et al., 2010; and Dolce et al., 2011).

Another important property of CXCR4 is to increase GBM cell resistance to apoptosis. Blockade of CXCR4 in glioma cells by the antagonist AMD3100 increased the rate of apoptosis, confirming the ability of CXCR4 to support tumor cell survival (do Carmo et al., 2010). This anti-apoptotic effect is associated with the activation of PI3K/Akt (do Carmo et al., 2010), an observation consistent with results obtained from a variety of tumors in which CXCR4 actively contributes to the resistance of tumor cells to apoptosis. Stimulation of CXCR4 activates NF-κB, which in turn inhibits radiation-induced TNF-α production by glioma cells and increases tumor cell survival. In addition to directly protecting tumor cells from radiation-induced apoptosis, CXCR4 indirectly promotes cell survival by increasing their adherence. For example, stimulation of CXCR4 promotes the adhesion of glioma cells to vitronectin, a glioma-derived extracellular matrix protein, and prevents tumor cell death (do Carmo et al., 2010). Taken together, published results support the conclusion that CXCR4 plays an important role in promoting the proliferation and survival of glioma cells.

3.3.2 CXCR4 promotes the production of angiogenic factors by glioma cells

The requirement of CXCR4 and CXCL12 for angiogenesis was revealed by the prenatal lethal phenotype of both CXCR4 and CXCL12 knockout mice due to defects in the vascular development of gastrointestinal tract and cardiogenesis (Tachibana et al., 1998). In vitro, activation of CXCR4 in ECs stimulates the formation of capillary-like tubules (Salvatore et al., 2010). ECs in gliomas have been shown to be genetically and functionally distinct from normal ECs, and exhibit higher expression of CXCR4 and its ligand CXCL12. Proliferating ECs in GBM are positive for CXCR4 and its ligand CXCL12, while ECs that form a single layer in the capillaries of the anaplastic astrocytoma appeared to be negative for these two molecules. The lower levels of CXCR4/CXCL12 expression in anaplastic astrocytoma may contribute to the lower density of proliferating microvasculature. Consistent with these observations, CXCR4 and CXCL12 are detected in both malignant glioma cells and vascular ECs are associated with increased cell survival (Salmaggi et al., 2004).

Interestingly, elevated CXCL12 levels by themselves in gliomas failed to induce significant vascularization. This was associated with the co-presence of low levels of VEGF, suggesting synergism of these angiogenic factors (Kryczek et al., 2005). In fact, although a major angiogenic factor in GBM, VEGF was detected only in a few cells or not at all in low-grade astrocytomas or in the normal brain tissue (Takano et al., 2010). Clinical and experimental evidence indicates that CXCR4 activation induces the production of VEGF in human glioma cells and glioma stem-like cells (Ping et al., 2007 and 2011). Therefore, CXCR4 may contribute to the production of VEGF by malignant glioma cells and the two pro-angiogenic factors synergistically promote angiogenesis in tumor. In addition to VEGF, the activation of CXCR4 in gliomas also is associated with increases the secretion of an angiogenic chemokine, CXCL8 (IL-8) (Ping et al., 2007). Interestingly, VEGF binds the receptors on ECs and leads to the up-regulation of the anti-apoptotic molecule Bcl-2 as well as the release of CXCL8 from ECs (Nör et al., 2001). CXCL8 then is capable of maintaining the angiogenic phenotype of ECs in an autocrine and paracrine manner (Nör et al., 2001; Heidemann et al., 2003). In addition, the activation of CXCR4 also results in NF-κB translocation in glioma cells, which elicits the production of other angiogenic chemokines, such as CXCL1, CXCL2, and CXCL5 (Richmond et al., 2002). Therefore, glioma angiogenesis is the result of a well-coordinated process participated in by multiple angiogenic factors among which CXCR4 appears to be an upstream initiator.

3.3.3 CXCR4/CXCL12 mediates vasculogenesis by mobilizing bone marrow derived progenitor cells

In addition to tumor angiogenesis, which is thought to be established by the sprouting of blood vessels through the division of normal differentiated host ECs present in the tissue adjacent to tumor, another way to generate tumor vessels is through the process of vasculogenesis, which is formed by the recruitment of circulating EC precursor cells or bone marrow-derived cells (BMDCs) (Garcia-Barros et al., 2003). Circulating EC progenitor cells mobilized from the bone marrow are normally present in the peripheral blood of several species and participate in the neovascularization in tumor and in ischemic tissues (Spaeth et al., 2009). CXCR4 has been demonstrated to guide prime stem cells to the sites of rapid vascular expansion during embryonic organogenesis (Napoli et al., 2010). The pivotal role of CXCR4 and its ligand CXCL12 in vasculogenesis has been demonstrated in gene deletion mice as discussed earlier.

Similar to the development of embryonic vessels, CXCR4 mediates tumor neovascularization by switching from angiogenesis in the recurrent malignant glioma to vasculogenesis. For instance, tumor growth supported mainly by angiogenesis from nearby normal vessels is abrogated by irradiation (Kioi et al., 2010). As a consequence, the growth of new tumor vasculature in irradiation animals will rely mainly on circulating blood EC progenitor cells from the bone marrow. Studies have demonstrated that CXCR4 is a key factor for the influx of BMDCs into the recurrent tumor after irradiation, since both the CXCR4 inhibitor AMD3100 and antibodies against CXCR4 are able to block the recruitment of BMDCs into tumor and prevent the restoration of the vasculature (Kioi et al., 2010). Hypoxia also mediates tumor vasculogenensis through CXCR4 in animal models. Irradiation results in a hypoxic microenvironment in the tumor resulting in the up-regulation of the transcription factor HIF-1 (Ahn and Brown, 2008) and enhanced production of CXCL12 and VEGF. CXCL12 then induces the homing of CD11b+ BMDCs into the tumor site to initiate the formation of new vasculature (Kioi et al., 2010).

4. CXCR7/CXCL12

4.1 CXCR7 expression in glioma

Although it was believed that CXCL12 uses CXCR4 as a sole receptor, recent studies have shown that CXCR7, a newly identified chemokine GPCR, acts as an alternate receptor for

CXCL12 and for another chemokine e.g. interferon-inducible T cell α chemoattractant (I-TAC; also known as CXCL11). CXCR7 is expressed in several tumors and plays an important role in preventing tumor cell apoptosis and promoting tumor cell adhesion to ECs, a key step for the development of blood-borne metastasis (Burns et al., 2006). In glioma specimens, CXCR7 is widely distributed in tumor cells, microglia and ECs. In contrast, CXCR4 seems to be restricted to certain subsets of glioma cells and tumor stem-like cell populations. While the CXCR4 level is significantly higher in GBM than in lower grade gliomas, no distribution difference was detected for CXCR7 (Hattermann et al., 2010). One study reported that in eight glioma cell lines tested, only one expresses CXCR4. However, CXCR7 is highly expressed in all glioma cell lines (Hattermann et al., 2010). Interestingly, tumor stem-like cells derived from GBM cell line express CXCR4, but not CXCR7. In addition, differentiated glioma cells often are found to express CXCR7, but not CXCR4. These observations suggest that there is a difference between the role of CXCR4 and CXCR7 in the function of glioma cells. In some tumors, CXCR7 and CXCL12 are co-localized and potentially cooperate in tumor progression (Hattermann et al., 2010).

4.2 CXCR7 may mediate glioma progression

Initially, CXCR7 was regarded as a decoy receptor that recognizes CXCL12 or a coreceptor that may form a heterodimeric complex with CXCR4 to enhance CXCL12 signaling in embryonic cells. Subsequently, CXCR7 was demonstrated to be functionally active in glioma cells. CXCR7 activation by CXCL12 stimulates a transient phosphorylation of ERK1/2 and inhibits the apoptosis of glioma cells induced by camptothecin and temozolomide, but did not increase tumor cell proliferation and migration (Hattermann et al., 2010). CXCR7 activation also did not elicit calcium mobilization in tumor cells, but increases their adhesion (Burns et al., 2006). The absence of ligand-induced calcium influx and cell migration distinguishes the CXCR7 signaling pathway from CXCR4 and other typical chemokine GPCRs. In cells transiently transfected with human CXCR7 and rat cells expressing CXCR7, the signaling of CXCR7 is not mediated by Gαi protein, but by β-arrestins associated with the phosphorylation of MAP kinases (Rajagopal et al., 2010). Based on these properties of CXCR7, it is assumed that some of the previously reported effects of CXCL12 on glioma cells, such as phosphorylation of kinases and prevention of apoptosis might be partially mediated by CXCR7. Since ECs isolated from GBM express high levels of CXCR7 mRNA, it is postulated that CXCR7 may be involved in the formation of glioma vasculature (Takano et al., 2010). Indeed, in many $CXCR7^{+}$ tumors, VEGF and CXCL8 (IL-8) are up-regulated. Therefore, CXCR7 is a novel chemokine GPCR that promotes glioma progression by supporting tumor cell survival, adhesion and possibly vessel formation.

4.3 Potential interactions between CXCR7 and CXCR4

Accumulating evidence suggests that CXCR7 and CXCR4 interact with each other in malignant tumors. In human rhabdomyosarcomas (Grymula et al., 2010), downregulation of CXCR7 expression by hypoxia was thought to increase CXCL12 signaling through CXCR4 thus rendered rhabdomyosarcoma cells more motile and prone to detach from the primary tumor. Confocal microscopy shows that in glioma cell lines, CXCR7 is mainly localized in the space between the plasma membrane and endosomal compartment, whereas CXCR4 is mostly present on the cell surface of membrane (Calatozzolo et al., 2011). The biological significance of the distinct pattern of CXCR7 and CXCR4 expression in glioma cells is not clear. However, in somatic cells, CXCR7 facilitates CXCR4-mediated migration of primordial germ cells by controlling the level of CXCL12 in the microenvironment to form a chemotactic gradient (Boldajipour et al., 2008). In HeLa cells, CXCR7 acts as a scavenger receptor for CXCL12, which results in the internalization of CXCL12 and the subsequent reduction of CXCR4 activity (Naumann et al., 2010). An alternative mechanism by which CXCR7 regulates CXCR4 activity may be its potential to form heterodimer with CXCR4. In fact, some studies have shown changes in CXCR4 signaling by heterodimerization with CXCR7. Although the precise mechanisms of interaction between CXCR7 and CXCR4 and the consequences in glioma progression remain to be determined, the available results suggest an important role for CXCR7 in regulating the activity of the more ubiquitously expressed CXCR4 in gliomas (Fig. 1B).

5. CX3CR1/CX3CL1 in glioma progression

Another chemoattractant GPCR CX3CR1 and its agonist CX3CL1 have also been reported to play a role in glioma progression. CX3CL1 is one of the most highly expressed chemokines in the brain (Bazan et al., 1997) and is a peculiar member of the chemokine family which can mediate both chemotaxis and adhesion of inflammatory cells via its highly selective receptor CX3CR1. CX3CR1 is overexpressed in gliomas at both mRNA and protein levels, regardless of tumor classification and clinical severity, while CX3CL1 expression is correlated with glioma grade and overall patient survival (Locatelli et al., 2010). CX3CL1 is more highly expressed in tumor area near sites of necrosis suggesting that necrosis may directly enhance CX3CL1 transcription in tumor cells, or indirectly via inflammatory cytokines released by necrotic cells, including TNFα, which is a potent stimulant of CX3CL1 transcription (Marchesi et al., 2010). The increased expression of CX3CL1 in higher grade gliomas implies the involvement of CX3CL1 and its receptor CX3CR1 in tumor progression. CX3CR1 and CX3CL1 contribute to glioma progression in two ways: (1) by affecting the host defense mediated by immune cells and (2) by directly promoting tumor cell proliferation.

5.1 The role of CX3CR1 in immune cell activation in the brain

In colorectal cancer patients, high expression of CX3CR1 in tumor tissue is correlated with increased density of tumor infiltrating lymphocytes, which is associated with more favorable prognosis (Dimberg et al., 2007). CX3CR1 deficient mice bearing B16 melanoma are reported to show increased lung tumor metastasis and cachexia as well as reduced recruitment of monocytes and NK cells into the tumor (Yu et al., 2007). Thus, CX3CR1 may promote the infiltration of immune cells with antitumor activity.

Glioma-infiltrating microglia/macrophages (GIMs) are the major component in the stroma of glioma tumors and these cells express CX3CR1. In vitro, activation of CX3CR1 in GIMs isolated from human glioma specimens increases these cell adhesion and migration in response to CX3CL1 (Held-Feindt et al., 2010). Blocking CX3CR1 by a specific antibody reduced the migration of GIMs in response to the conditioned medium containing CX3CL1 secreted by human GBM cell lines (Held-Feindt et al., 2010). However, GIMs in glioma stroma did not mediate antiglioma immune responses (Liu et al., 2008). In fact, GIMs are characterized by a phenotype that may potentially promote tumorigenesis, i.e., more likely functioning as type II macrophages. Also, CX3CR1 activation increases the expression of MMP2, 9 and 14 in GIMs, which may not only favor the migration and adhesion of GIMs, but also the infiltration of normal brain tissue by tumor cells (Markovic et al., 2005).

5.2 The direct effect of CX3CR1 on glioma cells

Since CX3CL1 and CX3CR1 are co-expressed by glioma cells, they are hypothesized to play a role in glioma growth in an autocrine loop. However, the interaction of CX3CR1 with

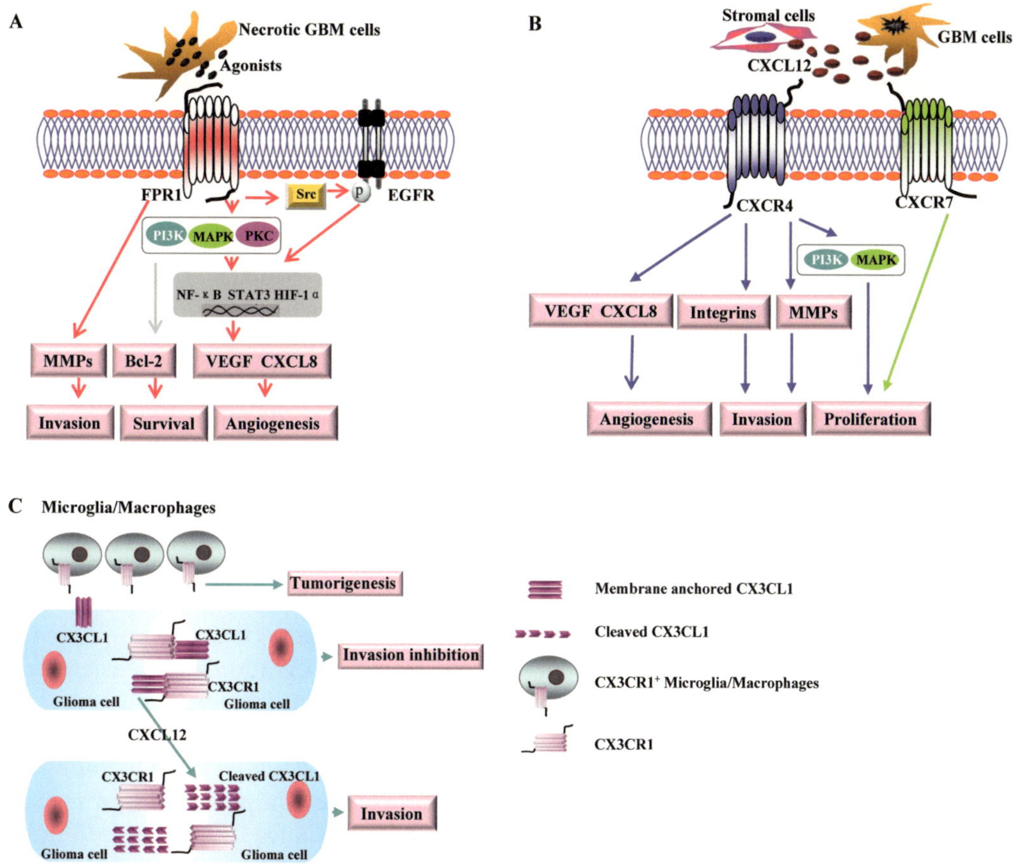

Fig. 1. The role of chemoattractant GPCRs in glioma progression. A. FPR1 and EGFR cooperate to exacerbate the progression of GBM. FPR1 in GBM cells was activated by agonists released by necrotic tumor cells to promote GBM cell survival, invasion and angiogenesis. The FPR1 function in GBM cells is mediated in part by transactivation of EGFR through a Src kinase pathway. B. Interaction of CXCR4 with CXCL12 produced by glioma cells and stromal cells promotes the proliferation, invasion and angiogenesis of tumor. The activity of CXCL12 may be partially mediated by another CXCL12 receptor CXCR7. C. CX3CL1 secreted by glioma cells increases the infiltration of microglia /macrophages expressing CX3CR1 and promotes tumor progression. Interaction of CX3CR1 with CX3CL1 produced by glioma cells increases cell-cell adhesion in tumor that inhibits the invasion of tumor cells. However tumor cells activated by CXCR4 ligand CXCL12 cleave CX3CL1 that increases the invasiveness of the individual tumor cells.

CX3CL1 has been shown to inhibit glioma cell invasion in vitro (Sciumè et al., 2010). This activity of CX3CR1 may be attributed to the peculiar structure of the agonist CX3CL1 and may account for its ability to directly promote cell-cell adhesion when expressed as a transmembrane protein therefore impeding cell motility. The effect of this CX3CR1 and CX3CL1 interaction was reduced by TGF-β1 (Sciumè et al., 2010), which is also produced by glioma cells and downregulates CX3CL1 expression. The in vivo role of CX3CR1 in glioma growth is more complex. CXCL12 constitutively expressed in the central nervous system (CNS) activates CXCR4 in glioma cells to promote the cleavage of CX3CL1 into a soluble form that reduces the intercellular adhesion and results in the dissemination of glioma cells (Cook et al., 2010). Thus, it is postulated that CX3CR1 in the CNS may favor the invasion of glioma cells into neighboring tissues. In support of this assumption, CX3CR1 and CX3CL1 have been reported to drive the neurotropic cancer cells to disseminate to peripheral nerves (Marchesi et al., 2010), a distinct but largely under appreciated route of metastasis, which has been shown in several tumors, including tumors of the brain, prostate, stomach, pancreas, bladder, and colorectum, as well as head and neck carcinoma. Thus, the balance between the transmembrane and soluble form plays an important role in the activity of CX3CL1 to either prevent or promote glioma progression (Fig. 1C).

6. Involvement of chemoattractant GPCRs in infiltration of gliomas by regulatory T cells (Tregs)

Tregs have been recognized as one of the major immune cell components that suppress host anti-tumor responses. Recruitment of Tregs into tumors contributes to tolerance by suppressing autoreactive T cells. It has been shown that Tregs infiltrate human brain tumors (Tran Tang et al., 2010) and preferentially accumulate in high grade malignant gliomas such as GBM. The importance of Tregs in the control of anti-tumor immune responses in experimental mouse glioma models is demonstrated by the observation that transient Treg depletion markedly augments the anti-tumor immunity (Tran Tang et al., 2010). Treg trafficking in vivo is facilitated by chemokine receptors. For instance, Treg accumulation in ovarian carcinoma is mediated by the chemokine receptor CCR4, which binds the ligand CCL22 produced in the tumor where specific T cell immunity is compromised (Curiel et al., 2004). Analysis of lymphocyte subsets in GBM from patients shows that tumor infiltrating Tregs highly express CCR4 (Jacobs et al., 2010) and the ligand CCL22 is produced by GBM cells. But unlike ovarian carcinoma in which Treg accumulation clearly correlates with reduced patient survival, there is no correlation between Tregs and overall survival of GBM patients. Regardless, post-surgical immunotherapy has been proposed as a potentially valid method to eliminate residual GBM cells while preserving surrounding healthy brain cells.

7. Chemoattractant GPCRs in gliomas as potential therapeutic targets

Given the broad range of functions of chemoattractant GPCRs in malignant glioma development, progression, invasion and angiogenesis, blockage of these receptors is considered a novel therapeutic approach in conjunction with conventional surgical resection, irradiation and chemotherapy. Based on the association of CXCR4 with the malignant behavior of glioma, anti-CXCR4 monoclonal antibody and specific low-molecular weight antagonist for CXCR4 have been tested for their effects on tumor cell growth in vitro and in vivo. As predicted, anti-CXCR4 monoclonal antibody is able to attenuate the migration and proliferation of human GBM cells induced by CXCL12 (Cheng et al., 2009). In addition, administration of the CXCR4 antagonist AMD3100 suppressed the growth of

xenograft tumors formed by human GBM cells transplanted intracranially into mice, with increased apoptosis of the transplanted GBM cells (Rubin et al., 2003).
Studies have also revealed the potential benefit of a combination of CXCR4 inhibitor with chemotherapy and radiotherapy in malignant glioma patients. In tests on a variety of GBM cell lines, a conventional cytotoxic chemotherapeutic agent, BCNU, in combination with the CXCR4 antagonist AMD3100 exhibits synergistic inhibition of tumor cell growth in vitro. In vivo in animal models, subtherapeutic doses of BCNU and AMD3100 also result in tumor regression, which is attributed to increased tumor cell apoptosis and decreased proliferation (Redjal et al., 2006). These effects of AMD3100 in conjunction with its capacity to reduce the recruitment of bone marrow EPCs to recurrent tumors post irradiation, suggest that targeting CXCR4 may not only directly inhibit tumor cell proliferation, but also indirectly abrogates neovascularization in GBMs (Kioi et al., 2010).
Considering targeting CXCR4 as a means of inhibiting glioma, the ability of the CXCR4 agonist CXCL12 to activate CXCR7 casts doubts about whether blockage of CXCR4 alone is sufficient without simultaneously inhibiting CXCR7. In fact, inhibition of CXCR4 only partially decreases the responsiveness of tumor cells to CXCL12 in several animal models. Studies have found that GSLCs express high levels of CXCR4 and low levels of CXCR7 (Hattermann et al., 2010). In contrast, differentiation of GSLCs markedly decreased CXCR4 expression but up-regulated CXCR7. It is therefore postulated that CXCR4 may mediate GSLC chemotaxis and survival, whereas differentiated glioma cells are protected from apoptosis by CXCR7 in response to CXCL12. It is therefore important to design strategies that target one or both CXCL12 receptors based on the stages of glioma cell differentiation.
Small molecule natural compounds constitute another source of inhibition of chemoattractant GPCRs with therapeutic potential for gliomas (Ping et al., 2007). One of such compounds is Nordy, a chiral mimetic of a natural lipoxygenase inhibitor nordihydroguaiaretic acid. Nordy has been shown to exhibit a broad inhibitory activity on chemoattractant GPCRs such as CXCR4 and FPR1 on GBM cells by downregulating receptor expression, interfering with their signal transduction pathways and reducing tumor cell production of angiogenic factors VEGF and the chemokine CXCL8 (Ping et al., 2007; Chen et al., 2006 and 2007). In addition, Nordy has been found to inhibit GBM cell proliferation and to promote tumor cell differentiation into a lesser malignant phenotype. Recently, Nordy was found to inhibit the self-renewal of glioma stem cells and growth of xenografts generated by the stem cells (Wang et al., 2011). However, the effect of Nordy may not be specific by targeting only chemoattractant GPCRs on GBM cells. Further studies are required to identify more specific receptor targeting natural compounds with minimal side effects on key physiological cell processes.

8. Conclusions

There is now mounting evidence that chemoattractant GPCRs play multiple roles in the progression of malignant gliomas, by mediating the tumor cell growth, invasion and angiogenesis (Table 1). However, further molecular epidemiologic and genetic studies are required to obtain a better understanding of the mechanisms of the function of these receptors in glioma cells. It is especially important not to single out a given receptor to study glioma biology, but rather, studies should consider the complex host environment in which many factors may drive the aberrant expression of chemoattractant GPCRs and ligands. In addition, the interaction of chemoattractant GPCRs such as CXCR4 and FPR1 with other growth factor receptors has been reported and in fact different types of the receptors cooperate to exacerbate the progression of malignant glioma. In addition to their direct effect on glioma progression, chemoattractant GPCRs expressed on immune cells also mediate host response to tumors by promoting recruitment of "suppresive" leukocytes including myeloid suppressor cells, type II macrophages and Tregs into the tumor and peripheral lymphoid organ to compromise anti-tumor defense. Therefore, recognition of the multifaceted role of chemoattractant GPCRs in gliomas and other malignant tumors in general is fundamental to elucidating the mechanisms of tumor progression and the development of novel therapeutic agents.

9. Acknowledgments

The author thanks Dr Joost J. Oppenheim of the National Cancer Institute, NIH, USA, for reviewing the manuscript. This project was supported in part by the National Basic Research Program of China (973 Program, No. 2010CB529403), the National Natural Science Foundation of China (NSFC, No. 30800421) and the Natural Science Foundation Project of CQ (CSTC, 2008BB5136). This project was also funded in part with Federal funds from the National Cancer Institute, National Institutes of Health, under Contract No. HHSN261200800001E and was supported in part by the Intramural Research Program of the NCI, NIH.

10. References

Adler, M.W., & Rogers, T.J. (2005). Are chemokines the third major system in the brain? J Leukoc Biol 78, 1204-1209.

Ahn, G.O., & Brown, J.M. (2008). Matrix metalloproteinase-9 is required for tumor vasculogenesis but not for angiogenesis: role of bone marrow-derived myelomonocytic cells. Cancer Cell 13, 193-205.

Ambrosini, E., & Aloisi, F. (2004). Chemokines and glial cells: a complex network in the central nervous system. Neurochem Res 29, 1017-1038.

Bajetto, A., Barbieri, F., Dorcaratto, A., et al. (2006). Expression of CXC chemokine receptors 1-5 and their ligands in human glioma tissues: role of CXCR4 and SDF1 in glioma cell proliferation and migration. Neurochem Int 49, 423-432.

Balkwill, F. (2004). Cancer and the chemokine network. Nat Rev Cancer, 4, 540-550.

Bar, E.E. (2011). Glioblastoma, cancer stem cells and hypoxia. Brain Pathol 21, 119-129.

Bazan, J.F., Bacon, K.B., Hardiman, G., et al. (1997). A new class of membrane-bound chemokine with a CX3C motif. Nature 385, 640-644.

Bian, X.W., Yang, S.X., Chen, J.H., et al. (2007). Preferential expression of chemokine receptor CXCR4 by highly malignant human gliomas and its association with poor patient survival. Neurosurgery 61, 570-578.

Boldajipour, B., Mahabaleshwar, H., Kardash, E., et al. (2008). Control of chemokine-guided cell migration by ligand sequestration. Cell 132, 463-473.

Brat, D.J., Bellail, A.C., & Van Meir, E.G. (2005). The role of interleukin-8 and its receptors in gliomagenesis and tumoral angiogenesis. Neuro Oncol 7, 122-133.

Burns, J.M., Summers, B.C., Wang, Y., et al. (2006). A novel chemokine receptor for SDF-1 and I-TAC involved in cell survival, cell adhesion, and tumor development. J Exp Med 203, 2201-2213.

Calatozzolo, C., Canazza, A., Pollo, B., et al. (2011). Expression of the new CXCL12 receptor, CXCR7, in gliomas. Cancer Biol Ther 11, 242-253.

Chen, J.H., Bian, X.W., Yao, X.H., et al. (2006). Nordy, a synthetic lipoxygenase inhibitor, inhibits the expression of formylpeptide receptor and induces differentiation of malignant glioma cells. Biochem Biophys Res Commun 342, 1368-1374.

Chen, J.H., Yao, X.H., Gong, W., et al. (2007). A novel lipoxygenase inhibitor Nordy attenuates malignant human glioma cell responses to chemotactic and growth stimulating factors. J Neurooncol 84, 223-231.

Cheng, Z., Zhou, S., Wang, X., et al. (2009). Characterization and application of two novel monoclonal antibodies against human CXCR4: cell proliferation and migration regulation for glioma cell line in vitro by CXCR4/SDF-1alpha signal. Hybridoma (Larchmt) 28, 33-41.

Cook, A., Hippensteel, R., Shimizu, S., et al. (2010). Interactions between chemokines: regulation of fractalkine/CX3CL1 homeostasis by SDF/CXCL12 in cortical neurons. J Biol Chem 285, 10563-10571.

Curiel, T.J., Coukos, G., Zou, L., et al. (2004). Specific recruitment of regulatory T cells in ovarian carcinoma fosters immune privilege and predicts reduced survival. Nat Med 10, 942-949.

Dimberg, J., Dienus, O., Löfgren, S., et al. (2007). Polymorphisms of Fractalkine receptor CX3CR1 and plasma levels of its ligand CX3CL1 in colorectal cancer patients. Int J Colorectal Dis 22, 1195-1200.

do Carmo, A., Patricio, I., Cruz, M.T., et al. (2010). CXCL12/CXCR4 promotes motility and proliferation of glioma cells. Cancer Biol Ther 9, 56-65.

Dolce, V., Cappello, A.R., Lappano, R., & Maggiolini, M. (2011). Glycerophospholipid synthesis as a novel drug target against cancer. Curr Mol Pharmacol Jan 11 [Epub ahead of print].

Ehtesham, M., Winston, J.A., Kabos, P., & Thompson, R.C. (2006). CXCR4 expression mediates glioma cell invasiveness. Oncogene 25, 2801-2806.

Furusato, B., Mohamed, A., Uhlén, M., & Rhim, J.S. (2010). CXCR4 and cancer. Pathol Int 60, 497-505.

Garcia-Barros, M., Paris, F., Cordon-Cardo, C., et al. (2003). Tumor response to radiotherapy regulated by endothelial cell apoptosis. Science 300, 1155-1159.

Grymula, K., Tarnowski, M., Wysoczynski, M., et al. (2010). Overlapping and distinct role of CXCR7-SDF-1/ITAC and CXCR4-SDF-1 axes in regulating metastatic behavior of human rhabdomyosarcomas. Int J Cancer 127, 2554-2568.

Hambardzumyan, D., Squatrito, M., Carbajal, E., & Holland, E.C. (2008). Glioma formation, cancer stem cells and akt signaling. Stem Cell Rev 4, 203-210.

Hart, S., Fischer, O.M., Prenzel, N., et al. (2005). GPCR-induced migration of breast carcinoma cells depends on both EGFR signal transactivation and EGFR-independent pathways. Biol Chem 386, 845-855.

Hartmann, T.N., Burger, M., & Burger, J.A. (2004). The role of adhesion molecules and chemokine receptor CXCR4 (CD184) in small cell lung cancer. J Biol Regul Homeost Agents 18, 126-130.

Hartmann, T.N., Burger, J.A., Glodek, A., Fujii, N., & Burger, M. (2005). CXCR4 chemokine receptor and integrin signaling co-operate in mediating adhesion and chemoresistance in small cell lung cancer (SCLC) cells. Oncogene 24, 4462-4471.

Hattermann, K., Held-Feindt, J., Lucius, R., et al. (2010). The chemokine receptor CXCR7 is highly expressed in human glioma cells and mediates antiapoptotic effects. Cancer Res 70, 3299-3308.

Heidemann, J., Ogawa, H., Dwinell, M.B., et al. (2003). Angiogenic effects of interleukin 8 (CXCL8) in human intestinal microvascular endothelial cells are mediated by CXCR2. J Biol Chem 278, 8508-8515.
Held-Feindt, J., Hattermann, K., Müerköster, S.S., et al. (2010). CX3CR1 promotes recruitment of human glioma-infiltrating microglia/macrophages (GIMs). Exp Cell Res 316, 1553-1566.
Huang, J., Hu, J., Bian, X., et al. (2007). Transactivation of the epidermal growth factor receptor by formylpeptide receptor exacerbates the malignant behavior of human glioblastoma cells. Cancer Res 67, 5906-5913.
Huang, J., Chen, K., Gong, W., et al. (2008). Receptor "hijacking" by malignant glioma cells: a tactic for tumor progression. Cancer Lett 267, 254-261.
Huang, J., Chen, K., Gong, W., et al. (2008). G-protein coupled chemoattractant receptors and cancer. Front Biosci 13, 3352-3363.
Huang, J., Chen, K., Chen, J., et al. (2010). The G-protein-coupled formylpeptide receptor FPR confers a more invasive phenotype on human glioblastoma cells. Br J Cancer 102, 1052-1060.
Huang, S., Chen, L.Y., Zuraw, B.L., et al. (2001). Chemoattractant-stimulated NF-kappaB activation is dependent on the low molecular weight GTPase RhoA. J Biol Chem 276, 40977-40981.
Jacobs, J.F., Idema, A.J., Bol, K.F., et al. (2010). Prognostic significance and mechanism of Treg infiltration in human brain tumors. J Neuroimmunol 225, 195-199.
Jahraus, C.D., & Friedman, A.H. (2010). Chemopotentiation by ultrafractionated radiotherapy in glioblastoma resistant to conventional therapy. Tumori 96, 771-775.
Kioi, M., Vogel, H., Schultz, G., et al. (2010). Inhibition of vasculogenesis, but not angiogenesis, prevents the recurrence of glioblastoma after irradiation in mice. J Clin Invest 120, 694-705.
Kouno, J., Nagai, H., Nagahata, T., et al. (2004). Up-regulation of CC chemokine, CCL3L1, and receptors, CCR3, CCR5 in human glioblastoma that promotes cell growth. J Neurooncol 70, 301-307.
Kryczek, I., Wei, S., Keller, E., Liu, R., & Zou, W. (2007). Stroma-derived factor (SDF-1/CXCL12) and human tumor pathogenesis. Am J Physiol Cell Physiol 292, C987-C995.
Kryczek, I., Lange, A., Mottram, P., et al. (2005). CXCL12 and vascular endothelial growth factor synergistically induce neoangiogenesis in human ovarian cancers. Cancer Re 65, 465-472.
Lappano, R., & Maggiolini, M. (2011). G protein-coupled receptors: novel targets for drug discovery in cancer. Nat Rev Drug Discov 10, 47-60.
Le, Y., Murphy, P.M., & Wang, J.M. (2002). Formyl-peptide receptors revisited. Trends Immunol 23, 541-548.
Le, Y., Zhou, Y., Iribarren, P., & Wang, J. (2004). Chemokines and chemokine receptors: their manifold roles in homeostasis and disease. Cell Mol Immunol 2, 95-104.
Liang, Y., Bollen, A.W., & Gupta, N. (2008). CC chemokine receptor-2A is frequently overexpressed in glioblastoma. J Neurooncol 86, 153-163.
Liu, C., Luo, D., Streit, W.J., & Harrison, J.K. (2008). CX3CL1 and CX3CR1 in the GL261 murine model of glioma: CX3CR1 deficiency does not impact tumor growth or infiltration of microglia and lymphocytes. J Neuroimmunol 198, 98-105.
Liu, C., Luo, D., Reynolds, B.A., et al. (2010). Chemokine receptor CXCR3 promotes growth of glioma. Carcinogenesis 32, 129-137.

Locatelli, M., Boiocchi, L., Ferrero, S., et al. (2010). Human glioma tumors express high levels of the chemokine receptor CX3CR1. Eur Cytokine Netw 21, 27-33.

Marchesi, F., Locatelli, M., Solinas, G., et al. (2010). Role of CX3CR1/CX3CL1 axis in primary and secondary involvement of the nervous system by cancer. J Neuroimmunol 224, 39-44.

Marchesi, F., Piemonti, L., Mantovani, A., & Allavena, P. (2010). Molecular mechanisms of perineural invasion, a forgotten pathway of dissemination and metastasis. Cytokine Growth Factor Rev 21, 77–82.

Markovic, D.S., Glass, R., Synowitz, M., Rooijen, N., & Kettenmann, H. (2005). Microglia stimulate the invasiveness of glioma cells by increasing the activity of metalloprotease-2. J Neuropathol Exp Neurol 64, 754-762.

Maru, S.V., Holloway, K.A., Flynn, G., et al. (2008). Chemokine production and chemokine receptor expression by human glioma cells: role of CXCL10 in tumour cell proliferation. J Neuroimmunol 199, 35-45.

Montuori, N., Bifulco, K., Carriero, M.V., et al. (2010). The cross-talk between the urokinase receptor and fMLP receptors regulates the activity of the CXCR4 chemokine receptor. Cell Mol Life Sci DOI 10.1007/s00018-010-0564-7.

Napoli, C., Hayashi, T., Cacciatore, F., et al. (2010). Endothelial progenitor cells as therapeutic agents in the microcirculation: An update. Atherosclerosis doi:10.1016/j.atherosclerosis.2010.10.039.

Naumann, U., Cameroni, E., Pruenster, M., et al. (2010). CXCR7 functions as a scavenger for CXCL12 and CXCL11. PLoS One 5, e9175.

Nör, J.E., Christensen, J., Liu, J., et al. (2001) Up-Regulation of Bcl-2 in microvascular endothelial cells enhances intratumoral angiogenesis and accelerates tumor growth. Cancer Res 61, 2183-2188.

Pan, Z.K., Chen, L.Y., Cochrane, C.G., & Zuraw, B.L. (2000). fMet-Leu-Phe stimulates proinflammatory cytokine gene expression in human peripheral blood monocytes: the role of phosphatidylinositol 3-kinase. J Immunol 164, 404-411.

Ping, Y.F., Yao, X.H., Chen, J.H., et al. (2007). The anti-cancer compound Nordy inhibits CXCR4-mediated production of IL-8 and VEGF by malignant human glioma cells. J Neurooncol 84, 21-29.

Ping, Y.F., Yao, X.H., Bian, X.W., et al. (2007). Activation of CXCR4 in human glioma stem cells promotes tumor angiogenesis. Zhonghua Bing Li Xue Za Zhi 36, 179-183. in Chinese.

Ping, Y.F., Jiang, J.Y., Zhao, L.T., et al. (2011). The chemokine CXCL12 and its receptor CXCR4 promote glioma stem cell-mediated VEGF production and tumor angiogenesis via PI3K/AKT signaling. J Pathol DOI: 10. 1002/path.2908.

Rajagopal, S., Kim, J., Ahn, S., et al. (2010). Beta-arrestin-but not G protein-mediated signaling by the "decoy" receptor CXCR7. Proc Natl Acad Sci USA 107, 628-632.

Ransohoff, R.M., Liu, L., & Cardona, A.E. (2007). Chemokines and chemokine receptors: multipurpose players in neuroinflammation. Int Rev Neurobiol 82, 187-204.

Raychaudhuri, B., & Vogelbaum, M.A. (2011). IL-8 is a mediator of NF-κB induced invasion by gliomas. J Neurooncol 101, 227-235.

Redjal, N., Chan, J.A., Segal, R.A., & Kung, A.L. (2006). CXCR4 inhibition synergizes with cytotoxic chemotherapy in gliomas. Clin Cancer Res 12, 6765-6771.

Richmond, A. (2002). NF-kappa B, chemokine gene transcription and tumour growth. Nat Rev Immunol 2, 664-674.

Rubin, J.B., Kung, A.L., Klein, R.S., et al. (2003). A small-molecule antagonist of CXCR4 inhibits intracranial growth of primary brain tumors. Proc Natl Acad Sci USA 100, 13513-13518.

Salmaggi, A., Gelati, M., Pollo, B., et al. (2004). CXCL12 in malignant glial tumors: a possible role in angiogenesis and cross-talk between endothelial and tumoral cells. J Neurooncol 67, 305-317.

Salvatore, P., Pagliarulo, C., Colicchio, R., & Napoli, C. (2010). CXCR4-CXCL12-dependent inflammatory network and endothelial progenitors. Curr Med Chem 17, 3019-3029.

Sciumè, G., Soriani, A., Piccoli, M., et al. (2010) CX3CR1/CX3CL1 axis negatively controls glioma cell invasion and is modulated by transforming growth factor-beta1. Neuro Oncol 12, 701-710.

Spaeth, E.L., Dembinski, J.L., Sasser, A.K., et al. (2009). Mesenchymal stem cell transition to tumor-associated fibroblasts contributes to fibrovascular network expansion and tumor progression. PLoS One 4, e4992.

Stojic, J., Hagemann, C., Haas, S., et al. (2008). Expression of matrix metalloproteinases MMP-1, MMP-11 and MMP-19 is correlated with the WHO-grading of human malignant gliomas. Neurosci Res 60, 40-49.

Sun, R., Iribarren, P., Zhang, N., et al. (2004). Identification of neutrophil granule protein cathepsin G as a novel chemotactic agonist for the G protein-coupled formyl peptide receptor. J Immunol 173, 428-436.

Tachibana, K., Hirota, S., Iizasa, H., et al. (1998). The chemokine receptor CXCR4 is essential for vascularization of the gastrointestinal tract. Nature 393, 591-594.

Takano, S., Yamashita, T., & Ohneda, O. (2010). Molecular therapeutic targets for glioma angiogenesis. J Oncol 2010, 351908.

Tran Thang, N.N., Derouazi, M., Philippin, G., et al. (2010). Immune infiltration of spontaneous mouse astrocytomas is dominated by immunosuppressive cells from early stages of tumor development. Cancer Res 70, 4829-4839.

Virchow, R. (1855). Editorial. Virchows Arch Pathol Anat Physiol Klin Med. 3, 23.

Wang, B., Yu, SC., Jiang, J.Y., et al. (2011). A novel inhibitor of arachidonate 5-lipoxygenase, Nordy, induces differentiation and inhibits self-renewal of glioma stem-like cells. Stem Cell Rev 7, 458-470.

Yao. X.H., Ping, Y.F., Chen, J.H., et al. (2008). Production of angiogenic factors by human glioblastoma cells following activation of the G-protein coupled formylpeptide receptor FPR. J Neurooncol, 86, 47-53.

Yao, X.H., Ping, Y.F., Chen, J.H., et al. (2008). Glioblastoma stem cells produce vascular endothelial growth factor by activation of a G-protein coupled formylpeptide receptor FPR. J Pathol 215, 369-376.

Yu, Y.R., Fong, A.M., Combadiere, C., et al. (2007). Defective antitumor responses in CX3CR1-deficient mice. Int J Cancer 121, 316-322.

Zhou, Y., Bian, X., Le, Y., et al. (2005). Formylpeptide receptor FPR and the rapid growth of malignant human gliomas. J Natl Cancer Inst 97, 823-835.

Zou, Y.R., Kottmann, A.H., Kuroda, M., Taniuchi, I., & Littman, D.R. (1998). Function of the chemokine receptor CXCR4 in haematopoiesis and in cerebellar development. Nature 393, 595-599.

Part 4

Glioma Immunology

14

Immune Connection in Glioma: Fiction, Fact and Option

Anirban Ghosh
Immunobiology Lab, Department of Zoology
Panihati Mahavidyalaya (West Bengal State University), West Bengal, India

1. Introduction

After the hypothesis of 'immune surveillance' in tumor proposed in 1970, several investigations showed the evidences of its existence where immune system is able to recognize the defects due to tumor onset (MacFarlan Burnet, 1970). But how far this surveillance is effective in the compartmentalized brain in case of glioma still remains a big uncertainty. Glioma is one of the deadliest types of cancer for its rapid growth, invasiveness and short life expectancy of the victim. So, figuring out of the extent of host immune efficiency in glioma is crucial. As glioma is able to create a hostile environment for the immune cells by releasing different soluble factors, expressing death receptors and by receptor camouflaging etc, the working situation for the host immunity becomes more difficult. Therefore, proper assessment of the role of brain immune connection in glioma is crucial to explore the probable level of support that can be extended by the immune defense mechanism against glioma. This immune resistance is also vital to support the present therapeutic modalities including adjuvants used for treating glioma.

2. Death of 'Privilege' myth: Immunocytes do not spare brain from their vigilance

2.1 'Immune privilege' of brain: A notion that prevailed more than 5 decades

At the beginning of 20th Century, brain was thought to be a separate organ mostly abandoned by the immune system. The initial evidences of immune compromise of the brain compartment were observed from 1920s with the tumor tissue transplantation studies. Rat sarcoma, when transplanted in mouse brain parenchyma, was found to grow better in comparison to its subcutaneous and intramuscular (systemic) transplantations (Shirai, 1921). On contrary, when portions of recipient spleen were co-transferred with tumor in brain parenchyma, inhibition in tumor growth occurred (Murphy and Sturm, 1923). Thus a weak or less efficient immune intervention in brain was conceptualized and the term 'immune privilege' was proposed by Billingham and Boswell (Billingham & Boswell, 1953).

With this, another set of observations in late 19th century and afterwards developed a concept of existence of a barrier between blood and CNS tissue. Basically, Paul Ehrlich's observation with the intravenous administration of vital dye in experimental animals showed infiltration of the dye in other organs except brain. That led him to propose a barrier between brain and blood stream (Ehrlich, 1885 & 1904). Goldmann's study showed that tracers injected in blood do not enter into the parenchyma proper in brain, but accumulated in the choroid plexus, perivascular space or lymphatic clefts (Obersteiner, 1870; Goldmann, 1913). The 'no entry' status of blood immunocytes was further fueled with the xeno- and allogenic tissue transplantation studies (Medawar, 1948; Barker & Billingham, 1977). In the following decades ultrastructural studies of the blood capillaries in brain showed the distinct cellular organization present in the interphase of blood and brain that prevent the flow of blood immunocytes and large molecular weight solvents into brain (Reese & Karnovsky, 1967; Engelhardt & Wolburg, 2002). Thus blood-brain-barrier (BBB) encapsulates the brain and seems to maintain the 'immune privilege' status. Till 1980s no direct lymphatic drainage from nervous system was detected. Negligible expression of MHC and undetected dendritic cells (DC) in brain indicated the inefficiency of antigen presentation in the organ (Sedgwick, 1995; Perry, 1998).

2.2 Detection of secret routes connecting brain with systemic circulation

But in last two decades a paradigm shift has occurred in this 'immune privilege' rank of brain. Basically, three obstacles that maintain the privilege are - i) lack of drainage of CNS antigens at least to cervical lymph node, ii) hindrance to easy access of T cells in the CNS parenchyma and iii) T cells require antigen presentation in the reaction site by the APCs which were thought to be scarce in brain. Initial experiments suggested that CNS antigens can drip outside passively by a different route along the olfactory nerves on to the cribriform plate which is connected to the lymphatics of nasal submucosa and finally to the cervical lymph node (Cserr & Knopf, 1992; Sedgwick, 1995). Tracer studies indicated CSF drainage to cervical lymph node (Boulton *et al*, 1999). CSF circulates from ventricles through subarachnoid spaces (a space between arachnoid and pial membrane filled with CSF and surround the brain and spinal cord) and it has access to Virchow-Robin space that surrounds blood vessels when they enter brain parenchyma [Figure - 1]. Ependymal lining of the ventricles lack 'tight junctions' and in other specialized perivascular spaces including Virchow-Robin's that porosity is also present, which help in clearance of interstitial fluid from brain parenchyma (Ransohoff *et al*, 2003; Piccio *et al*, 2002). So the protein antigens have the probable, though slightly difficult than other organs, access to the lymphoid tissue through CSF. This generates opportunity for the passage of immunocytes.

The afferent arm of CNS immune response is initiated with the antigen leakage from brain parenchyma to CSF; whereas the efferent arm is largely progressed with the migration of leukocytes to CNS into different routes. Ransohoff and colleagues identified three distinct routes which are - i) cells from blood extravasate through choroid plexus to the CSF, ii) leukocytes flowing through internal carotid artery cross the post capillary venules in the subarachnoid space and Virchow-Robin perivascular space and iii) finally leukocytes may cross the BBB deep into the brain to enter directly into the brain parenchyma (Ransohoff *et al*, 2003). Precisely speaking, BBB is a metaphor that describes the property of brain vasculatures restricting the entry of large molecules and cells (Bechmann *et al*, 2007). The perivascular spaces exist in the pre- and post-capillary segments in brain where a heterogeneous assembly of lymphocytic and monocytic cells are observed, more during inflammation. Both in the perivascular spaces and after entering into parenchyma they encounter antigen presenting cells (APCs) to continue the immune response in brain.

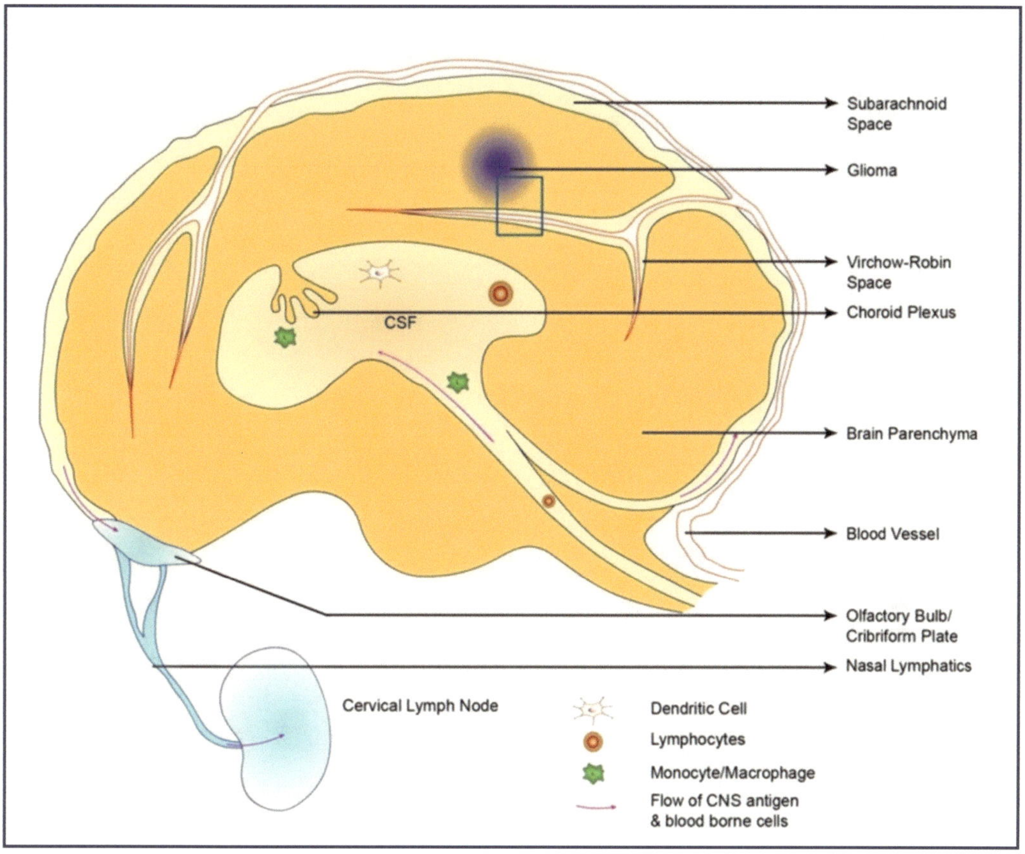

Fig. 1. This figure represents routes of CNS antigen escape and immune cell connection from brain to peripheral circulation. T cells initially are primed by the CNS antigen leaked from brain to the cervical lymph node or olfactory bulb or nasal mucosa, become activated and reach to the blood vessel, subarachnoid area, Virchow-Robin space or perivascular space and CSF in brain. There also a repriming of the glioma antigen specific lymphocytes occurs by the APC circulating or residing at those spaces. Choroid plexus is also a very important route of this CNS antigen escape and site of antigen presentation to lymphocytes by the local APCs. These specific glioma antigen primed activated lymphocytes enter into the brain parenchyma and invade towards glioma. [The box has been elaborated in Figure - 4]

2.3 Lymphocytes assess CNS antigen and enter into neuropil

2.3.1 T cells can pass into neuropil and interact with brain APCs

Early experiments showed that though graft rejection is comparatively slow in brain, once the graft is familiar to the immune system outside brain, the rejection occurs rapidly (Mason *et al*, 1986; Sedgwick, 1995). Simultaneously, Wekerle and colleagues demonstrated that activated or antigen primed T cell from the periphery can cross the BBB nonspecifically (Wekerle *et al*, 1986). Following experiments supported the fact when it was found that CD4+ T cell blasts of any specificity injected intravenous to experimental animals can pass into CNS tissue, although myelin antigen specific T cells are found to remain longer (Hickey *et al*, 1991). This delay of the myelin antigen specific T cells suggests some mechanism that holds them to process and react in brain parenchyma. The answer is the cross-talk between them and microglia (or brain APC). Microglia is found *ex-vivo* to induce IFN-γ and TNF production from CD4 T cells as their effector activation, but do not support proliferation by IL-2 and induce apoptosis. Interestingly, perivascular macrophages show activation with IL-2 mediated proliferation and survival of CD4+ T cells (Ford *et al*, 1996).

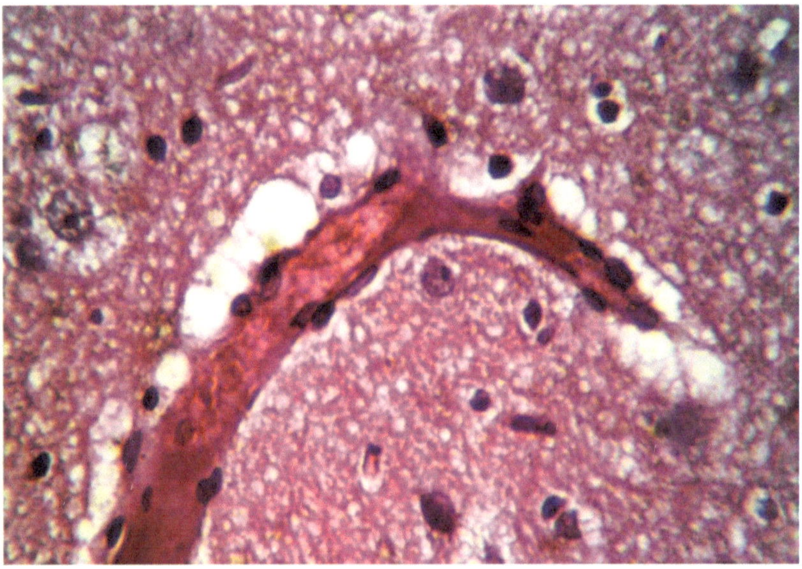

Fig. 2. This section of brain parenchyma shows a blood capillary containing leukocytes. Many of them are at the margin of the capillary, tethering the endothelium and extravaseting at the perivascular spaces. Perivascular microglia/macrophage are visible. Few infiltrated leukocytes are found scattered in brain parenchyma. At least one rod shaped ramified microglia is detectable in the parenchyma. A simple H/E staining section of brain furnishes these visual evidences of neuro-immune connection. (Magnification 1000X, oil immersion in Olympus CH20*i* Microscope and photographed by Olympus DSC)

The reverse is also visible in the GvHD affected CNS model where $CD4^+\alpha\beta TCR^+CD2^+$T cells infiltrat and scatter deep into neuropil or brain parenchyma. The microglial cells show activation with many fold increase in their CD11b/c, CD45 and MHC class II expression and cluster with intimate association with these T cells *in situ* that lead to microglial activation, proliferation and expansion (Sedgwick *et al*, 1998). Thus both microglia and infiltrated lymphocytes influence each other for their maturation and effector function in brain.

With the citations of entry of lymphocytes in brain, the role of CNS APCs started to come into surface. They are subdivided as microglia and perivascular macrophages based on their position, morphology, immunophenotype and functional priority (Sedgwick *et al*, 1991; Bechmann *et al*, 2001). Therefore entry of lymphocytes into neuropil through pre- and post-capillary vessels needs a two step process. Crossing the vessel endothelium, muscle layers and basement membranes lymphocytes and blood borne monocytes reside at the perivascular space encapsulated with glial limitans and pericytes. Next step is more restricted where the leukocytes cross the layer of glial limitans and step in to neuropil (Bechmann *et al*, 2007). To proceed for this step, brain APC associated with this limiting layer is crucial (Tran *et al*, 1998; Greter *et al*, 2005) [Figure - 2]. Then the infiltrated lymphocytes may come across the APC present in the brain parenchyma or at the site of pathogenesis. The T cell-microglia interactions in CNS autoimmune encephalomyelitis (EAE) or brain tumor; T cell secretion of Th1 cytokines to mature microglia as functional APC and resulting restimulation of leukocytes by them; counter regulation of this inflammation by Th2 induction by microglia etc had been detailed mostly on the functional studies committed so far (Aloisi *et al*, 2000; Ghosh & Chaudhuri, 2010).

2.3.2 Cell tracking experiments visualize leukocyte access in brain

But a new generation of cell tracking experiments and lebelling methods now provide us more direct evidences of the events occurring beneath the skull. GFP-labelled unspecifically activated CD4 T lymphocytes when injected into cortex and ventricle of mice brain, there path through the cross-section of entire head-neck region was monitored. Irrespective of the sites, it was visualized that they pass through the cribroid plate, reach to nasal mucosa and accumulate in the cervical lymph node (Goldmann *et al*, 2006). Shifting the focus on CD8+ T cells, it was recently found that selective traffic of antigen specific CD8 T cells occurs in brain. Using immunofluroscence and confocal micrographs it was found that the process is dependent on luminal expression of MHC class I by cerebral endothelium in response to intracerebral antigen injection. Significantly, the process is quite independent of perivascular macrophages and different from CD4+ T cell entry (Galea *et al*, 2007). After visualizing the entry and exit of T cells from brain their activities in the brain needs a close watching.

3. But glioma makes the immune system puzzled

Despite the efforts of host immune system, which Burnet and Thomas described as 'immune surveillance', malignant glioma can evade and overcome this defense to grow. There are several generalized strategies for the tumor cells to bypass the immune resistance. They can be simply categorized as follows -

a. Making the immune system ignorant about the tumor growth by lacking the tumor antigens in lymphoid organs, growing in immune privileged position, creating physical barriers by stoma, lacking adhesion molecules for cellular interactions etc.
b. Actively impairing and suppressing the immune system by down-regulating the expression of MHC genes or imposing defects in antigen processing, secreting suppressive cytokines like TGF-β, IL-10 etc and other factors like prostaglandins.
c. Inducing tolerance to immune system by minimizing costimulation that results into anergy and central tolerance to the tumor antigen as many of them produce self-antigens or mimic them. Regulatory T cell mediated inhibition of DC maturation and T cell activation in the tumor environment plays a crucial role for dampening the immune resistance.
d. Counter attacking the immune system by expressing different death receptor ligands like CD95L, decoy receptors, TRAIL family etc and expressing anti-apoptotic molecules for themselves.

Glioma adapt most of these mechanisms successfully with their additional advantage to grow in a position which has been visited or monitored by the peripheral immune cells less frequently and less aggressively.

3.1 Glioma drastically reduces immune efficiency

Different studies on a number of patients harboring glioma revealed that they suffered from impaired cell mediated immunity (Elliott *et al*, 1984). *In vitro* studies showed that peripheral blood lymphocytes (PBL) obtained from patients with gliomas proliferated poorly in response to mitogen and/or antigen stimulation *in vitro* and unresponsiveness to T-cell mitogens concanavalin A (ConA), phytohemagglutinin (PHA) and anti-CD3 mAb etc (McVicar *et al*, 1992). A number of potential mechanisms explaining the observed immune-suppression including qualitative or quantitative alterations in cell surface marker expression on T-cells, elevated suppressor cell activity or T-cell lymphopenia were explored. T-cells obtained from glioma patients have intrinsic defects, which synthesize and secrete less than normal levels of interleuken-2 (IL-2) required for T-cell proliferation. IL-2 mRNA synthesis is impaired with less production of IL-2 receptor (IL-2R), and they also are unable to enter G1 phase of cell cycle (Elliott *et al*, 1990). Additionally, the numbers of $CD4^+$ T-cells obtained from patients are reduced to a great extent than $CD8^+$ T-cells, which predominately infiltrate glioma, but are deprived from $CD4^+$ help. Based on their inability to produce and respond to IL-2 and lack of $CD4^+$ help, T-cells obtained from glioma patients appear to be anergic (Elliott *et al*, 1990; Giometto *et al*, 1996).
Wide level of T-cell signaling defects are observed in glioma patient derived T-cells. T-cells from glioma patients show reduced tyrosine phosphorylation compared to normal T cells, which is mostly reduced in PLCγ1. Additionally, both PLCγ1 and $p56^{lck}$ protein levels are found reduced dramatically and thus it causes the overall impairment of TCR/CD3-mediated signaling. Reduced $p56^{lck}$ and associated signals also resists the cells to make sufficient contact with APCs, reduced their appropriate stimuli and movements (Marford *et al*, 1997, Dix *et al*, 1999). Severe T-cells lymphopenia i.e. rapid depletion of the cells is an important feature of glioma patients. As $CD4^+$ T-cells are reduced in number and less responsive to mitogens and antigens, IL-2 and IFNγ production decreases further. Because both these cytokines are important for generation of LAK cells and CTL activity, they are responsible for impaired generation of antigen-stimulated, MHC-unrestricted cytotoxicity observed in glioma patients (Urbani *et al*, 1996; Dix *et al*, 1999). Even glioma condition facilitates to increase Th2 type IL-10 production and inhibit Th1 type IL-12 and TIL secrete predominantly Th2 type cytokines underscoring the Th1 effect. Glioma has been shown to synthesize and secrete multiple factors including TGFβ, PGE_2, IL-10 and gangliosides (Zou *et al*, 1999, Huettner *et al*, 1997). Gliomas synthesize and secrete $TGF\beta_{1,\ 2,\ \text{and}\ 3}$ which down-regulate monocyte surface marker expression, cytokine secretion, cytotoxicity and T-cell responsiveness. Gangliosides (GANGs) are components of human plasma with G_{M3} and G_{D3} being major constituents, and can bind to both plasma proteins and lipoproteins. The highest concentrations of GANGs are found in brain and mainly include G_{M1}, G_{D1a}, G_{D1b} and G_{T1b}. These are highly immunosuppressive by inhibiting T-cell proliferation, CD4 expression, generation of CTL and NK cell activity. In addition, GANGs may also suppress Ca^{2+} flux in T-cells (Ladisch *et al*, 1992; Zou *et al*, 1999; Dix *et al*, 1999).

3.2 The mechanism behind glioma immune evasion

Like any other tumors immune selective pressure on the glioma cells is also working to eradicate abnormal cells. Though the initial intensity is less and additional time is required to recognize and react, the precision is much higher against the neoplastic cells in brain (which will be discussed in the following sections). The genetic instability of glioma and their repeated exposure to immune selection act as the key to develop glioma cell variants with enhanced capacity to evade immune defense.

Glioma cells are capable to secret copious factors that influence the immune system negatively. Cyclooxygenase enzyme COX-2 derived prostaglandin E2 (PGE2) bind with its receptor EPI-4 on glioma cells and encourage them to invade by increasing motility. PGE2 downregulate Th1 cytokines like IL-2, IFNγ and TNFα, and upregulate Th2 cytokines like IL-4, IL-10 and IL-6 (Wang & Dubois, 2006). Glioma cells secrete IL-10 which inhibit IL-2 induced T cell proliferation, DC and macrophage activation (Grutz, 2005). IL-10 is expressed by Treg cells present in glioma vicinity (Sakaguchi, 2005). TGFβ with its three isoform (TGFβ1,2,3) is involved in regulating inflammation, angiogenesis and proliferation (Govinden and Bhoola, 2003). TGFβ is the dominant isoform expressed by glioblastoma. They inhibit maturation of professional APCs, obstruct the synthesis of cytotoxic molecules including perforin, granzymes, FasL in activated CTL (Thomas and Massague, 2005). This cytokine may also efficiently recruit T reg cells in glioma. Glioma shows a considerable level of resistance against Fas induced apoptosis. Decoy receptor 3 (DcR3) is expressed in brain tumor and prevents Fas mediated apoptosis as well as decreases infiltration of CD4 and CD8 T cells (Roth *et al*, 2001). Apoptosis inhibitory proteins (IAPs) are active in glioma which inhibit caspase activity (Gomez & Kruse, 2006). Some of the glioma cells express FasL to counteract with the immunocytes (Husain *et al*, 1998).

As cell to cell contact plays an important role to deliver the immune assault, glioma cells take the strategy to minimize or impair these adhesions. Cell adhesion interaction between glioma and immune cells was found to be prevented by a thick glycosaminoglycan coating and protect the neoplastic cells from CTL action (Dick *et al*, 1983). In glioma condition, ICAM-1/LFA-1 interaction is interrupted which inhibit target cell lysis by tumor specific T and NK cells (Schiltz *et al*, 2002; Fiore *et al*, 2002). The aberrant HLA class I expression in glioma helps them to evade T cell detection of transformed cells and subsequent cytotoxicity (Rosenberg *et al*, 2003). In glioma, B7-H1 (B7-homologue 1, a costimulatory molecule) inhibits allogenic T cell activation and associated cytokine secretion (Wilmotte *et al*, 2005).

Some other factors like Indoleamine 2,3-dioxygenase (IDO) expression in glioma cells cause T cells to starve for tryptophan, cell cycle arrest and tolerance (Uyttenhove *et al*, 2003). Interestingly, IFNγ stimulate IDO production in glioma, create a local tryptophan shortage and T cell tolerance (Shirey *et al*, 2006). The activation of STAT-3 is another trick for glioma. STAT-3 regulates the anti-apoptotic proteins like Bcl-2, Bcl-XL, Mcl-1, cFLIP, surviving etc in glioma (Rahaman *et al*, 2005; Akasaki *et al*, 2006). Glioma uses various factors including chemokines and matrix degrading enzymes secreted from the brain macrophage/microglia population for their migration and spread in brain (these will be discussed later).

4. Undaunted immune effort continues to resist transformed cells

4.1 T cells mature to effector state after local interaction with APCs in CNS, even in brain tumor

The experimental evidences furnished by Ford and his colleagues in 1996 revealed that the resident antigen presenting cell of brain i.e., microglia, interacts with the T cells to induce final effector function (Ford *et al*, 1996). Years' later studies with GFP-labeled encephalitogenic T cells specific for MBP ($T_{MBP-GFP}$ cells) showed that, with the onset of the disease, huge number of CD4+ effector cells infiltrate in CNS with upregulated chemokine receptors. But these infiltrated $T_{MBP-GFP}$ cells when recovered after 24 hrs from brain parenchyma or neuropil they showed fresh sign of reactivation with upregulation of OX-40 and IL-2R, and upregulated expression of IFNγ, TNFα, TGFβ, IL-2, IL-10, CD3 mRNA expression (Flugel *et al*, 2001). These observations suggested the importance of brain APC at the site of proper functioning of the recruited cells.

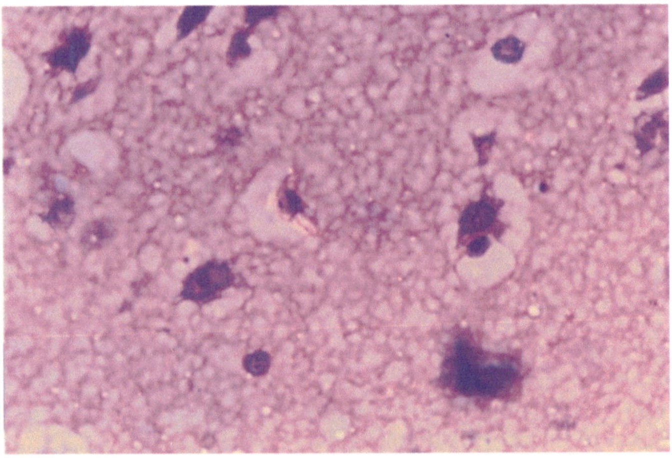

Fig. 3. The section shows that infiltrated lymphocytes in brain parenchyma interact with transformed oligodendroglial cells in a murine oligodendroglioma model and offer them the 'kiss of death'. One oligodendroglioma cell nucleus is protruded out of the cytoplasm and for the other cell, the lymphocyte is overlapping with it. One oligodendroglioma cell, one astrocyte and a free lymphocyte is visible in the field. (Magnification 1000X, oil immersion in Olympus CH20i Microscope and photographed by Olympus DSC)

The function of APC is now becoming more substantial in CNS as some new experimental evidences indicate that they are important to reshape and retain Ag-specific CTLs in the site of neuropathogenesis. In a series of experiments Walker and team addressed the issue with precision. Whether CNS retention of tumor specific MHC class I restricted $CD8^+$ T cells also require recognition of local APC cross-presenting tumor Ag was the problem under scrutiny. They used murine glioma transfected with cDNA encoding HLA-CW3 implanted in mice model. The observation was a massive expansion of $H2K^d/CW3_{170\text{-}179}$-specific CTL using BV10TCR after immunization with CW3. In that animal model the endogenous presentation was tactically avoided and due to the absence of MHC class II on MT-CW3 transfect, the CD4 arm is also avoided. Therefore any expansion of $H2K^d$ restricted CW3-specific CTL suggests the involvement of hosts APC at the tumor site. Detection of the localization of specific CTL, their cytotoxic efficacy and retention of effector functions in an antigen dependent manner speaks the importance of local APC within CNS (Calzascia *et al*, 2003). They are activated macrophage/microglia and cells with DC phenotype found infiltrated heavily in tumor. In subsequent studies they also provide support for the fact that T cell homing at the specific CNS tumor site is defined by the cross-presentating APCs there and not predetermined in the lymph nodes where initial priming occurs (Calzascia *et al*, 2005). In extended studies it was further found that Ag-experienced $CD8^+$ T cells further differentiate at the intracerebral tumor site with enhanced IFNγ and Granzyme-B expression and induction of $\alpha_E\beta_7$ integrin that facilitate their retention in brain (Masson *et al*, 2007). Thus cytotoxic activity of lymphocytes on glioma is not rare [Figure – 3].

4.2 Microglia, the local/resident APCs of brain accumulate in glioma

Microglia is designated as local or resident antigen presenting cell throughout the brain parenchyma or neuropil and its margin. Most emphatic efforts of microglial research in the last two decades were invested to explore its functional relevance in the brain tissue. The striking feature of microglia is its versatile ability to respond according to the CNS microenvironment. Functionally speaking, microglia is a hybrid between white blood cells and glial cells, which is intended to protect and support the neuronal environment in brain. Microglia can respond against an extensive list of biochemical factors ranging as diverse as glycoconjugates, neurotransmitters or cytokines/chemokines (Nakamura, 2002).

Nearly two decade of studies demonstrated the causative effects of chemokines in glioma microenvironment for macrophage/microglia infiltration. The C-C family chemokines, viz, monocyte chemotactic protein 1 (MCP-1) was first purified from glioma and Leung *et al*, 1997 found that with increased MCP-1 the macrophage/microglia infiltrates in glioma. Astrocytoma cells were found capable of producing MCP-1, and complementary receptor CCR2 was present and expressed on activated microglia (Leung *et al*, 1997). In 2003, evidence showed that, MCP-1 promoted the microglial migration in glioma and microglia infested glioma grew rapidly (Platten *et al*, 2003). The involvement of PI-3K/Akt pathway was assumed in the secretion of microglia derived factors that mediate glioma invasiveness (Joy *et al*, 2003; Pu *et al*, 2004). CSF-1 (colony stimulating factor 1), which acted as chemotactic and mitogenic factors for myeloid lineage cells, and its receptor, were long been detected in glioma, whereas microglia also possessed the option of secreting and receiving the factor from self and neighboring cells. Eventually from glioma G-CSF/GM-CSF (granulocytes and granulocytes macrophage colony stimulating factor) were secreted and influenced the differentiation and maturation process of microglia like other myeloid lineage cells. Badie *et al*, 1999, *in vitro* demonstrated the specific microglia attracting capacity of glioma by the hepatocyte growth factor/scatter factor (HGF/SF). HGF/SF signals the spectrum of mesenchymal cells for mitogenic stimulation, invasion and extravasation. Microglia possesses its receptor Met and can produce HGF/SF, whereas the glioma cells are capable of doing the same (Badie & Schartner, 2001). Thus, the balancing ratios of the factors in glioma microenvironment act as the determinant in the migration process of the cells.

In 2002, the 15.3 KDa heparin-binding peptide Pleiotrophin (PTN) was found to appear in adult human glioma, normally a mitogenic/angiogenic factor in embryonic stage. Uniquely, PTN did not help to proliferate the glioma cells by its own, rather influenced microglial accumulation by acting as strong chemotactic and mitogenic agent. Its action thus passively helped glioma growth by targeting endothelial and microglial cells (Mentlein & Held-Feindt, 2002). The question arose that what would be the interest of glioma to include microglia in its vicinity? In fact, the role of infiltrating macrophage/microglia in the process of angiogenesis in glioma was hinted previously when macrophage associated heme-oxygenase-1 (HO-1) enzyme was found to be correlated with the vascular density of human glioma (Nishie *et al* 1999). Another enzyme cyclooxygenase (COX)-2 was found to be produced in higher amount in microglia isolated from intracranial glioma which increased the prostaglandin E_2 (PGE_2) production. The study suggested that glioma infiltrating microglia contributed in developing fatal cerebral edema in glioma through COX-2 dependent pathway. It was reported that PGE_2 increased the permeability of vascular endothelium by cytoskeletal rearrangement where TNFα acted as positive inducer. In that case, microglia was the source of both COX-2 and TNFα probably playing a role in its own migration, leukocyte trafficking and in parallel, glioma invasiveness (Badie *et al*, 2003).

Contrary to the reports and assumptions, others demonstrated that TNF dependent action enhanced the macrophage/microglia recruitment in glioma where they form small cavities named microcysts and reduces the glioma growth (Villeneuve *et al*, 2005). A report stated that, the infiltrated macrophages ($CD11b^{+}CCR3^{-}CD45^{high}$) caused TNF induced apoptosis in GL261 glioma cells where related microglial cells ($CD11b^{+}CCR3^{+}CD45^{+}$) were negligible (Nakagawa *et al*, 2007). Actually the thin line of demarcation of cellular identity between macrophage and microglia could not exclude any of them from the function of TNF dependent glioma elimination. Opposing the recent believe of pro-tumoregenic role of macrophage population in different tumors, the reports raised question against application of anti-inflammatory drugs to suppress microglial action in glioma. To reestablish its role against glioma, the mechanism of their phagocytic recognition, killing machinery, and antigen presentation to CTL etc must have to be introspected more specifically.

4.3 Microglia protects host brain as well as support glioma: A bi-edged sword

Further findings showed that microglia helped glioma to invade by releasing matrix degrading enzymes. Even it was recently found that in rare Neurofibromatosis 1 (NF1), the heterozygote microglia had the role to promote glioma growth (Daginakatte & Gutmann, 2007). In 2005, it was found that metalloprotease-2 (MMP-2) activity was increased in microglia by the soluble factors released from glioma cells (Markovic *et al*, 2005). Thus glioma in turn influenced microglia to invade and migrate, which was utilized by neoplastic cells itself to spread and grow. Previously, a separate study hinted the process when the motility of GL261 mouse glioma cells was assessed in presence of microglia. Even the microglia stimulated with GM-CSF or LPS enhanced this migration (Bettinger *et al*, 2002). Adenosine mediated anti-inflammatory effects on macrophage cell lines by modulating the cytokine balance was observed. Additionally, macrophage and microglia both the cells were found to present adenosine receptors. In 2006, Synowtz and his team found the effect of nucleoside Adenosine on microglial cell and glioma. Deficiency of A1 adenosine receptor (A_1AR) on microglia helped to grow the GL261 glioblastoma cells and increased number of A_1AR expressing microglia in the site inhibited this growth. The mentioned study also hinted that adenosine signaling through the receptor depleted glioma influenced microglial MMP-2 release, which in turn restricted glioma growth and invasion (Synowitz *et al* 2006). Again, Kettenmann and colleagues observed that Microglia express membrane type 1 metalloprotease (MT1-MMP) in glioma condition, which helps to activate glioma released pro-MMP2 and thus promotes the spread of glioma in brain parenchyma (Markovic *et al*, 2009). Their most recent finding is that the antibiotic minocycline attenuates microglial MT1-MMP expression in glioma and as a result neoplastic cell expansion is reduced in glioma (Markovic *et al*, 2011).

Plasticity, its migration to the site of injury or inflammation, response and then departure from the site required a plausible explanation mostly for its movement. Microglia was found to express α6β1 integrin, which was the receptor for laminin expressed on the extracellular matrix constituent projections of astrocytes. This particular adhesion was for migration and under strict control of cytokine milieu (Milner & Campbell, 2002). It was found recently that another integrin α5β1 expressed both on glioma and microglial cells were capable of inhibiting glioma growth when attenuated. Remarkably it was found that, the attenuation process and resulting depletion of glioma required the presence of microglial cells (Färber *et al*, 2008). It might be probable that microglia secreting products had control over this integrin-laminin adhesion and migration of cell itself and invasive migration of glioma cells.

Regarding the cytokine microenvironment, the role of TGF-β was hinted in migration (Milner & Campbell, 2002). The specific importance of the cytokine was demonstrated by RNAi mediated gene silencing of TGF-β in promoting growth and invasiveness of glioma by integrin family adhesion molecule (Wesolowska *et al*, 2008). Recently it was found that cyclosporin A (CsA), an inhibitor of calcineurin and immunosuppressive in effect, could inhibit microglia mediated glioma invasion and cause to change morphological structure of microglia via MAPK signaling (Silwa *et al*, 2007).

In the present context, most of the studies demonstrated pro-tumerogenic action of microglia in glioma, which was facilitated by the secretary products, signaling molecules including cytokines, chemokines and receptors etc. In parallel, glioma cells favor microglial migration and encroachment in its vicinity. Though primarily macrophages/microglia are the cells to defend host tissue from faulty or malfunctioning cells or pathogens, their pro-glioma role leads to confusion. Remarkably, several findings also came with hopeful antagonistic results as already mentioned, where the roles of TNFα, TGFβ, A_1AR dependent MMP-2 inhibition etc were focused (Villeneuve *et al*, 2005; Nakagawa *et al*, 2007; Synowitz *et al* 2006; Wesolowska *et al*, 2008). In 2007, Galarneau and team demonstrated that macrophage/microglia depletion helped in glioma growth (Galarneau *et al*, 2007). The study hinted for a separate anti-tumor potential of the cells. These contradicting results present microglia with a double agent stature.

4.4 Glioma antigen presentation by microglia

To determine the antigen presenting role of microglia their MHC class II expression along with the co-stimulatory molecule like B7.1 (CD80) and B7.2 (CD86) had been evaluated. Badie and his team found the lower level of expression of these essential surface molecule for APC function in microglia freshly isolated from glioma invasive cells and that suggested suppressive effect on glioma microenvironment *in vivo* (Badie & Schartner, 2001). In a comparative study of different rodent glioma model viz., C6, 9L and RG2, the expression profile was found to vary significantly depending on the immunogenicity of the model. The costimulatory B7 molecule expression could be favored when microglia were rejuvenated by cytokines GM-CSF and IFN-γ *in vitro* (Badie *et al*, 2002). At the same time, Graeber with his colleagues scanned 97 glioma samples of different WHO grades and found no such simple relations of the MHC expression of the cell with tumor grades, rather found downregulation of MHC class II in tissue areas where dense glioblastoma cells were infested. According to them microglia were functional in astrocytic tumors, though might be subjected to suppression with T cell clonal anergy in that glioma microenvironment (Tran *et al*, 1998).

The stimulatory effect of the novel glycoprotein T11TS/SLFA-3 on microglial MHC class II expression was found. The dose-time dependent efficient MHC expression was found on microglia in rodent bearing experimental glioma when treated with T11TS (Begum *et al*, 2004). Chaudhuri and her team also identified another important costimulatory molecule CD2 on microglia, which could also be regulated by the glycoprotein dose in glioma condition (Begum *et al*, 2004; Chaudhuri & Ghosh, 2006). A separate study by her team found simultaneous co-expression of MHC class II and CD2 on microglia in glioma where both expressed in low quantity (Sarkar *et al*, 2004). This observation with others supported the view of immunosuppressive milieu offered to microglia in glioma mostly by TGFβ, IL-10, PGE_2, gangliosides etc (Zou *et al*, 1999; Graeber *et al*, 2002), which could also simultaneously cripple the infiltrated lymphocytes (Dix *et al*, 1999). In this regard, the fact that microglia was the source of that IL-10 in glioma, had been finally established by Wagner and team (Wagner *et al*, 1999).

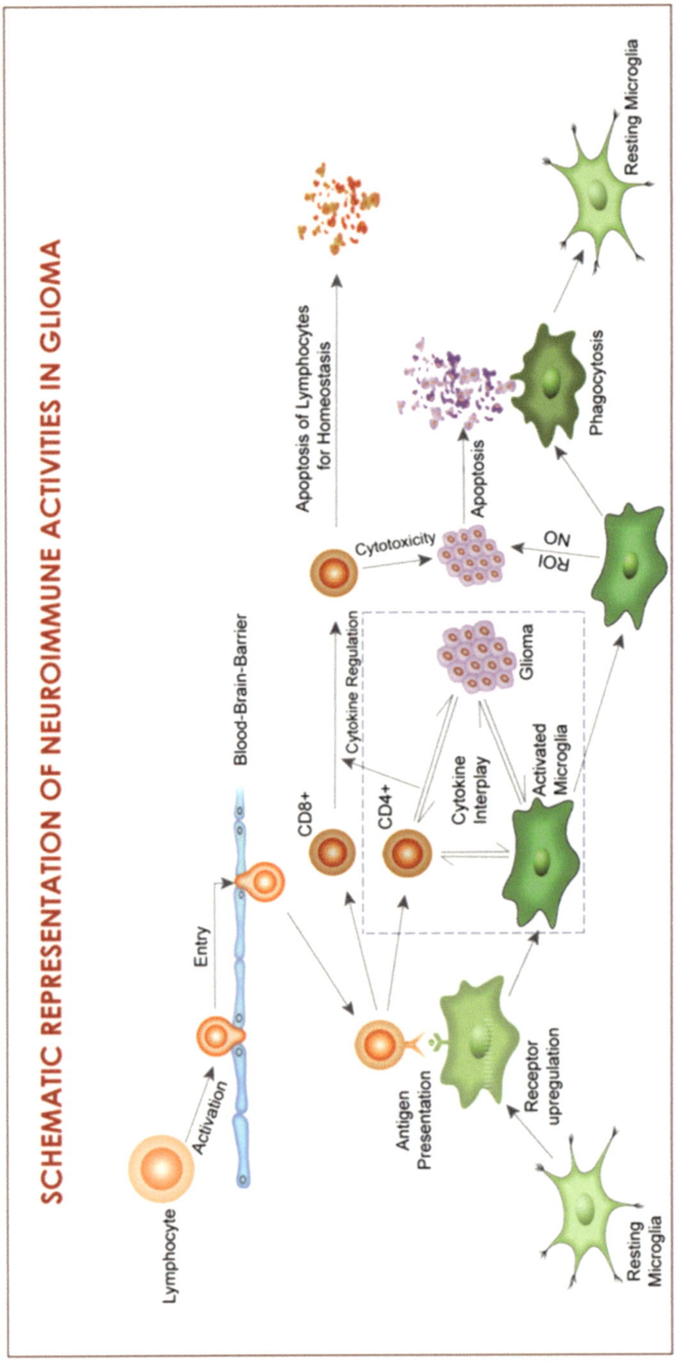

Fig. 4. This schematic diagram shows the activities of immune components in brain during glioma. After activated glioma antigen specific T cells enter into brain parenchyma they progressed towards glioma through parenchyma. Simultaneously, during glioma pathogenesis resident resting microglia get activated, upregulate their receptors, enhance

their local antigen presenting capacity and move towards glioma vicinity where astrocytic projections may assist this movement by providing the pavement for integrin-laminin interaction. At the glioma site, microglia locally represent antigens, produce cytokines and adhesion molecules to dialogue with lymphocytes which help them to mature and attain final effector function. At this point, a triangular complex interaction circuit become active between infiltrated lymphocytes, microglia and glioma cells when glioma tries to cripple the immune attack by applying many of its tricks (as discussed in the text). Overall cytokine, chemokine, growth factor and immunosuppressive factor become crucial to determine the success of immune defense or glioma. At the next step, cytotoxic T cells exert perforin, granzyme, FasL and other cytotoxic means to kill glioma and microglia uses its reactive oxygen and nitrogen intermediates to damage the abnormal or neoplastic cells. Target cells, intact, damaged or dead debris are scavenged by microglia. If the immune system manages to overcome the situation for a certain period they return to homeostasis. But aggressive glioma, after the initial arrest, overrules the immune defense by its rapid proliferation rate, immune evasion strategies and diverse modes for bypassing the attack. Gaining dominance during the triangular interaction phase marks the success of the party in the succeeding phases (Adopted from *Chaudhuri & Ghosh, 2006, CNSAMC*).

Hemiberger and colleagues studied the myeloid lineage cells in post-operative tissue samples in human glioma. Accepting the cellular identity crisis, these workers found macrophage/microglia and dendritic cell populations within the tumor tissue. In their higher grade glioma samples microglial population though found to express MHC class II, lacked co-stimulatory CD80, CD86 and CD40, crucial for T cell functioning. Activation of microglia via Toll-like receptors (TLRs) were also insignificant to augment tumoricidal activity (Hussain *et al*, 2006a). Particularly, proinflammatory cytokines including IL-1β, IL-6, TNF α could not be sufficiently released to launch substantial innate immune function against glioma, however their phagocytic function was not impaired and also exhibited low level of non-specific cytotoxicity (Hussain *et al*, 2006b). In rodent glioma model lack of proinflammatory cytokines IFN γ, IL-12 and IL-6, and conversely cumulative dominance of IL-4 and IL-10 favoring the suppression of immune response was recently observed (Ghosh *et al*, 2010). Microglial activity stature was also reflected in their morphometry in scanning electron microscopy (SEM), where their filapodial extensions, sizes and shapes had shown noticeable alterations (Begum *et al*, 2003).

4.5 Microglia can destroy glioma cells

The cytotoxic effector function is an important part of CNS microglia/macrophage population which mainly dependents on its phagocytic mode of action. For the purpose super oxide anion production is the major function of phagocytic cells, however microglia generate sufficient endogenous NO in addition (Beyer *et al*, 2000). When microglial effector function in rat glioma model was studied, it was found that microglia mostly depends on NO production than ROS generation for exerting effector activity, whereas peripheral macrophages mainly depends on ROS for their normal phagocytic functions (Ghosh *et al*, 2007). With tumoricidal actions NO plays certain role in complex signaling network of cytokine production, angiogenesis etc in brain microenvironment. Even microglia was found to release iNOS/NO from astrocytoma cells in contact. This was by IL-1β production of activated microglia and probably via p38 MAPK and NF-κB signaling pathway (Kim *et al*, 2006).

Expression of Fas ligand on a cell may cause damage to adjoining cells or infiltrated activated lymphocytes in the tissue by triggering the death pathway. In glioma, FasL expression was thought to be a means of immune escape, whereas, investigations found FasL expression also on microglial cells in glioma (Badie *et al*, 2001). Hence, it could be thought that microglia would play role in local immune suppression by limiting the lymphocyte populations; or it might express FasL to damage glioma cells, which in turn restricted or crippled the lymphocytes infiltrated locally. Microglia prefers to phagocytose the damaged cells rather than intact ones (Bohatschek *et al*, 2001). A study showed that after adoptive transfer of alloreactive cytotoxic T cells in rat 9L gliosarcoma infested brain, the CTL damaged glioma cells were removed by phagocytic scavenging activities of microglia, whereas undamaged ones were spared (Kulprathipanja & Kruse, 2004). In this process of either Fas or oxidative stress mediated cell death, externalization of phosphatidylserine was found to be crucial in corpse clearance by microglia. Experimental evidences revealed increasing PS externalization in correlation with cytotoxic effector functions of microglia and infiltrated lymphocytes. Additionally, the investigation showed that microglia population was more steady than infiltrated lymphocytes as Bcl-2 aided the cells to maintain that steady turnover rate and low apoptosis in brain microenvironment (Kagan *et al*, 2002 & Ghosh *et al*, 2007).

5. Conclusion: Future immuno-therapeutics must capitalize this resident and infiltrated immunocyte liaison to combat glioma

Now it can be clearly stated that lymphocytes can enter into the brain parenchyma. During their entry, they are checked by the antigen presenting cells for their glioma antigen specificity. APCs try to ensure this glioma specific T cell entry by restimulating the candidates presenting the glioma antigens mostly in perivascular space and allied blood brain interface (Engelherdt, 2010). After entering they migrate to glioma and again interact with the local APCs which help them to gain maturation and final effector function. In this process peripheral APC in brain and 'so called' resident microglia as well as DCs also play very important role. The role of local APC in glioma immunity has been detailed by Ghosh and Chaudhuri with a new outlook to explain the contradiction of glioma promoting role of microglia (Ghosh and Chaudhuri, 2010).These myeloid cell populations have the potential to act as chief immunomodulator in brain by surveillance in the tissue environment, guiding the leukocytes in CNS and simultaneously exerting effector function to neoplastic cells. The damaging activities of the cell are probably their own misfired 'goodness' or their potential that is misled by glioma cells. Thus, both the lymphocytes and local APC (predominantly microglia) are capable of exerting the immune effector function against glioma in spite of the immune-compromise in the brain and glioma immune evasion strategies [Figure - 4].

Now the success of immunotherapeutic approaches against glioma, largely as adjuvant therapeutic strategy, depends on the proper usages of this delicate immune defense against this detrimental threat. The battle becomes more interesting and challenging because the opponent is extremely clever. So development of immunotherapeutic strategies against glioma needs detailed and critical interpretation of the work-plan of immunity in glioma and its careful application. Basic findings are increasing the repertoire of information about immune activity deep into the brain during glioma which in turn provide us newer tactics or facilitate the amendment of old ones for better effects (Dietrich *et al*, 2010; Vauleon *et al*,

2010). Even some of the approaches interestingly propose microglia as an effective vehicle for gene therapy and drug delivery by using its predifferentiated cellular status (Neumann, 2006). Present immunotherapeutic advancements and limitations will be discussed in other chapters of this book and beyond the scope of this article. In this essay, the basic immune mechanisms, which are active in glioma, has been detailed. Further development of effective therapy needs this fundamental background knowledge for setting up a new immunotherapeutic intervention against glioma.

6. Acknowledgement

I am thankful to Prof Swapna Chaudhuri of School of Tropical Medicine, Kolkata who initiated my drive in this field and constantly supported me with valuable suggestions. I also admit the cooperation of Debasis Das to develop the illustrations and support of my colleagues and students to continue my work.

7. References

Akasaki Y, Liu G, Matundan HH *et al* (2006). A peroxisome proliferatoractivated receptor-gamma agonist, troglitazone, facilitates caspase-8 and -9 activities by increasing the enzymatic activity of protein-tyrosine phosphatase-1B on human glioma cells. J Biol Chem 281:6165–74.

Aloisi F, Serafini B, Adorini L (2000). Glia- T cell dialogue. J Neuroimmunol 107: 111-117.

Badie B and Schartner J (2001). Role of microglia in glioma biology. Microscopy Res Tech 54: 106-111.

Badie B, Schartner JM, Hagar AR *et al* (2003). Microglia cyclooxygenase-2 activity in experimental gliomas: possible role in cerebral edema formation. Clin Canc Res 9: 872-877.

Badie B, Bartley B, Schartner J (2002). Differential expression of MHC class II and B7 costimulatory molecules by microglia in rodent gliomas. J Neuroimmunol 133: 39-45.

Barker CF and Billingham RE (1977). Immunologically privileged sites. Adv Immunol 25:1–54.

Bechmann I, Galea I, Perry VH (2007). What is blood brain barrier (not)? Trends Immunol 28(1): 5-11.

Bechmann I, Kwidzinski E, Kovac AD *et al* (2001). Turnover of Rat Brain Perivascular Cells. Experimental Neurology 168, 242–249.

Begum Z, Sarkar S, Mukherjee J *et al* (2003). Evaluation of anti-tumor property of specific and nonspecific BRMS in experimental glioma by assessing the microglial cell functional and phenotypic modulations. Cancer Biol Ther 2(4): 356-363.

Begum Z, Ghosh A, Sarkar S *et al* (2004). Documentation of immune profile of microglia through cell surface marker study in glioma model primed by a novel cell surface glycopeptide T11TS/SLFA-3. Glycoconj J 20: 515-523.

Bettinger I, Thanos S, Paulus W (2002). Microglia promote glioma migration. Acta Neuropathol 103(4): 351-355.

Beyer M, Gimsa U, Eyupogiu IY *et al* (2000). Phagocytosis of neuronal or glial debris by microglial cells: upregulation of MHC class II expression and multinuclear giant cell formation in vitro. Glia 31: 262-266.

Billingham RE and Boswell T (1953). Studies on the problem of corneal homografts. Proc R Soc Lond B Biol Sci 141:392–406.

Bohatschek M, Kloss CUA, Kall R *et al* (2001). In vitro model of microglial deramification: ramified microglia transform into amoeboid phagocytes following addition of brain cell membranes to microglia-astrocyte cocultures. J Neurosci Res 64: 508-522.

Boulton M, Flessner M, Armstrong D *et al* (1999). Contribution of extracranial lymphatics and arachnoid villi to the clearance of a CSF tracer in rat. Am J Physiol 276: R818-R823.

Calzascia T, Di Berardino Besson W, Masson F *et al* (2005). Homing phenotypes of tumour-specific CD8 T cells are pre-determined at the tumour site by cross-presenting APCs. Immunity 22: 175-184.

Calzascia T, Di Berardino Besson W, Wilmotte R *et al* (2003). Cutting edge: Cross-presentation as a mechanism for efficient recruitment of tumor-specific CTL to the brain. J Immunol 171: 2187-2191.

Chaudhuri S and Ghosh A (2006). Glioma Therapy: A Novel Insight in the Immunotherapeutic Regime with T11TS/SLFA-3. Cent Nerv Syst Agents Med Chem 6(4): 245-270.

Cserr HF and Knopf PM (1992). Cervical lymphatics, the blood brain barrier and the immunoreactivity of the brain: a new view. Immunol Today 13: 507-512.

Daginakatte GC and Gutmann DH (2007). Neurofibromatosis-1 (Nf1) heterozygous brain microglia elaborate paracrine factors that promote Nf1-deficient astrocyte and glioma growth. Hum Mol Genet 16(9): 1098-1112.

Dick SJ, Macchi B, Papazoglou S *et al* (1983). Lymphoid cell glioma cell interaction enhances cell coat production by human gliomas: novel suppressor mechanism. Science 220: 739–42.

Dietrich PY, Dutoit V, Tran Thang NN *et al* (2010). T-cell immunotherapy for malignant glioma: towards a combined approach. Curr Opin Oncol 22(6): 604-10.

Dix AR, Brooks WH, Roszman TL *et al* (1999). Immune defects observed in patients with primary malignant brain tumors. J Neuroimmunol 100:216-232.

Ehrlich, P. (1885) Das Sauerstoff-Bedürfnis des Organismus. Eine farbenanalytische Studie. [On the oxygen consumption of the body. A study using intravital dyes.], Verlag von August Hirschwald, Berlin.

Ehrlich, P. (1904) Uben die Beziehungen chemischer constitution, Verheilung, and phanmdkologischen Wirkung. In:
Gesaammelte Arbeiten zur Immunitatsforschung, Berlin.

Elliott LH, Brooks WH, Roszman TL (1984). Cytokinetic basis for the impaired activation of lymphocytes from patients with primary intracranial tumors. J Immunol 132: 1208–1215.

Elliott LH, Brooks WH, Roszman TL (1990). Inability of mitogenactivated lymphocytes obtained from patients with malignant primary intracranial tumors to express high affinity interleukin 2 receptors. J Clin Invest 86: 80–86.

Engelhardt B (2010). T cell migration into the central nervous system during health and disease: Different molecular keys allow access to different central nervous system compartments. Clin Exp Neuroimmunol 1: 79-93.

Engelhardt, B. and Wolburg, H. (2004) Mini-review: Transendothelial migration of leukocytes: through the front door or around the side of the house? Eur. J. Immunol. 34, 2955–2963.

Färber K, Synowitz M, Zahn G *et al* (2008). An α5β1 integrin inhibitor attenuates glioma growth. Mol Cell Neurosci 39(4): 579-585.

Fiore E, Fusco C, Romero P *et al* (2002). Matrix metalloproteinase 9 (MMP-9/gelatinase B) proteolytically cleaves ICAM-1 and participates in tumor cell resistance to natural killer cell mediated cytotoxicity. Oncogene 21:5213–23.

Flügel A, Berkowicz T, Ritter T (2001). Migratory activity and functional changes of green fluorescent effector T cells before and during experimental autoimmune encephalomyelitis. Immunity 14:547–560.

Ford AL, Foulcher E, Lemckert FA *et al* (1996). Microglia induce CD4+ T lymphocyte final effector function and death. J Exp Med 184:1737-1745.

Galarneau H, Villeneuve J, Gowing G *et al* (2007). Increased Glioma Growth in Mice Depleted of Macrophages. Cancer Res 67(18): 8874-8881.

Galea I, Bernardes-Silva M, Forse PA et al (2007). An antigen-specific pathway for CD8 T cells across the blood-brain barrier. J Exp Med 204(9): 2023-30.

Ghosh A and Chaudhuri S (2010). Microglial action in glioma: A boon turns bane. Immunol Lett 131: 3-9.

Ghosh A, Mukherjee J, Bhattacharjee M *et al* (2007). T11TS/SLFA-3 Differentially Regulate The Population Of Microglia And Brain Infiltrating Lymphocytes To Reduce Glioma By Modulating Intrinsic Bcl-2 Expression Rather Than p53. Cent Nerv Syst Agents Med Chem 7(2): 145-155.

Ghosh A, Mukherjee J, Bhattacharjee M *et al* (2007). The Other Side of the Coin: Beneficiary Effect of 'Oxidative Burst' Upsurge with T11TS Facilitates the Elimination of Glioma Cells. Cell Mol Biol 53(5): 53-62.

Giometto B, Bozza F, Faresin F *et al* (1996). Immune infiltrates and cytokines in gliomas. Acta Neurochir 138: 50–56.

Goldmann J, Kwidzinski E, Brandt C et al (2006). T cells traffic from brain to cervical lymph nodes via the cribroid plate and the nasal mucosa. J Leukoc Biol 80(4): 797-801.

Goldmann, E. (1913) Vitalfärbungen am Zentralnervensystem. Beitrag zur Physio-Pathologie des Plexus Choroideus und der Hirnhäute. [Intravital labelling of the central nervous system. A study on the pathophysiology of the choroid plexus and the meninges.] Abhandlungen der kőniglich preußischen Akademie der Wissenschaften. Physikalisch-Mathematische Classe 1:1–64.

Gomez GG and Kruse CA (2006). Mechanisms of malignant glioma immune resistance and sources of immunosuppression. Gene Ther Mol Biol 10(A): 133–146.

Govinden R and Bhoola KD (2003). Genealogy, expression, and cellular function of transforming growth factor-β. Pharmacol Ther 98: 257–65.

Graeber MB, Scheithauer BW, Kreutzberg GW (2002). Microglia in brain tumors. Glia 40: 252-259.

Greter M, Heppner F, Lemos MP et al (2005). Dendritic cells permit immune invasion of the CNS in an animal model of multiple sclerosis. Nat Med 11: 328-34.

Grutz G (2005). New insights into the molecular mechanism of interleukin-10-mediated immunosuppression. J Leuk Biol 77:3–15.

Hickey WF, Hsu BL, Kimura H (1991). T-lymphocyte entry into the central nervous system. J Neurosci Res 28: 254-60.

Huettner C, Czub S, Kerkau S *et al* (1997). Interleukin 10 is expressed in human gliomas in vivo and increases glioma cell proliferation and motility in vitro. Anticancer Res 17: 3217–3224.

Husain N, Chiocca EA, Rainov N, Louis DN, Zervas NT (1998). Co-expression of Fas and Fas ligand in malignant glial tumors and cell lines. Acta Neuropathol (Berl) 95: 287–95.

Hussain SF, Yang D, Suki D *et al* (2006a). The role of human glioma-infiltrating microglia/macrophages in mediating antitumor immune responses. Neuro-Oncology 8: 261–227.

Hussain SF, Yang D, Suki D *et al* (2006b). Innate immune functions of microglia isolated from human glioma patients. J Trans Med 4(15): doi:10.1186/1479-5876-4-15.

Joy AM, Beaudry CE, Tran NL *et al* (2003). Migrating glioma cells activate the PI3-K pathway and display decreased susceptibility to apoptosis. J Cell Sci 116, 4409–17.

Kagan VE, Gleiss B, Tyurina YY *et al* (2002). A Role for Oxidative Stress in Apoptosis: Oxidation and Externalization of Phosphatidylserine Is Required for Macrophage Clearance of Cells Undergoing Fas-Mediated Apoptosis. J Immunol 169: 487–499.

Kim YJ, Hwang SY, Oh ES *et al* (2006). IL-1β, an immediate early protein secreted by activated microglia, induces iNOS/NO in C6 astrocytoma cells through p38 MAPK and NF-κB pathways. J Neurosci Res 84(5), 1037-46.

Kulprathipanja NV and Kruse CA (2004). Microglia phagocytose alloreactive CTL-damaged 9L gliosarcoma cells. J Neuroimmunol 153: 76-82.

Ladisch S, Becker H, Ulsh L (1992). Immunosuppression by human gangliosides: I. Relationship of carbohydrate structure to the inhibition of T cell responses. Biochim Biophys Acta 1125: 180–188.

Leung SY, Wong MP, Chung LP *et al* (1997). Monocyte chemoattractant protein-1 expression and macrophage infiltration in gliomas. Acta Neuropathol 93, 518-527.

MacFarlane Burnet (1970). Immunological Surveillance. Pergamon Press. Oxford. Pp 280.

Markovic DS, Glass R, Synowitz M *et al* (2005). Microglia stimulate the invasiveness of glioma cells by increasing the activity of metalloprotease-2. J Neuropathol Exp Neurol 64: 754–762.

Markovic DS, Vinnakota K, Chirasani S et al (2009). Gliomas induce and exploit microglial MT1-MMP expression for tumor expansion. PNAS 106(30):12530-5.

Markovic DS, Vinnakota K, van Rooijen N et al (2011). Minocycline reduces glioma expansion and invasion by attenuating microglial MT1-MMP expression. Brain Behav Immun. 25(4): 624-8.

Mason DW, Charlton HM, Jones AJ *et al* (1986). The fate of allogenic and xenogenic neuronal tissue transplanted into the third ventricle of rodents. Neurosci 19: 685-94.

Masson F, Calzascia T, Di Berardino-Besson W *et al* (2007). Brain Microenvironment Promotes the Final Functional Maturation of Tumor-Specific Effector CD8+ T Cells. J. Immunol 179: 845-853.

McVicar DW, Davis DF, Merchant RE (1992). In vitro analysis of the proliferative potential of T cells from patients with brain tumor: glioma-associated immunosuppression unrelated to intrinsic cellular defect. J Neurosurg 76: 251–260.

Medawar PB (1948). Immunity to homologous grafted skin. Brit J Exp Path 29:58–69.

Mentlein R and Held-Feindt J (2002). Pleiotrophin, an angiogenic and mitogenic growth factor, is expressed in human gliomas. J Neurochem 83(4): 747-753.

Milner R and Campbell IL (2002). Cytokines Regulate Microglial Adhesion to Laminin and Astrocyte Extracellular Matrix via Protein Kinase C-Dependent Activation of the α6β1 Integrin. J Neurosci 22(5): 1562-1572.

Morford LA, Elliott LH, Carlson SL *et al* (1997). T cell receptor-mediated signaling is defective in T cells obtained from patients with primary intracranial tumors. J Immunol 159: 4415–4425.

Murphy JB and Sturm E (1923). Conditions determining the transplantability of tissues in the brain. J Exp Med 38:183–197.

Nakagawa J, Saio M, Tamakawa N *et al* (2007). TNF expressed by tumor-associated macrophages, but not microglia, can eliminate glioma. Int J Oncol 30: 803-811.
Nakamura Y (2002). Regulating factors for microglial activation. Biol Pharm Bull 25: 945-953.
Neumann H (2006). Microglia: a cellular vehicle for CNS therapy. J Clin Invest 116(11): 2857-2860.
Nishie A, Ono M, Shono T *et al* (1999). Macrophage infiltration and heme oxygenase-1 expression correlate with angiogenesis in human gliomas. Clin Canc Res 5: 1107-1113.
Obersteiner, H. (1870). Űber einige Lymphraüme im Gehirn. [A study on lymphatic compartments of the brain.]. Sitzungsberichte der Mathematisch-Naturwissenschaftlichen Classe der Kaiserlichen Akademie der Wissenschaften 61: 57–67.
Perry VH (1998). A revised view of the central nervous system microenvironment and major histocompatibility complex class II antigen presentation. J Neuroimmunol 90: 113-121.
Piccio L, Rossi B, Scarpini E *et al* (2002). Molecular mechanisms involved in inflamed brain microvessels: critical roles for P-selectin glycoprotein ligand-1 and heterotrimeric G(i) linked receptors. J Immunol 168: 1940-1949.
Platten M, Kretz A, Naumann U *et al* (2003). Monocyte chemoattractant protein-1 increases microglial infiltration and aggressiveness of gliomas. Ann Neurol 54: 388–92.
Pu P, Kang C, Li J *et al* (2004). Antisense and dominant-negative AKT2 cDNA inhibits glioma cell invasion. Tumour Biol 25: 172–8.
Rahaman SO, Vogelbaum MA, Haque SJ (2005). Aberrant Stat3 signaling by interleukin-4 in malignant glioma cells: involvement of IL-13R alpha 2. Cancer Res 65: 2956–63.
Ransohoff RM, Kivisäkk P, Kidd G (2003). Three or more routes for leukocyte migration into the central nervous system. Nat Rev Immunol 3: 569-581.
Reese, T.S. and Karnovsky, M.J. (1967) Fine structural localization of a blood–brain barrier to exogenous peroxidase. J. Cell Biol. 34, 207–217.
Rosenberg SA, Yang JC, Robbins PF *et al* (2003). Cell transfer therapy for cancer: lessons from sequential treatments of a patient with metastatic melanoma. J Immunother 26: 385–93.
Roth W, Isenmann S, Nakamura M *et al* (2001). Soluble decoy receptor 3 is expressed by malignant gliomas and suppresses CD95 ligand induced apoptosis and chemotaxis. Cancer Res 61: 2759–65.
Sakaguchi S (2005). Naturally arising Foxp3-expressing CD25+CD4+ regulatory T cells in immunological tolerance to self and non-self. Nat Immunol 6:345–52.
Sarkar S, Ghosh A, Mukherjee J *et al* (2004). CD2-SLFA-3/T11TS interaction facilitates immune activation and glioma regression by T11TS. Cancer Biol Ther 3(11): 1121-1128.
Schiltz PM, Gomez GG, Read SB *et al* (2002). Effects of IFN-γ and interleukin-1β on major histocompatibility complex antigen and intercellular adhesion molecule-1 expression by 9L gliosarcoma: relevance to its cytolysis by alloreactive cytotoxic T lymphocytes. J Int Cyt Res 22:1209–16.
Sedgwick JD (1995). Immune surveillance and autoantigen recognition in the central nervous system. Aust NZ J Med 25: 784-792.
Sedgwick JD, Ford AL, Foulcher E *et al* (1998). Central nervous system microglial cell activation and proliferation follows direct interaction with tissue infiltrating T cell blasts. J Immunol 160:5320-5330.

Sedgwick JD, Schwender S, Imrich H *et al* (1991). Isolation and direct characterization of resident microglial cells from the normal and inflamed central nervous system. PNAS 88: 7438-42.

Shirai Y (1921). On the transplantation of the rat sarcoma in adult heterogenous animals. Jap Med World 1:14–15.

Shirey KA, Jung JY, Maeder GS *et al* (2006). Upregulation of IFN-gamma receptor expression by proinflammatory cytokines influences IDO activation in epithelial cells. J Int Cyt Res 26: 53–62.

Sliwa M, Markovic D, Gabrusiewicz K *et al* (2007). The invasion promoting effect of microglia on glioblastoma cells is inhibited by cyclosporin A. Brain 130: 476-489.

Synowitz M, Glass R, Färber K *et al* (2006). A1 Adenosine Receptors in Microglia Control Glioblastoma-Host Interaction. Cancer Res 66(17): 8550-8557.

Thomas DA and Massague J (2005). TGF-β directly targets cytotoxic T cell functions during tumor evasion of immune surveillance. Cancer Cell 8: 369–80.

Tran CT, Wolz P, Egensperger R *et al* (1998). Differential expression of MHC class II molecules by microglia and neoplastic astroglia: relevance for the escape of astrocytoma cells from immune surveillance. Neuropathol Appl Neurobiol 24(4): 293-301.

Tran EH, Hoekstra K, Van Rooijen N, Dijkstra CD, Owens T (1998). Immune invasion of the central nervous system parenchyma and experimental allergic encephalomyelitis, but not leukocyte extravasation from blood, are prevented in macrophage depleted mice. J Immunol 161:3767–75.

Urbani F, Maleci A, La Sala A *et al* (1995). Defective expression of interferon-gamma, granulocyte-macrophage colony-stimulating factor, tumor necrosis factor alpha, and interleukin-6 in activated peripheral blood lymphocytes from glioma patients. J Interferon Cytokine Res 15: 421–429.

Uyttenhove C, Pilotte L, Theate I *et al* (2003). Evidence for a tumoral immune resistance mechanism based on tryptophan degradation by indoleamine 2, 3-dioxygenase. Nat Med 9:1269–74.

Vauleon E, Avril T, Collet B *et al* (2010). Overview of cellular immunotherapy for patients with glioblastoma. Clin Dev Immunol Volume 2010: Article ID 689171, 18 pages, doi:10.1155/2010/689171.

Villeneuve J, Tremblay P and Vallières L (2005). Tumor necrosis factor reduces brain tumor growth by enhancing macrophage recruitment and microcyst formation. Cancer Res 65(9): 3928-3936.

Wagner S, Czub S, Greif M *et al* (1999). Microglial/macrophage expression of interleukin 10 in human glioblastomas. Int J Canc 82(1), 12-16.

Wang D and Dubois RN (2006). Prostaglandins and cancer. Gut 55: 115–22.

Wekerle H, Linington C, Lassmann H *et al* (1986). Cellular immune reactivity within the CNS. Trends Neurosci 19: 685-94.

Wesolowska A, Kwiatkowska A, Slomnicki L *et al* (2008). Microglia-derived TGF-β as an important regulator of glioblastoma invasion—an inhibition of TGF-β dependent effects by shRNA against human TGF-β type II receptor. Oncogene 27, 918–930.

Wilmotte R, Burkhardt K, Kindler V *et al* (2005). B7-homolog 1 expression by human glioma: a new mechanism of immune evasion. Neuroreport 16: 1081–5.

Zou JP, Morford LA, Chougnet C *et al* (1999). Human glioma-induced immunosuppression involves soluble factor (s) that alters monocyte cytokine profile and surface markers. J Immunol 162: 4882–4892.

15

Direct Antitumor Activity of Interferon-Induced Dendritic Cells of Healthy Donors and Patients with Primary Brain Tumors

Olga Leplina et al.*
Institute of Clinical Immunology SB RAMS
Russia

1. Introduction

Dendritic cells (DCs) are well known for their capacity to induce adaptive antitumor immune response through their unique ability to uptake, processing and presenting antigens (Ags), and tumor-specific T cell activation. In addition, cytokines produced by dendritic cells are able to regulate the direction and strength of immune response, activate the cytotoxic cells (NK-, NKT-cells) and participate in the coordination of the humoral immune response (Melief, 2008; Banchereau et al., 2000).

An increasing number of reports evidenced that besides this role, DCs may display additional antitumor effects. Indeed, DCs in vitro can inhibit proliferation and provide a direct cytotoxic effect on tumor cells. In this, human monocyte-derived DCs might exert antitumor activity through multiple TNF family members (i.e. TNF-α, lymphotoxin-α1β2, FasL, TRAIL), as well as perforin and/or granzyme (Wesa & Storkus, 2008; Chauvin & Josien, 2008).

Direct tumor cell killing by DCs themselves appear to be highly important since involves immediate presentation of tumor-associated Ags in the context of MHC molecules for recognition by cognate T cells, inducing a specific immune response. Importantly, pleiotropy in DC mechanisms of cytotoxicity allows DCs to overcome the resistance of tumor cells that are heterogeneous with regard to their sensitivity to the various death pathways. A number of evidence suggests that the direct antitumor effect of DCs is not purely in vitro phenomenon, and is implemented in vivo. First, DCs are present in the tumors, and their higher content correlates with a more favorable prognosis (Becker 1999). Second, intra-tumoral injection of intact DC (not loaded with tumor antigen) has been shown to correlate with reduced tumor growth and even regression (Becker et al., 2001; Ehtesham et al., 2003). Finally, it is shown that the intra-tumoral introduction of DCs improves the effectiveness of chemotherapy, which may be due to synergistic effects of cytostatics and DCs (Vanderheyde et al., 2004).

---

* Tamara Tyrinova[1], Marina Tikhonova[1], Ekaterina Shevela[1], Vyacheslav Stupak[2], Sergey Mishinov[2], Ivan Pendyurin[2], Mikhail Sadovoy[2], Alexander Ostanin[1] and Elena Chernykh[1]
[1]*Institute of Clinical Immunology SB RAMS, Russia*
[2]*Institute of Traumatology and Orthopedics,Russia*

Most studies on antitumor activity of DCs in humans were performed with myeloid DCs isolated from peripheral blood or generate in vitro from peripheral blood monocytes in the presence of granulocyte-macrophage colony-stimulating factor (GM-CSF) and interleukin-4 (IL-4). Cytotoxic activity of these DCs was found to be stronger after treatment with type I interferons (IFN) or IFNγ (Liu et al., 2001; Fanger et al., 1999). More recently, monocyte-derived DCs generated in the presence of GM-CSF and IFNα instead of IL-4 were described. Is also known that IFNα-DCs are characterized by a higher expression of some molecules (TRAIL, FasL), which may mediate the cytotoxic/cytostatic activity of DCs (Chauvin & Josien, 2008). Indeed, we have demonstrated that LPS-activated IFNα-DCs inhibit the growth of tumor cell line HEp-2 more efficiently than IL4-DCs (Leplina et al., 2010). However, the antitumor potential of DCs generated in the presence of IFNα, remain virtually unexplored.
Of great relevance is also an issue on safety of DC cytotoxic activity in cancer settings. Recently, we found that in patients with malignant gliomas IFNα-DCs generated in vitro are able to activate Th1 cells and induce an antitumor immune response (Leplina et al., 2007a). Nevertheless, these DCs exhibit several phenotypic and functional features, such as the moderate delay of differentiation/maturation and low capacity to induce the IFNγ-producing T-cells in mixt lymphocyte culture (MLC) (Leplina et al., 2007b). Given the data on the development of immune insufficiency and monocyte dysfunctions in patients with malignant brain tumors (Khonina et al., 2002) the study of various functions of DCs in this pathology is important not only in terms of understanding pathogenesis of the disease, but also to rationale the therapy with dendritic cells. In this article we investigated the cytotoxic potential of human monocyte-derived DCs generated under replacement of IL-4 with IFNα, and compared cytostatic/cytotoxic activities of IFNα-induced DCs in healthy donors and patients with brain tumors.

2. The text of the article

2.1 Materials and methods

2.1.1 Patients

The study was held in 32 healthy volunteers and 37 patients with brain tumors (21 men and 16 women; from 21 to 71 years; median age 37 years). Patients' group included 20 patients with histologically verified gliblastoma (Grade IV), 8 - with astrocytoma (Grade III) and 9 - with angioreticuloma, fibrilyarno-protoplasmic astrocytoma or meningioma (Grade I-II). All studies were performed after receiving a written informed consent.

2.1.2 In vitro differentiation and maturation of DCs

Peripheral blood mononuclear cells (MNCs) were obtained by density gradient centrifugation (Ficoll-Paque, Sigma-Aldrich) of heparinized whole blood samples. Dendritic cells were generated by culturing of plastic-adherent MNC fraction in 6-well plates (Nunclon, Denmark) in RPMI-1640 medium (Sigma-Aldrich), supplemented with 0,3 mg/ml L-glutamine, 5 mM HEPES buffer, 100 μg/ml gentamicin and 5% fetal calf serum (FCS, Sigma-Aldrich), in the presence of recombinant human (rh) GM-CSF (40 ng/ml, Sigma-Aldrich) and rhIFN-α (Roferon-A, 1000 U/ml, Roche, Switzerland) for 4 days (IFNα-DCs) or with rhGM-CSF (40 ng/ml) and IL-4 (40 ng/ml, Sigma-Aldrich) for 5 days (IL4-DCs). The resulting immature DCs were further exposed with 10 μg/ml lipopolysaccharide (LPS E.colli 0114: B4, Sigma-Aldrich) into IFNα-DC and IL4-DC cultures for additional 24h and 48h, respectively. For some experiments DC supernatans generated from LPS-activated IFNα-DCs were collected. The viability of obtained IFNα-DCs or IL4-DCs determined by Trypan blue exclusion was more than 93-95% in all cases.

2.1.3 Cell lines

Tumor cell lines used in this study included leukemia cell line Jurkat (T- lymphoblast cell leukemia) and solid tumor-derived cell lines: epithelial cells of human larynx carcinoma HEp-2 and glioblastoma U-87 were purchased from American Type Culture Collection (Manassas, VA). All cell lines were of human origin, mycoplasma free and were grown under standard cell culture conditions.

2.1.4 Cytotoxicity assay

Generated IFNα-DCs were tested for their cytotoxic activity against various tumor cell lines including Jurkat, HEp-2 and U-87. Before coculture, target cells were labeled with [^{3}H]thymidine (1 μCi/well) for 18 h at 37°C, washed and placed at 10^4/well in 96-well tissue culture plates in RPMI-1640 medium containing 10% FCS. Cell-free supernatants from DC cultures (30%, v/v) or different numbers of effector cells (DCs) were added to tumor cells at effector:target (E:T) ratios of 10:1, 20:1 and 40:1. In some experiments DCs were pre-incubated for 1 h with the following fusion proteins: rhTNFR1/TNFRSF1A Fc chimera (10 μg/ml), rhFas/TNFRSF6/CD95 Fc chimera (10 μg/ml), and rhTRAIL R2/TNFRSF10B Fc chimera (10 μg/ml; all reagents from R & D Systems, USA). After 18 h of culture cells were harvested and thymidine incorporation was measured on a Liquid Scintillation beta-Counter (Packard Instrument, Meriden, CT). Percentage of cytotoxicity was calculated by the formula:

[1 - (cpm in cocultures of tumor and effector cells or DC supernatans/ cpm in tumor cell cultures)] x 100%.

2.1.5 Cytostatic assay

Cytostatic activity of DCs was evaluated by their ability to suppress the proliferation of tumor line cells (HEp-2 and U-87). For this, the target cells (10^3/well) were incubated for 48 h in 96-well plates alone and in the presence of effector cells at E:T ratios about 10:1, 20:1 and 40:1. Cell proliferation was measured by [^{3}H]thymidine incorporation (1 μCi/well for last 24 h). The percentage of cytostatic activity was calculated by the formula:

[1 - (cpm in cultures with effector cells / cpm in control cultures)] x 100%.

2.1.6 Apoptosis detection

To determine the level of apoptosis, HEp-2 tumor cells were preliminary stained with vital dye CFSE (2 mM, Molecular probes, USA) for 15 min, then washed in RPMI-1640/10% FCS and incubated in 96-well tissue culture plates (10^4/well) in the presence of IFNα-DCs at a ratio 10:1 for 18 hours. The number of cell divisions was analyzed by flow cytometry (FACS Calibur, Becton Dickinson, USA) on channel FL1 (CFSE fluorescence) with the emission of 517 nm. The level of apoptosis was detected by DNA intercalating dye 7-AAD (Calboichem, Israel). Results were expressed as a percentage of positive cells to the total cell number in the region studied.

2.1.7 TNFα production

DC-free supernatants collected as deascribe above were measured for soluble TNFα by ELISA using a commercial kit (R & D Systems, USA) according to the manufacturer`s recommendations.

2.1.8 Statistical analysis

The data were expressed as mean ± SE. Statistica 6.0 software for Windows (StatSoft Inc. USA) was used for analysis of data. Statistical comparisons were performed using the nonparametric Mann-Whitney U test. P-values < 0,05 indicate significant differences.

2.2 Results

2.2.1 Cytotoxic activity of donor IFNα-DCs and DC supernatants against tumor cell lines

First, we assessed whether in vitro generated mature IFNα-DCs could lyse tumor cell lines. IFNα-DCs in our study possessed significant dose-dependent cytotoxic activity against [^{3}H]thymidine-labeled tumor cell lines HEp-2 and Jurkat. As illustrated in Fig.1A, Jurkat cells were lysed more efficiently at all E:T cell ratios. The most pronounced differences in cytotoxic activity of IFNα-DCs against Jurkat and HEp-2 were observed at a E:T ratio of 20:1 (35,17 ± 5,6% and 16,44 ± 4,01 %, respectively; P_U=0,027). High cytotoxic activity of IFNα-DCs was also manifested when human glioblastoma U-87 cells were used as targets (Fig.1B). In this case, the cytotoxic potential of DCs at 20:1 was two-fold higher than with HEp-2 cells (38,6 ± 8,3%; P_U=0,049). Taken together, these data indicate that i) mature IFNα-DCs mediated significant antitumor cytotoxic activity, effective at various E:T cell ratios, and ii) the cytotoxic activity of IFNα-DCs against tumor cell lines Jurkat and U-87 unlike HEp-2 cells was considerably higher.

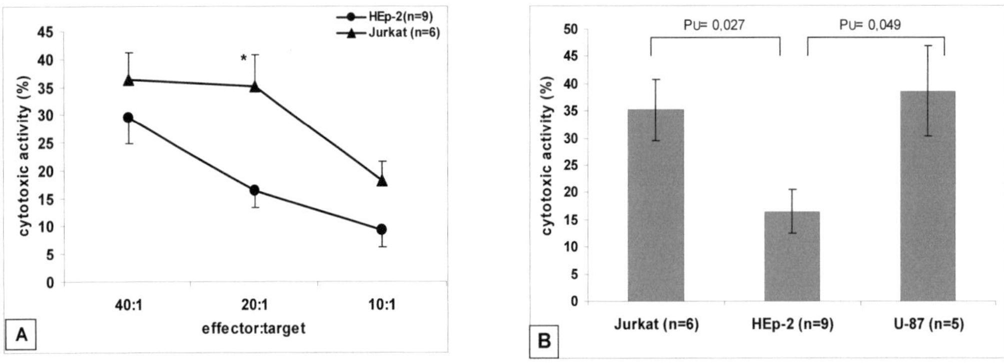

Fig. 1. Cytotoxic activity of donor IFNα-DCs against Jurkat, Hep-2, and U-87. A) The average values of IFNα-DC cytotoxic activity against tumor cell lines Jurkat and HEp-2 are presented. Effector cells (DCs) and [^{3}H]thymidine-labeled target cells (Jurkat and HEp-2) were cultured for 18 h at ratios indicated. B) Cytotoxic activity of IFNα-DCs against Jurkat, HEp-2 and U-87 tumor cells at E:T ratio of 20:1. Results are shown as mean ± SE of triplicate values. * - P_U <0,05 - between HEp-2 and Jurkat at E:T ratio of 20:1 (U - Wilcoxon's test, Mann-Whitney).

To examine the possible mechanisms underlying the cytotoxic activity of IFNα-DCs against tumor cells, we evaluated the cytotoxic activity associated with DC culture-conditioned medium. Contrary to DCs themselves, IFNα-DC culture-conditioned medium lacked cytotoxic activity or had a low ability to lyse tumor cells. Indeed, supernatants of DC cultures added to targets at 30% (v/v) were unable to lyse HEp-2 cells, and had some cytotoxic activity against Jurkat cell line (13,0 ± 1,7%) (Fig.2). These results showed that mediators of DC-associated antitumor activity are more likely cell membrane-bound molecules but not secreted proteins.

2.2.2 Induction of apoptosis of tumor cell line HEp-2 by IFNα-DCs

To investigate whether DC killer activity involved the induction of apoptosis, we next analyzed cell cycle in tumor cells HEp-2 pre-labeled with vital dye CFSE (Fig.3). Co-culturing of CFSE-labeled HEp-2 cells with IFNα-DCs resulted in significant increase in the level of apoptosis detected in tumor cells. In addition, the cultivation of tumor cells with IFNα-DCs was accompanied by a decrease in number of cycling tumor cells (S + G2M phases of the cell cycle). These results showed that DCs in vitro can efficiently induce death of tumor cells using an apoptotic mechanism.

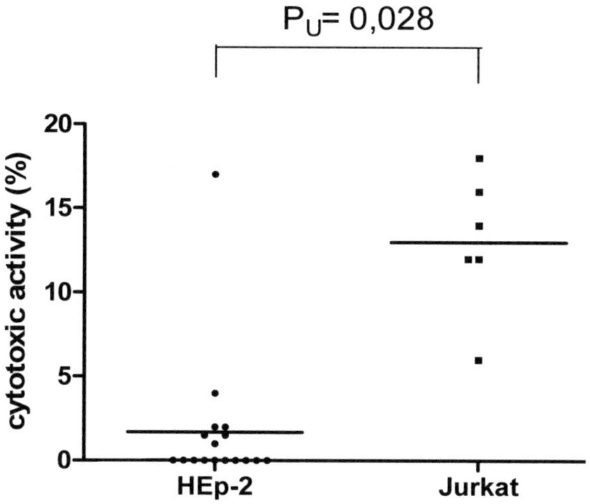

Fig. 2. Cytotoxic activity of DC culture-conditioned medium against Jurkat and HEp-2. The figure represents individual values of cytotoxic activity mediated by supernatants from cultures of healthy donor IFNα-DCs against tumor cell lines HEp-2 (n = 17) and Jurkat (n = 6). Jurkat cells and HEp-2 cells (10^4cells/well) were labeled with [^{3}H]thymidine and incubated with DC culture-conditioned medium (30%, v/v) for 18 hours.

2.2.3 Growth inhibition effect of IFNα-DCs on tumor cell lines HEp-2 and U-87

These data result in the suggestion that the cytotoxic activity of IFNα-DCs is conditioned by induction of apoptosis in tumor cells and that, along with a cytotoxic effect, IFNα-DCs apparently could block cell cycle in tumor cells, thereby providing cytostatic effect. Indeed, analysis of IFNα-DCs impact on the proliferation of tumor cells (Fig. 4) revealed a pronounced antiproliferative effect exerted by donor DCs against the cell line HEp-2.

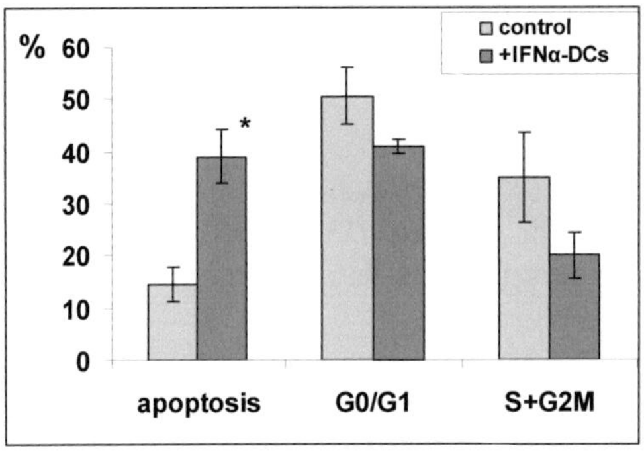

Fig. 3. Effect of IFNα-DCs from healthy donors on the cell cycle in HEp-2. The figure shows the relative content (%) of CFSE-labeled HEp-2 cells in cell cycle phases in the absence of DCs (control; n= 4) and in co-cultures with IFNa-DCs (n= 4) for 18 hours at E:T ratio of 10:1. The data are presented as M ± SE (%). * - P_U<0,01 (U - Wilcoxon's test, Mann-Whitney).

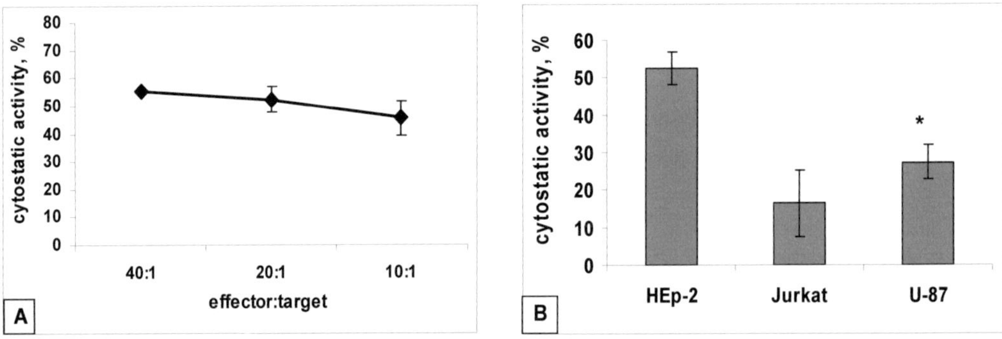

Fig. 4. Tumor-inhibiting activity of IFNα-DCs from healthy donors against HEp-2, Jurkat, and U-87. A) The graph shows the mean values (M ± SE) of cytostatic activity of IFNα-DCs against HEp-2 tumor cells (n = 8). Effector cells (DC) and target cells were cultured at ratios indicated for 24 hours, followed by the introduction of [^{3}H]thymidine for 24 hours. **B)** Cytostatic activity rendered by IFNα-DCs against HEp-2 (n = 8), Jurkat (n = 7) and U-87 (n = 5) in E:T ratio of 20:1. * - P_U <0,05 - between the cytostatic activity of DCs *vs* HEp-2 and U-87 (U - Wilcoxon's test, Mann-Whitney).

Importantly, DCs mediated potent inhibitory activity (45,4 ± 6,24%) even at a low E:T cell ratio (10:1). Moreover, IFNα-DCs also suppressed the proliferation of glioblastoma cell line U-87. However, in this case inhibition was almost two-fold lower, accounting for 27,4 ± 4,4% at E:T ratio of 20:1 *vs* 52,4 ± 4,4% in HEp-2 cultures (p <0,05). Thus, in our study IFNα-DCs were found to be cytostatic for tumor cell lines. Comparative analysis of cytotoxic and cytostatic activity mediated by IFNα-DCs showed no correlations between the level of DC cytotoxicity and their ability to inhibit the proliferation of HEp2 (r_S = 0,21; p = 0,7), U-87 (r_S = 0,5; p = 0,28) and Jurkat (r_S = 0,33; p = 0,5) tumor cell line. The lack of such a relationship was also indicated by the fact that in cultures of U-87 dendritic cells displayed the highest cytotoxic effect while their cytostatic effects were only moderate. Contrary, in cultures of HEp-2 DCs had a relatively low cytotoxic effect and pronounced anti-proliferative activity.

2.2.4 Role of TNFα, FasL and TRAIL in cytotoxic activity of IFNα-DCs

To get inside into the mechanism that could be responsible for DC tumoricidal activity, we have investigated the role of key molecules involved in the apoptosis pathway. Cytotoxic activity of DCs is attributed to the expression of some proapoptotic molecules such as TRAIL, FasL, perforin, granzymes A and B, TNF-α, lymphotoxin-α1, β2 (Chauvin & Josien, 2008). To further characterized the molecular mechanisms by which HEp-2 cell death results from interaction with DCs, we studied the effect of some soluble receptors at the DC-mediated cytotoxic activity. As evident from Fig. 5, pretreatment of IFNα-DCs with TNFR1: Fc resulted in almost complete neutralization of DC cytotoxic activity, whereas pretreatment with soluble forms of TRAIL-R2: Fc and Fas: Fc did not followed by suppression of DC killer activity.

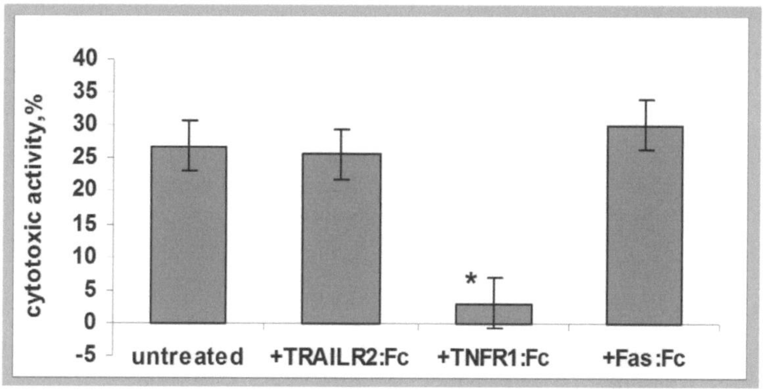

Fig. 5. Neutralization of DC cytotoxic function by soluble forms of R:Fc, specific for TNF-family ligands. [^{3}H]thymidine-labeled tumor cells HEp-2 (10^4 cells/well) were incubated for 18 hours with IFNα-DCs (at E:T ratio of 20:1) pre-treated for 1 h with TRAIL-R2: Fc fusion protein (10 µg/ml; n = 6), or TNFR1: Fc fusion protein (10 µg/ml; n = 6), or Fas: Fc fusion protein (10 µg/ml; n = 6). Data are presented as mean (M ± SE) of cytotoxic activity of IFNα-DCs *vs* HEp-2. * - P_U <0,01 - between intact DCs and DCs treated with TNFR1: Fc (U - Wilcoxon's test, Mann-Whitney).

Thus, our data suggest that lysis of HEp-2 cells is not related with TRAIL- and FasL-mediated cytotoxicity but occurs with the involvement of TNFα molecules, since blocking of TNFα/TNFR1 binding leads to almost full suppression of DC killer activity. Apparently, the involvement only a single of three described mechanisms of DC cytotoxicity is due to resistance of tumor cells HEp-2 to TRAIL-and FasL-mediated apoptosis and determines relatively low cytotoxic activity of DCs against HEp-2 cells compared to Jurkat and U-87 which are sensitive to FasL-and TRAIL-mediated apoptosis (Röhn et al., 2001; Hoves et al., 2003).

2.2.5 Cytotoxic activity of donor IL4-DCs in compared with IFNα-DCs

Since we proposed IFNα-DCs may have a more pronounced antitumor activity than DCs generated with GM-CSF and IL-4, we then investigated whether cytotoxic and cytostatic activities of these two types of LPS-activated DC were distinct. As seen in Fig.6, IFNα-DCs possessed the higher ability to lyse leukemia cells Jurkat (Fig. 6A) and comparable cytotoxic activity in HEp-2 cultures (Fig.6B). However, IFNα-DCs were found to be more effective in suppressing the growth of tumor cell line HEp-2 than IL4-DCs (45 ± 6% *vs* 29 ± 7%, respectively, at E:T ratio of 10:1, P_U <0,05).

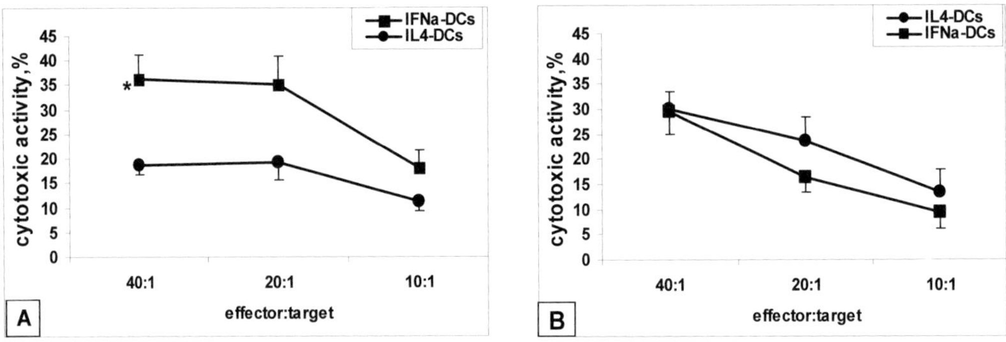

Fig. 6. Cytotoxic activity of IFNα-DCs and IL4-DCs of healthy donors against tumor lines Jurkat (A) and HEp-2 (B). Data are presented as mean (M ± SE) of cytotoxic activity. Effector cells (donor IFNα-DCs and IL4-DCs) were incubated with target cells ([^{3}H]thymidine-labeled tumor cell lines Jurkat and HEp-2) at ratios indicated for 18 h. *- P_U<0,05 – between IFNα-DCs and IL4-DCs against Jurkat (U - Wilcoxon's test, Mann-Whitney).

2.2.6 Cytotoxic activity of patient IFNα-DCs *vs* HEp-2

While donor DCs were found to be tumoricidal, evaluation of the cytotoxic activity of DCs generated in vitro from peripheral blood of brain glioma patients revealed they were significantly less cytotoxic against HEp-2 cells (Fig.7A). The decrease of cytotoxic activity was manifested at all E:T ratios which were analyzed. At the same time assessment of patient DC killer activity at E:T ratio of 20:1 (n=37) allowed to reveal significant heterogeneity for DC cytotoxic potential in patients with brain tumors (Fig.7B). Indeed, in 25 patients (67%) cytotoxic activity was completely absent, whereas remained relatively unaltered in another 12 patients (32%).

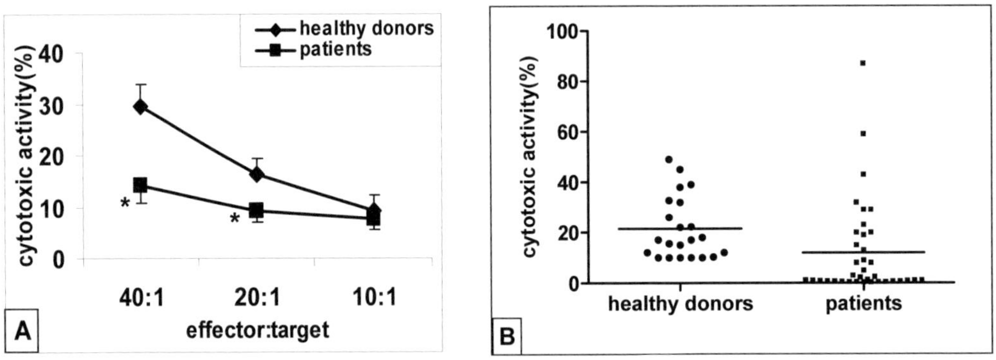

Fig. 7. Cytotoxic activity of IFNα-DCs of patients with brain tumors against HEp-2. **A)** Effector cells (donor and patient IFNα-DCs) were cultured with [^{3}H]thymidine-labeled target cells (HEp-2) for 18 h at ratios indicated. Results are shown as the mean ± SE of DC cytotoxic activity. *- P_U <0,01 - between donor and patient DCs (U - Wilcoxon's test, Mann-Whitney) at E:T ratio of 40:1 and 20:1. **B)** Individual values of cytotoxic activity mediated by IFNα-DCs of healthy donors and brain tumor patients against HEp-2 are presented. Effector cells (DC) were cultured with [^{3}H]thymidine-labeled target cells (HEp-2) for 18 h at ratio of 20:1.

Analysis of patients according to the degree of tumor malignancy demonstrated that the decrease in cytotoxic activity of DCs was typical for patients with high grade (III-IV) gliomas while patients with low grade (I-II) intracerebral gliomas were characterized by unaltered cytotoxic activity (Table 1).

E:T ratio = 20:1	Donors (n=22)	Patients with brain tumors	
		Grade I-II (n=9)	Grade III-IV (n=28)
M ± S.E	21,5 ± 2,6	22,56 ± 5,64	4,75 ± 1,95
Median	17,0	20,0	0
LQ-UQ	10,3- 32,0	13,0- 29,0	0- 4,0

Table 1. Cytotoxic activity of IFNα-DCs in patients with low and high grade glioma

Effector cells (IFNα-DCs) were generated from peripheral blood of healthy donors and patients with low grade (I-II) and high grade (III-IV) gliomas and cultured with [^{3}H]thymidine-labeled target cells (HEp-2) for 18 h at E:T ratio of 20:1. The average values (M ± SE), Median and interquartile range (from low to upper quartile, LQ-UQ) of cytotoxic activity are presented.

Figure 8 shows the individual examples of cytotoxic activity of IFNα-DCs of patients with Grade I-II (n=3) and III-IV (n=3) brain tumors.

2.2.7 Survival rates of patients with intact and reduced levels of IFNα-DC cytotoxic activity vs HEp-2 cells

Considering that the degree of malignancy is predictive factor of patient survival, we further questioned about the survival rates of patients with intact and reduced levels of DC cytotoxic activity against HEp-2 cells (Fig. 9). The criterion for division into such groups was the lower quartile range of cytotoxic activity mediated by donor IFNα-DCs against HEp-2 cells (LQ=10,3%).

Patients with decreased cytotoxic activity of IFNα-DCs (< 10,3%, 1 patient with Grade II and 15 patients with Grade III-IV) differed by a lower survival rate compared with patients of the opposite group. For example, a median of survival in patients with low DC cytotoxic activity was about 13 months, and in the group with unchanged cytotoxic activity of DCs all patients (5 patients with Grade I-II and 4 patients with Grade III) were followed alive.

2.2.8 Growth inhibition effect of patient IFNα-DCs on tumor cell line HEp-2

Next, we investigated whether DCs of patients with brain tumors could inhibit the growth of HEp-2 cells (Table 2). While donor DCs possessed the marked cytostatic activity, IFNα-DCs of patients with intracerebral gliomas were found to be incapable of suppressing the proliferation of HEp-2. Moreover, the addition of DCs led to 3-fold increased tumor cell proliferation. The index of DC impact ranged from 0,5 to 7,2, averaging about 3,06± 0,4. It should be noted that such a stimulatory effect of DCs on HEp-2 cell growth was detected both in patients with high grade III-IV (3,08 ± 0,65; n = 19) and low grade I-II (3,37 ± 1,49; n = 8) tumors, and unlike cytotoxic activity, was independent on the degree of malignancy.

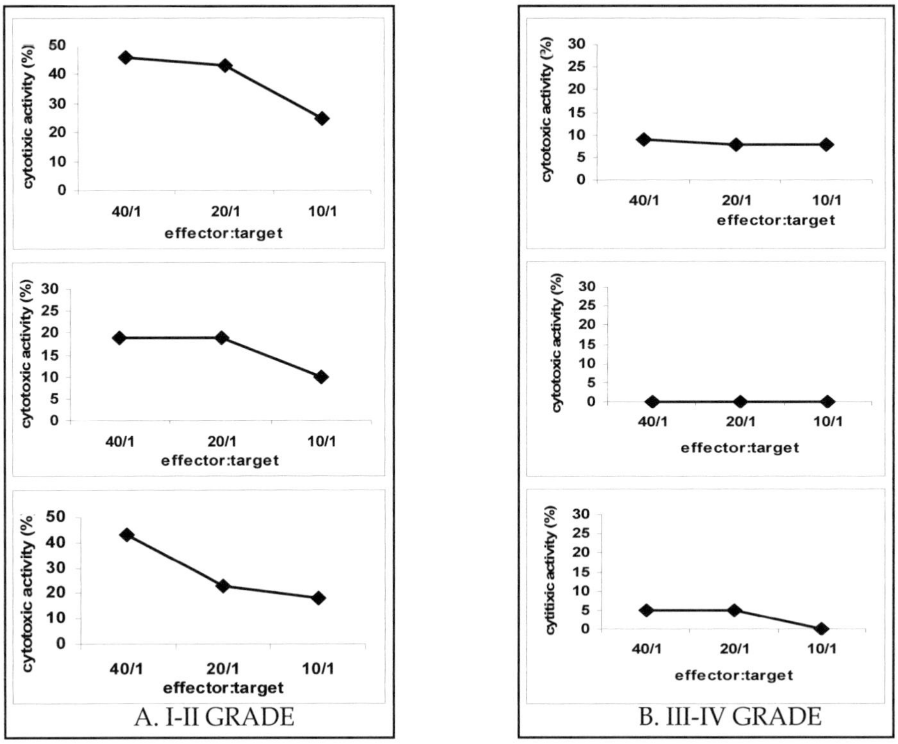

Fig. 8. Cytotoxic activity of IFNα-DCs of individual patients. Figure represents the individual values of cytotoxic activity of IFNα-DCs generated in vitro from peripheral blood of tumor patients against HEp-2. Effector cells (DCs) and [^{3}H]thymidine-labeled HEp-2 cells were co-cultured for 18 h at ratios indicated. Percentage of cytotoxicity was calculated as follows: [1 - (cpm in cultures with target and effector cells / cpm in control cultures without effector cells)] x 100%.

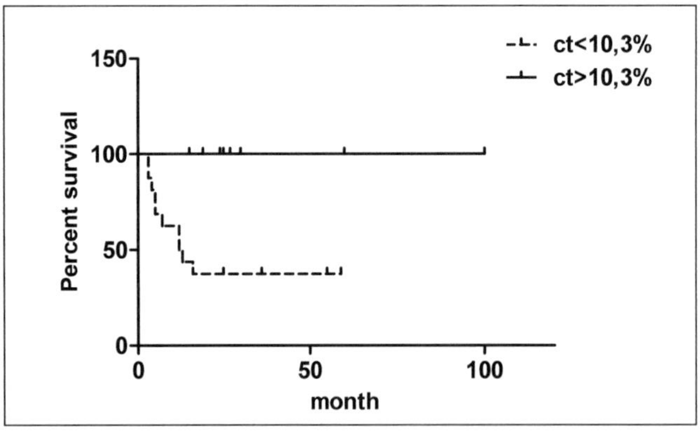

Fig. 9. Survival rates of patients with brain tumors based on the level of DC cytotoxic activity. Dotted line: cytotoxic activity of DCs of patients is below (<10,3%) donor lower quartile values. Solid line: cytotoxic activity of patient DCs is above 10,3%.

The table represents the individual values of indexes of IFNα-DC impact on proliferation of tumor cell line HEp-2. For this, effector cells (DCs) and targets were cultured at 20:1 for 24 hours, followed by the introduction of [^{3}H]thymidine for the next 24 hours. The index of DC impact was calculated by the formula: cpm in cultures with target and effector cells / cpm in control cultures without effector cells. * - P_U <0,01 between donors and patients (U - Wilcoxon's test, Mann-Whitney).

Patients	**Diagnosis**	**DC cytostatic activity (Indexes of DC impact)**
P 1, female, 60 years	Grade 1	5,6
P 2, female, 71 years	Grade 1	6,2
P 3, male, 53 years	Grade 1	0,9
P 4, female, 35 years	Grade 2	7,2
P 5, male, 42 years	Grade 2	3,4
P 6, female, 38 years	Grade 2	0,8
P 7, female, 36 years	Grade 2	0,5
P 8, female, 35 years	Grade 2	0,5
M±SE (n=8)		3,37 ± 1,49
P 9, male, 56 years	Grade 3	5,0
P 10, male, 25 years	Grade 3	3,5
P 11, male, 46 years	Grade 3	0,5
P 12, male, 29 years	Grade 3	2,3
P 13, female, 24 years	Grade 3	3,2
P 14, male, 32 years	Grade 4	3,1
P 15, female, 54 years	Grade 4	5,2
P 16, male, 48 years	Grade 4	3,2
P 17, male, 53 years	Grade 4	2,4
P 18, male,41 years	Grade 4	2,4
P 19, male, 34 years	Grade 4	1,8
P 20, male, 24 years	Grade 4	1,4
P 21, male, 38 years	Grade 4	0,8
P 22, male,47 years	Grade 4	2,3
P 23, female, 45 years	Grade 4	6,9
P 24, female, 58 years	Grade 4	6,5
P 25, female, 60 years	Grade 4	6,9
P 26, female, 71 years	Grade 4	0,8
P 27,female, 57 years	Grade 4	2,0
M±SE (n=19)		3,08 ± 0,645
Patients (n=27)		3,06 ± 0,4*
Healthy donors (n=14)		0,4 ± 0,04

Table 2. Effect of IFNα-DCs of patients with brain tumors on the proliferation of HEp-2 cells

2.2.9 Cytotoxic activity of patient IFNα-DCs vs U-87

In the next experiments, we investigated cytotoxic potential of patient IFNα-DCs towards TRAIL-sensitive tumor line U-87. Interestingly, we found no decrease in killer activity of patient DCs in this case. Furthermore, IFNα-DCs of patients with malignant tumors (Grade III-IV), unable to lyse HEp-2 cells, were highly cytotoxic against U-87 cells compared with healthy donors (Table 3). Further experiments demonstrated the ability of patient DCs to inhibit the proliferation of U-87 cell line which is also more expressed in patients than in donors (46,6 ± 7,5 and 27,4 ± 4,4%, respectively; $P_U < 0,01$). In this, we found a strong positive correlation between cytotoxic and cytostatic activities (r_S = 0,89; p = 0,001). Thus, impairment of cytotoxic and cytostatic activity of patient DCs was only revealed against HEp-2 cells.

Patients	**Diagnosis**	**DC cytotoxic activity (%)**	**DC cytostatic activity (%)**
P 1, male, 36 years	Grade 4	76	54
P 2, male, 24 years	Grade 4	55	28
P 3, female,69 years	Grade 4	39	40
P 4, female, 42 years	Grade 3	60	44
P 5, female, 71 years	Grade 3	57	40
P 6, female, 54 years	Grade 4	60	43
P 7, female, 46 years	Grade 4	56	12
P 8, male, 48 years	Grade 4	80	89
P 9, male, 24 years	Grade 3	69	69
Patients (n=9)		61,3 ± 4,1*	46,6 ± 7,5*
Healthy donors (n=5)		38,6 ± 8,3	27,4 ± 4,4

Table 3. Cytotoxic/cytostatic activity of DCs in patients with brain tumors against U-87. The table represents the individual and average values (M ± SE) of cytotoxic and cytostatic activities of patient and donor DCs. Cytotoxicity was measured by coculturing of DCs and [^{3}H]thymidine-labeled U-87 cells for 18 h at 20:1. For cytostatic activity evaluation, DCs and U-87 cells were cultured at 20:1 for 24 hours, followed by the introduction of [^{3}H]thymidine for 24 hours. * - P_U <0,01 between donors and patients (U - Wilcoxon's test, Mann-Whitney).

2.2.10 TNFα production by donor and patient IFNα-DCs

Since the cytotoxic activity of DCs against HEp-2 cells was related with TNF-mediated apoptosis, we further compared the ability of DCs of patients with malignant gliomas (Grade III-IV) and donors to produce TNFα. The concentration of TNFα was evaluated in 4-

day cultures of LPS-activated IFNα-DCs. As follows from Table 4, supernatants from patient DC cultures differed little from healthy donor culture-conditioned medium by the level of TNFα production. A slight decrease in production of TNFα was a tendency, which had no statistical significance.

Patients	Diagnosis	TNFa (pg/ml)
P 1, male, 39 years	Grade 4	856
P 2, female, 46 years	Grade 3	767
P 3, male, 35 years	Grade 3	800
P 4, male, 46 years	Grade 3	914
P 5, male, 24 years	Grade 4	918
P 6, female, 43 years	Grade 4	693
P 7, female, 38 years	Grade 2	256
P 8, male, 52 years	Grade 4	486
P 9, male, 68years	Grade 3	710
Patients (n=9) M ± SE		711 ± 82
Healthy donors (n=11) M ± SE		824 ± 59

Table 4. TNFα concentrations in cultures of donor and glioma patient IFNα-DCs. The table represents the individual and average values (M ± SE) of TNFα concentrations in culture supernatants of IFNα-DCs generated in vitro from peripheral blood of patients with malignant gliomas and healthy donors.

2.3 Discussion

The ability of DCs generated in vitro to inhibit the growth of human tumor cell lines and lyse tumor cells was first demonstrated by Chapoval (Chapoval et al., 2000). Thereafter, spontaneous cytotoxicity mediated by DCs without any stimulation was also described by other authors (Vanderheyde et al. 2004; Yang et al., 2001; Manna & Mohanakumar, 2002; Joo et al., 2002 ; Janjic et al., 2002), which revealed that the tumoricidal potential of DCs generated in the presence of GM-CSF and IL-4 was mediated by effector molecules such as FasL (Yang et al., 2001), TNF (Manna & Mohanakumar, 2002; Joo et al., 2002), lymphotoxin-α1, β2 (Lu et al., 2002) or TRAIL (Liu et al., 2001). The cytolytic properties of cultured human monocyte-derived DCs are enhanced by certain activation stimuli, such as LPS (Chapoval et al., 2000; Manna & Mohanakumar, 2002). While myeloid DCs being treated with IFN-γ exhibited upregulation of intracellular TRAIL and increased cytotoxic potential (Liu et al., 2001), study of antitumor activity of DCs generated in the presence of IFNα were not performed previously. In this study, we reported the novel data on cytostatic/cytotoxic activities of LPS-activated IFNα-DCs generated in vitro from peripheral blood monocytes of healthy donors and patients with brain tumors.

We report here that LPS-activated IFNα-DCs can lyse both NK-sensitive (Jurkat lymphoma cells) and NK-resistant (HEp-2, U-87) tumor cell lines. Such a cytotoxic effect requires cell contact, since the supernatants of IFNα-DCs either lack or possess the poor cytotoxic activity. Using HEp-2 tumor cells as targets, we revealed that DCs appear to promote the apoptosis and suppress cell cycle in tumor cells, thus having a cytostatic effect. Cytostatic activity was also confirmed by the tumor growth/proliferation inhibiting capacity realized by IFNα-DCs. When compare the cytotoxicity of IFNα-DCs and IL4-DCs, we revealed that IFNα-DCs expressed the higher ability to kill Jurkat tumor cells as well as comparable with IL4-DCs cytotoxic activity in HEp-2 cultures.

Since the highest cytotoxic activity of IFNα-DCs was manifested in U-87 and Jurkat tumor cell cultures, which are reported to be sensitive to TRAIL-induced apoptosis (Lee et al., 2003; Panner et al., 2005; Siegelin et al., 2009), it is reasonable to assume that this cytotoxicity could be due to the stimulative effect of IFNα on TRAIL expression (Riboldi et al., 2009). Indeed, as a further corroboration of the suggested cytotoxic capacity, our data demonstrated that LPS-activated IFNα-DCs were found to contain significantly higher amounts of cells expressing membrane-bound TRAIL compared with IL4-DCs (data not shown). Apparently, these data could also explain a higher cytotoxic activity of IFNα-DCs on Jurkat tumor cells.

There are a very few data on sensitivity of HEp-2 cells to the cytotoxic effect of DCs mediated by TNF family molecules. The tumoricidal activity was not mediated by FasL/Fas or TRAIL/TRAILR2 systems, whereas TNFα/TNFR1 blocking completely abolished the ability of DCs to lyse HEp-2 cells. Thus, tumor cell line HEp-2 cells can be considered as resistant to FasL- and TRAIL-induced apoptosis, but sensitive to cytotoxicity triggered by TNFα/TNFR1 pathway. At that, the fact that anti–TNFα antibody almost completely decreased cytotoxicity, while DC culture-conditioned medium containing quite high concentrations of TNFα lacked lytic activity (Leplina et al., 2007b), further implies that membrane-bound, not the soluble form, of TNFα partially contributes to the effect.

Our results are consistent with the reported data on TNFα expression by HEp-2 cells (Paland et al., 2008), as well as the resistance of this tumor cell line to FasL-induced apoptosis (Morton & Blaho, 2007). The lack of sensitivity HEp-2 cells to TRAIL/TRAILRII-induced death explains the absence of distinction in the cytotoxic activity of IFNα-DCs and IL4-DCs against HEp-2 cells.

Since we revealed no correlations between cytotoxic and cytostatic effects of IFNα-DCs on HEp-2 cells, then one can believe that cytotoxicity and cytostasis could be mediated by distinct mechanisms. Similar tendency was observed for IL4-DCs (Vanderheyde et al., 2004), where the authors have shown that LPS-stimulated IL4-DCs possess TNFα-associated cytostatic activity unrelated with cytotoxicity. Indeed, IL4-DCs inhibited the growth of modified Jurkat cells deficient in caspase-8 or overexpressing Bcl-2. On the other hand, supernatants of IL4-DCs suppressed the proliferation of non-modified Jurkat cells, but showed no cytotoxic activity. Evidently, cytostatic and cytotoxic activities of IFNα-DCs are also implemented through independent mechanisms. This hypothesis could be confirmed by the fact that a higher cytotoxic activity of IFNα-DCs against U-87 and Jurkat cells was associated with less pronounced DC cytostatic activity on these lines compared with HEp-2.

Investigation of the effector functions of IFNα-DCs in patients with intracerebral gliomas revealed impaired ability of these cells to lyse HEp-2 tumor cells. Importantly, such an impairment of DC cytotoxicity was identified mainly in patients with high grade (III-IV) brain tumors, while in low grade (I-II) tumors DCs were quite effective killers. Furthermore, patients with intact DC cytotoxic activity had a higher survival rate than patients with reduced killer activity. In addition, patient DCs regardless of tumor histology showed no cytotoxic activity against HEp-2 cells, whereas both cytotoxic and cytostatic activities of DCs against U-87 cells were found to be enhanced.

According to the data, glioblastoma cells U-87 are resistant to cytotoxicity mediated by TNFα (Sawada et al., 2004), and sensitive to TRAIL- (Knight et al., 2001) and Fas-induced apoptosis (Choi et al., 2004). As we have found, DC cytotoxicity on HEp-2 cells likely engaged TNF/TNFR1 pathway than TRAIL or FasL effects. Given these facts, the high cytotoxic activity of patient DCs against U-87 cells and dramatic decline of such activity against HEp-2 tumor cells could indicate a defect in TNFα-related mechanism of DC cytotoxicity in patients with malignant gliomas.

Our facts seemed to be important in several aspects. First, the defect in cytotoxic activity of DCs may be of interest in diagnosis and prognosis, since the expression of cytotoxic activity is associated with tumor malignancy and survival rates. Second, this phenomenon is of interest from the pathogenetic point of view. Malignant brain tumors induce a weak antigen-specific response due to tumor-induced immunosuppression, as well as localization of the tumor in the immunologically privileged brain tissues (Parney et al., 2000). We have previously shown that patient IFNα-DCs are characterized by intact antigen-presenting function, capable of activating T cells to produce Th1 cytokines and induce proliferation of T lymphocytes to antigens of tumor cell lysates (Chernykh et al., 2009). Then impairment of DC effector functions may inhibit the early induction of antigen-specific immune response being yet another reason for infringement of anti-tumor protection in patients with malignant brain tumors.

We can also assume that if tumoricidal potential of DCs is disturbed, cytoreductive therapy (radio-chemotherapy) becomes especially important, both in regard of direct elimination of tumor cells and release of tumor antigens required to start specific immune response.

However, whether IFNα-DCs could effectively destroy primary glioma cells and does this ability is disrupted in patients with malignant gliomas remains to find. Most of glioblastoma cell lines and primary cells gliomas are absolutely resistant to cytotoxic effect of certain proapoptogenic molecules, such as TRAIL (Eramo et al., 2005) and TNF. At that, the effective destruction of tumor lines by DCs requires the interaction of separate molecules. Besides, it is shown that some proapoptogenic molecules could induce the expression of receptors for another mediators of apoptosis. Such as, TNFα can induce the expression of Fas and sensitize glioma cells to FasL/Fas-mediated apoptosis (Weller et al., 1994).

The further elucidation of the DC cytotoxic/static activity mechanisms and the possible role of the defect of DC cytotoxic properties in patients with gliomas as weel as the studies on correlation between the antitumor activity of IFNα-DCs and clinical outcomes could probably explain the different sensitivity of cancer patients to the treatment, and justify new immunotherapeutic approaches to the treatment of malignant brain gliomas.

3. Conclusion

The capacity of IFNα-DCs to lyse tumor cell lines and inhibit their proliferation has been investigated. LPS-activated IFNα-DCs of healthy donors were shown to have dose-dependent cytotoxic and cytostatic activity against various tumor lines through the induction of apoptosis and arrest of cell cycle. DCs lysed both TRAIL-sensitive (Jurkat cells) and TRAIL-resistant (HEp-2) cells, and cytotoxic activity against HEp-2 line was mediated through the TNF-TNFR1 pathway. In contrast to healthy donors, DCs of patients with malignant glioma failed to inhibit growth, but stimulated proliferation of HEp-2 cells. In addition, patient DCs had significantly reduced cytotoxic activity against HEp-2 cells. Patients with decreased cytotoxic activity were characterized by significantly lower survival since defect of cytotoxic activity was associated with high-grade glioma. The defective cytotoxic activity of DCs noted against HEp-2 cells was not revealed against glioblastoma U-

87 line. The data obtained suggest that defect of antitumor activity of patient DCs may have diagnostic and prognostic significance. However, whether IFNα-DCs could effectively destroy primary glioma cells and does this ability play role in pathogenesis of brain glioma remains to be clarified.

4. Acknowledgment

We are grateful to our patients for their courage and faith in us.

5. References

Banchereau, J., Briere, F., Caux, C., Davoust, J., Lebecque, S., Liu, Y., Pulendran, B. & Palucka K. (2000). Immunobiology of dendritic cells. *Annual Review of Immunology*, Vol.18, pp.767-811

Becker, Y. (1993). Dendritic cell activity against primary tumors: an overview. *In Vivo*, Vol.7, pp. 187-191

Becker, Y., Tong, Y., Song, W. & Crystal, R. (2001). Combined intratumoral injection of bone marrow-derived dendritic cells and systemic chemotherapy to treat pre-existing murine tumors. *Cancer Research*, Vol.61, pp. 7530-7535

Chapoval, A., Tamada, K. & Chen, L. (2000). In vitro growth inhibition of a broad spectrum of tumor cell lines by actvated human dendritic cells. *Blood,* Vol..95, No.7, (April 2000), pp.2346-2351

Chauvin, C. & Josien, R. (2008). Dendritic cells as killers: mechanistic aspects and potential roles. *The Journal of Immunology*, Vol.181, pp.11–16

Chernykh, E., Leplina, O., Stupak, V., Pendurin, I., Nikonov S., Tikhonova, M. & Ostanin A. (2009). Cell technologies in the treatment of malignant brain gliomas. Cell technology. Theoretical and applied aspects, Kozlov, V., Sennikov, S., Chernykh, E., Ostanin, A. pp.240-276, *Nauka*, Novosibirsk, Russia

Choi, C., Jeong, E. & Benveniste, E. (2004). Caspase-1 Mediates Fas-Induced Apoptosis and is Up-Regulated by Interferon-γ in Human Astrocytoma Cells. *Journal of Neuro-Oncology,* Vol.67, No.1-2, pp. 167-176

Ehtesham, M., Kabos, M., Gutierrez, K., Samoto, K., Black, J. & Yu, S. (2003). Intratumoral dendritic cell vaccination elicits potent tumoricidal immunity against malignant glioma in rats. *Journal of Immunotherapy*, Vol.26, pp. 107-116

Eramo, A., Pallini, R., Lotti, F., Sette, G., Patti, M., Bartucci, M., Ricci-Vitiani, L., Signore, M., Stassi, G., Larocca, L., Crino, L., Peschle, C. & De Maria, R. (2005). Inhibition of DNA Methylation Sensitizes Glioblastoma for Tumor Necrosis Factor–Related Apoptosis-Inducing Ligand–Mediated Destruction. *Cancer Research,* Vol.65, No.24, (December), pp.11469-11477

Fanger, N., Maliszewski, C., Schooley, K. & Griffith, T. (1999). Human dendritic cells mediate cellular apoptosis via tumor necrosis factor-related apoptosis-inducing ligand (TRAIL). *Journal of Experimental Medicine*, Vol.190, pp.1155-1164

Hoves, S., Krause, S., Schölmerich, J. & Fleck, M. (2003). The JAM-assay: optimized conditions to determine death-receptor-mediated apoptosis. *Methods,* Vol.31, pp.127-134

Janjic, B., Lu, G., Pimenov, A., Whiteside, T., Storkus, W., & Vujanovic, N. (2002). Innate direct anticancer effector function of human immature dendritic cells. I.

Involvement of an apoptosis-inducing pathway. *The Journal of Immunology*, Vol.168, (February 2002) pp.1823-1830

Joo, H., Fleming, T., Tanaka, Y., Dunn, T., Linehan, D., Goedegebuure, P. & Eberlein, T. (2002). Human dendritic cells induce tumor-specific apoptosis by soluble factors. *International Journal of Cancer*, Vol.102, pp.20-28

Khonina, N., Tsentner, M., Leplina, O., Tikhonova, M., Stupak, V., Nikonov, S., Chernykh, E. & Ostanin, A. (2002). Characteristics and mechanisms of immune disorders in patients with malignant brain tumors. *Oncology issues*, Vol.48, No.2, pp.196-201

Knight, M., Riffkin, C., Muscat, A., Ashley, D. & Hawkins, C. (2001). Analysis of FasL and TRAIL induced apoptosis pathways in glioma cells. *Oncogene*, Vol.20, No.41, pp. 5789-5798

Lee, N., Cheong, H., Kim, S-J., Kim, S-E., Kim, C-K., Lee, K., Park, S., Baick, S., Hong, D., Park H. & Won, J. (2003). Ex vivo purging of leukemia cells using tumor-necrosis-factor-related apoptosis-inducing ligand in hematopoietic stem cell transplantation. *Leukemia*, Vol.17, pp. 1375–1383

Leplina, O., Stupak, V., Kozlov, Yu., Pendyurin, I., Nikonov, S., Tikhonova, M., Sycheva, N., Ostanin, A. & Chernykh, E. (2007). Use of Interferon-α-Induced Dendritic Cells in the Therapy of Patients with Malignant Brain Gliomas. *Cell Technologies in Biology and Medicine*, No.2, pp. 92-98 –a

Leplina, O., Tikhonova, M., Kozlov, Yu., Stupak, V., Ostanin, A. & Chernykh, E. (2007). Characteristics of IFNα-indused dendritic cells in malignant brain gliomas patients. *Bulletin of SB of RAMS*, Vol.124, pp.27-33- b

Leplina, O.,Tikhonova, M., Tyrinova, T., Ostanin, A., Bogachev, S. & Chernykh, E. (2010). Comparative characteristics of surface markers and cytokines produced in the populations of dendritic cells generated in the presence of interferon-alpha and interleukin-4. *Immunology in press*

Leplina, O., Tyrinova, T., Tikhonova, M., Stupak, V., Mishinov, S., Pendurin, I., Ostanin, A. & Chernykh, E. (2010). Anti-tumor activity of dendritic cells in healthy donors and patients with brain tumors *Medical Immunology*, Vol.12, No.3, pp.199-206

Liu, S., Yu, Y., Zhang, M., Wang, W. & Cao, X. (2001). The involvement of TNF-α- related apoptosis-inducing ligand in the enhanced cytotoxicity of IFN-β-stimulated human dendritic cells to tumor cells. *The Journal of Immunology*, Vol.166, pp.5407–5415

Lu, G., Janjic, B., Janjic, J., Whiteside, T., Storkus, W. & Vujanovic, N. (2002). Innate direct anticancer effector function of human immature dendritic cells. II. Role of TNF, lymphotoxin -1-2, Fas ligand, and TNF-related apoptosis-inducing ligand. *The Journal of Immunology*, Vol.168, pp.1831-1840

Manna, P.& Mohanakumar,T. (2002). Human dendritic cell mediated cytotoxicity against breast carcinoma cells in vitro. *Journal of Leukocyte Biology*, Vol.72, (August 2002), pp.312-320

Melief, C. (2008). Cancer immunotherapy by dendritic cells. *Immunity*, Vol.29, pp. 372-383

Morton, E. & Blaho, J. (2007). Herpes simplex virus blocks Fas-mediated apoptosis independent of viral activation of NF-kappaB in human epithelial HEp-2 cells. *Journal of Interferon Cytokine Research*, Vol.27, No.5, (May 2007), pp.365-376

Paland, T., Bohme, L., Gurumurthy, R., Maurer, A., Szczepek, A. & Rudel, T. (2008). Reduced Display of Tumor Necrosis Factor Receptor I at the Host Cell Surface

Supports Infection with Chlamydia trachomatis. *The Journal of Biological Chemistry*, Vol.283, No.10, (March 2008), pp. 6438–6448

Panner, A., James, C., Berger, M. & Piepe, R. (2005). mTOR controls FLIPS translation and TRAIL sensitivity in glioblastoma multiforme cells. *Molecular Cell Biology*, Vol.25, No.20, pp. 8809–8823

Parney, I., Hao, C. & Petruk, K. (2000). Glioma immunology and immunotherapy. *Neurosurgery*, Vol.46, pp.778-791

Riboldi, E., Daniele, R., Cassatella, M., Sozzani, S. & Bosisio D. (2009). Engagement of BDCA-2 blocks TRAIL-mediated cytotoxic activity of plasmacytoid dendritic cells. *Immunobiology*, Vol.214, pp.868–876

Röhn, T., Wagenknecht, B., Roth, W, Naumann, U., Gulbins, E., Krammer, P., Walczak, H. & Weller, M. (2001). CCNU-dependent potentiation of TRAIL/Apo2L-induced apoptosis in human glioma cells is p53-independent but may involve enhanced cytochrome c release. *Oncogene*, Vol.20, No.31, pp. 4128-4137

Sawada, M., Kiyono, T., Nakashima, S., Shinoda, J., Naganawa. T., Hara, S., Iwama, T. & Sakai, N. (2004). Molecular mechanisms of TNFα-induced ceramide formation in human glioma cells: P53-mediated oxidant stress-dependent and -independent pathways. *Cell Death and Differentiation*, Vol.11, pp.997–1008

Siegelin, M., Reuss, D., Habel, A., Rami, A. & von Deimling, A. (2009) Quercetin promotes degradation of survivin and thereby enhances death-receptor–mediated apoptosis in glioma cells. *Neuro-Oncology*, Vol.11, No.2 (April 2009), pp.122-131

Vanderheyde, N., Vandenabeele, P., Goldman M. & Willems F. (2004). Distinct mechanisms are involved in tumoristatic and tumoricidal activities of monocyte-derived dendritic cells. *Immunology Letters*, Vol.91, No. 2

Wesa, A. & Storkus, W. (2008). Killer dendritic cells: mechanisms of action and therapeutic implications for cancer. *Cell Death & Differentiation*, Vol.15, pp. 51-57

Weller, M., Frei, K., Groscurth, P., Krammer, P., Yonekawa, Y. & Fontana A. (1994). Anti-Fas/APO-1 antibody-mediated apoptosis of cultured human glioma cells. Induction and modulation of sensitivity by cytokines. *Journal of Clinical Investigation*, Vol. 94, No.3 (September 1994), pp. 954–964

Yang, R., Xu, D. Zhang, A. &. Gruber, A. (2001). Immature dendritic cells kill ovarian carcinoma cells by a FAS/FASL pathway, enabling them to sensitize tumor-specific CTLs. *International Journal of Cancer*, Vol.94, No.3, pp.407-413

Part 5

Glioma Model and Culture Systems

16

Animal Models of Glioma

Lijun Sun
Department of Neurosurgery, Tianjin Huanhu Hospital
P.R. China

1. Introduction

Gliomas are the most common primary tumors that arise from glial cells and their precursors in the central nervous system. Animal models always are important tool in the study of tumorigenesis, various therapy or preclinical trials for gliomas. It has been known since the 1970's that repetitive intravenous administration of nitrosourea compounds such as methynitrosourea (MNU) and N-ethyl-N-nitrosourea (ENU) produces glial-type neoplasms in immunocompetent rats. However, the long time required to induce neoplasms, and inconsistency of tumor development, led to a shift towards implantation of neoplastic cells propagated in vitro. Implantation of rodent glioma cells has proven an excellent intracranial brain tumor model due to their efficient tumorigenesis, reproducible and fast growth rates and accurate knowledge of the tumor location. Over the past few decades, several mouse glioma models have been generated based on human genetic abnormalities and the induced gliomas exhibit histological similarities to their human counterparts. More accurate animal models are required for research on the molecular and genetic bases of this disease. Here we expand on the existing animal models for gliomas with different strategies.

2. Classification

While there exist a multitude of methods for introducing glial-type neoplasms into the rodent central nervous system (CNS), which histologically mimic human primary tumors, these methods can be described as belonging to one of two groups: 1) Tumors created by methods which do not target a specific gene, and 2) Tumors created by targeted mutation of genes known to be mutated in human tumors.

2.1 Traditional animal models of glioma

While the majority of these models involve the use of rodent glioma cells injected in syngeneic hosts, it is also possible to use human glioma cells in vivo via their implantation in athymic mice. We will describe both of the two classes of glioma animal models, and eight commonly used rat brain tumor models and their application for the development of novel therapeutic and diagnostic modalities.

The rat has been one of the most widely used experimental animals, and rat brain tumor models have been used extensively since the mid 1970s. Here we will focus on rat brain tumor models and their utility in evaluating the efficacy of various therapeutic modalities. Until recently, murine models (Fomchenko & Holland, 2006) were used less frequently than rat models, but the ability to produce genetically engineered cell lines (Lampson, 2001) has increased the use of murine models over the past five years. The relative advantages of rat and murine tumor models are summarized in Table 1. Feline and canine models have been used less frequently (Kimmelman & Nalbantoglu, 2007), but nevertheless, still provide an intermediate between rodent models and humans.

2.1.1 Rat brain tumor models

It was first reported in the early 1970s that CNS tumors could be induced reproducibly and selectively in adult rats that had been given repeated, weekly intravenous injections of MNU or a single dose of ENU. These studies led to the development of a number of rat brain tumor models that were highly reproducible and did not require the toxic application of a chemical carcinogen to the brain (Candolfi et al, 2007).

	Advantages	Disadvantages
1.	Larger size of the rat brain (compared to the mouse brain ~1200 mg vs ~ 400 mg) permits more precise stereotactic implantation than in mice, a longer interval of time until death and a thicker skull essentially eliminates osseous invasion and s.c. growth.	Rat brain tumor models cannot be as easily genetically engineered and manipulated as mouse models in order to elucidate the importance of genetic factors, signaling pathways, cell types and stroma in tumor growth and invasion.
2.	Larger tumor size prior to death permits better in vivo localization and imaging by a variety of diagnostic modalities in the rat.	The potential to produce genetically engineered tumor cell lines is less in the rat than in the mouse.
3.	Larger tumor size prior to death permits the administration of larger amounts of various therapeutic agents, especially if administered i.c. by CED and more critical evaluation of their effectiveness.	There are a smaller number of mAbs directed against rat surface antigens and chemokines compared to the mouse.
4.	More extensive literature on in vitro and in vivo studies of rat brain tumors compared to mouse tumors.	Rats are more expensive to purchase and maintain than mice.

Table 1. Advantages and disadvantages of rat brain tumor models compared to mouse models.

The cellular signaling pathways important for the genesis of brain tumor are multiple, with feedback mechanisms that can dramatically affect the efficacy of molecularly targeted therapeutic strategies. The heterogeneous composition of human high grade gliomas, which consists of tumor stem cells and differentiated tumor cells with varying characteristics, further complicates their susceptibility to treatment. Brain tumors also can evolve within their microenvironment, adapting to changes that produce epigenetic effects thereby altering their biology, but concomitantly providing additional targets for therapeutic intervention. Finally, genetic variations between individuals can dictate how tumors initiate, progress, and respond to treatment. Rat brain tumor models have provided a wealth of information on the in vitro and in vivo responses to various therapeutic modalities. The larger rat brain (~1200 mg) compared to that of the mouse (~400 mg) allows for more precise tumor cell implantation, and relatively larger volumes (~20 µl) that can be injected versus mice (5 µl; Table 1). Mouse models, on the other hand, have allowed researchers to rigorously test hypotheses developed from examining human tumors by genetically manipulating them and controlling specific variables such as environmental influences, in order to better understand the roles of different pathways, cell types, stromal factors and genetic variation (Reilly et al, 2008). Mouse tumor models (Table 1) also have allowed researchers to test hypotheses derived from examining human tumors, in a controlled environment with specific genetic alterations and controlled environmental influences (Reilly et al, 2008). There is a general consensus that valid brain tumor models should fulfill the following criteria: (1) they should be derived from glial cells; (2) it should be possible to grow and clone them in vitro as continuous cell lines and propagate them in vivo by serial transplantation; (3) tumor growth rates should be predictable and reproducible; (4) the tumors should have glioma-like growth characteristics within the brain including neovascularization, alteration of the bloodbrain barrier (BBB), an invasive pattern of growth, and lack of encapsulation; (5) host survival time following i.c. tumor implantation should be of sufficient duration to permit therapy and determination of efficacy; (6) for therapy studies, the tumors should be either non or weakly immunogenic in syngeneic hosts; (7) they should not grow into the epidural space or extend beyond the brain and finally (8) their response or lack thereof to conventional treatment should be predictive of the response in human brain tumors.

In studies carried out prior to the 1970s, either cells or tumor fragments were injected i.c. using a free hand approach, which generally lacked reproducibility and precision. A stereotactic implantation procedure using suspensions of tissue-culture-derived brain tumor cells was more successful (Barker et al, 1973). This procedure was further improved by the use of concentrated cell suspensions in small volumes, improved injection needles, better stereotactic localization to structures deeper in the white matter such as the caudate nucleus, the use of slower injection rates (Landen et al, 2004), 0.5–1.0% low gelling agarose to prevent backflow of tumor cells through the injection track (Kobayashi et al, 1980) and cleansing of the operative field with a solution of Betadine. Finally, rinsing the surface of the brain with sterile water destroys extravasated tumor cells by osmosis prior to closure of the skull with bone wax has also been recommended. This implantation procedure resulted in high success rates of i.c. tumor growth with the elimination of spinal and extracranial dissemination. The implantation of plastic (Kobayashi et al, 1980)or metallic screws (Lal et al, 2000) with an entry port, which are permanently implanted in the skull to inject tumor cells, have been very useful (Saini et al, 2004). Such devices can be left in place either at the time of or after tumor cell implantation in order to facilitate future administration of therapeutic agents at the same location without further stereotactic surgery. These are well tolerated and non-irritating in rats, but they cannot be as easily used in mice due to the thinness of their skulls. Keeping these general principles of tumor cell implantation in mind, we will now discuss the currently available rat glioma models that have been used in immunocompetent animals.

The C6 glioma was produced by Benda et al. (Benda et al, 1968)and Schmidek et al. (Schmidek et al, 1971), in Sweet's laboratory at the Massachusetts General Hospital (MGH) by repetitively administering MNU to outbred Wistar rats over a period of approximately 8 months. When animals developed neurological signs, they were euthanized, and the tumors were excised and explanted into tissue culture. Among these was a tumor designated as "#6", which was subsequently cloned by Benda et al. and was shown to produce S-100 protein. Following cloning, it was redesignated "C6" (Pfeiffer et al, 1970). The C6 glioma is composed of a pleomorphic population of cells with variably shaped nuclei. There is focal invasion into contiguous normal brain (Fig. 1a). Initially, the tumor was histopathologically classified as an astrocytoma, and eventually it was designated as a glial tumor following accession by the American Type Culture Collection, Rockville, MD (ATCC# CCL-107). The cells have been reported to have a mutant p16/Cdkn2a/ Ink4a locus (Schlegel et al, 1999) with no expression of p16 and p19ARF mRNAs, and a wildtype p53 (Asai et al, 1994). More recent molecular characterization, which compared changes in gene expression between the C6 glioma and rat stem cell-derived astrocytes, revealed that the changes in gene expression observed in the C6 cell line were the most similar to those reported in human brain tumors (Sibenaller et al, 2005). Compared to astrocytes, they also had increased expression of the PDGFβ, IGF-1, EGFR and Erb3/Her3 genes, which are frequently overexpressed in human gliomas (Guo et al, 2003; Heimberger et al,2005). In a recent study, the significance of PDGF in gliomagenesis in adult rats was established by infecting white matter with a retrovirus encoding for PDGF and GFP. Within 2 weeks 100% of the animals had tumors derived from both infected and uninfected glial progenitors, thereby implicating PDGF in both autocrine and paracrine stimulation of glial progenitor cells (Assanah et al, 2006). Although, IGF-1 was overexpressed in C6 glioma cells, there was reduced expression of IGF-2, FGF-9 and FGF-10 relative to astrocytes. Similar to the increased activity of the Ras pathway observed in human gliomas (Nakada et al, 2005), C6 cells also had an increase in both Ras expression and Ras guanine triphosphate activator protein (Sibenaller et al, 2005). However, contrary to what has been reported for human GBM, there was an increase in expression of Rb in these cells (Sibenaller et al, 2005). A subclone of C6 cells, stably expressing β-galactosidase, subsequently was described (Lampson et al, 1993) and this has permitted in vivo immunohistochemical analysis of these tumors in the brain. This clone is available through the ATCC (# CRL-2303). However, it must be noted that the β-galactosidase marker protein itself can serve as a tumor antigen, and immunization of rats against the reporter gene protected the animals against tumor growth.

The C6 rat glioma model has been widely used in experimental neuro-oncology to evaluate the therapeutic efficacy of a variety of modalities, including chemotherapy (Doblas et al, 2008), antiangiogenic therapy (Solly F et al, 2008), proteosome inhibitors (Ahmed et al, 2008), treatment with toxins (Zhao et al, 2008), radiation therapy (Sheehan et al, 2008), photodynamic therapy (Mannino et al, 2008), oncolytic viral therapy (Yang et al, 2004) and gene therapy (Tanriover et al, 2008). Since this tumor arose in an outbred Wistar rat, however, there is no syngeneic host in which it can be propagated. This is a very serious limitation that diminishes its usefulness for survival studies since the tumor is immunogenic, even in Wistar rats. The C6 glioma has been demonstrated to be immunogenic in Wistar and BDX rats (Parsa et al, 2000), and it therefore is not useful for evaluating the efficacy of immunotherapy. This problem is exemplified by prior studies in which C6 glioma cells were transfected with an antisense cDNA expression vector that downregulated the constitutive production of IGF-1 (Trojan et al, 1993). Not recognizing that the tumor was of Wistar origin, the authors unfortunately used BD IX rats, which they thought was the strain of origin, due to some ambiguity in the literature. Subsequently, it was reported that BD IX rats, which had been immunized with the C6 anti-sense IGF-1 transfected cells, were resistant to both s.c. and i.c. challenge of the C6 glioma. Similarly, Wistar rats, bearing C6 gliomas (s.c. or i.c.), developed potent humoral and cellular immune

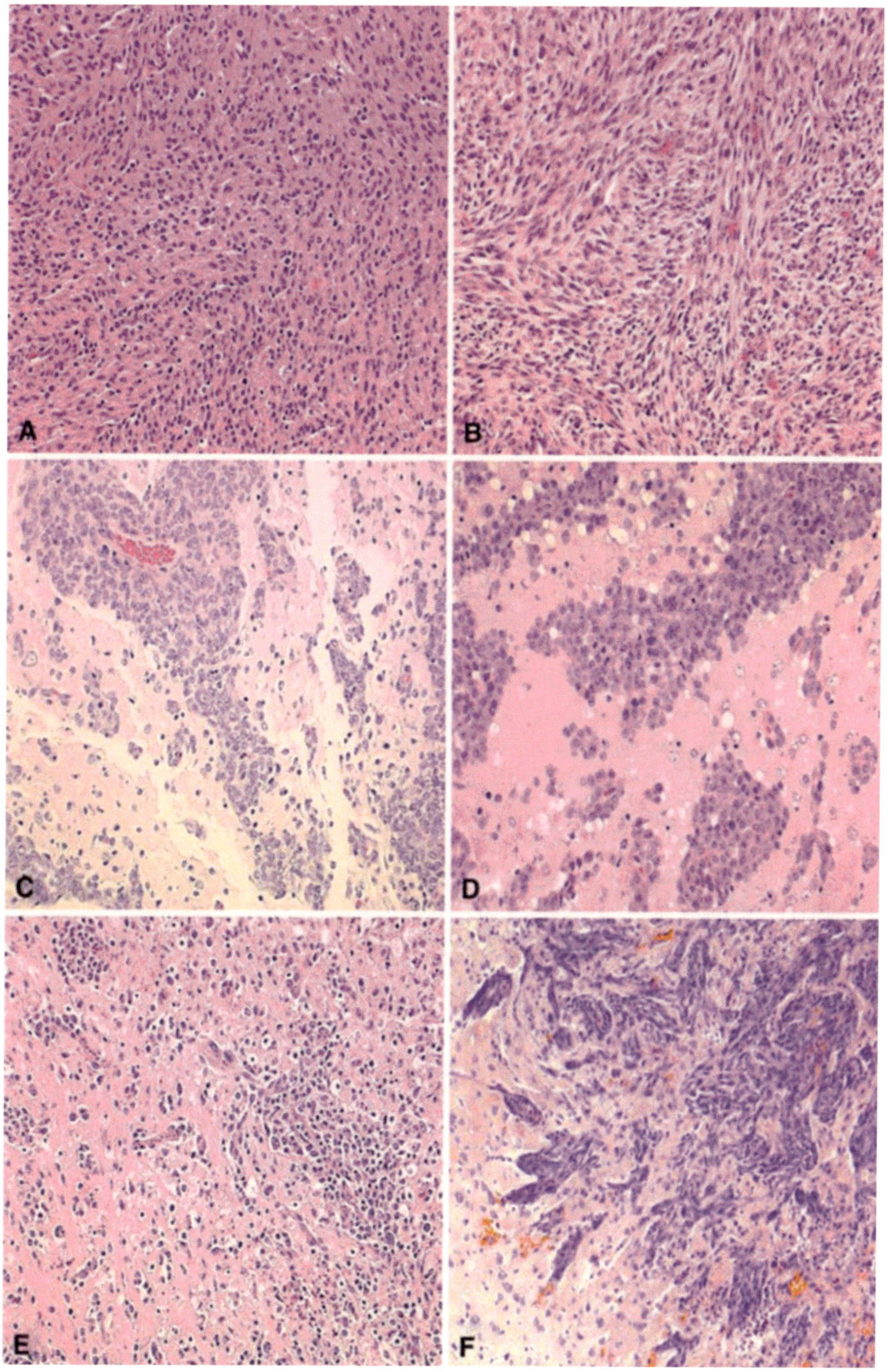

Fig. 1. Histopathologic features of the C6, 9L, RG2, F98, CNS-1, and BT4C brain tumors. A The C6 glioma is composed of a pleomorphic population of cells with nuclei ranging from round to oblong. A herring-bone pattern of growth is seen in some areas and there is focal invasion of contiguous normal brain. There are scattered foci of necrosis with pseudo-palisading of tumor

cells at the periphery. B The 9L gliosarcoma is composed of spindle-shaped cells with a sarcomatoid appearance. A whorled pattern of growth is seen with sharp delineation of the margins of the tumor with little invasion of contiguous normal brain. C The RG2 glioma is very similar in appearance to the F98 glioma and also has a highly invasive pattern of growth. D The F98 glioma is composed of a mixed population of spindle-shaped cells with fusiform nuclei, frequently forming a whorled pattern of growth, and a smaller subpopulation of polygonal cells with round to oval nuclei. There is extensive invasion of contiguous normal brain with islands of tumor cells at varying distances from the main tumor mass, which form perivascular clusters. Usually, there is a central area of necrosis filled with tumor cell ghosts. E The CNS-1 glioma is composed of a pleomorphic population of cells that show great variation in size and shape. There is extensive invasion of contiguous normal brain with dense infiltrates in some areas and in others, more circumscribed clusters of tumor cells. Small foci of hemorrhage are scattered through the tumor. F The BT4C glioma is composed of a pleomorphic population of tumor cells with a sarcomatous pattern of growth. Scattered tumor giant cells are seen and mitotic figures are frequent. The tumor grows expansively and invades the surrounding normal brain along perivascular tracts and occasional tumor cell nests are seen in the surrounding normal brain. There is neo-vascularization, especially in the tumor periphery, where microhemorrhages are frequent. Central necrosis is usually not present but occasionally scattered areas of necrosis may be seen in larger tumors. All photomicrographs are at a magnification of 200×, except for F

responses to the tumor, and rats challenged simultaneously with s.c. and i.c. tumors, had a survival rate of 100% (Parsa et al, 2000). Since C6 glioma cells are allogeneic in all inbred strains, this should provide a strong cautionary note for studies employing this tumor model and they should not be used for immunotherapy studies. Despite this limitation, the C6 glioma model continues to be used for a variety of studies related to brain tumor biology (Karmakar et al, 2007). These have included studies on tumor growth, invasion, migration, BBB disruption, neovascularization, growth factor regulation and production, and biochemical studies (Assadian et al, 2008). Finally, single-cell clonal analysis has revealed that C6 cells also have cancer stem cell-like characteristics, including self-renewal, the potential for multi-lineage differentiation in vitro and tumor formation in vivo (Shen et al, 2008).

The 9L gliosarcoma has been the most widely used experimental rat brain tumor model. It was produced in Fisher 344 rats by the intravenous injection of 5 mg/kg of MNU for 26 weeks (Benda et al, 1971). The original tumor was designated as tumor #9, which subsequently was cloned at the Brain Tumor Research Center, University of California, San Francisco, and then was designated "9L". These tumor cells could be propagated in vitro, which made them very useful for in vivo studies to investigate the effects of various therapeutic modalities on brain tumors. 9L cells can be implanted i.c. into syngeneic Fischer rats, following which they give rise to rapidly growing tumors. These are composed of spindle-shaped cells with a sarcomatoid appearance. The tumor margins are sharply delineated with little obvious invasion into the contiguous normal brain (Fig. 1b). The 9L gliosarcoma has a mutant p53 gene (Asai et al, 1994), but there is normal expression of p16 and p19ARF mRNAs, indicating that there is a wild type p16/Cdkn2a/INK4α locus (Schlegel et al, 1999). Molecular characterization of the 9L relative to rat stem cell derived astrocytes revealed an increased expression of the genes encoding TGFα and its receptor, EGFR (Sibenaller et al, 2005). Interestingly, decreased expression of FGF-2, FGF-9, and FGFR-1 and PDGFRβ also was noted (Sibenaller et al, 2005). Recently, cancer stem-like cells

(CSLCs) have been demonstrated in the 9L cell line. These CSLCs grow as neurospheres in chemically defined medium and express the neural stem cell markers Nestin and Sox2. They are self-renewable and differentiate in vitro into neuron- and glial-like cells (Ghods et al, 2007). The neurospheres have a lower proliferation rate and express several anti-apoptotic and drug related genes. Furthermore, these cells form tumors that are more aggressive than the parental 9L tumor (Ghods et al, 2007), which could be an important property in future studies. The 9L gliosarcoma model has been used extensively to investigate mechanisms and development of drug resistance (Barcellos-Hoff et al, 2006), transport of drugs across the blood-brain and bloodtumor barrier (Black et al, 2008), imaging of brain tumors including radiological techniques such as magnetic resonance imaging (MRI) and positron emission tomography (PET) and imaging to evaluate tumor hypoxia and metabolism (Bansal et al, 2008), pharmacokinetic studies of nitrosourea (Warnke et al, 1987), mechanisms and effects of anti-angiogenic drugs (Yang et al, 2007), effects of radiation (Regnard et al, 2008), chemotherapy (Bencokova et al, 2008), gene therapy (Kumar et al, 2008), cancer stem cells (Ghods et al, 2007), immunotoxin treatment, immunotherapy and cytokine therapy (Liu et al, 2007) and oncolytic viral therapy (Madara et al, 2005). A number of these studies have yielded impressive therapeutic results, including apparent cures of tumor bearing animals. However, it must be emphasized that this tumor has been shown to be highly immunogenic. Animals immunized with X-irradiated 9L cells were resistant to both subcutaneous (s.c.) as well as i.c. tumor challenge, compared to 100% tumor takes in immunologically naïve animals (Blume et al, 1974). This report was first published in the proceedings of a meeting, which did not receive wide circulation, but subsequent studies have confirmed the immunogenicity of this model (Morantz et al, 1979). Expression of the s-Myc gene under the control of a CMV promotor resulted in complete suppression of 9L tumor growth, as well as rejection of subsequent challenges of tumor cells. Histological examination of the tumors after s-Myc therapy revealed massive mononuclear cell infiltration with CD8 + T lymphocytes, which accounted for >70% of these infiltrating cells. These observations suggested that tumor rejection was due to a potent T-cell mediated, anti-tumor immune response. This, and several more recent studies, have underscored the significance of the anti-tumor immune response following gene therapy induced tumor eradication observed with 9L model. It is now recognized that in vivo bystander cell killing (Chen et al, 1995), which has been observed with the 9L gliosarcoma following delivery of the Herpes simplex virus thymidine kinase gene (hsv-tk), (Moolten et al, 1986) followed by treatment with ganciclovir, was due in part to an anti-tumor immune response. The immunogenicity of the 9L glioma must be kept in mind when utilizing this model to evaluate the efficacy of novel therapeutic agents. Early studies employing radiation or chemotherapy alone were largely unsuccessful in curing the 9L tumor. However, the success obtained by boron neutron capture therapy and gene therapy highlights the importance of utilizing anti-tumor treatments that can destroy individual cancer cells and simultaneously spare host immune effector cells that can eradicate residual tumor cells (Moriuchi et al, 2002).

Despite the fact that the 9L arose in a Fischer rat, 9L gliosarcoma cells also can form i.c. tumors in allogeneic Wistar rats (Stojiljkovic et al, 2003). Histopathological evaluation revealed that these tumors formed circumscribed masses that were not infiltrative and did not spread into the subarachnoid space or ventricles. Immunostaining of the tumors revealed the presence of glial fibrillary acidic protein (GFAP)-positive, infiltrating astrocytic cells, and activated ED1 positive macrophages/ microglia. Higher numbers of K(ATP) and K(Ca) channels have been observed in 9L tumors grown in allogeneic Wistar rats compared to those grown in syngeneic Fischer rats. Furthermore, the allogeneic tumors showed a greater increase in brain tumor permeability upon treatment with potassium channel agonists, compared to those grown in syngeneic hosts. The 9L tumor model also has been used following treatment to study the effect of BBB disruption, implantation of devices for repeated intratumoral delivery and imaging (Bhattacharya et al, 2007).

The 9L gliosarcoma model also has been used to develop a model for brainstem tumors (Jallo et al, 2006). Progression to hemiparesis with the onset of symptoms occurred 17 days postimplantation into the brainstem. This model has been used to evaluate the efficacy of convection enhanced delivery (CED) of carboplatin to the brainstem, and to study the response of recurrent, chemo-resistant gliomas. Two bis-chloroethyl nitrosourea (BCNU) resistant cell lines were derived from 9L cells by treating them with BCNU in vitro or in vivo. Both of these cell lines formed tumors in a 100% of the animals following i.c. implantation, and were much more invasive than the parental 9L cells (Saito et al, 2004). The 9L gliosarcoma also has been used as a model to evaluate drug-resistant and invasive recurrent gliomas (Schepkin et al, 2006), but as previously indicated, caution must be used in evaluating results obtained with such a highly immunogenic tumor.

Although not fully appreciated, the **T9 glioma** was at one time, and still may be the same as the 9L gliosarcoma. The original stock of T9 cells was obtained from Sweet's laboratory at the MGH by Denlinger, and Koestner, and it was renamed T9 by them. Similar to the immunogenicity of the 9L gliosarcoma, the T9 glioma also was found to be highly immunogenic. Kida et al. found that rats immunized with irradiated T9 cells or T9 cells mixed with C. parvum rejected subsequent s.c. implants of T9 glioma cells (Kida et al, 1983). However, in order to immunize against intracranial tumors, rats initially had to reject intradermal T9 cells. As might have been predicted, these results indicated that, similar to the 9L gliosarcoma, the T9 glioma also was immunogenic. The T9 cell line subsequently has been shared among numerous investigators and has been used for many studies, including the evaluation of antiangiogenic (Jeffes et al, 2005), and chemotherapeutic agents (Pietronigro et al, 2003), immunotherapy (Shibuya et al, 1984), and gene therapy with interferon-β(Harada et al, 1995). Although tumor specific or tumor associated antigens have yet to be identified, for the 9L gliosarcoma and T9 glioma, it is only a matter of time before they are identified.

The RG2 glioma (ATCC #CRL-2433) was produced in Koestner's laboratory at The Ohio State University by the i.v. administration of ENU (50 mg/kg body weight) to a pregnant Fischer 344 rat on the 20th day of gestation. Subsequently, the in vitro growth and morphology of the F98 glioma was described in detail (Ko et al, 1980), and based on its histopathology it was classified as an anaplastic or undifferentiated glioma. The progeny of ENU-injected rats subsequently developed tumors, and following cloning by Wechsler in Germany, one of these clones was designated as "RG2" (rat glioma 2). The same clone was called the "D74-RG2" or "D74" in Koestner's laboratory at The Ohio State University. The RG2 glioma (Fig. 1c) is similar in microscopic appearance to the F98 glioma (Fig. 1d), and also has a highly invasive pattern of growth, which has made it a good representative model for GBM (Weizsacker et al, 1982). Gene expression profiling of these cells established that they had increased gene expression of PDGFβ, IGF-1, Ras, Erb3/HER3 precursor mRNA and cyclin D2. They express a wildtype p53 and a concurrent loss in the expression of the p16/Cdkn2a/Ink4 gene locus. It has been used for a variety of preclinical studies to evaluate changes in vascular permeability (Ferrier et al, 2007), disruption of the BBB (Ningaraj et al, 2002), anti-angiogenic therapy (Zagorac et al, 2008), gene therapy, chemotherapy (Miknyoczki et al, 2007) and radionuclide therapy (Shen et al, 2004).

The RG2 glioma is non-immunogenic in syngeneic Fischer rats and has low levels of MHC-1 expression compared to the C6 and 9L gliomas (Oshiro et al, 2001). However, in vitro treatment with IFN-γ upregulated MHC class I antigen expression and also resulted in a significant in vivo anti-tumor immune response with increased survival of treated animals. More recently, the RG2 glioma has been stably transfected with human Herpes virus Entry Mediator C (HveC) to facilitate HSV infection and has been used to study the therapeutic effects of oncolytic Herpes simplex virus-1 treatment (Kurozumi et al, 2007). The transfected cells retained their tumorigenicity following i.c. implantation in Fischer rats, and transfection of the HveC gene did not affect i.c. tumor growth (Wakimoto et al, 2004). However, it has not been determined if HveC can cause these cells to become immunogenic, and therefore, this must be taken into account when using the RG2 for immunotherapy studies.

The F98 glioma (ATCC # CRL-2397) was produced by Wechsler in Koestner's laboratory at the same time as the RG2 glioma. It is composed of a mixed population of spindle-shaped cells, the majority of which have fusiform nuclei, and a smaller number of polygonal cells with round to oval nuclei. There is extensive invasion of contiguous normal brain with islands of tumor cells at varying distances from the tumor mass, many of which form perivascular clusters (Fig. 1d). Similar to human GBM, these cells overexpress PDGFβ, and Ras along with an increase in EGFR, cyclin D1 and cyclin D2 expression relative to rat astrocytes (Sibenaller et al, 2005). Like the C6 glioma, they also have increased expression of Rb relative to rat astrocytes. Immunofluorescence studies of F98 cells also revealed low expression of BRCA1, and a lack of radiation and cisplatin induced BRCA1 foci in these cells (Bencokova et al, 2008). Usually, there is a necrotic core, scattered mitotic cells and non-glomeruloid neovascular proliferation. The tumor is GFAP and vimentin positive with negligible staining for CD3 + T cells (Mathieu et al, 2007). Since it simulates the behavior of human GBMs in a number of important ways, such as its highly invasive pattern of growth and low immunogenicity, it has been used to evaluate the efficacy of a variety of experimental therapeutic agents. It is refractory to a number of therapeutic modalities, including systemic chemotherapy with paclitaxel, and carboplatin (von Eckardstein et al, 2005), and it is poorly responsive to photon-irradiation alone, which in part may be related to its functionally impaired BRCA1 status that can favor genomic instability and impaired DNA repair. Recently, it has been shown to be responsive to a combination of synchrotron radiation with cisplatin (Biston et al, 2004), and to convection enhanced delivery (CED) of carboplatin in combination with 6 MV photon-irradiation in rats bearing i.c. tumors (Rousseau et al, 2008). This model has been used extensively by Barth et al. to evaluate the efficacy of boron neutron capture therapy (BNCT) (Yang et al, 2008). Elleaume and her coworkers have evaluated cisplatin, carboplatin and iodine enhanced synchrotron stereotactic radiotherapy (Cho et al, 2002) in F98 glioma bearing rats (Adam et al, 2005). It has also been used to evaluate non-invasive MRI to visualize tumor growth, diffusion tensor imaging (Zhang et al, 2007), tumor angiogenesis and the tumor tropism of mesenchymal stem cells (Wu et al, 2008).

The F98 glioma is very weakly immunogenic (Tzeng et al, 1991) and transfection with the gene encoding B7.1 co-stimulatory molecule (Paul et al, 2000), or syngeneic cellular vaccination combined with GMCSF, did not enhance its immunogenicity (Clavreul et al,

2006). This makes it a very attractive model to investigate the mechanisms underlying glioma resistance to immunotherapy. It has also been used to study the molecular genetic alterations in GBMs (Hanissian et al, 2005), effects of infusion rates on drug distribution in i.c. tumors, and for suicide gene therapy with Herpes simplex virus-1 thymidine kinase (HSV-TK) (von Eckardstein et al, 2001). Like the 9L gliosarcoma, F98 cells also have been injected into the pontine tegmentum of the brainstem of Fischer rats to produce a model for brainstem tumors. The histopathological and radiobiological characteristics of these tumors were comparable to aggressive, primary human brainstem tumors, which could facilitate preclinical testing of therapeutics to treat these lethal tumors.

F98 cells have been stably transfected with expression vectors encoding for wildtype EGFR and EGFRvIII, and the resulting cell lines have been designated F98EGFR (ATCC# CRL-2948) and F98npEGFRvIII (ATCC# CRL-2949). They each express $\sim10^{5}$ non-functional (i.e. nonphosphorylatable) receptor sites per cell. This is below the threshold number of 10^{6} sites per cell that can evoke a xeno-immune response against human EGFR in rats. These cell lines have been used in Fischer rats for studies on molecular targeting (Yang et al, 2005) to evaluate the therapeutic efficacy of boronated mAbs and EGF for neutron capture therapy (NCT) (Wu et al, 2007). The boronated mAbs, L8A4, which is specific for EGFRvIII, and cetuximab, which recognizes wild type EGFR, specifically targeted their respective receptor positive i.c. tumors after CED and they were therapeutically effective following NCT.

A bioluminescent F98 cell line recently was constructed by stably transfecting F98 cells with the luciferase gene. When implanted i.c. into the brains of Fischer rats, tumor size could be monitored by measuring luminescence. This model should permit rapid, non-invasive imaging of i.c. tumor growth to evaluate novel therapeutic modalities (Bryant et al, 2008). Finally, F98 cells also are capable of growing as i.c. xenografts in cats (Ernestus et al, 1992), but since these cells can evoke a xenoimmune response, this model is of limited usefulness. It is important to note that, what may be therapeutically effective in the rat, may not be in the human. However, it probably is safe to say that if a particular therapeutic approach is ineffective in a rat model, it is even more unlikely to be so in humans.

The CNS-1 glioma was derived from an inbred Lewis rat that had received weekly i.v. injections of MNU for 6 months (Kruse et al, 1994). Following i.c. implantation into Lewis rats, it demonstrated an infiltrative pattern of growth with leptomeningeal, perivascular, and periventricular spread and extension of the tumor into the choroid plexus. Histologically, these tumors exhibited hypercellularity, nuclear atypia and pleomorphism, and had necrotic foci. These were surrounded by glioma cells arranged in a pseudopalisading pattern (Fig. 1e), although to a lesser extent than that seen in human GBM. These tumors are weakly immunogenic. Like human GBMs, these also were infiltrated with macrophages and T-cells, but did not have extensive glomeruloid endothelial/microvascular proliferation. Kielian et al. identified the constitutive expression of monocyte chemotactic factor 1 (MCP-1) by CNS-1 cells (Kielian et al, 2002). In vivo, CNS-1 tumors also showed extensive infiltration by macrophages, which might confer a growth advantage (Platten et al, 2003). This model has been useful to study glioma invasion (Owens et al, 1998), changes in the biology of glioma cells and their extracellular matrix (Lapointe et al, 2004), and gene therapy (Biglari et al, 2004). It also has been used to study the efficacy of immunotherapy as a potential treatment for human GBM (Ali et al, 2004) although its immunogenicity has not been studied in great detail.

The BT4C glioma was derived by giving a single transplacental administration of N-ethyl-Nnitrosourea (ENU) to pregnant BD IX rats. Dissociated brain tumor cells from one of these animals were propagated in vitro and after 200 days in culture they became tumorigenic. The cells subsequently were implanted s.c. into BD IX rats and the resulting tumors contained a mixture of multipolar glia-like cells and flattened cells with fewer and shorter cytoplasmic processes and occasional giant cells (Laerum et al, 1977). BT4C glioma-derived tumors show high cellularity and have pleomorphic nuclei and numerous mitotic figures and the tumor blood vessels are irregular, dilated and show areas of proliferation (Fig. 1f) (Stuhr et al, 2007). At the molecular level, BT4C cells express VEGF, tPA, uPA and MVD in the periphery of the growing tumor and are S100 positive by immunohistochemistry (M. Johansson, Personal communication). This model has been useful to test novel chemotherapeutic targeting strategies (Pulkkinen et al, 2008), antitumor effects of gene therapy (Raty JK et al, 2004), anti-angiogenic agents alone (Huszthy et al, 2006) and in combination with radiation and temozolomide (Sandstrom et al, 2008). BT4C gliomas also have been used to investigate the impact of hyperoxia on tumor bearing rats. This resulted in slower growth accompanied by increased apoptosis of tumor cells and reduced microvessel density (MVD). Apart from studies to evaluate therapeutic efficacy, the BT4C glioma model also has been used to study the molecular and biological changes induced by chemotherapy (Vallbo et al, 2002), radiation therapy (Andersson et al, 2002) and suicide gene therapy (Griffin et al, 2003). BT4C cells, stably transfected with cDNA encoding β-galactosidase, have been used to evaluate the migration of single migrating tumor cell glioma spheroids and fetal brain aggregate coculture systems in vitro and in rat brains in vivo (Garcia-Cabrera et al, 1996;).

Avian sarcoma virus induced and RT-2 glioma. The induction of experimental brain tumors by the injection of Rous sarcoma virus has been described in canines, rats, and monkeys. Tumors were induced by inoculating neonatal Fischer rats i.c. with purified avian sarcoma virus (ASV) suspensions (Copeland et al, 1976). All of the animals developed tumors within 2 weeks following ASV injection, 94% of which were anaplastic astrocytomas, and the remainder were low grade gliomas or sarcomas (Prabhu et al, 2000). This model has been used to study the effects of chemo- and radiotherapy, BBB disruption, tumor permeability, and if de novo tumor induction is an important requirement. The response to immunotherapy indicated that these tumors were immunogenic, and expressed a variety of virally encoded tumor specific antigens. A continuous cell line, designated "RT-2", was derived from an ASV-induced Fischer rat tumor, and this has been used to study tumor growth, photochemotherapy, cytotoxic gene therapy (Valerie et al, 2001) and radio-sensitization (Valerie et al, 2000). The RT2 tumor appears to be immunogenic, as evidenced by its ability to evoke a CD8 + T cell-mediated anti-tumor immune response (Shah et al, 2003), and this must be taken into account if it is used for immunotherapy studies. RT-2 cells expressing GFP have been used for quantitative assessment of glioma invasion in the rat brain (Mourad et al, 2003). The RT-2 glioma model also has been used to evaluate the therapeutic efficacy of oncolytic adenoviruses. Although they can be efficiently infected they do not permit efficient replication of E1- attenuated adenoviruses. These cells also have been transfected with cDNA encoding heat shock protein 72 (HSP72), which was thought to be necessary for replication of E1 deleted adenoviruses. These transfectants have been found to be permissive for replication of E1- deleted, conditionally replication-competent adenoviruses. The inherent immunogenicity of the RT-2 glioma may limit its usefulness for survival studies, but nevertheless it still may be a useful model for other types of studies.

Rat brain tumor models have provided a wealth of information on the biology, biochemistry, imaging and experimental therapeutics of brain tumors in experimental neuro-oncology, and there is every reason to believe that they will continue to do so. However, it is essential to recognize the limitations of each of the models that have been described, and depending on the nature of the study to be conducted, it is important that the appropriate model be selected. It now has become clear that immunogenic tumors such as the C6, 9L and T9 are not good choices for studies in immunocompetent rats, if the endpoint is prolongation of survival time or cure of the tumor. Destruction of tumor cells in these models, which have tumor infiltrating host immune effector cells within the tumor, can lead to significant amplification of an antitumor response. This may be the single most important in vivo contributor to the bystander effect that has been observed with gene therapy of the C6 and 9L gliomas following transfection with the HSV-tK gene and the lack of such immune amplification with the weakly immunogenic RG2 glioma. Anti-tumor immune response following transfection with suicide genes such as HSV-tK initially was unanticipated, but it is an important effect associated with both gene therapy and boron neutron capture therapy, but not with conventional chemo- and radiotherapy of the 9L gliosarcoma. Since human high grade brain tumors generally are regarded as being either non- or weakly immunogenic, therapeutic exploitation of this using modalities that spare tumor infiltrating host immune effector cells could have important therapeutic implications. Undoubtedly other rat brain tumor models will be developed, especially cell lines derived from genetically engineered rats that will expand the types of studies that can be carried out in this very important laboratory animal.

2.1.2 Human glioma xenografts implanted in immunocompromised mice

Xenograft models of malignant astrocytoma have been extensively used to assess the function of various signaling molecules or matrix proteins in glioma growth and invasion (Hingtgen et al, 2008). Xenograft models that transplant human malignant astrocytoma/glioma cells into the brains of immunocompromised mice (athymic nude or SCID) have the advantage of being relatively rapid models with which to assess the role of a particular molecule in positively or negatively regulating proliferation and/or regulating invasion in vivo. Also, these models are very useful for the initial evaluation of novel imaging techniques as well as new therapies for GBM, including antiangiogenic therapy chemotherapy, radiotherapy, targeted toxins, cytotoxic or conditionally replicative oncolytic viruses. One disadvantage of human xenograft models is that most human glioma cell lines are not invasive when propagated in vivo (Curtin et al, 2008). Another disadvantage is that the propagation of human malignant astrocytoma/glioma cell lines in culture can result in their loss of key genetic alterations, such as expression of the mutant EGFR (Tsurushima et al, 2007), that are the most likely to be important in gliomagenesis. This limitation has been overcome by propagating primary human GBM tumors in the nude mouse (either subcutaneously or intracerebrally) instead of in culture; when these tumors are propagated in vivo, the genetic alterations found in the patients biopsy are retained (Ozawa et al, 2005). For xenograft models it is also important to propagate the tumors for experimental analysis in an orthotopic environment (the brain) because the microenvironment in the brain (i.e., the extracellular matrix, growth factors, and stromal cells) is different from that found in the subcutaneous tissue.

2.2 Gene trgeted animal models

Recently, transgenic technology has allowed investigators to alter the function of specific genes of interest and thus exploit defined genetic lesions to produce more biologically correct models of CNS cancers that result from activation and/or inactivation of endogenous genes in rodent genomes.

- p53,
- INK4a/ARF,
- Phosphatase and Tensin Homolog (PTEN),
- Epidermal Growth Factor Receptor (EGF-R),
- Platelet Derived Growth Factor (PDGF)

These models support the concept that the genetic alterations in human tumors, such as p53 loss and loss of PTEN function, are probably important in the development of astrocytomas (Grades II and III). Rodent models of GBM tumors are also available. In a somatic gene-transfer model, simultaneous retroviral expression of constitutively active Ras and Akt gives rise to the formation of high-grade gliomas that are morphologically similar to human GBM tumors (Holland et al, 2000). Although Ras mutations are uncommon in GBM tumors, one study (Sharma et al, 2005) suggests that Ras activity is increased in human GBM biopsies due to a point mutation. In mice, the combination of EGFR amplification and either loss of p53 plus CDK4 overexpression or loss of INK4a-ARF is sufficient to induce glioma tumor formation that resembles that of human GBM tumors (Zhu et al, 2009). In an EGFR transgenic mouse model, LOH of p16INK4a, p19ARF, and PTEN cooperates with the amplification of EGFR to induce a highly infiltrative GBM tumor. Also, simultaneous deletion of p53 and PTEN in the mouse central nervous system generates an acute-onset, high-grade malignant glioma tumor that is histologically similar to human GBM tumors (Zheng et al, 2008). A new model of GBM tumor has been created by retroviral expression of PDGF-B in adult rat neural progenitor cells (Assanah et al, 2006). In this model, intracranial injection of retrovirus containing PDGF-B alone or in combination with PDGFRα results in the development of GBM-like tumors. To date, individual disruption or LOH of a single gene regulating the cell cycle, such as p53, INK4a, or ARF, has been insufficient to initiate gliomagenesis in vivo (Holland et al, 2001). Taken together, these studies suggest that alterations in neural progenitor cells probably give rise to at least some high-grade gliomas. There are limitations in the use of the above-discussed models. These include the facts that the tumor cells are not of human origin and that the rodents can in some instances require several months to reliably develop glioma tumors.

Over the past two decades, scientists have developed a greater understanding of the molecular and genetic basis of brain tumorigenesis (Zhu et al, 2002). Evidence of the downregulation of tumor suppressor genes such as p53 and PTEN as well as elevated expression of growth factors, and their cognate tyrosine kinase receptors, such as PDGF and EGFR are found in a high percentage of human GBM tumors (Schwartzbaum et al, 2006). Researchers have exploited the role of these molecular pathways in brain tumor development to induce endogenous brain tumors in rodents. Thus, genetic engineering of mouse genes or intracranial delivery of oncogenic transgenes in adult mice and rats have been attempted in order to trigger the development of endogenous brain tumor in rodents. Germline deletion of the tumor suppressor genes p53 and NF1 increased the susceptibility of mice to develop astrocytomas (Reilly KM, 2009). These mice exhibit a wide range of astrocytoma stages, with tumor growth detected in 50-70% of the mice and median survival times of 6-8 months. This model is a valuable tool to study the development of secondary glioblastoma upon loss of p53. Germline deletion of other tumor suppressor genes, such as PTEN and Rb has also been attempted (Begemann et al, 2002). However, deletion of certain genes can lead to embryonic lethality or to the generation of tumors in other organs, limiting the utility of these models.

Tissue specific overexpression of putative oncogenes of interest, using methods which link the gene of interest to a glial specific promoter such as GFAP, S100β, or Nestin, provides an appealing approach towards the creation of spontaneously occurring brain tumors in animals seen in many germline knockout animals. Tissue targeted models involving deletion of tumor suppressor genes is more difficult. Conditional knockout models represent a promising new attempt to eliminate tumor suppressor function in a cell specific manner. These techniques have recently been utilized to create of variety of transgenic brain tumor models using targeted conditional knockouts of p53, PTEN, Ptc, and Rb. Frequently, conditional knockouts used in combination with oncogenes overexpressed on tissue specific promoters or introduced using viral vectors can create a localized tumor genetically similar to human cancer in an immune competent animal.

Transgenic mice that display cell type-specific overexpression of oncogenes have been employed to study genetic abnormalities in astrocytes and neural progenitors. This has proven useful to establish the role of oncogenes in the tumorgenesis and progression of GBM (Ding et al, 2001). Overexpression of the transcription factor E2F1 under the transcriptional control of the GFAP promoter led to the formation of astrocytomas in p53 KO mice, suggesting a role for E2F1 as an oncogene in the formation of brain tumors (Olson et al, 2007). Considering that cell typespecific expression of certain genes is lethal during early development, oncogene overexpression has also been approached by delivery of gene therapy vectors into the brain of pre-natal or adult rodents, leading to the formation of endogenous brain tumors. These tumors harbor the genetic abnormalities found in human GBM, as well as the histopathological hallmarks of human GBM, including the aggressive invasive behavior. The use of viral or plasmid based vectors to introduce genetic aberrations permits the tight anatomical restriction of tumor-forming genetic events to specific areas of the brain. Furthermore, viral and plasmid vectors allow for the delivery of multiple tumorigenic genes in any combination, thereby reducing the amount of time required to generate germline transgenic mouse models. Thus, endogenous rodent GBM models constitute a very promising and stringent animal model of GBM which recapitulates the most salient histopathological features, molecular attributes, and heterogeneity of human GBM in a syngeneic rodent background. However, the applicability of the endogenous brain tumor models to assess the pre-clinical efficacy of experimental therapeutics is still limited due to the long latency and the variable reproducibility of these models.

Extensive evidence from across this developing field suggests that formation of endogenous brain tumors using viral vectors or plasmid systems to deliver oncogenes is somewhat variable. The degree of penetrance, tumor latency, and histopathological characteristics are dependant on the species and age of animals, the identity of specific genetic alterations and the vector system used to deliver them, and the anatomical location of genetic alterations. Retroviral- mediated delivery of PDGF into the adult rat white matter leads to formation of brain tumors with histopathological features that resemble human GBM; 100% of the animals succumb due to tumor burden 14-20 days after injection (Assanah et al, 2006). However, when retro-PDGF is delivered into the brain of newborn mice brain tumor formation only occurred in ~40% of the animals within 14-29 weeks. The incidence and grade of brain tumor formation in mice has been suggested to be dependant on the levels of expression of PDGF. Newborn mice were administered with retroviral vectors encoding a PDGF gene that lacks its regulatory sequences, which leads to higher levels of PDGF expression. Within 4-12 weeks, 100% of these mice developed invasive glioblastoma that exhibited neo-vascularization and tumor cell infiltration throughout the brain parenchyma (Shih et al, 2004).

In order to mimic the multiple genetic lesions encountered in human GBM, retroviral vectors that encode growth factors and a cycline-dependent kinase (cdk) were injected in the brain of neo-natal mice harboring additional mutations in tumor suppressor genes. Delivery of a constitutively active form of epidermal growth factor receptor gene (EGFR) in combination with basic fibroblast growth factor (bFGF) or ckd4 into the brain of neo-natal mice that are deficient in INK4a–ARF or p53 tumor suppressor genes led to formation of GBM in ~50% of the animals, while single mutations were unable of generating tumors (Holland et al, 1998). These findings support the notion that combination of genetic lesions is required for the induction of endogenous GBM in mice. Additionally, combined genetic aberrations can be targeted to specific cell populations by the development of transgenic mice that express the retroviral receptor under the control of cell-type specific promoters, such as the progenitor nestin promoter or the astrocyte GFAP promoter (Dai et al, 2001). This system is very functional because it allows cell-type-specific transfer of oncogenes expressed within retroviral vectors under any type of promoter.

Lentiviral vectors have recently been employed to deliver oncogenes into the mouse brain. Considering that lentiviral vectors can transduce both dividing and non-dividing cells, these vectors constitute an attractive vehicle to deliver oncogenes to the brain of adult rodents (Singer O, Verma IM, 2008). In order to recapitulate the initiation of GBM, which is thought to arise upon genetic mutations in a few cells, oncogenic transgenes were delivered in a small population of cells in adult mouse brain by region-specific injection of lentiviral vectors encoding H-Ras or AKT. To target astrocytes the Cre-LoxP-controlled lentiviruses were injected in the cortex, hippocampus and subventricular zone of GFAP-Cre mice. Again, administration of single oncogenes did not induce formation of tumors for up to 10 months. However, when Ras and AKT were delivered together in the hippocampal area ~30% of mice exhibited brain tumors that exhibit a high degree of invasiveness within 3-5 months post injection. Only one mouse developed a tumor following transduction in the sub-ventricular zone, and no animals had tumors following transduction into the cortex. Combined delivery of H-Ras and AKT into p53 KO mice greatly increased the tumorigenesis of these vectors leading to 75 and 100% of the mice injected in the subventricular zone and hippocampus, respectively. These tumors also exhibited a much shorter tumor latency with many histopathological characteristics found in human GBM (Marumoto et al, 2009). These findings indicate that lentiviral vectors are useful tools to induce endogenous GBM in adult mice when several genetical abnormalities are induced in combination in the appropriate area of the brain.

Another recent approach to induce endogenous GBM in mice is the use of the Sleeping Beauty (SB) transposable element to achieve integration of oncogenes in the genome of brain cells of neo-natal immune competent mice (Ohlfest et al, 2005). SB is a synthetic transposable element composed of a transposon DNA substrate and a transposase enzyme. SB transposase mediates excision and insertion of transposon DNA into the host genome, leading to long term expression (Ohlfest et al, 2004). Spontaneous brain tumors were induced by injecting SB-dependent plasmid harboring up to three genetic alterations (AKT, N-RAS, EGRFvIII, and/or shRNA specific for p53) into the lateral cerebral ventricle of neonatal mice of three different strains (Wiesner et al, 2009). The histological characteristics of the tumors were dependant of the combination of genetic lesions introduced to the mice, although most resembled human astrocytoma or GBM. In some mice, multifocal tumors, another hallmark of human GBM, was observed. The combination of N-RAs, EGFRvIII, and

p53 silencing was the most robust combination of genes with a 100% penetrance and a median survival of 83 days. These tumors were highly invasive and immunoreactive for nestin and GFAP indicating heterogeneity in the tumor mass. The SB is a very attractive and versatile system to induce endogenous brain tumors, allowing integration of large transposons (<10 kb) into the genome of many strains of mice.
In summary, endogenous rodent brain tumor models that recapitulate the genetic aberrations found in human GBM are very useful for the study of gliomagenesis; however, their variable tumor formation rate and long latency limits their use for testing preclinical treatments. Nevertheless, the use of imaging techniques to confirm tumor formation before the treatment would allow rigorous evaluation of novel therapies in these models, which resemble hystologically and genetically the human disease.

2.3 Other models

Dogs bearing spontaneous GBM constitute a valuable tool in preclinical brain cancer research. GBM is the most common primary brain tumor in dogs, and brachycephalic breeds such as Boston terriers and Boxers (Heidner et al, 1991) are predisposed to develop spontaneous GBM (Stoica et al, 2004). Dog GBM exhibits the same histopathological characteristics of the human disease, including necrosis with pseudopalizading, neovascularization and endothelial proliferation. The presence of pseudopalisading necroses and endothelial proliferation that closely resemble those found in human GBMs suggest the presence of a hypoxic environment in dog GBM, as described in human patients (Rong et al, 2006). Importantly, canine GBM is highly invasive and exhibits the classical patterns of human GBM invasion, which makes it a very valuable tool to test not only the efficacy of novel therapies, but also their toxicity to the normal brain. The large size of the dog brain would be useful for preclinical assessment of doses and volumes in order to optimize treatment protocols before the translation into the clinic. Also, the detection of therapy-induced toxicity and side effects, as well as behavioral abnormalities are technically very well developed in dogs and constitutes a routine assessment in clinical veterinary practice. Moreover, the individual variability of outbreed dogs could help to better predict the clinical outcomes in human patients. Clinical signs and prognosis of dogs with spontaneous GBM are very similar to those in human, and there is a high correlation of neuro-imaging features seen with MRI in canine and human GBM, which is also used as a diagnostic tool for canine GBM (Lipsitz et al, 2003). The standard care of treatment in dogs with GBM is very similar to that used in human patients, consisting of surgical resection followed by radiation therapy and chemotherapy which leads to a median survival of 8.5-10 months. This allows performing preclinical trials that will mimic more closely the clinical scenario, in which new therapies are applied in patients that simultaneously undergo traditional treatment. Candolfi and others have previously demonstrated the feasibility of delivering therapeutic transgenes to dog GBM cells in vitro and dog brain cells in vivo upon intracranial injection of gene therapy vectors, such as type 5 adenoviral vectors (Candolfi et al, 2007), adeno-associated viral vectors (Ciron et al, 2006), plasmid DNA/polyethylenimine (PEI) complexes (Oh et al, 2007), which suggests that dogs bearing spontaneous GBM would be a suitable model to test novel gene therapy approaches. Importantly, the availability of canine GBM J3T (Rainov et al, 2000) and W&W (Garcia-Escudero et al, 2008) cell lines allows in vitro screening of novel therapeutic agents before moving to preclinical trials in dogs bearing spontaneous GBM. Also, the characterization of cancer stem cells from a GBM in a Boxer has been recently reported (Stoica et al, 2009). These cells exhibit cancer stem markers

and have highly proliferative rate, and ability of self-renewal and differentiation. In vitro they form neurospheres and in vivo they growth intracranially in the brain of nude mice, forming GBMs that exhibit histopathological features of dog GBM.
In summary, canine GBM emerges as an attractive animal model for testing novel therapies in a spontaneous tumor in the context of a large brain. The features of dog GBM make it a unique large animal model for preclinical cancer research with therapeutic outcomes which could better predict their efficacy in human trials. In spite of these attractive features, dogs are very expensive to treat and scarce, therefore the routine testing on novel therapeutics in these animals would be unfeasible.

3. Application and future projection

As a prelude to the implementation of gene therapy clinical trials for glioblastoma multiforme, it is critical to test potential novel therapies in relevant animal models of this disease. The ideal brain tumor model should exhibit predictable and reproducible intracranial growth patterns, have histopathological and biochemical resemblance to human GBMs and be nonimmunogenic. There are several models available in which it is feasible to study the efficacy and toxicity of different therapeutic approaches for this disease, i.e., anti-angiogenic agents, proapoptotic molecules, immunotherapy, etc. these glioma models help unravel the biology of tumorigenesis and etiology of human central nervous system tumors. These mouse-modeling experiments may identify essential targets for therapy and provide test animals for preclinical trials of mechanistically designed therapeutics.

4. Conclusion

Main glioma animal models are murine implantation models traditionally, in this chapter, 9 rat models are described in detail. The most widely used model C6 rat glioma arose in an outbred Wistar rat, is non-syngeneic. Since the tumor is immunogenic, even in Wistar rats, the C6 glioma is not suitable for study of immunotherapy. Syngeneic murine models, i.e. CNS-1 cells in Lewis rats, F98 and RG-2 cells in Fisher rats, GL26 cells in C57BL6 mice, SMA-560 cells in VMDK mice, are non-immunogenic, constituting an excellent tool. Human glioma xenografts implanted in immunocompromised mice have been extensively employed in preclinical brain cancer research. Although their xenogeneic nature impairs the study of immune-mediated anti-tumor strategies, they allow assessing the efficacy of therapeutic approaches in human GBM cells in the context of normal brain tissue. In fact, human xenografts exhibit histopatological features that resemble the human GBM and retain gene amplifications detected in the in situ tumors.
Recently, transgenic technique and gene knock-out technique rapidly developed, new animal models of gliomas were created. Central nervous system–specific inactivation of the genes encoding the tumor suppressors p53 and Nf1 leads to the spontaneous onset of Grade II and III astrocytoma tumors, as well as to GBM tumors in mice. This gliomagenesis can be accelerated by haploinsufficiency of the PTEN gene, and in neural progenitor cells conditional inactivation of p53 coordinates with a haploinsufficiency of PTEN and Nf1 to induce tumor formation. p53, INK4a/ARF, PTEN, EGFR, PDGF are the most popular genes in glioma research. Viral vectors or plasmid systems are used to deliver oncogenes. By means of linking the gene of interest to a glial specific promoter such as GFAP, S100β, or Nestin, transgenic mice that display cell type-specific overexpression of oncogenes. When large animal models are necessary, dog glioma models are available for alternative.

	Tumorigenesis Method	Technique	Tumor	Animal
Implantation	9 L Gliosarcoma	Syngeneic Graft	GS	Rat
	C6	Syngeneic Graft	GBM	Rat
	T9	Syngeneic Graft	GS	Rat
	RG2	Syngeneic Graft	GBM	Rat
	F98	Syngeneic Graft	GBM	Rat
	RT-2	Syngeneic Graft	GBM	Rat
	CNS-1	Syngeneic Graft	GBM	Rat
	GL261	Syngeneic Graft	GBM	Mouse
	Human Tumor Cells (U87, U251)	Xenograft	GBM	Mouse
Genetic	p53 +/-, NF-1 +/-	Germline mutations	Astro	Mouse
	GFAP- p53 +/-, NF-1 +/-	Conditional KO	Astr o	Mouse
	GFAP- p53 +/-, NF-1 +/-, PTEN-/-	Conditional KO	Astro	Mouse
	GFAP- p53 +/-, PTEN-/-	Conditional KO	Astro	Mouse
	INK4a/ARF -/-, PDGF Overexpression	Germline mutation, RCAS	Astro	Mouse
	INK4a/ARF -/-, EGF-R overexpression	Germline mutation, RCAS	Astro	Mouse
	INK4a/ARF -/-, Ras, Akt overexpression	Germline mutation, RCAS	Astro	Mouse
	Ras, Akt overexpression	RCAS	Astro	Mouse
	Ras, Akt overexpression, PTEN -/-	RCAS, Conditional KO	Astro	Mouse
	GFAP-V12 Ras, EGFRvIII	Astrocyte targeted mutation, Adenovirus	Astro	Mouse
	GFAP-V12 Ras, PTEN -/-	Astrocyte targeted mutation, Germline mutation	Astro	Mouse
	RAS, EGF-R targeted overexpression	Astrocyte targeted mutations	Astro	Mouse
	PDGF-B overexpression	MMLV retrovirus	ODG	Mouse
	PDGF-B overexpression	RCAS	ODG	Mouse
	Rb inactivation, PTEN -/-	GFAP-Cre targeted conditional KO	ODG	
	INK4a/ARF -/-, PDGF overexp., PTEN -/-	Germline mutation, RCAS, Conditional KO	ODG	Mouse
	P53 +/-, S100β promoter driven-v-erbB	Germline mutation, Oligodendrocyte mutation	ODG	Mouse
	INK4a-ARF +/-, S100β promoter v-erbB	Germline mutation, Oligodendrocyte mutation	ODG	Mouse
	p53 +/-, EGF-R overexpression	Germline mutation, Oligodendrocyte mutation	ODG	Mouse
	Ptc +/-	Germline mutation or Conditional KO	MB	Mouse
	Ptc +/-, p53 -/-	Germline mutations	MB	Mouse
	Shh, n-Myc	RCAS	MB	Mouse
	Rb +/-, p53 +/-	GFAP-conditional KO	MB	Mouse
	BRCA2 -/-, p53 +/-	Nestin-conditional KO	MB	Mouse
	Xrcc4 -/-, p53 -/-	Nestin-conditional KO	MB	Mouse
	SmoM2	GFAP-conditional KO MB		Mouse

Abbreviations (GS-Gliosarcoma, GBM-glioblastoma multiforme, Astro-astrocytoma, ODG-oligodendroglioma, MB-Medulloblastoma, KO-knockout)

Table 2. A summary of existing animal models of brain tumors

5. References

Adam JF, Joubert A, Biston MC, et al. (2006). Prolonged survival of Fischer rats bearing F98 glioma after iodine-enhanced synchrotron stereotactic radiotherapy. *International journal of radiation oncology,* Vol. 64, pp. 603- 611, ISSN 0360-3016

Ahmed AE, Jacob S, Nagy AA, et al. (2008). Dibromoacetonitrile-induced protein oxidation and inhibition of proteasomal activity in rat glioma cells. *Toxicology letters,* Vol. 179, pp. 29–33, ISSN 0378-4274

Ali S, Curtin JF, Zirger JM, et al. (2004). Inflammatory and anti-glioma effects of an adenovirus expressing human soluble Fms-like tyrosine kinase 3 ligand (hsFlt3L): treatment with hsFlt3L inhibits intracranial glioma progression. *Molecular therapy,* Vol. 10, pp. 1071–1084, ISSN 1525-0016

Andersson U, Grankvist K, Bergenheim AT, et al. (2002). Rapid induction of long-lasting drug efflux activity in brain vascular endothelial cells but not malignant glioma following irradiation. *Medical oncology,* Vol. 19, pp. 1–9, ISSN 1357-0560

Asai A, Miyagi Y, Sugiyama A, et al. (1994). Negative effects of wild-type p53 and s-myc on cellular growth and tumorigenicity of glioma cells. Implication of the tumor suppressor genes for gene therapy. *Journal of neuro-oncology,* Vol. 19, pp. 259–268, ISSN 0167-594X

Assadian S, Aliaga A, Del Maestro RF, et al. (2008). FDG-PET imaging for the evaluation of antiglioma agents in a rat model. *Neuro-oncology,* Vol. 10, pp. 292–299, ISSN 1522-8517

Assanah M, Lochhead R, Ogden A, Bruce J, Goldman J & Canoll P. (2006). Glial progenitors in adult white matter are driven to form malignant gliomas by platelet-derived growth factor–expressing retroviruses. *Journal of clinical neuroscience,* Vol. 26, pp. 6781–90. ISSN 0270-6474

Assanah M, Lochhead R, Ogden A, et al. (2006). Glial progenitors in adult white matter are driven to form malignant gliomas by platelet-derived growth factor-expressing retroviruses. *Journal of clinical neuroscience,* Vol. 26, pp. 6781–90, ISSN 0270-6474

Bansal A, Shuyan W, Hara T, et al. (2008). Biodisposition and metabolism of [(18)F]fluorocholine in 9L glioma cells and 9L glioma-bearing Fisher rats. *European journal of nuclear medicine and molecular imaging,* Vol. 35, pp. 1192- 1203, ISSN 1619-7070

Barcellos-Hoff MH, Linfoot PA, Marton LJ, et al. (1992). Production of stable phenotypes from 9L rat brain tumor multicellular spheroids treated with 1, 3-bis(2-chloroethyl)-1-nitrosourea. *International journal of cancer,* Vol. 52, pp. 409–413, ISSN 0020-7136

Barker M, Hoshino T, Gurcay O, et al. (1973). Development of an animal brain tumor model and its response to therapy with 1, 3-bis(2-chloroethyl)-1-nitrosourea. *Cancer research,* Vol. 33, pp. 976–986, ISSN 0008-5472

Begemann M, Fuller GN & Holland EC. (2002). Genetic modeling of glioma formation in mice. *Brain pathology,* Vol. 12, pp. 117–32, ISSN 1015-6305

Bencokova Z, Pauron L, Devic C, et al. (2008). Molecular and cellular response of the most extensively used rodent glioma models to radiation and/or cisplatin. *Journal of neuro-oncology,* Vol. 86, pp. 13–21, ISSN 0167-594X

Benda P, Lightbody J, Sato G, et al. (1968). Differentiated rat glial cell strain in tissue culture. *Science,* Vol. 161, pp. 370–371, ISSN 0193-4511

Benda P, Someda K, Messer J, et al. (1971). Morphological and immunochemical studies of rat glial tumors and clonal strains propagated in culture. *Journal of neurosurgery,* Vol. 34, pp. 310–323, ISSN 0022-3085

Bhattacharya P, Chekmenev EY, Perman WH, et al. (2007). Towards hyperpolarized (13)C-succinate imaging of brain cancer. *Journal of magnetic resonance,* Vol. 186, pp. 150–155, ISSN 1090-7807

Biglari A, Bataille D, Naumann U, et al. (2004). Effects of ectopic decorin in modulating intracranial glioma progression in vivo, in a rat syngeneic model. *Cancer gene therapy,* Vol. 11, pp. 721–732, ISSN 0929-1903

Biston MC, Joubert A, Adam JF, et al. (2004). Cure of Fischer rats bearing radioresistant F98 glioma treated with cis-platinum and irradiated with monochromatic synchrotron X-rays. *Cancer research,* Vol. 64, pp. 2317–2323, ISSN 0008-5472

Black KL, Yin D, Konda BM, et al. (2008). Different effects of KCa and KATP agonists on brain tumor permeability between syngeneic and allogeneic rat models. *Brain Research,* Vol. 1227, pp. 198–206, ISSN 0006-8993

Blume, MR.; Wilson, CP. & Vasquez, DA. (1974). Immune response to a transplantable intracerebral glioma in rats. In: Sane, K.; Ishi, S.; Le Vey, D., editors. Recent progress in neurological surgery. *Excerpta Medica; Amsterdam,* pp. 129-134, ISSN 0927-2798

Bryant MJ, Chuah TL, Luff J, et al. (2008). A novel rat model for glioblastoma multiforme using a bioluminescent F98 cell line. Journal of clinical neuroscience, Australasia, Vol. 15, pp. 545–551, ISSN 0270-6474

Candolfi M, Curtin JF, Nichols WS, et al. (2007). Intracranial glioblastoma models in preclinical neurooncology: neuro-pathological characterization and tumor progression. *Journal of neuro-oncology,* Vol. 85, pp. 133– 148, ISSN 0167-594X

Candolfi M, Kroeger KM, Pluhar GE, et al. (2007). Adenoviral-mediated gene transfer into the canine brain in vivo. *Neurosurgery,* Vol. 60, pp. 167–77, discussion 78, ISSN 0148-396X

Candolfi M, Pluhar GE, Kroeger K, et al. (2007). Optimization of adenoviral vector-mediated transgene expression in the canine brain in vivo, and in canine glioma cells in vitro. *Neuro-oncology* , Vol. 9, pp. 245– 58, ISSN 1522-8517

Chen CY, Chang YN, Ryan P, et al. (1995). Effect of herpes simplex virus thymidine kinase expression levels on ganciclovir-mediated cytotoxicity and the "bystander effect". *Human Gene Therapy,* Vol. 6, pp. 1467– 1476, ISSN 1043-0342

Cho JY, Shen DH, Yang W, et al. (2002). In vivo imaging and radioiodine therapy following sodium iodide symporter gene transfer in animal model of intracerebral gliomas. *Gene therapy,* Vol. 9, pp. 1139– 1145, ISSN 0969-7128

Ciron C, Desmaris N, Colle MA, et al. (2006). Gene therapy of the brain in the dog model of Hurler's syndrome. *Annals of neurology,* Vol. 60, pp. 204–13, ISSN0364-5134

Clavreul A, Delhaye M, Jadaud E, et al. (2006). Effects of syngeneic cellular vaccinations alone or in combination with GM- CSF on the weakly immunogenic F98 glioma model. *Journal of neuro-oncology,* Vol. 79, pp. 9–17, ISSN 0167-594X

Copeland DD, Talley FA & Bigner DD. (1976). The fine structure of intracranial neoplasms induced by the inoculation of avian sarcoma virus in neonatal and adult rats. *American Journal Pathology,* Vol. 83, pp. 149–176, ISSN 0002-9440

Curtin JF, Candolfi M, Xiong W, Lowenstein PR & Castro MG. (2008). Turning the gene tap off; implications of regulating gene expression for cancer therapeutics. *Molecular cancer therapeutics,* Vol. 7, pp. 439–48, ISSN 1535-7163

Dai C, Celestino JC, Okada Y, et al. (2001). PDGF autocrine stimulation dedifferentiates cultured astrocytes and induces oligodendrogliomas and oligoastrocytomas from neural progenitors and astrocytes in vivo. *Genes and Devlopment,* Vol. 15, pp. 1913–25, ISSN 0890-9369

Ding H, Roncari L, Shannon P, et al. (2001). Astrocyte-specific expression of activated p21-ras results in malignant astrocytoma formation in a transgenic mouse model of human gliomas. *Cancer research,* Vol. 61, pp. 3826–36, ISSN 0008-5472

Doblas S, Saunders D, Kshirsagar P, et al. (2008). Phenyl-tert-butylnitrone induces tumor regression and decreases angiogenesis in a C6 rat glioma model. *Free radical biology & medicine,* Vol. 44, pp. 63–72, ISSN 0891-5849

Ernestus RI, Wilmes LJ & Hoehn-Berlage M. (1992). Identification of intracranial liqor metastases of experimental stereotactically implanted brain tumors by the tumor-selective MRI contrast agent MnTPPS. *Clinical & experimental metastasis,* Vol. 10, pp. 345–350, ISSN 0262-0898

Ferrier MC, Sarin H, Fung SH, et al. (2007). Validation of dynamic contrast-enhanced magnetic resonance imaging-derived vascular permeability measurements using quantitative autoradiography in the RG2 rat brain tumor model. *Neoplasia,* Vol. 9, pp. 546–555, ISSN 1522-8002

Fomchenko EI & Holland EC. (2006). Mouse models of brain tumors and their applications in preclinical trials. *Clinical cancer research,* Vol. 12, pp. 5288–5297, ISSN 1078-0432

Garcia-Cabrera I, Edvardsen K, Tysnes BB, et al. (1996). The lac-z reporter gene: a tool for in vitro studies of malignant glioma cell invasion. *Invasion & Metastasis,* Vol. 16, pp. 107–115, ISSN 0251-1789

Garcia-Escudero V, Gargini R & Izquierdo M. (2008). Glioma regression in vitro and in vivo by a suicide combined treatment. *Molecular Cancer Research,* Vol. 6, pp. 407–17, ISSN 1541-7786

Ghods AJ, Irvin D, Liu G, et al. (2007). Spheres isolated from 9L gliosarcoma rat cell line possess chemoresistant and aggressive cancer stem-like cells. *Stem Cells,* Vol. 25, pp. 1645–1653, ISSN 1066-5099

Griffin JL, Lehtimaki KK, Valonen PK, et al. (2003). Assignment of 1H nuclear magnetic resonance visible polyunsaturated fatty acids in BT4C gliomas undergoing ganciclovir-thymidine kinase gene therapy-induced programmed cell death. *Cancer research,* Vol. 63, pp. 3195–3201, ISSN 0008-5472.

Guo P, Hu B, Gu W, et al. (2003). Platelet-derived growth factor-B enhances glioma angiogenesis by stimulating vascular endothelial growth factor expression in tumor endothelia and by promoting pericyte recruitment. *American Journal Pathology,* Vol. 162, pp. 1083–1093, ISSN 0002-9440

Hanissian SH, Teng B, Akbar U, Janjetovic Z, Zhou Q, Duntsch C & Robertson JH. (2005). Regulation of myeloid leukemia factor-1 interacting protein (MLF1IP) expression in glioblastoma. *Brain Res,* Vol. 1047, pp. 56–64, ISSN 0006-8993

Harada K, Yoshida J, Mizuno M, et al. (1995). Growth inhibition of intracerebral rat glioma by transfectioninduced human interferon-beta. *Journal of Surgical Oncology,* Vol. 59, pp. 105–109, ISSN 0022-4790

Heidner GL, Kornegay JN, Page RL, Dodge RK & Thrall DE. (1991). Analysis of survival in a retrospective study of 86 dogs with brain tumors. *Journal of veterinary internal medicine,* Vol. 5, pp. 219–26, ISSN 0891-6640

Heimberger AB, Suki D, Yang D, et al. (2005). The natural history of EGFR and EGFRvIII in glioblastoma patients. *Journal of translational medicine,* Vol. 3, pp. 38, ISSN 1479-5876

Hingtgen S, Ren X, Terwilliger E, et al. (2008). Targeting multiple pathways in gliomas with stem cell and viral delivered S-TRAIL and Temozolomide. *Molecular cancer therapeutics,* Vol. 7, pp. 3575–85, ISSN 1535-7163

Holland EC, Celestino J, Dai C, Schaefer L, Sawaya RE & Fuller GN. (2000). Combined activation of Ras and Akt in neural progenitors induces glioblastoma formation in mice. *Nature Genetics,* Vol. 25, pp. 55–57, ISSN 1061-4036

Holland EC, Hively WP, DePinho RA & Varmus HE. A constitutively active epidermal growth factor receptor cooperates with disruption of G1 cell-cycle arrest pathways to induce glioma-like lesions in mice. *Genes and Development,* (1998). Vol. 12, pp. 3675–85, ISSN 0890-9369

Holland EC. (2001). Animal models of cell cycle dysregulation and the pathogenesis of gliomas. *Journal of neuro-oncology,* Vol. 51, pp. 265–76, ISSN 0167-594X

Huszthy PC, Brekken C, Pedersen TB, et al. (2006). Antitumor efficacy improved by local delivery of species-specific endostatin. *Journal of neurosurgery,* Vol. 104, pp. 118–128, ISSN 0022-3085

Jallo GI, Volkov A, Wong C, et al. (2006). A novel brainstem tumor model: functional and histopathological characterization. *Child's nervous system,* Vol. 22, pp. 1519–1525, ISSN 0256-7040

Jeffes EW, Zhang JG, Hoa N, et al. (2005). Antiangiogenic drugs synergize with a membrane macrophage colony-stimulating factor-based tumor vaccine to therapeutically treat rats with an established malignant intracranial glioma. *Journal of immunology,* Vol. 174, pp. 2533–2543, ISSN0022-1767

Karmakar S, Olive MF, Banik NL, et al. (2007). Intracranial stereotaxic cannulation for development of orthotopic glioblastoma allograft in Sprague-Dawley rats and histoimmunopathological characterization of the brain tumor. *Neurochemical research,* Vol. 32, pp. 2235–2242, ISSN 0364-3190

Kida Y, Cravioto H, Hochwald GM, et al. (1983).Immunity to transplantable nitrosourea-induced neurogenic tumors. II. Immunoprophylaxis of tumors of the brain. *Journal of neuropathology and experimental neurology,* Vol. 42, pp. 122– 135, ISSN 0022-3069

Kielian T, van Rooijen N, Hickey WF. (2002). MCP-1 expression in CNS-1 astrocytoma cells: implications for macrophage infiltration into tumors in vivo. *Journal of neuro-oncology,* Vol. 56, pp. 1–12, ISSN 0167-594X

Kimmelman J & Nalbantoglu J. (2007). Faithful companions: a proposal for neurooncology trials in pet dogs. *Cancer research,* Vol. 67, pp. 4541–4544, ISSN 0008-5472

Ko L, Koestner A & Wechsler W. (1980). Morphological characterization of nitrosourea-induced glioma cell lines and clones. *Acta neuropathologica,* Vol. 51, pp. 23–31, ISSN 0001-6322

Kobayashi N, Allen N, Clendenon NR, et al. An improved rat brain-tumor model. Journal of neurosurgery 1980;53:808–815. ISSN 0022-3085

Kruse CA, Molleston MC, Parks EP, et al. (1994). A rat glioma model, CNS-1, with invasive characteristics similar to those of human gliomas: a comparison to 9L gliosarcoma. *Journal of neuro-oncology,* Vol. 22, pp. 191– 200, ISSN 0167-594X

Kumar S, Brown SL, Kolozsvary A, et al. (2008). Efficacy of suicide gene therapy in hypoxic rat 9L glioma cells. *Journal of neuro-oncology,* Vol. 90, pp. 19–24, ISSN 0167-594X

Kurozumi K, Hardcastle J, Thakur R, et al. (2007). Effect of tumor microenvironment modulation on the efficacy of oncolytic virus therapy. *Journal of the National Cancer Institute,* Vol. 99, pp. 1768–1781, ISSN 0027-8874

Laerum OD, Rajewsky MF, Schachner M, et al. (1977). Phenotypic properties of neoplastic cell lines developed from fetal rat brain cells in culture after exposure to ethylnitrosourea in vivo. *Zeitschrift für Krebsforschung und klinische Onkologie. Cancer research and clinical oncology,* Vol. 89, pp. 273–295, ISSN 0084-5353

Lal S, Lacroix M, Tofilon P, et al. (2000). An implantable guide-screw system for brain tumor studies in small animals. *Journal of neurosurgery,* Vol. 92, pp. 326–333, ISSN 0022-3085

Lampson LA, Lampson MA & Dunne AD. (1993). Exploiting the lacZ reporter gene for quantitative analysis of disseminated tumor growth within the brain: use of the lacZ gene product as a tumor antigen, for evaluation of antigenic modulation, and to facilitate image analysis of tumor growth in situ. *Cancer research,* Vol. 53, pp. 176–182, ISSN 0008-5472

Lampson LA. (2001). New animal models to probe brain tumor biology, therapy, and immunotherapy: advantages and remaining concerns. *Journal of neuro-oncology,* Vol. 53, pp. 275–287, ISSN 0167-594X

Landen JW, Hau V, Wang M, et al. (2004). Noscapine crosses the blood-brain barrier and inhibits glioblastoma growth. *Clinical cancer research,* Vol. 10, pp. 5187–5201, ISSN 1078-0432

Lapointe M, Lanthier J, Moumdjian R, et al. (2005). Expression and activity of l-isoaspartyl methyltransferase decrease in stage progression of human astrocytic tumors. *Brain research Molecular brain research,* Vol. 135, pp. 93–103, ISSN 0169-328X

Lipsitz D, Higgins RJ, Kortz GD, et al. (2003). Glioblastoma multiforme: clinical findings, magnetic resonance imaging, and pathology in five dogs. *Veterinary Pathology,* Vol. 40, pp. 659–69, ISSN 0300-9858

Liu Y, Wang Q, Kleinschmidt-DeMasters BK, et al. (2007). TGF-beta2 inhibition augments the effect of tumor vaccine and improves the survival of animals with pre-established brain tumors. *Journal of neuro-oncology,* Vol. 81, pp. 149–162, ISSN 0167-594X

Madara J, Krewet JA & Shah M. (2005). Heat shock protein 72 expression allows permissive replication of oncolytic adenovirus dl1520 (ONYX-015) in rat glioblastoma cells. *Molecular Cancer,* Vol. 4, pp. 12, ISSN1476-4598

Mannino S, Molinari A, Sabatino G, et al. (2008). Intratumoral vs systemic administration of metatetrahydroxyphenylchlorin for photodynamic therapy of malignant gliomas: assessment of uptake and spatial distribution in C6 rat glioma model. *International journal of immunopathology and pharmacology,* Vol. 21, pp. 227–231, ISSN 0394-6320

Marumoto T, Tashiro A, Friedmann-Morvinski D, et al. (2009).Development of a novel mouse glioma model using lentiviral vectors. *Nature Medicine,* Vol. 15, pp. 110–6, ISSN1078-8956

Mathieu D, Lecomte R, Tsanaclis AM, et al. (2007). Standardization and detailed characterization of the syngeneic Fischer/F98 glioma model. *The Canadian journal of neurological sciences,* Vol. 34, pp. 296–306, ISSN 0317-1671

Miknyoczki S, Chang H, Grobelny J, et al. (2007). The selective poly(ADP-ribose) polymerase-1(2) inhibitor, CEP-8983, increases the sensitivity of chemoresistant tumor cells to temozolomide and irinotecan but does not potentiate myelotoxicity. *Molecular cancer therapeutics,* Vol. 6, pp. 2290–2302, ISSN 1535-7163

Moolten FL. (1986). Tumor chemosensitivity conferred by inserted herpes thymidine kinase genes: paradigm for a prospective cancer control strategy. *Cancer research,* Vol. 46, pp. 5276–5281, ISSN 0008-5472

Morantz RA, Wood GW, Foster M, et al. (1979). Macrophages in experimental and human brain tumors. Part 1: Studies of the macrophage content of experimental rat brain tumors of varying immunogenicity. *Journal of neurosurgery,* Vol. 50, pp. 298–304, ISSN 0022-3085

Moriuchi S, Wolfe D, Tamura M, et al. (2002). Double suicide gene therapy using a replication defective herpes simplex virus vector reveals reciprocal interference in a malignant glioma model. *Gene therapy,* Vol. 9, pp. 584–591, ISSN 0969-7128

Mourad PD, Farrell L, Stamps LD, et al. (2003). Quantitative assessment of glioblastoma invasion in vivo. *Cancer Letters,* Vol. 192, pp. 97–107, ISSN 0304-3835

Nakada M, Niska JA, Tran NL, et al. (2005). EphB2/R-ras signaling regulates glioma cell adhesion, growth, and invasion. *American Journal Pathology,* Vol. 167, pp. 565–576, ISSN 0002-9440

Namba H, Tagawa M, Miyagawa T, et al. (2000). Treatment of rat experimental brain tumors by herpes simplex virus thymidine kinase gene-transduced allogeneic tumor cells and ganciclovir. *Cancer gene therapy,* Vol. 7, pp. 947–953, 0929-1903

Ningaraj NS, Rao M, Hashizume K, et al. (2002). Regulation of blood-brain tumor barrier permeability by calcium-activated potassium channels. *The Journal of pharmacology and experimental therapeutics,* Vol. 301, pp. 838–851, ISSN 0022-3565

Oh S, Pluhar GE, McNeil EA, et al. (2007). Efficacy of nonviral gene transfer in the canine brain. *Journal of neurosurgery,* Vol. 107, pp. 136–44, ISSN 0022-3085

Ohlfest JR, Freese AB & Largaespada DA. (2005). Nonviral vectors for cancer gene therapy: prospects for integrating vectors and combination therapies. *Current Gene Therapy,* Vol. 5, pp. 629–41, ISSN 1566-5232

Ohlfest JR, Lobitz PD, Perkinson SG & Largaespada DA. (2004). Integration and long-term expression in xenografted human glioblastoma cells using a plasmid-based transposon system. *Molecular therapy,* Vol. 10, pp. 260–8, ISSN 1525-0016

Olson MV, Johnson DG, Jiang H, et al. (2007). Transgenic E2F1 expression in the mouse brain induces a human-like bimodal pattern of tumors. *Cancer research,* Vol. 67, pp. 4005–9, ISSN 0008-5472

Oshiro S, Liu Y, Fukushima T, et al. (2001). Modified immunoregulation associated with interferon-gamma treatment of rat glioma. *Neurological research,* Vol. 23, pp. 359–366, ISSN 0161-6412

Owens GC, Orr EA, DeMasters BK, et al. (1998). Overexpression of a transmembrane isoform of neural cell adhesion molecule alters the invasiveness of rat CNS-1 glioma. *Cancer research,* Vol. 58, pp. 2020- 2028, ISSN 0008-5472

Ozawa T, Hu JL, Hu LJ, et al. (2005). Functionality of hypoxia-induced BAX expression in a human glioblastoma xenograft model. *Cancer gene therapy,* Vol. 12, pp. 449–55, ISSN 0929-1903

Parsa AT, Chakrabarti I, Hurley PT, et al. (2000). Limitations of the C6/Wistar rat intracerebral glioma model: implications for evaluating immunotherapy. *Neurosurgery,* Vol. 47, pp. 993- 999, discussion 999–1000, ISSN 0148-396X

Paul DB, Barth RF, Yang W, et al. (2000). B7.1 expression by the weakly immunogenic F98 rat glioma does not enhance immunogenicity. *Gene therapy,* Vol. 7, pp. 993–999, ISSN 0969-7128

Pfeiffer SE, Herschman HR, Lightbody J, et al. (1970). Synthesis by a clonal line of rat glial cells of a protein unique to the nervous system. *Journal of cellular physiology,* Vol. 75, pp. 329–339, ISSN 0021-9541

Pietronigro D, Drnovsky F, Cravioto H & Ransohoff J. (2003). DTI-015 produces cures in T9 gliosarcoma. *Neoplasia,* Vol. 5, pp. 17–22, ISSN 1522-8002

Platten M, Kretz A, Naumann U, et al. (2003). Monocyte chemoattractant protein-1 increases microglial infiltration and aggressiveness of gliomas. *Annals of neurology,* Vol. 54, pp. 388–392, ISSN 0364-5134

Prabhu SS, Broaddus WC, Oveissi C, et al. (2000). Determination of intracranial tumor volumes in a rodent brain using magnetic resonance imaging, Evans blue, and histology: a comparative study. *IEEE transactions on bio-medical engineering,* Vol. 47, pp. 259–265, ISSN 0018-9294

Pulkkinen M, Pikkarainen J, Wirth T, et al. (2008). Three-step tumor targeting of paclitaxel using biotinylated PLA-PEG nanoparticles and avidin-biotin technology: formulation development and in vitro anticancer activity. *European journal of pharmaceutics and biopharmaceutics,* Vol. 70, pp. 66–74, ISSN 0939-6411

Rainov NG, Koch S, Sena-Esteves M & Berens ME. (2000). Characterization of a canine glioma cell line as related to established experimental brain tumor models. *J ournal of neuropathology and experimental neurology,* Vol. 59, pp. 607–13, ISSN 0022-3069

Raty JK, Airenne KJ, Marttila AT, et al. (2004). Enhanced gene delivery by avidin-displaying baculovirus. *Molecular therapy,* Vol. 9, pp. 282–291, ISSN 1525-0016

Regnard P, Le Duc G, Brauer-Krisch E, et al. (2008). Irradiation of intracerebral 9L gliosarcoma by a single array of microplanar x-ray beams from a synchrotron: balance between curing and sparing. *Physics inmedicine and biology,* Vol. 53, pp. 861–878, ISSN 0031-9155

Reilly KM, Rubin JB, Gilbertson RJ, et al. (2008). Rethinking brain tumors: the fourth mouse models of human cancers consortium nervous system tumors workshop. *Cancer research,* Vol. 68, pp. 5508– 5511, ISSN 0008-5472

Reilly KM. (2009). Brain tumor susceptibility: the role of genetic factors and uses of mouse models to unravel risk. *Brain pathology,* Vol. 19, pp. 121–31, ISSN 1015-6305

Rong Y, Durden DL, Van Meir EG & Brat DJ. (2006). 'Pseudopalisading' necrosis in glioblastoma: a familiar morphologic feature that links vascular pathology, hypoxia, and angiogenesis. *Journal of neuropathology and experimental neurology,* Vol. 65, pp. 529–39, ISSN 0022-3069

Rousseau R, Barth RF, Moeschberger ML, et al. (2008). Efficacy of intracerebral delivery of carboplatin in combination with photon irradiation for treatment of F98 glioma bearing rats. *International journal of radiation oncology, biology, physics,* Vol. 73, pp. 530–536, ISSN 0360-3016

Saini M, Roser F, Samii M, et al. (2004). A model for intra-tumoural chemotherapy in the rat brain. *Acta Neurochirurgica (Wien)* , Vol. 146, pp. 731–734, ISSN 0001-6268

Saito R, Bringas J, Mirek H, et al. (2004). Invasive phenotype observed in 1, 3-bis(2-chloroethyl)-1- nitrosourea-resistant sub-lines of 9L rat glioma cells: a tumor model mimicking a recurrent malignant glioma. *Journal of neurosurgery*, Vol. 101, pp. 826–831, ISSN 0022-3085

Sandstrom M, Johansson M, Bergstrom P, et al. (2008). Effects of the VEGFR inhibitor ZD6474 in combination with radiotherapy and temozolomide in an orthotopic glioma model. *Journal of neuro-oncology*, Vol. 88, pp. 1–9, ISSN 0167-594X

Schepkin VD, Lee KC, Kuszpit K, et al. (2006). Proton and sodium MRI assessment of emerging tumor chemotherapeutic resistance. *NMR in biomedicine*, Vol. 19, pp. 1035–1042, ISSN 0952-3480

Schlegel J, Piontek G, Kersting M, Schuermann M, Kappler R, Scherthan H, Weghorst C, Buzard G & Mennel H. (1999). The p16/Cdkn2a/Ink4a gene is frequently deleted in nitrosourea-induced rat glial tumors. *Pathobiology*,Vol. 67, pp. 202–206, ISSN 1015-2008

Schmidek HH, Nielsen SL, Schiller AL, et al. (1971). Morphological studies of rat brain tumors induced by N-nitrosomethylurea. *Journal of neurosurgery*, Vol. 34, pp. 335–340, ISSN 0022-3085

Schwartzbaum JA, Fisher JL, Aldape KD & Wrensch M. (2006). Epidemiology and molecular pathology of glioma. Nature clinical practice. *Neurology*, Vol. 2, pp. 494–503, ISSN 1745-834X

Shah MR & Ramsey WJ. (2003). CD8 + T-cell mediated anti-tumor responses cross-reacting against 9L and RT2 rat glioma cell lines. *Cellular immunology*, Vol. 225, pp. 113–121, ISSN 0008-8749

Sharma MK, Zehnbauer BA, Watson MA & Gutmann DH. (2005). RAS pathway activation and an oncogenic RAS mutation in sporadic pilocytic astrocytoma. *Neurology*, Vol. 65, pp. 1335–36, ISSN 0028-3878

Sheehan J, Ionescu A, Pouratian N, et al. (2008). Use of trans sodium crocetinate for sensitizing glioblastoma multiforme to radiation: laboratory investigation. *Journal of neurosurgery*, Vol. 108, pp. 972–978, ISSN 0022-3085

Shen DH, Marsee DK, Schaap J, et al. (2004). Effects of dose, intervention time, and radionuclide on sodium iodide symporter (NIS)-targeted radionuclide therapy. *Gene therapy*, Vol. 11, pp. 161–169, ISSN 0969-7128

Shen G, Shen F, Shi Z, et al. (2008). Identification of cancer stem-like cells in the C6 glioma cell line and the limitation of current identification methods. *In vitro cellular & developmental biology. Animal* , Vol. 44, pp. 280– 289, ISSN 1071-2690

Shibuya N, Hochgeschwender U, Kida Y, et al. (1984). Immunity to transplantable nitrosourea-induced neurogenic tumors. III. Systemic adoptive transfer of immunity. *Journal of neuropathology and experimental neurology*, Vol. 43, pp. 426–438 ISSN 0022-3069

Shih AH, Dai C, Hu X, et al. (2004). Dose-dependent effects of platelet-derived growth factor-B on glial tumorigenesis. *Cancer research*, Vol. 64, pp. 4783–9, ISSN 0008-5472

Sibenaller ZA, Etame AB, Ali MM, et al. (2005). Genetic characterization of commonly used glioma cell lines in the rat animal model system. *Neurosurgical focus*, Vol. 19, E1. 10. pp. 3171 ISSN 1092-0684

Singer O & Verma IM. (2008). Applications of lentiviral vectors for shRNA delivery and transgenesis. *Current Gene Therapy*, Vol. 8, pp. 483–8, ISSN 1566-5232

Smilowitz HM, Micca PL, Nawrocky MM, et al. (2000). The combination of boron neutron-capture therapy and immunoprophylaxis for advanced intracerebral gliosarcomas in rats. *Journal of neuro-oncology*, Vol. 46, pp. 231– 240, ISSN 0167-594X

Solly F, Fish R, Simard B, et al. (2008). Tissue-type plasminogen activator has antiangiogenic properties without effect on tumor growth in a rat C6 glioma model. *Cancer gene therapy,* Vol. 15, pp. 685- 692, ISSN 0929-1903

Stoica G, Kim HT, Hall DG & Coates JR. (2004). Morphology, immunohistochemistry, and genetic alterations in dog astrocytomas. *Veterinary Pathology,* Vol. 41, pp. 10–9, ISSN 0300-9858

Stoica G, Lungu G, Martini-Stoica H, et al. (2009). Identification of cancer stem cells in dog glioblastoma. *Veterinary Pathology,* Vol. 46, pp. 391–406, ISSN 0300-9858

Stojiljkovic M, Piperski V, Dacevic M, et al. (2003). Characterization of 9L glioma model of the Wistar rat. *Journal of neuro-oncology,* Vol. 63, pp. 1–7, ISSN 0167-594X

Stuhr LE, Raa A, Oyan AM, et al. (2007). Hyperoxia retards growth and induces apoptosis, changes in vascular density and gene expression in transplanted gliomas in nude rats. *Journal of neuro-oncology,* Vol.85, pp. 191–202, ISSN 0167-594X

Tanriover N, Ulu MO, Sanus GZ, et al. (2008). The effects of systemic and intratumoral interleukin-12 treatment in C6 rat glioma model. *Neurological research,* Vol. 30, pp. 511–517, ISSN 0161-6412

Trojan J, Johnson TR, Rudin SD, et al. (1993). Treatment and prevention of rat glioblastoma by immunogenic C6 cells expressing antisense insulin-like growth factor I RNA. *Science,* Vol. 259, pp. 94–97, ISSN 0193-4511

Tsurushima H, Yuan X, Dillehay LE & Leong KW. (2007). Radioresponsive tumor necrosis factor-related apoptosis-inducing ligand (TRAIL) gene therapy for malignant brain tumors. *Cancer gene therapy,* Vol. 14, pp. 706–16, ISSN0929-1903

Tzeng JJ, Barth RF, Orosz CG, et al. (1991). Phenotype and functional activity of tumor-infiltrating lymphocytes isolated from immunogenic and nonimmunogenic rat brain tumors. *Cancer research,* Vol. 51, pp. 2373–2378, ISSN 0008-5472

Valable S, Lemasson B, Farion R, et al. (2008). Assessment of blood volume, vessel size, and the expression of angiogenic factors in two rat glioma models: a longitudinal in vivo and ex vivo study. *NMR in biomedicine,* Vol. 21, pp. 1043–1056, ISSN 0952-3480

Valerie K, Brust D, Farnsworth J, et al. (2000). Improved radio-sensitization of rat glioma cells with adenovirus-expressed mutant herpes simplex virus-thymidine kinase in combination with acyclovir. *Cancer gene therapy,* Vol. 7, pp. 879–884, ISSN 0929-1903

Valerie K, Hawkins W, Farnsworth J, et al. (2001). Substantially improved in vivo radiosensitization of rat glioma with mutant HSV-TK and acyclovir. *Cancer gene therapy,* Vol.8, pp. 3–8, ISSN 0929-1903

Vallbo C, Bergenheim T, Hedman H, et al. (2002). The antimicrotubule drug estramustine but not irradiation induces apoptosis in malignant glioma involving AKT and caspase pathways. *Journal of neuro-oncology,* Vol. 56, pp. 143–148, ISSN 0167-594X

von Eckardstein KL, Patt S, Kratzel C, et al. (2005), Local chemotherapy of F98 rat glioblastoma with paclitaxel and carboplatin embedded in liquid crystalline cubic phases. *Journal of neuro-oncology,* Vol. 72, pp. 209- 215, ISSN 0167-594X

von Eckardstein KL, Patt S, Zhu J, et al. (2001). Short-term neuropathological aspects of in vivo suicide gene transfer to the F98 rat glioblastoma using liposomal and viral vectors. *Histology and histopathology,* Vol. 16, pp. 735–744, ISSN 0213-3911

Wakimoto H, Fulci G, Tyminski E, et al. (2004). Altered expression of antiviral cytokine mRNAs associated with cyclophosphamide's enhancement of viral oncolysis. *Gene therapy,* Vol.11, pp. 214–2230969-7128

Warnke PC, Blasberg RG & Groothuis DR. (1987). The effect of hyperosmotic blood-brain barrier disruption on blood-to-tissue transport in ENU-induced gliomas. *Annals of neurology*, Vol. 22, pp. 300–305, ISSN 0364-5134

Weizsacker M, Nagamune A, Winkelstroter R, et al. (1982). Radiation and drug response of the rat glioma RG2. *European journal of cancer & clinical oncology*, Vol. 18, pp. 891–895, ISSN 0277-5379

Wiesner SM, Decker SA, Larson JD, et al. (2009). De novo induction of genetically engineered brain tumors in mice using plasmid DNA. *Cancer research*, Vol. 69, pp. 431–9, ISSN 0008-5472

Wu G, Yang W, Barth RF, et al. (2007). Molecular targeting and treatment of an epidermal growth factor receptor-positive glioma using boronated cetuximab. *Clinical cancer research*, Vol. 13, pp. 1260– 1268, ISSN1078-0432

Wu X, Hu J, Zhou L, et al. (2008). In vivo tracking of super-paramagnetic iron oxide nanoparticle-labeled mesenchymal stem cell tropism to malignant gliomas using magnetic resonance imaging. Laboratory investigation. *Journal of neurosurgery*, Vol. 108, pp. 320–329, ISSN 0022-3085

Yang H, Chopp M, Zhang X, et al. (2007). Using behavioral measurement to assess tumor progression and functional outcome after antiangiogenic treatment in mouse glioma models. *Behavioural brain research*, Vol. 182, pp. 42–50, ISSN 0166-4328

Yang W, Barth RF, Wu G, et al. (2005). Development of a syngeneic rat brain tumor model expressing EGFRvIII and its use for molecular targeting studies with monoclonal antibody L8A4. *Clinical cancer research*, Vol. 11, pp. 341–350, ISSN 1078-0432

Yang W, Wu G, Barth RF, et al. (2008). Molecular targeting and treatment of composite EGFR and EGFRvIII-positive gliomas using boronated monoclonal antibodies. *Clinical cancer research*, Vol. 14, pp. 883– 891, ISSN 1078-0432

Yang WQ, Lun X, Palmer CA, et al. (2004). Efficacy and safety evaluation of human reovirus type 3 in immunocompetent animals: racine and nonhuman primates. *Clinical cancer research*, Vol. 10, pp. 8561– 8576, ISSN 1078-0432

Zagorac D, Jakovcevic D, Gebremedhin D, et al. (2008). Anti-angiogenic effect of inhibitors of cytochrome P450 on rats with glioblastoma multiforme. *Journal of cerebral blood flow and metabolism*, Vol. 28, pp. 1431–1439, ISSN 0271-678X

Zhang J, van Zijl PC, Laterra J, et al. (2007). Unique patterns of diffusion directionality in rat brain tumors revealed by high-resolution diffusion tensor MRI. *Magnetic resonance in medicine*, Vol. 58, pp. 454–462, ISSN 0740-3194

Zhao S, Zhang X, Zhang J, et al. (2008). Intravenous administration of arsenic trioxide encapsulated in liposomes inhibits the growth of C6 gliomas in rat brains. *Journal of chemotherapy*, Vol. 20, pp. 253–262, ISSN 1120-009X

Zheng H, Ying H, Yan H, Kimmelman AC, Hiller DJ, et al. (2008). p53 and Pten control neural and glioma stem/progenitor cell renewal and differentiation. *Nature*, Vol.455, pp. 1129–33, ISSN 0028-0836

Zhu H, Acquaviva J, Ramachandran P, Boskovitz A, Woolfenden S, et al. (2009). Oncogenic EGFR signaling cooperates with loss of tumor suppressor gene functions in gliomagenesis. *Proceedings of the National Academy of Sciences of the United States of America USA*; Vol.106, pp. 2712–1, ISSN 0027-8424

Zhu Y. & Parada LF. (2002). The molecular and genetic basis of neurological tumours. *Nature review Cancer*, Vol.2, pp. 616–26, ISSN 1474-175X

17

Three-Dimensional In Vitro Models in Glioma Research – Focus on Spheroids

Stine Skov Jensen, Charlotte Aaberg-Jessen, Ida Pind Jakobsen, Simon Kjær Hermansen, Søren Kabell Nissen and Bjarne Winther Kristensen
Department of Pathology, Odense University Hospital, Institute of Clinical Research
University of Southern Denmark
Denmark

1. Introduction

In the field of glioma research, in vitro models are widely used to investigate tumor biology as well as tumor response to chemotherapy and radiation. There is an increasing need to improve these in vitro models in order to meet the new challenges arising in drug discovery. It is thus important that development of new drugs is based on the latest knowledge about glioma biology such as for example the recent discovery of tumor stem cells (Reya et al., 2001). When investigating glioblastomas in vitro - and especially the supposed tumor stem cells - three dimensional multicellular spheroid models have recently come into focus.

The aim of this chapter is to review the development as well as the most recent aspects of the three-dimensional glioma in vitro models focusing on glioma spheroids. The implementation of these models in current and in future in vitro glioma research will be discussed putting emphasis on the themes described below.

Cell lines cultured as monolayers have been the in vitro model of choice for many years (Ponten & Macintyre, 1968). However, the three-dimensional aspect came into focus in the 1970's, where scientists started to grow tumor cells from cell lines as multicellular spheroids (Yuhas et al., 1977). Over the years the spheroid model has been improved by deriving spheroids from cells obtained from dissociated primary glioblastoma tissue (Mackillop et al., 1985) as well as by using organotypic primary spheroids derived from small tumor fragments (Bjerkvig et al., 1990).

In general, most in vitro studies are performed with cells cultured in conventional serum-containing medium. Recently - as the tumor stem cell theory has evolved - the culturing medium has come into focus. It has thus been demonstrated that the use of serum-free medium for culturing of cell line-derived spheroids preserved the in vivo-like features as well as the tumor stem cell-like phenotype suggesting crucial importance of the use of serum-free medium in tumor stem cell research (Lee et al., 2006).

Identification of the glioma stem cells is still a matter of discussion. The most used marker in the field has been the cell surface marker CD133. Expression of this putative tumor stem cell marker in gliomas has been studied in several papers demonstrating clusters or niches of CD133 positive tumor cells as well as CD133 positive single cells dispersed in the tumor

(Christensen et al., 2008; Hermansen et al., 2011). These important tumor stem cell niches are preserved in primary glioma spheroids in contrast to cell line spheroids (Christensen et al., 2010).

Another important aspect in culturing of glioma stem cells is hypoxia, since several studies have shown that hypoxia influences radiation resistance. This may be explained by effects of hypoxia in vitro on proliferation of the tumor cells, spheroid formation and expression of stem cell markers, suggesting that also this aspect should be taken into consideration (Heddleston et al., 2009; Kolenda et al., 2010; McCord et al., 2009; Soeda et al., 2009).

Several studies have used the different types of spheroids mentioned above for investigating the effects of chemotherapy and radiation on the tumor cells and in particular on the tumor stem-like cells (Bao et al., 2006; Bauman et al., 1999; Fehlauer et al., 2005; Fehlauer et al., 2006; Fehlauer et al., 2007; Genc et al., 2004; Gliemroth et al., 2003; Haas-Kogan et al., 1996; Johannessen et al., 2009; Kaaijk et al., 1997; Khaitan et al., 2009; Sunayama et al., 2010; Terzis et al., 1997; Terzis et al., 1998; Wakimoto et al., 2009; Wang et al., 2010). After such treatments cell viability and cell proliferation assays as well as secondary spheroid formation assays have been used to evaluate induced effects. Moreover, expression of apoptosis and proliferation markers and for example stem cell markers have been investigated immunohistochemically in paraffin embedded spheroids (Christensen et al., 2010). The advantages using this panel of methods will be an important part of this chapter.

High grade gliomas are known to be highly invasive and new knowledge concerning tumor cell invasion also incorporating the tumor stem cell aspect is urgently needed. In our laboratory we have worked to improve in vitro models when investigating the invasive features of gliomas. This led to establishment of an in vivo-like model of invasion, where spheroids are implanted into organotypic brain slice cultures.

Taken together the three-dimensional multicellular spheroid model is the three dimensional model of choice for in vivo-like glioma in vitro studies. However, at the same time this model is under ongoing development to become an even more in vivo-like model in order to meet the new challenges of glioma research and drug development. The use of spheroids in especially tumor stem cell research has been fast increasing in recent years making spheroids an important tool also in future glioma research.

2. Establishment and development of the spheroid model

In the field of cancer research it is important to continuously develop in vitro models mimicking in vivo conditions as much as possible. By isolating cells from tumor tissue, tumor cell lines can be established from almost any kind of tumor including brain tumors such as glioblastomas. Glioblastoma cell lines are traditionally cultured as adherent monolayers but can also be cultured as single cell suspensions or spheroids. One of the most used cell lines in glioblastoma research is the cell line U87MG established by Pontén and Macintyre in 1968 (Ponten & Macintyre, 1968). This cell line was established from an astrocytic tumor with necrosis, which corresponds to this tumor being a glioblastoma multiforme according to WHO (World Health Organization) guidelines 2007 (Louis et al. 2007). U87MG was originally established in a traditional serum containing medium and the cells were described as large, extremely bizarre and very slowly growing. Today U87MG can be described as having only limited pleomorphism as well as being fast growing, clearly indicating that such cell lines change over time. U87MG has been used in a variety of glioma studies and is still used. Since the cell line has been cultured in different laboratories for over 40 years new genomic mutations have arisen capable of giving rise to different phenotypic subpopulations in different laboratories. It is also well known that the phenotypic characteristics and genetic aberrations found within in vitro cells passaged repeatedly for about 10 times in serum containing medium often show only little resemblance with the original primary tumor (Lee et al., 2006). It is therefore not surprising that the U87MG cell line is known to have a highly aberrant genomic structure as visualized by karyotyping (Galli et al., 2004). Galli et al. (Galli et al., 2004) demonstrated loss of chromosome 1, 9, 10, 11, 12, 13, 14, 16, 19, 20, 22 and X. Furthermore, 11 unidentified abnormal chromosomes were found, whereas no gains of chromosomes were seen. In addition to this, Clark et al (Clark et al., 2010) have sequenced the genome of U87MG in order to further characterize it. They identified 35 interchromosomal translocation events, 1,315 structural variations (>100 bp), 191,743 small (< 21 bp) insertions and deletions as well as 2,384,470 single nucleotide variations. Protein coding sequences were disrupted predominantly by small insertions and deletions as well as larger deletions and translocations and 512 genes were homozygously mutated. Surprisingly, the study by Clark et al. also indicated that although this U87MG cell line has been cultured for more than 40 years, the cell line has now been relatively stable for years and is not rapidly changing anymore. This relative stability could be an advantage when using the U87MG cell line. In addition, the use of this cell line for four decades has resulted in a very well characterized cell line.

In general, there are many advantages when using cell lines. When first established, they are easy to handle in the laboratory and a large number of cells can be obtained in a short period of time, making it feasible to conduct large scale studies. In addition, cell lines are relatively easy to manipulate genetically by transfection and knock-down etc. establishing subpopulations with specific gene expression. These cell lines are important tools in the field of basic research investigating cellular pathways involved in tumor biology and response to different drugs. In addition to the obvious advantages, there will always be challenges when working with cell lines. As mentioned above, tumor cell lines are very likely to acquire new mutations and chromosome damage when undergoing cell division, because of the unstable genome in the tumor cells. The longer cultures are maintained and passaged the more changes accumulate (Lee et al., 2006) leading to changes in tumor cell behaviour. This is one of the main problems by culturing cell lines for many years. There will always be a possibility that the cells further mutate and several subpopulations will arise. This is important to keep in mind, when comparing results obtained with the same commercial cell line but in different laboratories at different time points.

Another obstacle to overcome when using cell lines is the heterogeneity seen in tumors like glioblastomas. It is not possible to maintain the high degree of heterogeneity in long term cell cultures. In order to improve models using cell lines, short term cultures prepared from fresh tumor biopsies can be an alternative (Kolenda et al., 2010; Potter et al., 2009). The use of short term cultures may reduce differences between the tumor of origin and the cultured cells. In a study by Potter et al. (Potter et al., 2009) short term cultures from 6 pediatric pilocytic astrocytomas and 3 adult glioblastomas were established and cultured in conventional medium containing fetal calf serum. Gene expression profiles of the derived short term cell cultures harvested below passage 8 and their respective original biopsies were performed. They demonstrated that although short term cultures more resemble in situ gliomas than homogenous long term cultures, significant changes in gene expression were found between the biopsies and the derived short term cultures. The most significant functions differing for the glioblastomas were associated with cell structure, shape, motility, proliferation, cellular development, cell death, cellular assembly and organization, cell-to-cell signaling and interaction, as well as cell cycle.

As our knowledge of tumor cells expands, there is a need to establish more advanced models to mimic the tumor in situ. One of the main problems is the fact, that the cells are removed from their natural environment, dissociated and cultured as single cells. It may therefore be important to prevent this in order to be able to mimic the natural environment as much as possible. Moreover in the recent years, the use of serum containing cell culturing medium has come into focus. The composition of serum has not been fully understood for many years, but it is known that it supplies the cells with nutrients, vitamins, hormones, and growth-, differentiation-, and attachment-factors. These factors may affect the cells in ways we are not fully aware of. It is also well known that there are differences between batches of serum (Fisher & Wieser, 1983). Another important issue is the fact that only a small fraction of cells in the organism is in direct contact with serum. This may be a problem in glioma research, since the brain and brain tumor tissues are not among these cells. In this context, it is also worth highlighting that neural stem cells should be cultured under serum-free conditions similar to what has been found for the so called glioblastoma tumor stem cells.

The three-dimensional glioma spheroid model came into focus in the 1970's, where scientists started to grow tumor cells as multicellular spheroids using tumor cells from conventional monolayer cultures (Yuhas et al., 1977). Such spheroids are usually formed by aggregation of cells growing into the larger three-dimensional spheroids. They are believed to be a better model than monolayer cultures due to a three-dimensional structure with more in vivo-like intercellular contacts. This model was later on further improved by deriving spheroids from single cells obtained from dissociated primary glioblastoma tissue (Mackillop et al., 1985). In order to obtain an even more in vivo-like model the primary organotypic spheroids were introduced (Bjerkvig et al., 1990). Organotypic means that the properties characteristic of the tissue of origin is maintained. These spheroids are derived from freshly removed glioma tissue and have been shown to be a valid tumor model providing a biological system that mimics the original glioma in vivo.

When deriving primary spheroids from glioma biopsies, it is important to process the tumor tissue as soon as it is removed. As we have published earlier (Christensen et al., 2010) the glioma tissue should be collected directly in the operation theatre, where the tissue is placed in a tube with Hanks' Balanced Salt Solution supplemented with 0.9 % glucose and transported to the laboratory. The tumor tissue can then be processed according to the study by Bjerkvig et al. (Bjerkvig et al., 1990), where small tumor fragments of approximately 200-400 µm in diameter are obtained after sectioning the tumor tissue manually using scalpels. These fragments are then transferred to 0.75% agar-coated culture flasks of 75 cm^2 with pre-warmed medium. The cultures should be kept in a standard tissue culture incubator (95% humidity, 95% air, and 5% CO_2) and the following day the culturing medium should be changed in order to remove dead blood cells and cellular debris. The tumor fragments should then be examined under a light microscope every day, until they round up to form spheroids within 5-15 days.

The main advantages by primary organotypic spheroids are the preservation of the original intercellular contacts and the tumor heterogeneity. However, because of this heterogeneity it is important to include a larger number of spheroids in in vitro studies using primary spheroids in order to obtain reproducible results. In a study by Bjerkvig et al., (Bjerkvig et al., 1990) it was shown that when culturing small tumor fragments from astrocytic brain tumors of increasing grade, small primary spheroids were formed for the majority of the tumors within 3-5 days. The spheroids were analyzed by light microscopy as well as transmission- and scanning electron microscopy (TEM and SEM, respectively) after 3 and 10 weeks of culture, showing the unique preservation of cell- to cell interaction, blood vessels, extracellular matrix, and macrophages. It was moreover demonstrated that the primary spheroids could be cultured for 70 days with preservation of the histology of the spheroids. In a similar study in our laboratory, glioma tissue was collected from 11 patients. The tissue pieces from 7 of these patients formed vital spheroids within a week. Thereafter, the spheroids were fixed, paraffin embedded and investigated immunohistochemically as described later in this chapter. Areas of necrosis were seen in some of the spheroids, whereas blood vessels were present in the majority of the glioma-derived spheroids.

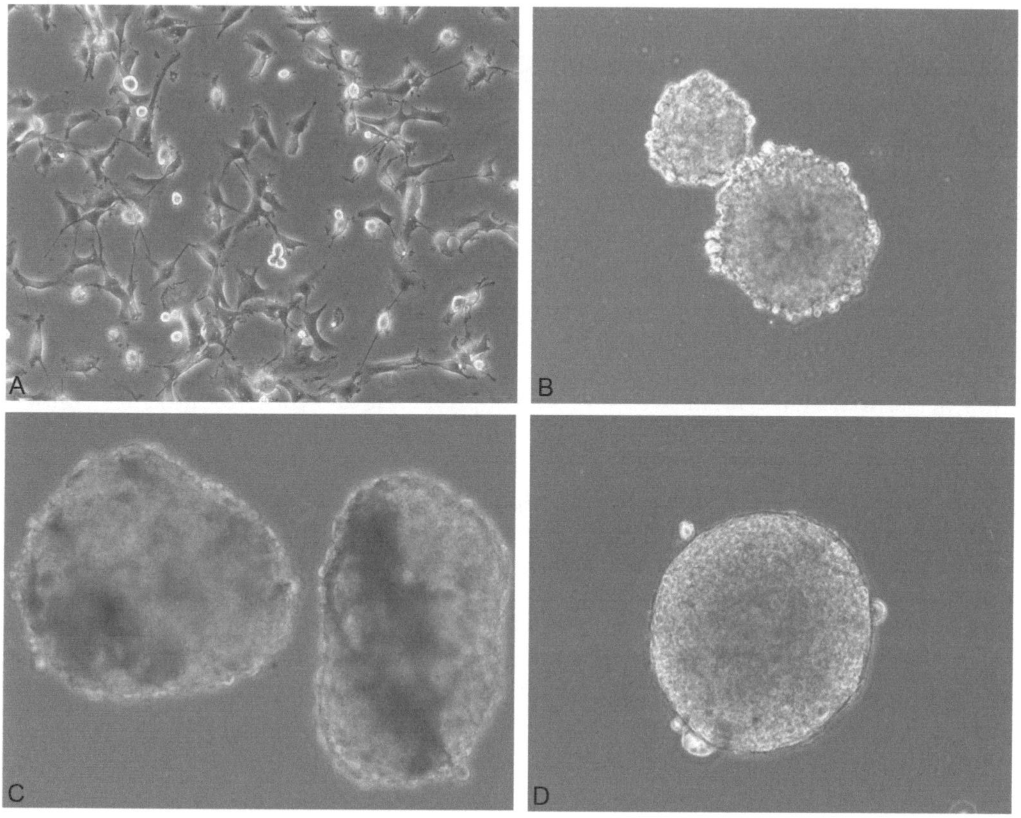

Fig. 1. Adherent monolayer cells and free floating spheroids. U87MG grows as an adherent monolayer when the cells are cultured in serum containing medium (A). However, in serum-free medium U87MG grows as spheroids (B). Tissue derived from freshly removed glioblastoma (C) and cells from a glioblastoma short term culture (D) also grow as spheroids when cultured in a serum-free medium. The organotypic spheroids (C) can be grown in serum containing medium as well and preserves in both media some of the characteristics found in the primary tumor such as tumor necrosis and blood vessels, whereas the short term culture spheroid in (D) has lost these characteristics.

1. Collect tissue and transport the freshly removed tumor tissue in Hanks' Balanced Salt Solution supplemented with 0.9% glucose
2. Place the tissue in a sterile petri dish
3. Section the tumor tissue manually using two scalpels until tumor fragments of 50-400 μm in diameter are obtained
4. Culture fragments in 0.75% agar coated culture flasks containing 20 ml medium
5. Incubate the cultures in 36°C humidified air containing 5% CO_2 and 95% atmospheric air
6. Change the medium the next day
7. Change the medium twice a week in 10-15 days until the fragments round up and form spheroids

Box 1. Preparation of organotypic primary spheroids

3. The tumor stem cell paradigm and the spheroid model

The tumor stem cell paradigm proposes that only a small subset of cells - the so-called tumor stem cells - within the tumor cell population is able to initiate and sustain tumor growth (Ward & Dirks, 2007). These tumor stem cells have been found in a variety of different cancers such as leukaemia (Bonnet & Dick, 1997), colon cancer (Daidone et al., 2004), breast cancer (Al-Hajj et al., 2003) and brain cancer (Singh et al., 2004). With the discovery of the neural stem cells (Reynolds & Weiss, 1992) it also became plausible that brain tumors could be derived from the transformation of neural stem cells or progenitor cells (Singh et al., 2004). The neural stem cells were first isolated by Reynolds and Weiss in 1992 (Reynolds & Weiss, 1992). They found a small population of cells isolated from the adult striatum in mouse brain that were able to proliferate and differentiate. They cultured these cells in a serum-free environment supplemented with the growth factors EGF (epidermal growth factor) and bFGF (basic fibroblast growth factor), and the cells grew as neurospheres. When dissociating the neurospheres and re-plating them as single cells new neurospheres developed. Under these serum-free conditions most differentiating and differentiated cells died, whereas the neural stem cells responded to the growth factors and proliferated to form neurospheres (Vescovi et al., 2006). By applying the same conditions to human glioblastoma cells, it was possible to isolate a population of cells that formed tumorspheres. These cells were capable of differentiation and self-renewal (Galli et al., 2004; Ignatova et al., 2002; Lee et al., 2006; Singh et al., 2003). Furthermore, the cells from the tumorspheres gave rise to tumors resembling the primary tumor when injected into the brains of immunodeficient mice, suggesting that a population of the cells isolated were brain tumor-initiating stem-like cells.

When culturing putative tumor stem cells, spheroid models are often used. Especially the clonogenic neurosphere assay is used for preserving tumor stem-like cells in serum-free medium (Lee et al., 2006). In this assay, primary human brain tumor tissue form spheroids after repeated dissociation into single cells. However, cell-to-cell interactions are interrupted and this might affect experimental results obtained with the tumor stem cell line-derived spheroids. This could be particularly important in tumor stem cell research, since the suggested close relationship between brain tumor stem cells and adjacent endothelial cells (Bao et al., 2006; Calabrese et al., 2007) is lost in these spheroids. In addition, the culturing medium has come into focus when performing studies focusing on tumor stem cells. As mentioned earlier, normal neural stem cells are cultured under serum-free conditions, since it is well known that serum causes irreversible differentiation of neural stem cells (Gage et al., 1995). Lee et al. (Lee et al., 2006) cultured glioblastoma short term cultures in a serum-free medium similar to the medium used for culturing neural stem cells in order to preserve and select for tumor stem-like cells. This serum-free medium consisted of neurobasal medium supplemented with EGF and bFGF, because EGF and bFGF earlier seemed to select for tumor stem-like cells by inducing proliferation of multipotent, self-renewing, and expandable tumor stem cells (Galli et al., 2004; Ignatova et al., 2002; Lee et al., 2006). In the study by Lee et al., (Lee et al., 2006) dissociated glioblastoma cells, cultured as short term cultures, formed spheroids expressing putative tumor stem cell markers but when culturing the selected cells in serum containing medium, they irreversibly differentiated into neural and glial cell lineages. Interestingly, this is in line with the irreversible differentiation of neural stem cells under the same conditions (Gage et al., 1995).

In the search for improvement of in vitro models we performed a study in our laboratory (Christensen et al., 2010), where organotypic primary spheroids were cultured in serum-free medium. In terms of the tumor stem cell concept, culturing of these organotypic primary spheroids in serum-free conditions may be closer to the in vivo situation than using tumor stem cell line-derived spheroids, especially regarding studies of radiation and chemo-sensitivity. We investigated the influence of serum-containing medium and serum-free medium on the phenotype of primary glioma spheroids. The aim was to elucidate whether serum-free medium also favors the presence of tumor cells expressing stem cell markers in these spheroids, when investigated immunohistochemically. The results based on seven malignant astrocytomas WHO Grade III–IV, supported the hypothesis that putative brain tumor stem cells are better preserved in serum-free culture medium with EGF and bFGF. When comparing spheroids from both media, we found increased CD133 expression when culturing primary glioma spheroids in serum-free medium compared to serum-containing medium, which is in line with the study by Lee et al. (Lee et al., 2006) using short term cultures. In contrast to Lee, who found a drastic decrease in Sox2, Bmi-1, and Nestin when culturing short term cultures in serum, we only found a slightly decreased expression of Sox2, whereas Bmi-1 and Nestin were equally expressed in both media. This better preservation of stem cell marker expression in serum-containing medium in primary glioma spheroids (Christensen et al., 2010) may be explained by primary spheroids preserving an intact microenvironment, whereas Lee et al. (Lee et al., 2006) repeatedly dissociated the spheroids. Another interesting observation was that primary glioma spheroids cultured in serum-free medium contained more blood vessels than in serum-containing medium, and furthermore, many blood vessels were hyperplastic. The immunohistochemical comparison showed more CD34 and VWF, but less CD31 in serum-free medium compared to serum-containing medium. This increase was accompanied with more CD133 positive cells, thus suggesting that the close relationship between blood vessels and tumor stem-like cells may be better preserved in serum-free medium.

As it is clear from the tumor stem cell research field, markers specific for tumor stem cells are of crucial importance. This has resulted in the development of a great number of antibodies against tumor stem cell-related proteins. Some of the most important markers in the field of brain tumors have been (table 1) CD133 (Bandopadhyay et al. 2010; Bidlingmaier et al., 2008; Christensen et al., 2008; Dell'albani, 2008; Fargeas et al., 2007; Griguer et al., 2008; Jaszai et al., 2007; Mizrak et al., 2008; Pfenninger et al., 2007; Wang et al., 2008; Zeppernick et al., 2008), A2B5 (Balik et al., 2009; Merzak et al., 1994; Ogden et al., 2008; Piepmeier et al.,

1993; Tchoghandjian et al., 2009), Podoplanin (Goodman et al. 2009; Grau et al., 2008; Mishima et al., 2006; Nakamura et al., 2006; Ogasawara et al., 2008; Ordonez, 2006; Shibahara et al., 2006), Nestin (Dahlstrand et al., 1992a; Dahlstrand et al., 1992b; Dell'albani, 2008; Ehrmann et al., 2005; Ma et al., 2008; Maderna et al., 2007; Strojnik et al., 2007; Wan et al., 2011), Mushashi-1 (Kanemura et al., 2001; Ma et al., 2008; Okano et al., 2005; Sakakibara & Okano, 1997; Thon et al., 2010; Toda et al., 2001), Bmi-1 (Bruggeman et al., 2007; Hayry et al., 2008; Park et al., 2004; Zencak et al., 2005) and Sox2 (Gangemi et al., 2009; Ma et al., 2008; Phi et al., 2008) and new upcoming markers such as ID1 (Kamalian et al., 2008; Maw et al., 2009; Nam & Benezra, 2009; Schindl et al., 2001; Schindl et al., 2003; Schoppmann et al., 2003; Tang et al., 2009), NG2 (Brekke et al., 2006; Chekenya et al., 1999; Chekenya et al., 2002a; Chekenya et al., 2002b; Chekenya et al., 2008; Chekenya & Immervoll, 2007; Chekenya & Pilkington, 2002; Joo et al., 2008; Petrovici et al., 2010; Stallcup & Huang, 2008) and CD15 (Capela & Temple, 2002; Capela & Temple, 2006; Read et al., 2009; Ward et al., 2009). Until now, the most widely used marker in brain tumors has been CD133 (Bidlingmaier et al., 2008; Christensen et al., 2008; Dell'albani, 2008; Fargeas et al., 2007; Griguer et al., 2008; Jaszai et al., 2007; Mizrak et al., 2008; Pfenninger et al., 2007; Wang et al., 2008; Zeppernick et al., 2008).

Markers	Short introduction	References
CD133	CD133 is a cell membrane glycoprotein with five transmembrane domains. CD133 has been found in a variety of non-pathogen human tissues including the brain. However, the function remains unknown. It was identified as a marker of hematopoietic stem cells in 1997 and later as a marker of human neural stem cells. Since 2004, CD133 has been widely used for identifying tumor stem cells in brain tumors. However, some results suggest that CD133 is not specific for tumor stem cells. Downregulation of CD133 in glioma cell lines has been suggested to influence migration, spheroid formation and resistance to chemotherapeutics.	Bandopadhyay et al. 2010; Bidlingmaier et al., 2008; Christensen et al., 2008; Dell'albani, 2008; Fargeas et al., 2007; Griguer et al., 2008; Jaszai et al., 2007; Mizrak et al., 2008; Pfenninger et al., 2007; Wang et al., 2008; Zeppernick et al., 2008
A2B5	A2B5 is a cell surface ganglioside found on white matter progenitors of the oligodendrocyte lineage. A2B5 has been found in gliomas in a population of cells, which are distinct from the CD133+ population but have the capacity to initiate tumors. A2B5 might be involved in glioma cell invasion in vitro, probably because of adhesion of the molecule to basement membrane components.	Balik et al., 2009; Merzak et al., 1994; Ogden et al., 2008; Piepmeier et al., 1993; Tchoghandjian et al., 2009
Podoplanin	Podoplanin is a mucin-type transmembrane glycoprotein found in several normal tissues but not in mature astrocytes, oligodendrocytes	Goodman et al. 2009; Grau et al., 2008; Mishima et al., 2006; Nakamura et al., 2006;

Markers	Short introduction	References
	or neurons. A high expression of Podoplanin has been found in high grade astrocytomas. However, no protein has been detected in diffuse astrocytomas or in normal brain tissue. Podoplanin has been suggested to be expressed in human glioma stem cells. This podoplanin positive cell population formed neurospheres in vitro and tumors in vivo. Moreover, these cells showed increased resistance to radiation.	Ogasawara et al., 2008; Ordonez, 2006; Shibahara et al., 2006
Nestin	Nestin is a protein belonging to the class VI of intermediate filaments and it appears after neurulation in the CNS stem cells. In the normal adult brain, nestin is only expressed in the neural stem cells lining the ventricular wall and the central canal. It is believed to be a marker of proliferating and migrating cells. Nestin has been found in several tumor types including gliomas. The expression of nestin may be related to a dedifferentiated tumor stem cell status, enhanced cell motility, invasive potential and increased malignancy.	Dahlstrand et al., 1992a; Dahlstrand et al., 1992b; Dell'albani, 2008; Ehrmann et al., 2005; Ma et al., 2008; Maderna et al., 2007; Strojnik et al., 2007; Wan et al., 2011
Musashi-1	Musashi-1 belongs to a family of evolutionary well conserved neural RNA-binding proteins. Musashi-1 is found in neural stem cells and progenitor cells in the adult human brain and plays important roles in cell fate decision, including the maintenance of the stem cell state, differentiation, and tumorigenesis. Musashi-1 has been found in a variety of tumors including gliomas.	Kanemura et al., 2001; Ma et al., 2008; Okano et al., 2005; Sakakibara & Okano, 1997; Thon et al., 2010; Toda et al., 2001
Bmi-1	Bmi-1 (B lymphoma Mo-MLV insertion region) is a *Polycomb* group transcription repressor, thought to be essential for self-renewal of neural stem cells and maintenance of the stem cell population by preventing premature senescence. Bmi-1 is found mainly around the ventricles in the subventricular zone and *in vitro* in cortical neural stem cells as well as in progenitor cells. Bmi-1 has been found to be highly expressed in human brain tumors including glioblastomas.	Bruggeman et al., 2007; Hayry et al., 2008; Park et al., 2004; Zencak et al., 2005
Sox2	Sox2 (SRY (sex determining region Y)-box 2) is a transcription factor that plays a role in sustaining self-renewal and maintaining	Gangemi et al., 2009; Ma et al., 2008; Phi et al., 2008

Markers	Short introduction	References
	neuronal stem cell fate. It is found in the ventricular and sub-ventricular zone in fetal brains, but only in the ependymal cells in the human adult brain. It has been found to be highly expressed in glioblastoma cells compared to normal human brain and is believed to be involved in proliferation and tumorigenesis.	
ID1	ID1 (inhibitor of DNA binding 1) belongs to a class of transcription factors known as helix-loop-helix (HLH) proteins. The Id gene family is involved in regulation of cell-cycle status and differentiation during embryogenesis and has been found in a rare type of neural stem cells, the B1 type, where it is necessary for self-renewal. Expression of Id proteins has been demonstrated in a variety of human tumors including gliomas and has been investigated as a potential proto-oncogene. Overexpression of Id1 in human tumor cells induces cell proliferation and invasion, and also protects cells against drug-induced apoptosis.	Kamalian et al., 2008; Maw et al., 2009; Nam & Benezra, 2009; Schindl et al., 2001; Schindl et al., 2003; Schoppmann et al., 2003; Tang et al., 2009
NG2	NG2 is a transmembrane proteoglycan that interacts with the ECM to mediate cell adhesion and proliferation. It is expressed on oligodendrocyte precursor cells in the adult CNS. It has been found in human acute myeloid leukemia and in gliomas, where it in the latter seems to increase tumor cell proliferation in vitro and promote angiogenesis in vivo.	Brekke et al., 2006; Chekenya et al., 1999; Chekenya et al., 2002a; Chekenya et al., 2002b; Chekenya et al., 2008; Chekenya & Immervoll, 2007; Chekenya & Pilkington, 2002; Joo et al., 2008; Petrovici et al., 2010; Stallcup & Huang, 2008
CD15	CD15 (leukocyte cluster of differentiation 15) also known as LeX or stage-specific embryonic antigen 1, SSEA-1, is an extracellular matrix-associated carbohydrate. CD15 is secreted by neural progenitor cells including stem cells into the stem cell niche, where it binds factors such as WNT-1 that are important for progenitor proliferation and self-renewal. It is highly expressed on pluripotent stem cells and has been found in CNS germinal zones. It has been found in various normal tissues but also in different cancers including gliomas.	Capela & Temple, 2002; Capela & Temple, 2006; Read et al., 2009; Ward et al., 2009

Table 1. Some of the most used stem cell markers in the field of brain tumors.

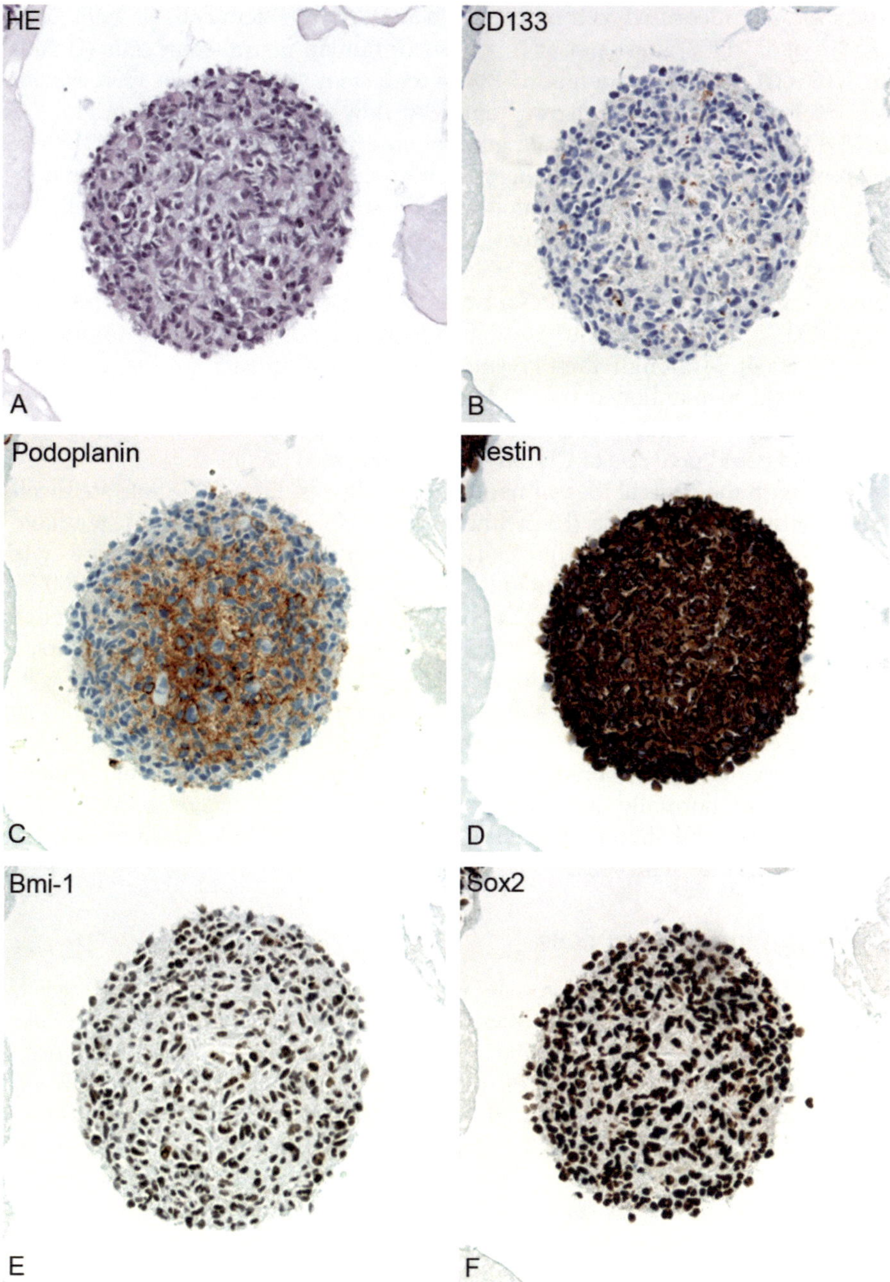

Fig. 2. Spheroids derived from a glioblastoma short term culture were stained immunohistochemically with a panel of stem cell markers. After culturing, the spheroids were formalin fixed, paraffin embedded and sectioned in 3 μm thin sections followed by immunohistochemical staining. The section in (A) was stained with hematoxylin and eosin (HE) which is widely used in histology to identify cell nucleus and cytoplasm. Moreover, sections were immunohistochemically stained with the stem or tumor stem cell markers CD133 (B), Podoplanin (C), Nestin (D), Bmi-1 (E) and Sox2 (F).

CD133 was initially identified as a marker of hematopoietic stem cells in 1997 (Miraglia et al., 1997; Yin et al., 1997) and later as a marker of human neural stem cells (Uchida et al., 2000). In 2003 a CD133+ subpopulation of cells with stem cell properties were isolated from medulloblastomas and pilocytic astrocytomas by flow cytometry (Singh et al., 2003). The isolated CD133+ cells formed primary neurospheres in vitro, whereas the CD133- cells did not. As previously mentioned, the sphere forming capability is believed to be a stem cell hallmark. In 2004 the same group isolated CD133+ subpopulations from medulloblastomas and glioblastomas and showed that they also exhibited stem cell properties in vivo. The CD133+ population could initiate phenotypically similar tumors, when injected intracranially into NOD/SCID mice in numbers as few as 100 CD133+ cells. This was not the case for CD133- cells, where up to 100,000 cells could not initiate new tumor formation (Singh et al., 2004). Although these results had a great impact on the field of glioma research, it should be mentioned that today controversies exist in this area. An important paper contributing to this controversy was a paper showing that also CD133- cells were tumorigenic and could give rise to CD133+ cells (Wang et al., 2008).

In accordance with the general idea of neural stem cells residing in discrete stem cell niches in the adult subventricular zone (Riquelme et al., 2008; Zhu et al., 2005), we have found CD133+ cells in this particular zone (Hermansen et al., 2011). In line with this, immunohistochemical studies performed by different groups (Calabrese et al., 2007; Thon et al., 2010; Zeppernick et al., 2008) including our group (Christensen et al., 2008; Hermansen et al., 2011) have shown that CD133 is located in clusters or niches in brain tumors, some of which are perivascular. The size of the niches varies from large positive areas to small perivascular niches comprising only a few cells. Several studies, including studies from our group (Christensen et al., 2008; Hermansen et al., 2011; Immervoll et al., 2008) have, however, also reported a widespread CD133 expression pattern in areas of various normal tissues, which is not normally associated with stem cells. This suggests that CD133 is not specific for stem cells and should be used in combination with other stem or progenitor cell markers to isolate tumor stem cells.

4. Hypoxia and tumor stem cells

Several studies associate tumor hypoxia with poor patient outcome and resistance to therapies (Bar, 2011; Li et al., 2009; Mashiko et al., 2011). In line with this, one of the hallmarks of glioblastomas is the presence of necrosis, occurring as a consequence of poor oxygenation and nutrition because of rapid tumor growth and formation of vessel thrombosis (Hulleman & Helin, 2005; Louis et al., 2007; Preusser et al., 2006). The hypoxia-inducible factors (HIFs) are transcription factors upregulated at low oxygen levels. These factors mediate the cellular hypoxia response influencing angiogenesis, cell survival, chemotherapy and radiation resistance, invasion and metastasis (Bar, 2011).

Usually culturing of cells is performed at 21 % O_2, but with the knowledge that the physiological oxygen concentration in the healthy brain ranges between 2.5 % and 12.5 % O_2 and in glioblastomas is even lower (Bar, 2011), it is worth considering culturing cells at lower oxygen concentrations. Spheroids of large sizes become hypoxic even if cultured in normoxia because of a diffusion gradient. However, a study by Glicklis et al. (Glicklis et al., 2004) has described that hepatocyte spheroids with diameters up to 100 μm have a good oxygenation status. Other studies by Fehlauer et al. (Fehlauer et al., 2005; Fehlauer et al., 2006; Fehlauer et al., 2007) have reported that by using glioma spheroids with diameters of 200-250 μm, there are only few hypoxic cells and no central necrosis present.

Low oxygen levels in different tumor types are believed to increase the population of tumor stem cells and to promote a stem-like state (Bar et al., 2010; Heddleston et al., 2009; Saigusa et al., 2011; Soeda et al., 2009; Wang et al., 2011; Xing et al., 2011; Yeung et al., 2011). This is similar to results obtained for embryonic stem cells showing that low oxygen levels promote maintenance of pluripotent potential, and maintenance of the cells in an undifferentiated stem cell state (Ezashi et al., 2005; Heddleston et al., 2009). The existence of tumor stem cells has been suggested to be restricted to perivascular niches and hypoxic areas within the tumor (Heddleston et al., 2009) explaining the poor outcome and therapeutic resistance seen in these hypoxic tumors. In addition to obtaining a more in vivo like metabolic milieu when culturing cells in hypoxic conditions, hypoxia also seems to promote the existence and propagation of tumor stem cells (Heddleston et al., 2009; McCord et al., 2009; Seno et al., 2009; Soeda et al., 2009). Several studies thus reported an increase in spheroid diameter, cell proliferation and number of spheroids (Heddleston et al., 2009; McCord et al., 2009; Soeda et al., 2009) when culturing spheroids in hypoxic compared to normoxic conditions. In a study from our group (Kolenda et al., 2010), spheroids obtained from a glioblastoma short term culture and the commercial glioblastoma cell line U87MG were cultured in both normoxia and hypoxia. Interestingly, a significant increase in the expression of the proposed stem cell markers CD133, Podoplanin and Bmi-1 was found in both types of spheroids when cultured in hypoxia. Furthermore, a study by Heddelston et al. (Heddleston et al., 2009) proposed that a phenotypic shift from non-stem to stem-like cells was obtained when culturing tumor cells in hypoxia. On the more mechanistic level, the spheroid formation in hypoxia has been shown to be affected by the hypoxia inducible factors as shown in studies by Li et al. (Li et al., 2009) and Méndez et al. (Mendez et al., 2010). Knockdown of HIF altered spheroid formation in glioma spheroids, resulting in smaller and fewer spheroids. Overall these findings suggest that culturing of cells in hypoxia as spheroids provides important in vivo-like conditions that are optimal when studying the stem cell biology of brain tumors.

5. Primary spheroids and radiotherapy

In the last three decades radiotherapy has been the standard treatment or part of the standard treatment for newly diagnosed glioblastoma patients (Stupp et al., 2009) providing a significant survival benefit (Laperriere et al., 2002). However, due to resistance to the current treatment of a subset of cells, it remains palliative. Primary spheroids obtained from glioma tissue have for years been reported to be a useful model for investigating in vitro radiobiology due to the preserved cellular organization. Features existing in these spheroids such as cell-cell contact, variation in the cell cycle distribution, diffusion effects, altered metabolism and hypoxia may influence the outcome of treatment, contributing to a better resemblance of the in vivo situation than obtained with a monolayer model (Olive & Durand, 1994; Sutherland & Durand, 1972). One feature of particular importance in these spheroids is possibly the low oxygen status being partly responsible for the increased radioresistance of the spheroid tumor cells (Blazek et al., 2007; Hsieh et al., 2010; Sutherland, 1998). Ionising radiation causes the formation of reactive oxygen species (ROS) (Brahme & Lind, 2010; 2008) and oxygen has therefore long been known to be a potent radiosensitizer (Vlashi et al., 2009). ROS causes damage to cellular components including DNA damage (Nishikawa, 2008) and are critical for irradiation-induced killing of tumor cells (Diehn et al., 2009). However, there have also been reports of no evident correlation between hypoxia and radioresistance (Buffa et al., 2001; Gorlach & Acker, 1994; Sminia et al., 2003) A study by

Sminia et al. (Sminia et al., 2003) found that both hypoxic and well-oxygenated organotypic multicellular spheroids derived from glioblastoma specimens showed high resistance to irradiation.
A study by Kaaijk et al. (Kaaijk et al., 1997) described the observation of only minor histological changes including a few shrunken nuclei, but no major histological damage in normoxic organotypic multicellular glioblastoma spheroids after a single dose of 50 Gy. This is in line with a study by Bauman et al. (Bauman et al., 1999), where C6 astrocytoma spheroids were implanted into a collagen type I gel. Following irradiation with 12 and 25 Gy, neither the hypoxic core nor the rim of the spheroids experienced a significant increase in the fraction of apoptotic cells. Similar to this, U87MG monolayer cultures irradiated with 8 and 20 Gy showed no considerable apoptosis five days after treatment and remained viable ten weeks after a 40 Gy dose was administered. However, in fact Kaaijk et al. reported that proliferation in three investigated organotypic multicellular spheroids was decreased 7-20 fold relative to untreated controls one week after hypofractionated radiation with a total of 40 Gy. Moreover, Fehlauer et al. (Fehlauer et al., 2005; Fehlauer et al., 2006) described in two studies a decrease in the percentage of MIB-1 positive proliferative cells in organotypic multicellular spheroids following irradiation with 20 Gy.
It has also been suggested that tumor stem cells might show increased radioresistance compared to more differentiated cells (Bao et al., 2006; Phillips et al., 2006; Rich, 2007). Bao et al. (Bao et al., 2006) thus showed that CD133+ cells survived ionizing radiation better than CD133- cells and that the fraction of CD133+ cells was enriched in gliomas after radiotherapy, suggesting that the CD133+ cellular population of gliomas is contributing to glioma radioresistance and could be the source of tumor repopulation after radiation. Liu et al. (Liu et al., 2006) investigated mRNA levels of various markers including BCRP1 (breast cancer resistance protein), MGMT (O-6-methylguanine-DNA methyltransferase), anti-apoptosis proteins and inhibitors of apoptosis protein families in CD133+ cells isolated by FACS. These markers are involved in treatment resistance and elevated mRNA levels were shown in CD133+ cells compared to CD133- cells. A significant degree of resistance towards chemotherapeutics such as temozolomide, carboplatin, paclitaxel and etoposide were demonstrated in the CD133+ cells (Liu et al., 2006). In line with these results Liu et al. showed enrichment of CD133+ cells in five recurrent gliomas when compared to the respective newly diagnosed tumors. Furthermore, results obtained in our laboratory have shown a much more pronounced reduction in the secondary spheroid formation capacity of irradiated spheroids derived from recently established glioma spheroids with stem cell characteristics compared to U87MG derived spheroids without these characteristics (Jakobsen et al. 2011).

6. Spheroids and chemotherapy

Besides irradiation and surgery, the treatment of glioblastomas consists of chemotherapy. Although the introduction of temozolomide as standard chemotherapeutic in 2005 (Stupp et al., 2005) has increased the overall patient survival, new and more efficient chemotherapeutics or targeted therapies are urgently needed. Here spheroids also have an important role to play.
Investigations of the specific effects of chemotherapeutics and other drugs on glioma spheroids are often done by investigating the size and number of spheroids as well as the

viability and the proliferation of cells in the spheroids, including the ability of the cells to form secondary spheroid.

Frequently used assays for measuring the viability of the cells after treatment is tetrazolium-based cell proliferation assays. Several variations of this assay exists (XTT, MTT, MTS or WST-1) (Berridge et al., 2005), but all utilize the conversion of tetrazolium salts by active mitochondria into dark red formazan that can be monitored by absorbance measurements (Berridge et al., 2005). Usually these assays are used on adherent monolayer cultures, which consist of uniform cell populations. However, these assays have also been used on spheroids consisting of more heterogenous cell populations. In one study (Johannessen et al., 2009) the doxorubicin sensitivity was determined in high and low passage spheroids by a MTS-assay. This was done by placing one spheroid per well in a 96 well plate, measuring viability relative to size after incubation with doxorubicin for 96 hours. After the viability measurements, the spheroids were allowed to adhere to the bottom of the plastic plates resulting in cell migration from the spheroids. Immunostaining of the migratory cells were performed using the neural stem cell markers Nestin, Vimentin and Musashi-1.

Another widely used assay is the lactate dehydrogenase assay (LDH-assay), measuring cell death. The LDH-assay indirectly measures plasma membrane damage, which is related to cell death. Due to membrane damage, LDH leaks to the culture medium, where it participates in the conversion of tetrazolium salts to formazan. The amount of formazan produced is directly proportional to the amount of LDH in the culture medium, which in turn is directly proportional to the number of dead or damaged cells (Korzeniewski & Callewaert, 1983).

The size of spheroids after drug treatment has also been used as a measure of cell viability (Fehlauer et al., 2007; Johannessen et al., 2009; Khaitan et al., 2009; Yamaguchi et al., 2010). Khaitan et al. (Khaitan et al., 2009) investigated the effect of the glycolytic inhibitor 2-deoxy-D-glucose on spheroids derived from a human glioma cell line by measuring the size of the spheroids after drug exposure. In a stem cell context, number and size of primary and secondary spheroids have also been widely used as measures of the self-renewal potential, which is one of the hallmarks of stem cells. Especially the traits that are attributable to tumor stem cells are of interest, as the tumor stem cell hypothesis states that the tumor stem cells need to be targeted specifically in order to improve cancer treatment. In the so called spheroid formation assays or clonogenic assays, the ability of the cells to form spheroids is investigated. In many studies (Sunayama et al., 2010; Wakimoto et al., 2009; Wang et al., 2010; Zhu et al., 2010) this is primarily done after treatment of the cells, thereby investigating the effect of a given drug on the ability of the cells to self-renew. Different experimental setups have been employed using different cell densities, probably resulting in two different assays - one assay with high cell densities for evaluation of proliferation and another assay with small so-called clonal cell densities for evaluation of self-renewal or clonogenic capabilities of the cells. High cell densities often result in cell and spheroid fusion due to a high motility of the spheroids (Singec et al., 2006) and it is therefore not possible to investigate the self-renewal mechanism in this assay. A plating density of 20 cells/µl has been considered as clonal conditions in terms of neurosphere formation (Singec et al., 2006). In glioma studies cell densities ranging between 0.15 cells/µl to 300 cells/µl have been used (Kolenda et al., 2010; Sunayama et al., 2010; Wakimoto et al., 2009; Wang et al., 2010; Zhu et al., 2010) when studying spheroid formation.

7. An in vivo-like in vitro model of glioma invasion

Gliomas are known to be highly invasive and new knowledge concerning tumor cell invasion also incorporating the tumor stem cell aspect is urgently needed. In our laboratory we have worked to improve in vitro models when investigating the invasive features of glioblastoma cells. This led to establishment of an in vivo-like model of invasion, where spheroids are implanted into organotypic brain slice cultures.

The organotypic brain slice cultures became very popular research tools especially with the development of the roller-tube technique by Gähwiler in 1981 (Gahwiler, 1981) and the inter-face culturing method developed by Stoppini in 1991 (Stoppini et al., 1991). These cultures preserve many of the basic structural and connective tissue structures present in the tissue, when it is localized in the brain (Gahwiler, 1988). By implanting the organotypic spheroids into the organotypic brain slice cultures, it is possible to establish an organotypic spheroid-based slice-culture invasion assay, suitable for following tumor cell invasion into the brain tissue in vitro.

The investigation of glioma invasion has been performed since the 1980's but the models used have improved during the years. Different assays have been used to address the invasive capacities of the tumor cells. A frequently used migration assay allows spheroids to adhere to the bottom of coated plastic plates, and after a period of time the distance of migrating cells from the spheroid can be measured (Gliemroth et al., 2003; Narla et al., 1998; Terzis et al., 1997; Terzis et al., 1998). Another extensively used invasion assay is the Boyden or Boyden-like chamber-based assays. The Boyden chamber was first introduced by Boyden in order to investigate the chemotactic effect of mixtures of antibody and antigen on leukocytes (Boyden, 1962). The principle in the Boyden chambers is cell migration into a microporous membrane, often made of matrigel (Deryugina et al., 1997; Paulus & Tonn, 1994; Schichor et al., 2005). The membrane is placed in between two medium-filled compartments; the upper compartment containing cells whereas the lower compartment may contain a chemotactic agent. After an incubation period, the cells migrating through the microporous membrane can be stained and counted (Chen, 2005). In a variation of the Boyden Chamber assay, slices of porcine white and gray matter were placed on top of a filter between the two compartments facilitating the cells to migrate through the porcine brain slice, making this assay a combination of the Boyden Chamber and the organotypic co-culture system (Schichor et al., 2005).

In the first real invasion studies, tissue aggregates from rat brain or chick heart were (Lund-Johansen et al., 1990) placed next to the tumor tissue, but first with the development of the organotypic brain slice culture, it was possible to preserve the brain architecture and organization in an optimal way, thereby creating the conditions necessary for a more in vivo-like model of glioma invasion. Several groups have been using this model to investigate the invasion of glioma cell into organotypic brain slice cultures (Aaberg-Jessen et al. 2011; Caspani et al., 2006; De et al., 2002; Eyupoglu et al., 2005; Guillamo et al., 2009; Jensen et al. 2010; Matsumura et al., 2000; Ohnishi et al., 1998; Palfi et al., 2004; Stoppini et al., 1991). In one study using this model, invasion was shown to be associated with the histological type and grade of the tumor (Palfi et al., 2004) and in another study invasion and tumor-induced neurotoxicity was shown to be associated (Eyupoglu et al., 2005). Most interestingly, quantitative analysis of invasion has also been performed (De et al., 2002) using confocal laser scanning microscopy and a three-dimensional visualization after having followed invasion over several weeks (Matsumura et al., 2000).

Besides investigating tumor invasion into the brain tissue, the model offers several other applications. Guillamo et al. (Guillamo et al., 2009) investigated the invasion, proliferation and angiogenesis of six human malignant glioma spheroids implanted into organotypic brain slice cultures, when these co-cultures were treated with gefinitib. Some of the tumors implanted had EGFR amplifications resulting in more pronounced invasion than tumors without EGFR amplification. Upon treatment with gefinitib only tumor cell invasion from tumors with EGFR amplification was inhibited, whereas vascular density was decreased in all tumors. In another study, Caspani et al. (Caspani et al., 2006) used the co-culture model to investigate the re-organization of the cytoskeleton in migrating glioblastoma cells. Cells transfected with green fluorescent protein were introduced into collagen gels, brain slice cultures and in vivo into mice brains and the re-organization and motility of the glioblastoma cells in the different models were monitored by confocal microscopy.

Organotypic brain slice cultures from rodents have been used in a variety of different studies using tissue obtained from different areas in the brain. The organotypic brain slice cultures used in the invasion studies varied from explants from spinal cord (Caspani et al., 2006), brain slices cut in the sagittal plane (Caspani et al., 2006) and the coronal plane (De et al., 2002; Guillamo et al., 2009; Matsumura et al., 2000; Ohnishi et al., 1998; Palfi et al., 2004) as well as entorhinohippocampal slice cultures (Eyupoglu et al., 2005). Since glioblastomas are often located in the subcortical white matter of the cerebral hemisphere and tumor infiltration often extends into the adjacent cortex and through corpus callosum (Louis et al., 2007) we have used organotypic corticostriatal brain slice cultures with cortex, striatum and corpus callosum for our studies of the invasive features of the glioblastoma cells. Such corticostriatal slice cultures should be cultured by the interface method placing the brain slices at the interface between air and culturing medium on a porous, transparent and low-protein binding membrane. This allows the cultures to be oxygenated on one site, while receiving nutrients from the other site. In the following text our approach is described in details.

The corticostriatal slice cultures are prepared from newborn Wistar rat pups by a method slightly modified from Kristensen et al. (Kristensen et al., 1999). The brain is aseptically removed from the pup and placed in a petri dish under a stereomicroscope, where the meninges are carefully removed. Hereafter the brain is sectioned coronally in 400 µm slices on a McIlwain tissue Chopper and the slices are transferred to a petri dish containing Hanks' Balanced Salt Solution supplemented with 0.9% glucose. The brain slices are separated from each other and the sections containing cortex and striatum are divided into the two hemispheric parts resulting in the final brain slices. These slices are randomly moved to the insert membranes with four cultures on each membrane. Finally, the membrane inserts are placed in a 6-well plate in 1 ml preheated medium, and incubated in 36°C humidified air containing 5% CO_2 and 95% atmospheric air.

Cell line spheroids or organotypic primary spheroids are implanted into organotypic brain slice cultures in the corpus callosum area between cortex and striatum, whereby a co-culture is established. In order to identify and follow tumor cells when they invade the slice, the spheroids can be labeled with the fluorescent dye, DiI (1,1'-Dioctadecyl-3,3,3',3'-tetramethylindocarbocyanine perchlorate) for 24 h before implantation, enabling confocal microscopy. The labeled spheroids are prepared by adding a DiI solution to the medium with spheroids, achieving a concentration of 25 µg/ml. Before implantation the spheroids are washed in medium to avoid bringing excess dye onto the brain slice cultures. Spheroids around 200-400 µm in diameter are captured using a denudation pipette and thereafter carefully placed next to corpus callosum between cortex and striatum in the brain slice cultures. The culturing plates are placed in the incubator in 36°C humidified air containing 5% CO_2 and 95% atmospheric air, whereafter the medium is changed twice a week. By monitoring the co-culture with confocal time-lapse microscopy, tumor cell invasion into the surrounding rat brain tissue can be visualized. Using a confocal microscope, a z-stack can be made consisting of thin sections at different levels of the culture. This makes it possible to follow invasion from all parts of the spheroid in different layers of the brain slice culture, whereby a three-dimentional movie and image can be constructed or alternatively an accumulated two-dimensional image based on overlay of all the images from one z-stack.

1. Decapitate a newborn rat pup
2. Aseptically remove the brain
3. Remove the meninges
4. Section the brain coronally in 400 μm slices on a McIlwain tissue Chopper
5. Separate the brain slices and choose the slices containing cortex and striatum
6. Divide these slices into the two identical halves for obtaining the final brain slice cultures
7. Move slices randomly to a transparent insert membrane
8. Place the insert membranes in a 6-well culturing plate with 1 ml preheated medium
9. Incubate the cultures in 36°C humidified air containing 5% CO_2 and 95% atmospheric air
10. Change the medium twice a week
11. Label organotypic spheroids or spheroids derived from short term cultures with 25μg/ml DiI for 24 h before implantation
12. Wash the spheroids 3 times with medium before implantation
13. Use spheroids in the size range from 200-400 μm
14. Place the spheroids in the area between cortex and striatum next to corpus callosum by a denudation pipette
15. Incubate the co-cultures in 36°C humidified air containing 5% CO_2 and 95% atmospheric air
16. Monitor the DiI-labeled spheroids using confocal microscopy

Box 2. Preparation of organotypic corticostriatal brain slice cultures and implantation of spheroids.

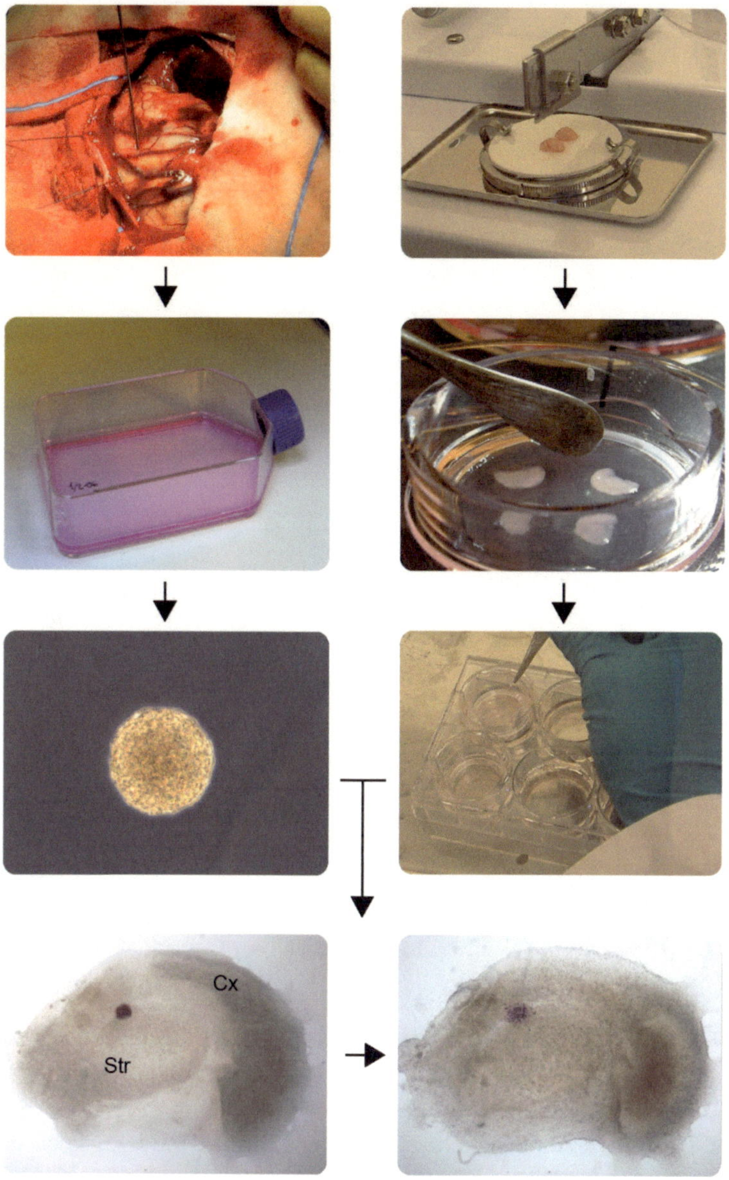

Fig. 3. Schematic overview of the implantation of glioma spheroids into organotypic rat corticostriatal brain slice cultures. Glioma tissue is obtained from patients and collected in the operation theatre. Thereafter, it is processed and cultured in the laboratory until spheroids are formed. Alternatively, spheroids from established short term cultures or cell lines can be used. Simultaneously, brain slice cultures from newborn rats are prepared and cultured by the interface method. The spheroids are labeled with the fluorescent dye DiI and implanted into the brain slice cultures in the corpus callosum area between cortex and striatum, here illustrated by a phase contrast image of a spheroid immediately after implantation and after 14 days of culturing. Note the less marked edge of the spheroid as the cells migrate into the surrounding brain tissue (Cx- cortex and Str-striatum).

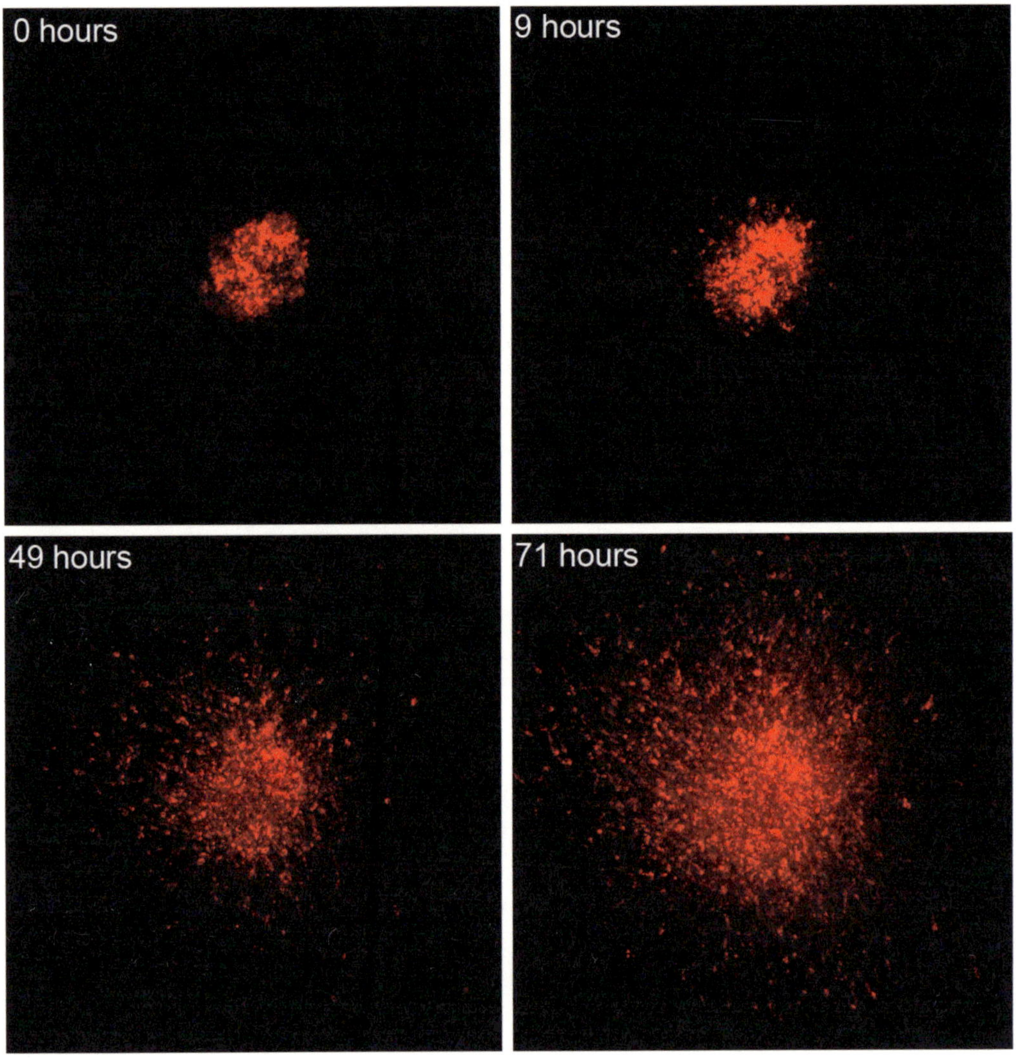

Fig. 4. Confocal images of an invasive DiI-labeled glioma spheroid implanted into an organotypic rat brain slice culture. The spheroid is followed by confocal timelapse microscopy for a period of 72 hours. The images are accumulated images based on overlay of all the images from one z-stack. A z-stack consists of several images obtained at different levels of the co-culture.

8. Conclusion

We conclude that the three-dimensional spheroid models offers advantages in glioma research taking tumor biology and microenvironment into account. Especially, when using the organotypic models, where the structure and organization of the tissue is preserved, features close to the in vivo situation are supposed to be obtained. In tumor stem cell research, the spheroids are a necessary tool as this culture method seems to promote the existence of these cells. This is especially the case when culturing the spheroids in a hypoxic environment. As discussed in the chapter, spheroids have been used in a wide range of experiments investigating radiation responses, effects of chemotherapy and effects of different types of experimental drugs as well as in migration and invasion studies. The experimental setups may be somewhat more difficult than by using monolayer cultures, but since the spheroid models are supposed to be closer to the in vivo situation, the results and answers obtained are also supposed to be closer to what it true for the corresponding tumors in the human brain. However, efforts should be made to develop these three-dimensional models to become even more in vivo-like, in order to meet new challenges in glioma research and drug development. The use of spheroids in especially tumor stem cell research has been fast increasing in recent years making spheroids an important tool also in future glioma research.

9. References

Aaberg-Jessen, C., Nørregaard, A., Christensen, K. G., Jensen, S. S., Andersen, C., & Kristensen, B. W. (2011). Invasion of primary glioma- and cell line-derived spheroids implanted into corticostriatal slice cultures, *Proceedings of American Association of Cancer Research 102nd annual meeting,* Orlando, Florida, USA, April 2011

Al-Hajj, M., Wicha, M. S., ito-Hernandez, A., Morrison, S. J., & Clarke, M. F. (2003). Prospective identification of tumorigenic breast cancer cells. *Proc. Natl.Acad. Sci. U.S.A.* Vol. 100, No. 7, pp. 3983-3988

Balik, V., Mirossay, P., Bohus, P., Sulla, I., Mirossay, L., & Sarissky, M. (2009). Flow cytometry analysis of neural differentiation markers expression in human glioblastomas may predict their response to chemotherapy. *Cell Mol. Neurobiol.* Vol. 29, No. 6-7, pp. 845-858

Bandopadhyay, G., Grabowska, A., Coyle, B., & Watson, S. (2010). Functional roles of CD133 in glioblastoma multiforme, *Proceedings of 22nd EORTC-NCI-AACR symposium on "Molecular targets and Cancer Therapeutics"*, Berlin, Germany, November 2010

Bao, S., Wu, Q., McLendon, R. E., Hao, Y., Shi, Q., Hjelmeland, A. B., Dewhirst, M. W., Bigner, D. D., & Rich, J. N. (2006). Glioma stem cells promote radioresistance by preferential activation of the DNA damage response. *Nature.* Vol. 444, No. 7120, pp. 756-760

Bao, S., Wu, Q., Sathornsumetee, S., Hao, Y., Li, Z., Hjelmeland, A. B., Shi, Q., McLendon, R. E., Bigner, D. D., & Rich, J. N. (2006). Stem cell-like glioma cells promote tumor angiogenesis through vascular endothelial growth factor. *Cancer Res.* Vol. 66, No. 16, pp. 7843-7848

Bar, E. E. (2011). Glioblastoma, cancer stem cells and hypoxia. *Brain Pathol.* Vol. 21, No. 2, pp. 119-129

Bar, E. E., Lin, A., Mahairaki, V., Matsui, W., & Eberhart, C. G. (2010). Hypoxia increases the expression of stem-cell markers and promotes clonogenicity in glioblastoma neurospheres. *Am.J.Pathol.* Vol. 177, No. 3, pp. 1491-1502

Bauman, G. S., Fisher, B. J., McDonald, W., Amberger, V. R., Moore, E., & Del Maestro, R. F. (1999). Effects of radiation on a three-dimensional model of malignant glioma invasion. *Int.J.Dev.Neurosci.* Vol. 17, No. 5-6, pp. 643-651

Berridge, M. V., Herst, P. M., & Tan, A. S. (2005). Tetrazolium dyes as tools in cell biology: new insights into their cellular reduction. *Biotechnol. Annu. Rev.* Vol. 11, No. 127-152

Bidlingmaier, S., Zhu, X., & Liu, B. (2008). The utility and limitations of glycosylated human CD133 epitopes in defining cancer stem cells. *J.Mol.Med.* Vol. 86, No. 9, pp. 1025-1032

Bjerkvig, R., Tonnesen, A., Laerum, O. D., & Backlund, E. O. (1990). Multicellular tumor spheroids from human gliomas maintained in organ culture. *J.Neurosurg.* Vol. 72, No. 3, pp. 463-475

Blazek, E. R., Foutch, J. L., & Maki, G. (2007). Daoy medulloblastoma cells that express CD133 are radioresistant relative to C. *Int.J.Radiat.Oncol.Biol.Phys.* Vol. 67, No. 1, pp. 1-5

Bonnet, D. & Dick, J. E. (1997). Human acute myeloid leukemia is organized as a hierarchy that originates from a primitive hematopoietic cell. *Nat.Med.* Vol. 3, No. 7, pp. 730-737

Boyden, S. (1962). The chemotactic effect of mixtures of antibody and antigen on polymorphonuclear leucocytes. *J.Exp.Med.* Vol. 115, No. 453-466

Brahme, A. & Lind, B. K. (2010). A systems biology approach to radiation therapy optimization. *Radiat.Environ.Biophys.* Vol. 49, No. 2, pp. 111-124

Brekke, C., Lundervold, A., Enger, P. O., Brekken, C., Stalsett, E., Pedersen, T. B., Haraldseth, O., Kruger, P. G., Bjerkvig, R., & Chekenya, M. (2006). NG2 expression regulates vascular morphology and function in human brain tumours. *Neuroimage.* Vol. 29, No. 3, pp. 965-976

Bruggeman, S. W., Hulsman, D., Tanger, E., Buckle, T., Blom, M., Zevenhoven, J., van, T. O., & van, L. M. (2007). Bmi1 controls tumor development in an Ink4a/Arf-independent manner in a mouse model for glioma. *Cancer Cell.* Vol. 12, No. 4, pp. 328-341

Buffa, F. M., West, C., Byrne, K., Moore, J. V., & Nahum, A. E. (2001). Radiation response and cure rate of human colon adenocarcinoma spheroids of different size: the significance of hypoxia on tumor control modelling. *Int.J.Radiat.Oncol.Biol.Phys.* Vol. 49, No. 4, pp. 1109-1118

Calabrese, C., Poppleton, H., Kocak, M., Hogg, T. L., Fuller, C., Hamner, B., Oh, E. Y., Gaber, M. W., Finklestein, D., Allen, M., Frank, A., Bayazitov, I. T., Zakharenko, S. S., Gajjar, A., Davidoff, A., & Gilbertson, R. J. (2007). A perivascular niche for brain tumor stem cells. *Cancer Cell.* Vol. 11, No. 1, pp. 69-82

Capela, A. & Temple, S. (2002). LeX/ssea-1 is expressed by adult mouse CNS stem cells, identifying them as nonependymal. *Neuron.* Vol. 35, No. 5, pp. 865-875

Capela, A. & Temple, S. (2006). LeX is expressed by principle progenitor cells in the embryonic nervous system, is secreted into their environment and binds Wnt-1. *Dev.Biol.* Vol. 291, No. 2, pp. 300-313

Caspani, E. M., Echevarria, D., Rottner, K., & Small, J. V. (2006). Live imaging of glioblastoma cells in brain tissue shows requirement of actin bundles for migration. *Neuron Glia Biol.* Vol. 2, No. 2, pp. 105-114

Chekenya, M., Enger, P. O., Thorsen, F., Tysnes, B. B., Al-Sarraj, S., Read, T. A., Furmanek, T., Mahesparan, R., Levine, J. M., Butt, A. M., Pilkington, G. J., & Bjerkvig, R. (2002a). The glial precursor proteoglycan, NG2, is expressed on tumour neovasculature by vascular pericytes in human malignant brain tumours. *Neuropathol.Appl.Neurobiol.* Vol. 28, No. 5, pp. 367-380

Chekenya, M., Hjelstuen, M., Enger, P. O., Thorsen, F., Jacob, A. L., Probst, B., Haraldseth, O., Pilkington, G., Butt, A., Levine, J. M., & Bjerkvig, R. (2002b). NG2 proteoglycan promotes angiogenesis-dependent tumor growth in CNS by sequestering angiostatin. *FASEB J.* Vol. 16, No. 6, pp. 586-588

Chekenya, M. & Immervoll, H. (2007). NG2/HMP proteoglycan as a cancer therapeutic target. *Methods Mol.Biol.* Vol. 361, No. 93-117
Chekenya, M., Krakstad, C., Svendsen, A., Netland, I. A., Staalesen, V., Tysnes, B. B., Selheim, F., Wang, J., Sakariassen, P. O., Sandal, T., Lonning, P. E., Flatmark, T., Enger, P. O., Bjerkvig, R., Sioud, M., & Stallcup, W. B. (2008). The progenitor cell marker NG2/MPG promotes chemoresistance by activation of integrin-dependent PI3K/Akt signaling. *Oncogene*. Vol. 27, No. 39, pp. 5182-5194
Chekenya, M. & Pilkington, G. J. (2002). NG2 precursor cells in neoplasia: functional, histogenesis and therapeutic implications for malignant brain tumours. *J.Neurocytol.* Vol. 31, No. 6-7, pp. 507-521
Chekenya, M., Rooprai, H. K., Davies, D., Levine, J. M., Butt, A. M., & Pilkington, G. J. (1999). The NG2 chondroitin sulfate proteoglycan: role in malignant progression of human brain tumours. *Int.J.Dev.Neurosci.* Vol. 17, No. 5-6, pp. 421-435
Chen, H. C. (2005). Boyden chamber assay. *Methods Mol.Biol.* Vol. 294, No. 15-22
Christensen, K., Aaberg-Jessen, C., Andersen, C., Goplen, D., Bjerkvig, R., & Kristensen, B. W. (2010). Immunohistochemical expression of stem cell, endothelial cell, and chemosensitivity markers in primary glioma spheroids cultured in serum-containing and serum-free medium. *Neurosurgery*. Vol. 66, No. 5, pp. 933-947
Christensen, K., Schrøder, H. D., & Kristensen, B. W. (2008). CD133 identifies perivascular niches in grade II-IV astrocytomas. *J.Neurooncol.* Vol. 90, No. 2, pp.157-70
Clark, M. J., Homer, N., O'Connor, B. D., Chen, Z., Eskin, A., Lee, H., Merriman, B., & Nelson, S. F. (2010). U87MG decoded: the genomic sequence of a cytogenetically aberrant human cancer cell line. *PLoS.Genet.* Vol. 6, No. 1, pp. e1000832
Dahlstrand, J., Collins, V. P., & Lendahl, U. (1992a). Expression of the class VI intermediate filament nestin in human central nervous system tumors. *Cancer Res.* Vol. 52, No. 19, pp. 5334-5341
Dahlstrand, J., Zimmerman, L. B., McKay, R. D., & Lendahl, U. (1992b). Characterization of the human nestin gene reveals a close evolutionary relationship to neurofilaments. *J.Cell Sci.* Vol. 103 (Pt 2), No. 589-597
Daidone, M. G., Costa, A., Frattini, M., Balestra, D., Bertario, L., & Pierotti, M. A. (2004). Correspondence re: T. Zhang et al., Evidence that APC regulates survivin expression: a possible mechanism contributing to the stem cell origin of colon cancer. Cancer Res., 61: 8664-8667, 2001. *Cancer Res.* Vol. 64, No. 2, pp. 776-777
De, B. S., Christov, C., Guillamo, J. S., Kassar-Duchossoy, L., Palfi, S., Leguerinel, C., Masset, M., Cohen-Hagenauer, O., Peschanski, M., & Lefrancois, T. (2002). Invasion of human glioma biopsy specimens in cultures of rodent brain slices: a quantitative analysis. *J.Neurosurg.* Vol. 97, No. 1, pp. 169-176
Dell'albani, P. (2008). Stem Cell Markers in Gliomas. *Neurochem.Res.* Vol. 33, No.12, pp. 2407-2415
Deryugina, E. I., Luo, G. X., Reisfeld, R. A., Bourdon, M. A., & Strongin, A. (1997). Tumor cell invasion through matrigel is regulated by activated matrix metalloproteinase-2. *Anticancer Res.* Vol. 17, No. 5A, pp. 3201-3210
Diehn, M., Cho, R. W., Lobo, N. A., Kalisky, T., Dorie, M. J., Kulp, A. N., Qian, D., Lam, J. S., Ailles, L. E., Wong, M., Joshua, B., Kaplan, M. J., Wapnir, I., Dirbas, F. M., Somlo, G., Garberoglio, C., Paz, B., Shen, J., Lau, S. K., Quake, S. R., Brown, J. M., Weissman, I. L., &

Clarke, M. F. (2009). Association of reactive oxygen species levels and radioresistance in cancer stem cells. *Nature*. Vol. 458, No. 7239, pp. 780-783

Ehrmann, J., Kolar, Z., & Mokry, J. (2005). Nestin as a diagnostic and prognostic marker: immunohistochemical analysis of its expression in different tumours. *J.Clin.Pathol.* Vol. 58, No. 2, pp. 222-223

Eyupoglu, I. Y., Hahnen, E., Heckel, A., Siebzehnrubl, F. A., Buslei, R., Fahlbusch, R., & Blumcke, I. (2005). Malignant glioma-induced neuronal cell death in an organotypic glioma invasion model. Technical note. *J.Neurosurg.* Vol. 102, No. 4, pp. 738-744

Ezashi, T., Das, P., & Roberts, R. M. (2005). Low O2 tensions and the prevention of differentiation of hES cells. *Proc.Natl.Acad.Sci.U.S.A.* Vol. 102, No. 13, pp. 4783-4788

Fargeas, C. A., Huttner, W. B., & Corbeil, D. (2007). Nomenclature of prominin-1 (CD133) splice variants - an update. *Tissue Antigens.* Vol. 69, No. 6, pp. 602-606

Fehlauer, F., Muench, M., Rades, D., Stalpers, L. J., Leenstra, S., van, d., V, Slotman, B., Smid, E. J., & Sminia, P. (2005). Effects of irradiation and cisplatin on human glioma spheroids: inhibition of cell proliferation and cell migration. *J.Cancer Res.Clin.Oncol.* Vol. 131, No. 11, pp. 723-732

Fehlauer, F., Muench, M., Richter, E., & Rades, D. (2007). The inhibition of proliferation and migration of glioma spheroids exposed to temozolomide is less than additive if combined with irradiation. *Oncol.Rep.* Vol. 17, No. 4, pp. 941-945

Fehlauer, F., Muench, M., Smid, E. J., Slotman, B., Richter, E., van, d., V, & Sminia, P. (2006). Combined modality therapy of gemcitabine and irradiation on human glioma spheroids derived from cell lines and biopsy tissue. *Oncol.Rep.* Vol. 15, No. 1, pp. 97-105

Fisher, G. , Wieser, R. J.1983). *Hormonally Defined Media. A Tool in Cell Biology*, Springer-Verlag, 3-540-12668-6, Berlin Heidelberg, Germany

Gage, F. H., Ray, J., & Fisher, L. J. (1995). Isolation, characterization, and use of stem cells from the CNS. *Annu.Rev.Neurosci.* Vol. 18, No. 159-192

Gahwiler, B. H. (1981). Organotypic monolayer cultures of nervous tissue. *J Neurosci.Methods.* Vol. 4, No. 4, pp. 329-342

Gahwiler, B. H. (1988). Organotypic cultures of neural tissue. *Trends Neurosci.* Vol. 11, No. 11, pp. 484-489

Galli, R., Binda, E., Orfanelli, U., Cipelletti, B., Gritti, A., De, V. S., Fiocco, R., Foroni, C., Dimeco, F., & Vescovi, A. (2004). Isolation and characterization of tumorigenic, stem-like neural precursors from human glioblastoma. *Cancer Res.* Vol. 64, No. 19, pp. 7011-7021

Gangemi, R. M., Griffero, F., Marubbi, D., Perera, M., Capra, M. C., Malatesta, P., Ravetti, G. L., Zona, G. L., Daga, A., & Corte, G. (2009). SOX2 silencing in glioblastoma tumor-initiating cells causes stop of proliferation and loss of tumorigenicity. *Stem Cells.* Vol. 27, No. 1, pp. 40-48

Genc, M., Castro, K. N., Barten-van, R. A., Stalpers, L. J., & Haveman, J. (2004). Enhancement of effects of irradiation by gemcitabine in a glioblastoma cell line and cell line spheroids. *J.Cancer Res.Clin.Oncol.* Vol. 130, No. 1, pp. 45-51

Glicklis, R., Merchuk, J. C., & Cohen, S. (2004). Modeling mass transfer in hepatocyte spheroids via cell viability, spheroid size, and hepatocellular functions. *Biotechnol.Bioeng.* Vol. 86, No. 6, pp. 672-680

Gliemroth, J., Zulewski, H., Arnold, H., & Terzis, A. J. (2003). Migration, proliferation, and invasion of human glioma cells following treatment with simvastatin. *Neurosurg.Rev.* Vol. 26, No. 2, pp. 117-124

Goodman, L. D., Le, T. T., Love, P., Gumin, J., Lang, F. F., Colman, H., Aldape, K., & Sulman, E. P. (2009). Glioma cancer stem cells expressing podoplanin exhibit a unique gene expression signature, even in the absence of CD133, *Proceedings of American association of Cancer research 100th annual meeting,* Denver, Colorado, USA, April 2009

Gorlach, A. & Acker, H. (1994). pO2- and pH-gradients in multicellular spheroids and their relationship to cellular metabolism and radiation sensitivity of malignant human tumor cells. *Biochim.Biophys.Acta.* Vol. 1227, No. 3, pp. 105-112

Grau, S. J., Trillsch, F., von, L., I, Nelson, P. J., Herms, J., Tonn, J. C., & Goldbrunner, R. H. (2008). Lymphatic phenotype of tumour vessels in malignant gliomas. *Neuropathol.Appl.Neurobiol.* Vol. 34, No. 6, pp. 675-679

Griguer, C. E., Oliva, C. R., Gobin, E., Marcorelles, P., Benos, D. J., Lancaster, J. R., Jr., & Gillespie, G. Y. (2008). CD133 is a marker of bioenergetic stress in human glioma. *PLoS.One.* Vol. 3, No. 11, pp. e3655

Guillamo, J. S., De, B. S., Valable, S., Marteau, L., Leuraud, P., Marie, Y., Poupon, M. F., Parienti, J. J., Raymond, E., & Peschanski, M. (2009). Molecular mechanisms underlying effects of epidermal growth factor receptor inhibition on invasion, proliferation, and angiogenesis in experimental glioma. *Clin.Cancer Res.* Vol. 15, No. 11, pp. 3697-3704

Haas-Kogan, D. A., Dazin, P., Hu, L., Deen, D. F., & Israel, A. (1996). P53-independent apoptosis: a mechanism of radiation-induced cell death of glioblastoma cells. *Cancer J.Sci.Am.* Vol. 2, No. 2, pp. 114-121

Hayry, V., Tynninen, O., Haapasalo, H. K., Wolfer, J., Paulus, W., Hasselblatt, M., Sariola, H., Paetau, A., Sarna, S., Niemela, M., Wartiovaara, K., & Nupponen, N. N. (2008). Stem cell protein BMI-1 is an independent marker for poor prognosis in oligodendroglial tumours. *Neuropathol.Appl.Neurobiol.* Vol. 34, No. 5, pp. 555-63

Heddleston, J. M., Li, Z., McLendon, R. E., Hjelmeland, A. B., & Rich, J. N. (2009). The hypoxic microenvironment maintains glioblastoma stem cells and promotes reprogramming towards a cancer stem cell phenotype. *Cell Cycle.* Vol. 8, No. 20, pp.

Hermansen, S. K., Christensen, K. G., Jensen, S. S., & Kristensen, B. W. (2011). Inconsistent immunohistochemical expression patterns of four different CD133 antibody clones in glioblastoma. *J.Histochem.Cytochem.* Vol. 59, No. 4, pp. 391-407

Hsieh, C. H., Lee, C. H., Liang, J. A., Yu, C. Y., & Shyu, W. C. (2010). Cycling hypoxia increases U87 glioma cell radioresistance via ROS induced higher and long-term HIF-1 signal transduction activity. *Oncol.Rep.* Vol. 24, No. 6, pp. 1629-1636

Hulleman, E. & Helin, K. (2005). Molecular mechanisms in gliomagenesis. *Adv.Cancer Res.* Vol. 94, No. 1-27

Ignatova, T. N., Kukekov, V. G., Laywell, E. D., Suslov, O. N., Vrionis, F. D., & Steindler, D. A. (2002). Human cortical glial tumors contain neural stem-like cells expressing astroglial and neuronal markers in vitro. *Glia.* Vol. 39, No. 3, pp. 193-206

Immervoll, H., Hoem, D., Sakariassen, P. O., Steffensen, O. J., & Molven, A. (2008). Expression of the "stem cell marker" CD133 in pancreas and pancreatic ductal adenocarcinomas. *BMC.Cancer.* Vol. 8, No.48

Jakobsen, I. P., Aaberg-Jessen, C., Jensen, S. S., Nielsen, M., Halle, D., & Kristensen, B. W. (2011). Effects of irradiation on glioblastoma spheroids cultured in stem cell medium, *Proceedings of American Association of Cancer Research 102nd annual meeting,* Orlando, Florida, USA, April 2011

Jaszai, J., Fargeas, C. A., Florek, M., Huttner, W. B., & Corbeil, D. (2007). Focus on molecules: prominin-1 (CD133). *Exp.Eye Res.* Vol. 85, No. 5, pp. 585-586

Jensen, S. S., Aaberg-Jessen, C., Nørregaard, A., & Kristensen, B. W. (2011). An in vivo-like tumor stem cell-related glioblastoma in vitro model for drug discovery, *Proceedings of American Association of Cancer Research 102nd annual meeting,* Orlando, Florida, USA, April 2011

Johannessen, T. C., Wang, J., Skaftnesmo, K. O., Sakariassen, P. O., Enger, P. O., Petersen, K., Oyan, A. M., Kalland, K. H., Bjerkvig, R., & Tysnes, B. B. (2009). Highly infiltrative brain tumours show reduced chemosensitivity associated with a stem cell-like phenotype. *Neuropathol.Appl.Neurobiol.* Vol. 35, No. 4, pp. 380-393

Joo, N. E., Watanabe, T., Chen, C., Chekenya, M., Stallcup, W. B., & Kapila, Y. L. (2008). NG2, a novel proapoptotic receptor, opposes integrin alpha4 to mediate anoikis through PKCalpha-dependent suppression of FAK phosphorylation. *Cell Death.Differ.* Vol. 15, No. 5, pp. 899-907

Kaaijk, P., Troost, D., Sminia, P., Hulshof, M. C., van der Kracht, A. H., Leenstra, S., & Bosch, D. A. (1997). Hypofractionated radiation induces a decrease in cell proliferation but no histological damage to organotypic multicellular spheroids of human glioblastomas. *Eur.J.Cancer.* Vol. 33, No. 4, pp. 645-651

Kamalian, L., Gosney, J. R., Forootan, S. S., Foster, C. S., Bao, Z. Z., Beesley, C., & Ke, Y. (2008). Increased expression of Id family proteins in small cell lung cancer and its prognostic significance. *Clin.Cancer Res.* Vol. 14, No. 8, pp. 2318-2325

Kanemura, Y., Mori, K., Sakakibara, S., Fujikawa, H., Hayashi, H., Nakano, A., Matsumoto, T., Tamura, K., Imai, T., Ohnishi, T., Fushiki, S., Nakamura, Y., Yamasaki, M., Okano, H., & Arita, N. (2001). Musashi1, an evolutionarily conserved neural RNA-binding protein, is a versatile marker of human glioma cells in determining their cellular origin, malignancy, and proliferative activity. *Differentiation.* Vol. 68, No. 2-3, pp. 141-152

Khaitan, D., Chandna, S., & Dwarakanath, S. B. (2009). Short-term exposure of multicellular tumor spheroids of a human glioma cell line to the glycolytic inhibitor 2-deoxy-D-glucose is more toxic than continuous exposure. *J.Cancer Res.Ther.* Vol. 5 Suppl 1, No. S67-S73

Kolenda, J., Jensen, S. S., Aaberg-Jessen, C., Christensen, K., Andersen, C., Brunner, N., & Kristensen, B. W. (2010). Effects of hypoxia on expression of a panel of stem cell and chemoresistance markers in glioblastoma-derived spheroids. *J.Neurooncol.* Vol. 103, No. 1, pp. 43-58

Korzeniewski, C. & Callewaert, D. M. (1983). An enzyme-release assay for natural cytotoxicity. *J.Immunol.Methods.* Vol. 64, No. 3, pp. 313-320

Kristensen, B. W., Noraberg, J., Jakobsen, B., Gramsbergen, J. B., Ebert, B., & Zimmer, J. (1999). Excitotoxic effects of non-NMDA receptor agonists in organotypic corticostriatal slice cultures. *Brain Res.* Vol. 841, No. 1-2, pp. 143-159

Laperriere, N., Zuraw, L., & Cairncross, G. (2002). Radiotherapy for newly diagnosed malignant glioma in adults: a systematic review. *Radiother.Oncol.* Vol. 64, No. 3, pp. 259-273

Lee, J., Kotliarova, S., Kotliarov, Y., Li, A., Su, Q., Donin, N. M., Pastorino, S., Purow, B. W., Christopher, N., Zhang, W., Park, J. K., & Fine, H. A. (2006). Tumor stem cells derived from glioblastomas cultured in bFGF and EGF more closely mirror the phenotype and genotype of primary tumors than do serum-cultured cell lines. *Cancer Cell*. Vol. 9, No. 5, pp. 391-403

Li, Z., Bao, S., Wu, Q., Wang, H., Eyler, C., Sathornsumetee, S., Shi, Q., Cao, Y., Lathia, J., McLendon, R. E., Hjelmeland, A. B., & Rich, J. N. (2009). Hypoxia-inducible factors regulate tumorigenic capacity of glioma stem cells. *Cancer Cell*. Vol. 15, No. 6, pp. 501-513

Liu, G., Yuan, X., Zeng, Z., Tunici, P., Ng, H., Abdulkadir, I. R., Lu, L., Irvin, D., Black, K. L., & Yu, J. S. (2006). Analysis of gene expression and chemoresistance of CD133+ cancer stem cells in glioblastoma. *Mol.Cancer*. Vol. 5, No. 67-

Louis, D. N., Ohgaki, H., Wiestler, O. D., & Cavenee, W. K. (2007). *WHO Classification of Tumours of the Central Nervous System*, IARC Press, 978-92-832-2430-2, Lyon, France

Lund-Johansen, M., Engebraaten, O., Bjerkvig, R., & Laerum, O. D. (1990). Invasive glioma cells in tissue culture. *Anticancer Res*. Vol. 10, No. 5A, pp. 1135-1151

Ma, Y. H., Mentlein, R., Knerlich, F., Kruse, M. L., Mehdorn, H. M., & Held-Feindt, J. (2008). Expression of stem cell markers in human astrocytomas of different WHO grades. *J.Neurooncol*. Vol. 86, No. 1, pp. 31-45

Mackillop, W. J., Blundell, J., & Steele, P. (1985). Short-term culture of pediatric brain tumors. *Childs Nerv.Syst*. Vol. 1, No. 3, pp. 163-168

Maderna, E., Salmaggi, A., Calatozzolo, C., Limido, L., & Pollo, B. (2007). Nestin, PDGFRbeta, CXCL12 and VEGF in glioma patients: different profiles of (pro-angiogenic) molecule expression are related with tumor grade and may provide prognostic information. *Cancer Biol.Ther*. Vol. 6, No. 7, pp. 1018-1024

Mashiko, R., Takano, S., Ishikawa, E., Yamamoto, T., Nakai, K., & Matsumura, A. (2011). Hypoxia-inducible factor 1alpha expression is a prognostic biomarker in patients with astrocytic tumors associated with necrosis on MR image. *J.Neurooncol*. Vol. 102, No. 1, pp. 43-50

Matsumura, H., Ohnishi, T., Kanemura, Y., Maruno, M., & Yoshimine, T. (2000). Quantitative analysis of glioma cell invasion by confocal laser scanning microscopy in a novel brain slice model. *Biochem.Biophys.Res.Commun*. Vol. 269, No. 2, pp. 513-520

Maw, M. K., Fujimoto, J., & Tamaya, T. (2009). Overexpression of inhibitor of DNA-binding (ID)-1 protein related to angiogenesis in tumor advancement of ovarian cancers. *BMC.Cancer*. Vol. 9, No. 430-

McCord, A. M., Jamal, M., Shankavaram, U. T., Lang, F. F., Camphausen, K., & Tofilon, P. J. (2009). Physiologic oxygen concentration enhances the stem-like properties of CD133+ human glioblastoma cells in vitro. *Mol.Cancer Res*. Vol. 7, No. 4, pp. 489-497

Mendez, O., Zavadil, J., Esencay, M., Lukyanov, Y., Santovasi, D., Wang, S. C., Newcomb, E. W., & Zagzag, D. (2010). Knock down of HIF-1alpha in glioma cells reduces migration in vitro and invasion in vivo and impairs their ability to form tumor spheres. *Mol.Cancer*. Vol. 9, No. 133-

Merzak, A., Koochekpour, S., & Pilkington, G. J. (1994). Cell surface gangliosides are involved in the control of human glioma cell invasion in vitro. *Neurosci.Lett*. Vol. 177, No. 1-2, pp. 44-46

Mettler, F. A. & Upton, A. C. (2008). *Medical effects of ionizing radiation*, Saunders/Elsevier, 978-0-7216-0200-4, Philadelphia, Pa

Miraglia, S., Godfrey, W., Yin, A. H., Atkins, K., Warnke, R., Holden, J. T., Bray, R. A., Waller, E. K., & Buck, D. W. (1997). A novel five-transmembrane hematopoietic stem cell antigen: isolation, characterization, and molecular cloning. *Blood*. Vol. 90, No. 12, pp. 5013-5021

Mishima, K., Kato, Y., Kaneko, M. K., Nishikawa, R., Hirose, T., & Matsutani, M. (2006). Increased expression of podoplanin in malignant astrocytic tumors as a novel molecular marker of malignant progression. *Acta Neuropathol.* Vol. 111, No. 5, pp. 483-488

Mizrak, D., Brittan, M., & Alison, M. R. (2008). CD133: molecule of the moment. *J.Pathol.* Vol. 214, No. 1, pp. 3-9

Nakamura, Y., Kanemura, Y., Yamada, T., Sugita, Y., Higaki, K., Yamamoto, M., Takahashi, M., & Yamasaki, M. (2006). D2-40 antibody immunoreactivity in developing human brain, brain tumors and cultured neural cells. *Mod.Pathol.* Vol. 19, No. 7, pp. 974-985

Nam, H. S. & Benezra, R. (2009). High levels of Id1 expression define B1 type adult neural stem cells. *Cell Stem Cell*. Vol. 5, No. 5, pp. 515-526

Narla, R. K., Liu, X. P., Klis, D., & Uckun, F. M. (1998). Inhibition of human glioblastoma cell adhesion and invasion by 4-(4'-hydroxylphenyl)-amino-6,7-dimethoxyquinazoline (WHI-P131) and 4-(3'-bromo-4'-hydroxylphenyl)-amino-6,7-dimethoxyquinazoline (WHI-P154). *Clin.Cancer Res.* Vol. 4, No. 10, pp. 2463-2471

Nishikawa, M. (2008). Reactive oxygen species in tumor metastasis. *Cancer Lett.* Vol. 266, No. 1, pp. 53-59

Ogasawara, S., Kaneko, M. K., Price, J. E., & Kato, Y. (2008). Characterization of anti-podoplanin monoclonal antibodies: critical epitopes for neutralizing the interaction between podoplanin and CLEC-2. *Hybridoma (Larchmt.)*. Vol. 27, No. 4, pp. 259-267

Ogden, A. T., Waziri, A. E., Lochhead, R. A., Fusco, D., Lopez, K., Ellis, J. A., Kang, J., Assanah, M., McKhann, G. M., Sisti, M. B., McCormick, P. C., Canoll, P., & Bruce, J. N. (2008). Identification of A2B5+CD133- tumorinitiating cells in adult human gliomas. *Neurosurgery*. Vol. 62, No. 2, pp. 505-514

Ohnishi, T., Matsumura, H., Izumoto, S., Hiraga, S., & Hayakawa, T. (1998). A novel model of glioma cell invasion using organotypic brain slice culture. *Cancer Res.* Vol. 58, No. 14, pp. 2935-2940

Okano, H., Kawahara, H., Toriya, M., Nakao, K., Shibata, S., & Imai, T. (2005). Function of RNA-binding protein Musashi-1 in stem cells. *Exp.Cell Res.* Vol. 306, No. 2, pp. 349-356

Olive, P. L. & Durand, R. E. (1994). Drug and radiation resistance in spheroids: cell contact and kinetics. *Cancer Metastasis Rev.* Vol. 13, No. 2, pp. 121-138

Ordonez, N. G. (2006). Podoplanin: a novel diagnostic immunohistochemical marker. *Adv.Anat.Pathol.* Vol. 13, No. 2, pp. 83-88

Palfi, S., Swanson, K. R., De, B. S., Chretien, F., Oliveira, R., Gherardi, R. K., Kros, J. M., Peschanski, M., & Christov, C. (2004). Correlation of in vitro infiltration with glioma histological type in organotypic brain slices. *Br.J.Cancer*. Vol. 91, No. 4, pp. 745-752

Park, I. K., Morrison, S. J., & Clarke, M. F. (2004). Bmi1, stem cells, and senescence regulation. *J.Clin.Invest.* Vol. 113, No. 2, pp. 175-179

Paulus, W. & Tonn, J. C. (1994). Basement membrane invasion of glioma cells mediated by integrin receptors. *J.Neurosurg.* Vol. 80, No. 3, pp. 515-519

Petrovici, K., Graf, M., Hecht, K., Reif, S., Pfister, K., & Schmetzer, H. (2010). Use of NG2 (7.1) in AML as a tumor marker and its association with a poor prognosis. *Cancer Genomics Proteomics*. Vol. 7, No. 4, pp. 173-180

Pfenninger, C. V., Roschupkina, T., Hertwig, F., Kottwitz, D., Englund, E., Bengzon, J., Jacobsen, S. E., & Nuber, U. A. (2007). CD133 is not present on neurogenic astrocytes in the adult subventricular zone, but on embryonic neural stem cells, ependymal cells, and glioblastoma cells. *Cancer Res.* Vol. 67, No. 12, pp. 5727-5736

Phi, J. H., Park, S. H., Kim, S. K., Paek, S. H., Kim, J. H., Lee, Y. J., Cho, B. K., Park, C. K., Lee, D. H., & Wang, K. C. (2008). Sox2 expression in brain tumors: a reflection of the neuroglial differentiation pathway. *Am.J.Surg.Pathol.* Vol. 32, No. 1, pp. 103-112

Phillips, T. M., McBride, W. H., & Pajonk, F. (2006). The response of CD24(-/low)/CD44+ breast cancer-initiating cells to radiation. *J.Natl.Cancer Inst.* Vol. 98, No. 24, pp. 1777-1785

Piepmeier, J. M., Fried, I., & Makuch, R. (1993). Low-grade astrocytomas may arise from different astrocyte lineages. *Neurosurgery.* Vol. 33, No. 4, pp. 627-632

Ponten, J. & Macintyre, E. H. (1968). Long term culture of normal and neoplastic human glia. *Acta Pathol.Microbiol.Scand.* Vol. 74, No. 4, pp. 465-486

Potter, N. E., Phipps, K., Harkness, W., Hayward, R., Thompson, D., Jacques, T. S., Harding, B., Thomas, D. G., Rees, J., Darling, J. L., & Warr, T. J. (2009). Astrocytoma derived short-term cell cultures retain molecular signatures characteristic of the tumour in situ. *Exp.Cell Res.* Vol. 315, No. 16, pp. 2835-2846

Preusser, M., Haberler, C., & Hainfellner, J. A. (2006). Malignant glioma: neuropathology and neurobiology. *Wien.Med.Wochenschr.* Vol. 156, No. 11-12, pp. 332-337

Read, T. A., Fogarty, M. P., Markant, S. L., McLendon, R. E., Wei, Z., Ellison, D. W., Febbo, P. G., & Wechsler-Reya, R. J. (2009). Identification of CD15 as a marker for tumor-propagating cells in a mouse model of medulloblastoma. *Cancer Cell.* Vol. 15, No. 2, pp. 135-147

Reya, T., Morrison, S. J., Clarke, M. F., & Weissman, I. L. (2001). Stem cells, cancer, and cancer stem cells. *Nature.* Vol. 414, No. 6859, pp. 105-111

Reynolds, B. A. & Weiss, S. (1992). Generation of neurons and astrocytes from isolated cells of the adult mammalian central nervous system. *Science.* Vol. 255, No. 5052, pp. 1707-1710

Rich, J. N. (2007). Cancer stem cells in radiation resistance. *Cancer Res.* Vol. 67, No. 19, pp. 8980-8984

Riquelme, P. A., Drapeau, E., & Doetsch, F. (2008). Brain micro-ecologies: neural stem cell niches in the adult mammalian brain. *Philos.Trans.R.Soc.Lond B Biol.Sci.* Vol. 363, No. 1489, pp. 123-137

Saigusa, S., Tanaka, K., Toiyama, Y., Yokoe, T., Okugawa, Y., Koike, Y., Fujikawa, H., Inoue, Y., Miki, C., & Kusunoki, M. (2011). Clinical Significance of CD133 and Hypoxia Inducible Factor-1alpha Gene Expression in Rectal Cancer after Preoperative Chemoradiotherapy. *Clin.Oncol.(R.Coll.Radiol.).* Vol. 23, No. 5, pp. 323-332

Sakakibara, S. & Okano, H. (1997). Expression of neural RNA-binding proteins in the postnatal CNS: implications of their roles in neuronal and glial cell development. *J.Neurosci.* Vol. 17, No. 21, pp. 8300-8312

Schichor, C., Kerkau, S., Visted, T., Martini, R., Bjerkvig, R., Tonn, J. C., & Goldbrunner, R. (2005). The brain slice chamber, a novel variation of the Boyden Chamber Assay, allows time-dependent quantification of glioma invasion into mammalian brain in vitro. *J Neurooncol.* Vol. 73, No. 1, pp. 9-18

Schindl, M., Oberhuber, G., Obermair, A., Schoppmann, S. F., Karner, B., & Birner, P. (2001). Overexpression of Id-1 protein is a marker for unfavorable prognosis in early-stage cervical cancer. *Cancer Res.* Vol. 61, No. 15, pp. 5703-5706

Schindl, M., Schoppmann, S. F., Strobel, T., Heinzl, H., Leisser, C., Horvat, R., & Birner, P. (2003). Level of Id-1 protein expression correlates with poor differentiation, enhanced malignant potential, and more aggressive clinical behavior of epithelial ovarian tumors. *Clin.Cancer Res.* Vol. 9, No. 2, pp. 779-785

Schoppmann, S. F., Schindl, M., Bayer, G., Aumayr, K., Dienes, J., Horvat, R., Rudas, M., Gnant, M., Jakesz, R., & Birner, P. (2003). Overexpression of Id-1 is associated with poor clinical outcome in node negative breast cancer. *Int.J.Cancer.* Vol. 104, No. 6, pp. 677-682

Seno, T., Harada, H., Kohno, S., Teraoka, M., Inoue, A., & Ohnishi, T. (2009). Downregulation of SPARC expression inhibits cell migration and invasion in malignant gliomas. *Int.J.Oncol.* Vol. 34, No. 3, pp. 707-715

Shibahara, J., Kashima, T., Kikuchi, Y., Kunita, A., & Fukayama, M. (2006). Podoplanin is expressed in subsets of tumors of the central nervous system. *Virchows Arch.* Vol. 448, No. 4, pp. 493-499

Singec, I., Knoth, R., Meyer, R. P., Maciaczyk, J., Volk, B., Nikkhah, G., Frotscher, M., & Snyder, E. Y. (2006). Defining the actual sensitivity and specificity of the neurosphere assay in stem cell biology. *Nat.Methods.* Vol. 3, No. 10, pp. 801-806

Singh, S. K., Clarke, I. D., Hide, T., & Dirks, P. B. (2004). Cancer stem cells in nervous system tumors. *Oncogene.* Vol. 23, No. 43, pp. 7267-7273

Singh, S. K., Clarke, I. D., Terasaki, M., Bonn, V. E., Hawkins, C., Squire, J., & Dirks, P. B. (2003). Identification of a cancer stem cell in human brain tumors. *Cancer Res.* Vol. 63, No. 18, pp. 5821-5828

Singh, S. K., Hawkins, C., Clarke, I. D., Squire, J. A., Bayani, J., Hide, T., Henkelman, R. M., Cusimano, M. D., & Dirks, P. B. (2004). Identification of human brain tumour initiating cells. *Nature.* Vol. 432, No. 7015, pp. 396-401

Sminia, P., Acker, H., Eikesdal, H. P., Kaaijk, P., Enger, P., Slotman, B., & Bjerkvig, R. (2003). Oxygenation and response to irradiation of organotypic multicellular spheroids of human glioma. *Anticancer Res.* Vol. 23, No. 2B, pp. 1461-1466

Soeda, A., Park, M., Lee, D., Mintz, A., Androutsellis-Theotokis, A., McKay, R. D., Engh, J., Iwama, T., Kunisada, T., Kassam, A. B., Pollack, I. F., & Park, D. M. (2009). Hypoxia promotes expansion of the CD133-positive glioma stem cells through activation of HIF-1alpha. *Oncogene.* Vol. 28, No. 45, pp. 3949-59

Stallcup, W. B. & Huang, F. J. (2008). A role for the NG2 proteoglycan in glioma progression. *Cell Adh.Migr.* Vol. 2, No. 3, pp. 192-201

Stoppini, L., Buchs, P. A., & Muller, D. (1991). A simple method for organotypic cultures of nervous tissue. *J.Neurosci.Methods.* Vol. 37, No. 2, pp. 173-182

Strojnik, T., Rosland, G. V., Sakariassen, P. O., Kavalar, R., & Lah, T. (2007). Neural stem cell markers, nestin and musashi proteins, in the progression of human glioma: correlation of nestin with prognosis of patient survival. *Surg.Neurol.* Vol. 68, No. 2, pp. 133-143

Stupp, R., Hegi, M. E., Mason, W. P., van den Bent, M. J., Taphoorn, M. J., Janzer, R. C., Ludwin, S. K., Allgeier, A., Fisher, B., Belanger, K., Hau, P., Brandes, A. A., Gijtenbeek, J., Marosi, C., Vecht, C. J., Mokhtari, K., Wesseling, P., Villa, S., Eisenhauer, E., Gorlia, T., Weller, M., Lacombe, D., Cairncross, J. G., & Mirimanoff, R. O. (2009). Effects of radiotherapy with concomitant and adjuvant temozolomide versus radiotherapy alone on survival in glioblastoma in a randomised phase III study: 5-year analysis of the EORTC-NCIC trial. *Lancet Oncol.* Vol. 10, No. 5, pp. 459-466

Stupp, R., Mason, W. P., van den Bent, M. J., Weller, M., Fisher, B., Taphoorn, M. J., Belanger, K., Brandes, A. A., Marosi, C., Bogdahn, U., Curschmann, J., Janzer, R. C., Ludwin, S. K., Gorlia, T., Allgeier, A., Lacombe, D., Cairncross, J. G., Eisenhauer, E.,

& Mirimanoff, R. O. (2005). Radiotherapy plus concomitant and adjuvant temozolomide for glioblastoma. *N.Engl.J.Med.* Vol. 352, No. 10, pp. 987-996

Sunayama, J., Sato, A., Matsuda, K., Tachibana, K., Suzuki, K., Narita, Y., Shibui, S., Sakurada, K., Kayama, T., Tomiyama, A., & Kitanaka, C. (2010). Dual blocking of mTor and PI3K elicits a prodifferentiation effect on glioblastoma stem-like cells. *Neuro.Oncol.* Vol. 12, No. 12, pp. 1205-1219

Sutherland, R. M. (1998). Tumor hypoxia and gene expression--implications for malignant progression and therapy. *Acta Oncol.* Vol. 37, No. 6, pp. 567-574

Sutherland, R. M. & Durand, R. E. (1972). Cell contact as a possible contribution to radiation resistance of some tumours. *Br.J.Radiol.* Vol. 45, No. 538, pp. 788-789

Tang, R., Hirsch, P., Fava, F., Lapusan, S., Marzac, C., Teyssandier, I., Pardo, J., Marie, J. P., & Legrand, O. (2009). High Id1 expression is associated with poor prognosis in 237 patients with acute myeloid leukemia. *Blood.* Vol. 114, No. 14, pp. 2993-3000

Tchoghandjian, A., Baeza, N., Colin, C., Cayre, M., Metellus, P., Beclin, C., Ouafik, L., & Figarella-Branger, D. (2009). A2B5 Cells from Human Glioblastoma have Cancer Stem Cell Properties. *Brain Pathol.* Vol. 20, No. 1, pp. 211-21

Terzis, A. J., Pedersen, P. H., Feuerstein, B. G., Arnold, H., Bjerkvig, R., & Deen, D. F. (1998). Effects of DFMO on glioma cell proliferation, migration and invasion in vitro. *J.Neurooncol.* Vol. 36, No. 2, pp. 113-121

Terzis, A. J., Thorsen, F., Heese, O., Visted, T., Bjerkvig, R., Dahl, O., Arnold, H., & Gundersen, G. (1997). Proliferation, migration and invasion of human glioma cells exposed to paclitaxel (Taxol) in vitro. *Br.J.Cancer.* Vol. 75, No. 12, pp. 1744-1752

Thon, N., Damianoff, K., Hegermann, J., Grau, S., Krebs, B., Schnell, O., Tonn, J. C., & Goldbrunner, R. (2010). Presence of pluripotent CD133+ cells correlates with malignancy of gliomas. *Mol.Cell Neurosci.* Vol. 43, No. 1, pp. 51-59

Toda, M., Iizuka, Y., Yu, W., Imai, T., Ikeda, E., Yoshida, K., Kawase, T., Kawakami, Y., Okano, H., & Uyemura, K. (2001). Expression of the neural RNA-binding protein Musashi1 in human gliomas. *Glia.* Vol. 34, No. 1, pp. 1-7

Uchida, N., Buck, D. W., He, D., Reitsma, M. J., Masek, M., Phan, T. V., Tsukamoto, A. S., Gage, F. H., & Weissman, I. L. (2000). Direct isolation of human central nervous system stem cells. *Proc.Natl.Acad.Sci.U.S.A.* Vol. 97, No. 26, pp. 14720-14725

Vescovi, A. L., Galli, R., & Reynolds, B. A. (2006). Brain tumour stem cells. *Nat.Rev.Cancer.* Vol. 6, No. 6, pp. 425-436

Vlashi, E., McBride, W. H., & Pajonk, F. (2009). Radiation responses of cancer stem cells. *J.Cell Biochem.* Vol. 108, No. 2, pp. 339-342

Wakimoto, H., Kesari, S., Farrell, C. J., Curry, W. T., Jr., Zaupa, C., Aghi, M., Kuroda, T., Stemmer-Rachamimov, A., Shah, K., Liu, T. C., Jeyaretna, D. S., Debasitis, J., Pruszak, J., Martuza, R. L., & Rabkin, S. D. (2009). Human glioblastoma-derived cancer stem cells: establishment of invasive glioma models and treatment with oncolytic herpes simplex virus vectors. *Cancer Res.* Vol. 69, No. 8, pp. 3472-3481

Wan, F., Herold-Mende, C., Campos, B., Centner, F. S., Dictus, C., Becker, N., Devens, F., Mogler, C., Felsberg, J., Grabe, N., Reifenberger, G., Lichter, P., Unterberg, A., Bermejo, J. L., & Ahmadi, R. (2011). Association of stem cell-related markers and survival in astrocytic gliomas. *Biomarkers.* Vol. 16, No. 2, pp. 136-143

Wang, J., Sakariassen, P. O., Tsinkalovsky, O., Immervoll, H., Boe, S. O., Svendsen, A., Prestegarden, L., Rosland, G., Thorsen, F., Stuhr, L., Molven, A., Bjerkvig, R., &

Enger, P. O. (2008). CD133 negative glioma cells form tumors in nude rats and give rise to CD133 positive cells. *Int.J.Cancer*. Vol. 122, No. 4, pp. 761-768
Wang, J., Wakeman, T. P., Lathia, J. D., Hjelmeland, A. B., Wang, X. F., White, R. R., Rich, J. N., & Sullenger, B. A. (2010). Notch promotes radioresistance of glioma stem cells. *Stem Cells*. Vol. 28, No. 1, pp. 17-28
Wang, Y., Liu, Y., Malek, S. N., Zheng, P., & Liu, Y. (2011). Targeting HIF1alpha Eliminates Cancer Stem Cells in Hematological Malignancies. *Cell Stem Cell*. Vol. 8, No. 4, pp. 399-411
Ward, R. J. & Dirks, P. B. (2007). Cancer stem cells: at the headwaters of tumor development. *Annu.Rev.Pathol*. Vol. 2, No. 175-189
Ward, R. J., Lee, L., Graham, K., Satkunendran, T., Yoshikawa, K., Ling, E., Harper, L., Austin, R., Nieuwenhuis, E., Clarke, I. D., Hui, C. C., & Dirks, P. B. (2009). Multipotent CD15+ cancer stem cells in patched-1-deficient mouse medulloblastoma. *Cancer Res*. Vol. 69, No. 11, pp. 4682-4690
Xing, F., Okuda, H., Watabe, M., Kobayashi, A., Pai, S. K., Liu, W., Pandey, P. R., Fukuda, K., Hirota, S., Sugai, T., Wakabayshi, G., Koeda, K., Kashiwaba, M., Suzuki, K., Chiba, T., Endo, M., Mo, Y. Y., & Watabe, K. (2011). Hypoxia-induced Jagged2 promotes breast cancer metastasis and self-renewal of cancer stem-like cells. *Oncogene*. April 18, Epub ahead of print.
Yamaguchi, S., Kobayashi, H., Narita, T., Kanehira, K., Sonezaki, S., Kubota, Y., Terasaka, S., & Iwasaki, Y. (2010). Novel photodynamic therapy using water-dispersed TiO2-polyethylene glycol compound: evaluation of antitumor effect on glioma cells and spheroids in vitro. *Photochem.Photobiol*. Vol. 86, No. 4, pp. 964-971
Yeung, T. M., Gandhi, S. C., & Bodmer, W. F. (2011). Hypoxia and lineage specification of cell line-derived colorectal cancer stem cells. *Proc.Natl.Acad.Sci.U.S.A*. Vol. 108, No. 11, pp. 4382-4387
Yin, A. H., Miraglia, S., Zanjani, E. D., Almeida-Porada, G., Ogawa, M., Leary, A. G., Olweus, J., Kearney, J., & Buck, D. W. (1997). AC133, a novel marker for human hematopoietic stem and progenitor cells. *Blood*. Vol. 90, No. 12, pp. 5002-5012
Yuhas, J. M., Li, A. P., Martinez, A. O., & Ladman, A. J. (1977). A simplified method for production and growth of multicellular tumor spheroids. *Cancer Res*. Vol. 37, No. 10, pp. 3639-3643
Zencak, D., Lingbeek, M., Kostic, C., Tekaya, M., Tanger, E., Hornfeld, D., Jaquet, M., Munier, F. L., Schorderet, D. F., van, L. M., & Arsenijevic, Y. (2005). Bmi1 loss produces an increase in astroglial cells and a decrease in neural stem cell population and proliferation. *J.Neurosci*. Vol. 25, No. 24, pp. 5774-5783
Zeppernick, F., Ahmadi, R., Campos, B., Dictus, C., Helmke, B. M., Becker, N., Lichter, P., Unterberg, A., Radlwimmer, B., & Herold-Mende, C. C. (2008). Stem cell marker CD133 affects clinical outcome in glioma patients. *Clin.Cancer Res*. Vol. 14, No. 1, pp. 123-129
Zhu, X., Bidlingmaier, S., Hashizume, R., James, C. D., Berger, M. S., & Liu, B. (2010). Identification of internalizing human single-chain antibodies targeting brain tumor sphere cells. *Mol.Cancer Ther*. Vol. 9, No. 7, pp. 2131-2141
Zhu, Y., Guignard, F., Zhao, D., Liu, L., Burns, D. K., Mason, R. P., Messing, A., & Parada, L. F. (2005). Early inactivation of p53 tumor suppressor gene cooperating with NF1 loss induces malignant astrocytoma. *Cancer Cell*. Vol. 8, No. 2, pp. 119-130

18

Endogenous Experimental Glioma Model, Links Between Glioma Stem Cells and Angiogenesis

Susana Bulnes[1], Harkaitz Bengoetxea[2], Naiara Ortuzar[2], Enrike G. Argandoña[3] and José Vicente Lafuente[2]

[1]*Laboratory of Clinical and Experimental Neuroscience (LaNCE), Department of Nursing I, University of the Basque Country, Leioa*

[2]*Laboratory of Clinical and Experimental Neuroscience (LaNCE), Department of Neuroscience, University of the Basque Country, Leioa,*

[3]*Unit of Anatomy, Department of Medicine, University of Fribourg, Fribourg,*

[1,2]*Spain*

[3]*Switzerland*

1. Introduction

Glioblastomas (GBM) are the most malignant solid tumours (grade IV) of CNS. They are glial lineage neoplasias with a high proliferative and invasive capacity, reaching to occupy an entire lobe of the brain (Kleihues et al., 2007). According with their genesis, they can be differentiated between primary and secondary glioblastoma. The primary is the most common glioblastoma. This is a new generated tumour after a brief medical history (three months), with no evidence of a less malignant lesion. On the other hand, secondary glioblastoma develops from diffuse astrocytoma, anaplastic astrocytoma or oligodendroglioma and malignant progression. Its development time is about five years. It is thought that both types of glioblastomas may be generated from neoplastic cells with characteristic of stem cells (Ohgaki & Kleihues, 2009). In addition, these cancer stem cells called "glioma stem cells" (GSCs) may be the responsible for glioma recurrences due to chemo-and radio resistance (Bao et al., 2006; Rich, 2007). Glioma stem cells (GSCs) are a subpopulation of neoplastic cells identified in glioma sharing properties with neural stem cells (self-renewal, high proliferation rate, undifferentiating, and neurospheres conformation) and the capacity for leading the tumourigenesis and tumour malignancy. The proliferation and the invasion into adjacent normal parenchyma have been attributed to glioma stem cells as well. Indeed, they were related to the angiogenesis process needed for the growth and survival of the neoplasia.

The microvascular network in gliomas has to get adapt to metabolic tissue requirements (Folkman, 2000). When the vascular network cannot satisfy cell requirements (Oxygen pressure of 5-10 mm Hg) tissue hypoxia occurs. This situation triggers the synthesis of pro-angiogenic factors as matrix metalloprotease (MMP-2), angiopoietin-1, phosphoglycerate kinase (PGK), erythropoietin (EPO), and vascular endothelial growth factor (VEGF)-A (Fong, 2008).

Vascular endothelial growth factor (VEGF) is a major regulator of tumour angiogenesis (Bulnes & Lafuente, 2007; Lafuente et al., 1999; Machein & Plate, 2004; Marti et al., 2000).

VEGF acts as mitogen, survival, antiapoptotic and vascular permeability factor (VPF) for the endothelial cells (Dvorak, 2006). The increase of this pro-angiogenic factor, secreted either by neoplastic cells or by cells of the tumour microenvironment, induces the start of angiogenesis, the called "angiogenic switch" (Bergers & Benjamin, 2003). This event results in the transition from avascularised hyperplasia to outgrowing vascularised tumour and eventually to malignant progression. It has been shown in human glioma biopsies that VEGF overexpression correlates directly to proliferation, vascularization and degree of malignancy, and therefore inversely to prognosis (Ke et al., 2000; Lafuente et al., 1999; Plate, 1999). The synthesis of VEGF is mediated by the Hypoxia-Inducible Factor (HIF-1), a critical step for the formation of new blood vessels and for the adaptation of microenvironment to the growth of gliomas (Jin et al., 2000; Marti et al., 2000; Semenza, 2003). Recent researches have reported that glioma stem cells play a pivotal role inducing the angiogenesis via HIF-1/VEGF (Bao et al., 2006). By the other hand, hypoxia has been related to clones selection of tumour cells. These clones adapted to the tumour microenvironment have acquired the phenotype of tumour stem cell with increased proliferative and infiltrative capacity (Heddleston et al., 2009; Li et al., 2009). Invasion of adjacent normal parenchyma has been attributed to glioma stem cells as well.

Due to these evidences, GSCs are currently being considered as a potential therapeutic target of the tumours. Recent studies have been focused on the identification of GSCs. In human glioblastomas they have been identified using CD133 marker (Ignatova et al., 2002). However, little is known about their genesis during glioma progression, especially during the early stages.

Some authors have previously reported the induction of glial tumour in rats by transplacentary administration of the carcinogen ethylnitrosourea (ENU) as a suitable method for studying the natural development of glioma (Bulnes-Sesma et al., 2006; Zook et al., 2000). In addition to this, it has been reported that ENU glioma model is a representative model for human glioma due to its location and also to its similar cellular, molecular and genetic alterations (Kokkinakis et al., 2004). Our experience with this model has proven to be useful to study many aspects of tumourigenesis and neoangiogenesis. In previous researches we reported the progression of tumour malignancy associated with vascular structural alterations and blood brain barrier (BBB) disturbances (Bulnes & Lafuente, 2007; Bulnes et al., 2009). ENU induced glioma permitted us to identify tumour development stages following microvascular changes. In addition, it was possible to study the angiogenesis process. Recently, we have used this model to study the relationship between glioma stem cells and angiogenesis process during the neoplasia development.

Many evidences corroborate the hypothesis that "glioma stem cells" have a close relationship with angiogenesis process, intratumour hypoxia and neoplastic microvascular network. In this chapter we centred to show this relationship from early to advanced stages of glioma using ENU-model.

2. Endogenous glioma model

Over the years, different methods have been employed to induce experimental tumours in the Central Nervous System of animals. Exposure to radiation, inoculation of carcinogenic virus, xenografts of tumour cell lines or tumour fragments in nude rats or mice, administration of chemical substances (Bulnes-Sesma et al., 2006) and genetically engineered mouse models have been used to replicate CNS tumours. The administration of chemical substances as nitroso compounds is one of the most commonly-used methods to induce experimental CNS neoplasm. There is strong experimental data showing that nitrosamides (R1NNO-COR2), a type of N-nitroso compounds (NOC), are potent neuro-carcinogens when administered transplacentally. N-nitrosoureas MNU and ENU (a class of nitrosamides) have been demonstrated to be carcinogenic in animals, and particularly related to the development of CNS tumours. N-ethyl-N-nitrosourea (ENU) acts alkylating the O_6 in the guanine (G:C---T:A transition) and the O_2 in the thymine (T:A---A:T transversion). The accumulation of these successive DNA mutations seems to be responsible of the neurooncogenic effect of ENU (Bulnes-Sesma et al., 2006; O'Neill, 2000). Recently it has been reported that ENU exposure affects primitive neuroepithelial cells of the subventricular plate (SVZ) and germinative zone (VZ). ENU prenatal exposure affects the differentiation of these cells generating glial lineage tumours (Burger, 1988; Vaquero et al., 1994; Yoshimura et al., 1998) and its exposure in adult affects the neurogenesis of the SVZ (Capilla-Gonzalez et al., 2010). In previous studies we found that gliomas induced in offspring were similar to the human gliomas (Kokkinakis et al., 2004). Therefore, ENU brain induced tumours have allowed the study of several aspects of glioma behaviour, for example, microvascular organization (Schlageter et al., 1999; Yoshimura et al., 1998); neoplastic cell dedifferentiation (Jang et al., 2004); gene mutations (Bielas & Heddle, 2000; O'Neil, 2000); microcirculation and angiogenesis process (Bulnes & Lafuente, 2007; Bulnes et al., 2009) or experimental therapeutic agents (Kish et al., 2001).

In our model, the glioma induction was performed by prenatal exposure of Sprague Dawley rats to ENU. Briefly, pregnancy rats, on the 15th day of gestation, were given a single i.p. injection of 80 mg of ENU/kg body weight (Bulnes et al., 2009; Bulnes et al., 2010). Offspring rats exposed to ENU were reared in standard laboratory conditions and the study was performed from 5 months to one year of age. The identification of ENU-Gliomas was performed by T2-w and postcontrast T1-weighted NMR images and by histopathology diagnosis from H&E staining and immunophenotypic study as previously described (Bulnes & Lafuente 2007) (Figure 1, 2). Following our results, ENU-glioma starts from the fifth month of offspring rat age and becomes GBM at 10 months of age (Bulnes-Sesma et al., 2006). ENU-glioma starts as cellular proliferation growing near ventricles in association with subcortical white matter. Over 6 months of extrauterine life, this tumour proliferation become nodular and rats display neurological signs (Figure 1). Around one year they grow as a GBM toward the contralateral hemisphere (Figure 2). Following our findings, we have identified three stages of ENU-glioma development: initial, intermediate and advanced. The advanced stage corresponds to anaplastic oligodendroglioma or glioblastoma (GBM) similar to the human. ENU-GBM may reach to infiltrate whole cerebral hemisphere, showing malignant histopathological features such as: high tissue heterogeneity, aberrant angioarchitecture, macro-haemorrhages, macrocysts or palisade necrosis (Klehiues et al., 2007). Thanks to this model we could isolate early glioma stages, which is impossible to carry out in human brain.

3. Stem cells and cancer stem cells

Stem cells are functionally defined as self-renewing and multipotent cells that exhibit multilineage differentiation (Till & McCulloch, 2011). Nowadays they have been proposed to be an important tool in regenerative therapy being used to regenerate tissue in many diseases like heart stroke, neurodegenerative diseases, etc (Nadig, 2009). However, in oncology and especially in cerebral gliomas, the presence of the stem cells has been related to a poor prognosis. Recent investigations in glioblastomas have reported that these cancer stem cells called glioma stem cells (GSCs) have tumourigenic capacities like tumour malignant process, peripheral tissue infiltration and angiogenesis induction (Hadjipanayis & Van Meir, 2009; Rich, 2007).

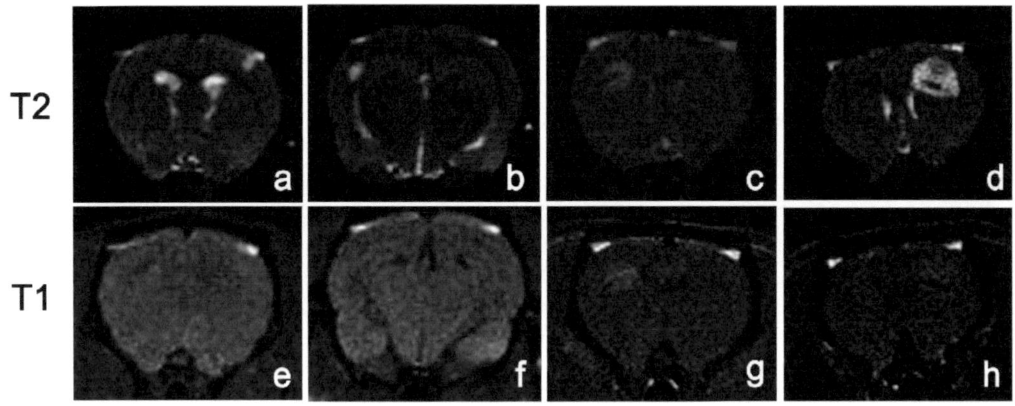

Fig. 1. Coronal sections of rat brains displaying ENU-glioma showed by MRI on T2-w and T1-w after injection of gadolinium. a, b) Small neoplastic mass growing on the cerebral cortex with an homogeneous hyperintense signal on T2-w images. These neoplastic masses correspond to initial stage of ENU-glioma. e, f) Both masses display an isointense signal on T1-w. c, d) ENU-glioma tumour with nodular shape showed on T2-w hyperintense signal that represents intermediate stage. g, h) At this stage there is a gadolinium contrast enhancement observed as homogeneous soft hyperintense signal on T1-w image.

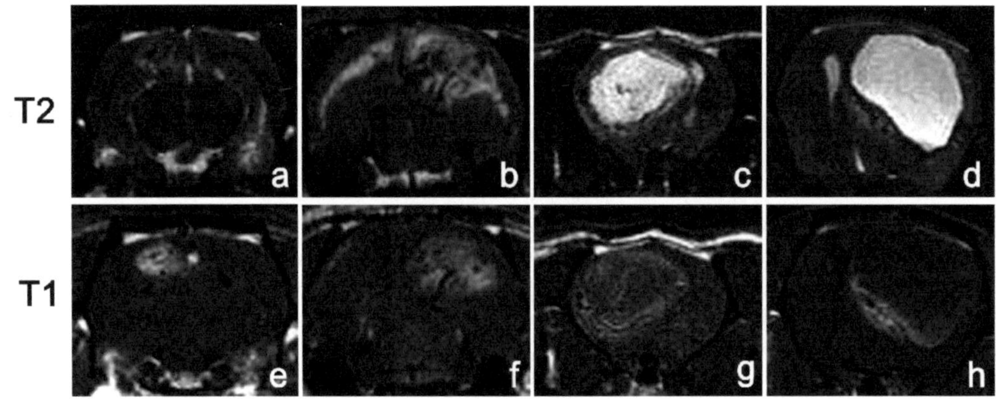

Fig. 2. Coronal sections of rat brains with ENU-glioma of advanced stage showed by MRI on T2-w and T1-w after injection of gadolinium. All of these anaplastic gliomas display heterogeneous hyperintense signal on T2 (a-d) and on T1-w (e-h). This heterogeneity is due to the presence of histopathology features of malignity. c-d) ENU-GBMs high-proliferative covering a whole cerebral hemisphere. The T2-w images reveal an intratumour hyperintense signal corresponding with intratumour oedema or macrocysts. g-h). Gadolinium enhancement of this T1-w image adopts a rim shape bordering the neoplastic mass. This rim represents the microvascular proliferation with dysfunction of Blood Brain Barrier.

In the middle of the 60s, Altman and Das reported the first evidences about stem cells in adult brain. They observed stem cells in the hippocampus and olfactory bulb of rats, and it supposed the first sign of division of stem cells. Later on they were called Neural Stem Cells (NSCs). NSCs were considered the unique population of Central Nervous System cells characterized by self-renewal and multilineage differentiation properties (Muller et al., 2006). They can form neurospheres (Reynolds & Weiss, 1992) and differentiate in vitro into the three neuroectodermal lineages astrocytes, oligodendrocytes and neurons (Alvarez-Buylla & Garcia-Verdugo, 2002). Furthermore, when they are transplanted in vivo in the cerebellum, they can generate neurons and glial cells (Lee et al., 2005). Also, after transplantation into nude mice they can differentiate into neuroblasts (Tamaki et al., 2002). NSCs reside in the germinal layers of the developing brain, initially in the early neuroepithelium, later in the ventricular (VZ) and subventricular zone (SVZ) during embryogenesis (Götz & Huttner, 2005). In adult brain, three areas are supposed to harbour neural stem cells: dentate gyrus of hippocampus, SVZ (Doetsch et al., 1999; Eriksson et al., 1998) and the fibbers connecting olfactory bulb to lateral ventricle (Lois & Alvarez-Buylla, 1994; Whitman & Greer, 2009). In recent times, they were also isolated in the subcortical white matter (Nunes et al., 2003).

In the 1960s, evidence emerged supporting the presence of stem cells in tumours. Bergsagel and Valeriote (1968) showed that only certain cells within a tumour had the capacity to generate a new tumour; they termed these cells "tumour stem cells". After this, tumour stem cells were identified in breast tumour (Al-Hajj et al., 2003), pancreatic tumour (Esposito et al., 2002) etc.

The first concept of cancer stem cell, later on also called tumour initiating cells, appeared in the beginning of the 90s. Bonnet and Dick (1977) describe how some cells, isolated from leukaemia patient´s blood, had proliferation and differentiation capacities in vivo. Fan et al. (2007) described cancer stem cells as the cellular subpopulation capable of tumour regeneration within a permissive environment. Rich and collaborators reported that cancer stem cells have tumourigenic, infiltration and angiogenesis properties as well as radio/chemo-resistance (Rich, 2007; Hadjipanayis & Van Meir, 2009).

The relation between stem cells and cancer stem cells was studied. The results explained that both cellular types share the previously mentioned characteristics, as well as many cell signalling pathways as oncogene bcl-2, Sonic hedgehog (Shh) and Wnt signalling cascade (Reya et al., 2001). Both types of stem cells also share common markers like CD133, Nestin (Dahlstrand et al., 1992) and transcription factor Sox2 (Gangemi et al., 2009). However, there are differences between stem cells and cancer stem cells, such as expression of different markers, chromosomal alterations and tumourigenic capacity. Holland et al. (2000) published that cancer stem cells could develop from modified neural stem cells. They have been described many pathways that can lead to cancer stem cell formation like Notch (Takebe & Ivy 2010), Akt (Germano et al., 2010) activation or p53 pathway alteration.

3.1 Glioma stem cells (GSCs)

Dahlstrand et al. (1992) identified a cancer stem cells subtype inside glial lineage brain tumours which were called Glioma Stem Cells (GSCs). These GSCs may be responsible for maintenance of the entire tumour and also they have the potential, when injected in immunodeficient mice, to generate gliomas similar to the original tumours (Heddleston et al., 2009).

GSCs indeed of share properties of somatic or embryonic stem cells (high proliferation rate, undifferentiating, formation of neurospheres) are chemo-and radio resistant (Bao et al., 2006, Rich, 2007). Their radiotherapy resistance may be thanks to a more efficient DNA reparation mechanism and protein kinases phosphorilation Chk1 and Chk2 (Bao et al., 2006). The resistance to chemotherapeutic drugs is through membrane transporters that bomb the drugs outside the cell (Donnenberg & Donnenberg, 2005).

The first GSCs identification was found in the tumour advanced stage corresponding with human-GBM (Ignatova et al., 2000). However, the first moment of GSCs expression remains unknown, as well as their role in early stages of tumour development. It is very important to identify and explain GSCs apparition in early glioma stages to research about future tumour therapy.

The discovery of GSCs in gliomas involved the creation of a new glioma-genesis hypothesis called "hierarchical hypothesis". Before GSCs discovery, glioma development was explained by the "stochastic theory". Stochastic theory is based on all neoplastic cells are clones from a single undifferentiated cell and they have the same genetic alterations (Hadjipanayis & Van Meir, 2009). Nowadays the "hierarchical theory" explains that only a few neoplastic cells can adapt to the tumour environment and are able to start the tumourigenic process. Even though the low proliferation of GSCs, they guide the tumour growth giving raise to more mature cells with limited proliferation capacity (Shen et al., 2008).

After the glioma stem cells finding, the research about glioma development has been centred in the identification of them. So far markers as CD133/Promonin-1, presents in glioma stem cells (Dell'Albani, 2008), Nestin, a protein found in neural stem cells in SVZ and other markers of neuroepithelial stem cells (Jang et al., 2004) including Musashi-1, Sox-2, GFAP, Map-2, Neural-tubulin, Neurofilament O4 and Noggin were used in order to identify tumour stem cells. But the lack of a specific marker makes it very difficult to identify (Hadjipanayis & Van Meir, 2009; Li et al., 2009).

Nestin is an intermediate filament protein typical for neural precursor cells. It has been extensively used as a marker for neural stem cells. It is expressed in primitive neuroepithelial cells of all regions of CNS during the development. In adult its expression is restricted to the ventricular wall (SVZ) and the central canal. In pathological conditions like brain trauma, CNS ischemia, neurotoxicity, neoplastic transformation and in response to cellular stress, the nestin over-expression was showed (Holmin et al., 1997, Jang et al., 2004). In primary malignant tumours of CNS high amounts of cells positive for Nestin have been reported. Nestin has been described as a marker of GSCs in astroglial tumours (Singh et al., 2003), indicating undifferentiating and malignance degree (Schiffer et al., 2010), but it is not specific for glioma stem cells (Hadjipanayis & Van Meir, 2009). Indeed, Nestin expression has been described to appear since the first stages in glioma models (Jang et al., 2004).

CD133 (prominin-1) was the first identified member of the prominin family of pentaspan membrane proteins which acts as a marker of hematopoietic progenitor cells. It is a cell surface marker used for the identification and isolation of stem/progenitor cells in several tissues, for instance, endothelium, brain, bone narrow, liver, prostate, pancreas and foreskin (Mizrak et al., 2008). CD133 was originally described as an hematopoietic stem cell marker and was subsequently related to number of progenitor cells including neuroepithelium (Corbeil et al., 2000) as well as cancer stem cells in various tumours such as prostate and colon cancer (Cheng et al., 2009; Collins et al., 2005; O'Brien et al., 2007). In human glioblastoma, CD133 expression has been associated to GSCs and bad prognosis of the tumour (Germano et al., 2010).

4. Tumour angiogenesis

Gliomas proliferate in the brain, a privileged organ from the point of view of blood supply. The exchange of metabolites between blood and cerebral tissue occurs essentially in the brain capillaries. The diameter of brain capillaries in the adult human is between 5 and 7 microns. These microvessels feed to the cells that are 10-20 microns away. Although the distance between cells and microvessels is lesser than 20 µm, the growth and survival of the gliomas depend on vascular remodelling and angiogenesis (Folkman, 2006). Along the early stages of small gliomas the metabolic demand is supplied by the vast microvascular network but when the metabolic supply has been exceeded, new formation of vessels becomes necessary (Carmeliet & Jain, 2000; Yancopoulos et al., 2000). The genesis of the new vessels from pre-existing ones is called angiogenesis in opposite to vasculogenesis refereed to the formation of vessels from hemopoietic niches (Carmeliet, 2003; Risau & Falmme 1995; Risau, 1997).

Angiogenesis is a complex process that requires proteolytic and mitogenic activity of endothelial cells and interaction of these with the extracellular matrix molecules and cells of peri-endothelial support cells (pericytes and smooth muscle cells). Many molecules and pathways are involved in this process, such as VEGF, its receptors VEGFR-1 and VEGFR-2, the endothelial receptor tyrosine kinase tie-1 and tie-2 and the angiopoietin ligands 1 and 2. Many other molecules as PDGF and TGF-β, integrin receptors, are very important (Millauer et al., 1993; Neufeld et al., 1999).

Angiogenesis requires some angiogenic stimulus, such as hypoxia, new metabolic requirements or tumour growth to start. Intratumour hypoxia occurs at the time when there is an imbalance between supply and demand oxygen due to the irregular and chaotic blood flow (Jensen, 2006). The relative tissue hypoxia triggers the production of hypoxia inducible factor-1α, upregulating the expression of VEGF. In addition to this, it was reported that hypoxia plays a fundamental role in the induction of cell phenotype neoplastic to the undifferentiated state of GSCs. According to recent research, hypoxia selects tumour cell clones that have adapted to the tumour microenvironment and have acquired the phenotype tumour stem cell, with its capabilities of proliferation and infiltration (Heddleston et al., 2009; Li et al., 2009).

Heddleston et al. (2009) observed how in cultures of human glioma neoplastic cells exposed to hypoxia reverted to a state of tumour stem cells. Griguer et al. (2008) related the appearance of CD133 + cells with oxygen stress in gliomas. On the other hand, it was observed a decrease in the expression of CD133 when reverted to conditions of normoxia. Furthermore, studies of human GBM have described the relationship between the gradient of intratumour oxygen and the appearance of the phenotype tumour stem cell (Pistollato et al., 2010). As above, only a cluster of neoplastic cells resists to the conditions of hypoxia and intratumoural ischemia. This group of cells may be stem cell precursors, and after adapting to the new microenvironment, are transformed to GSCs.

4.1 Vascular endothelial growth factor (VEGF)

Vascular endothelial growth factor (VEGF) is a major regulator of angiogenesis in development (Bengoetxea et al., 2008; Ferrara et al., 2003; Ment et al., 1997) and pathological disease (Bulnes & Lafuente, 2007; Lafuente et al., 1999; Marti et al., 2000; Plate, 1992). However, the role of VEGF in nervous tissue is even more extensive. Previous studies showed that VEGF also has strong neuroprotective, neurotrophic and neurogenic properties (Jin et al., 2002; Ortuzar et al., 2011; Rosenstein & Krum, 2004; Storkebaum et al., 2004).

Although the synthesis of this proangiogenic cytokine is associated to tumour cells and endothelial cells, it has been described in others, such as: neurons, astrocytes, pericytes, smooth muscle cells, macrophages, lymphoid cells, platelets and fibroblasts (Zagzag et al., 2000). The VEGF family consists of five different homologous factors, VEGF-A, VEGF-B, VEGF-C, VEGF-D and placental growth factor (PIGF) (Ferrara et al., 2003). VEGF-A (VEGF) is the predominant form and is a hypoxia-inducible 45 KDa homodimeric glycoprotein.

VEGF-A acts as mitogen, survival and antiapoptotic factor for the endothelial cells from arteries, veins and lymphatics. Faced with increased secretion of VEGF and its binding to receptors on the surface of endothelial cells, VEGF is a signal transduction leading to production of molecules including enzymes for the degradation of extracellular matrix and increase of vascular permeability. This will facilitate cell proliferation, survival and migration of endothelial cells. It is also known as the vascular permeability factor (VPF) (Dvorak, 2006) on the basis of its ability to induce leakage through the blood brain barrier in some pathological situations (Ferrara, 2001; Lafuente et al., 1999; Lafuente et al., 2002). Helmlinger et al. (2000) stated that in the vasodilatation process the VEGF induced the elongation of endothelial cells but not their proliferation. In the angiogenesis process, VEGF works in line with other factors such as angiopoietin and ephrins (Tonini et al., 2003). It has been shown in human biopsies that VEGF overexpression in gliomas correlates directly to proliferation, vascularization and degree of malignancy, and therefore inversely to prognosis (Ke et al., 2000; Lafuente et al., 1999; Plate, 1999).

5. ENU glioma microvascular adaptation

Along the glioma progression, there is a transition from the homogeneous capillary network to an anarchic angioarchitecture. Microvessels have to adapt in order to maintain blood perfusion and metabolic support in adverse conditions, constituting a peculiar tissular microenvironment in response to hypoxia (Blouw et al., 2003). Glioma microvascular remodelling consists in a process of vascular aberration along the neoplasia development. Vascular development process led to microvascular proliferations that are a histopathological hallmark of glioblastoma (Kleihues et al., 2007). Some authors consider the core of a high-grade glioma as an avascular zone, since it has scarce capillaries with wide lumen and a fragmented basal membrane, being rather inefficient for metabolic exchange (Vajkoczy & Menger, 2004).

Tumour blood vessels have multiple abnormalities that result in a heterogeneous environment. They are disorganized, tortuous, sinusoidal, branchy and leaky, the diameter is irregular and the walls are thinner than those found in healthy brain tissue (Bigner et al., 1998). Following our results obtained by LEA and Butyrylcholinesterase (BChE) histochemistry (Bulnes et al., 2009) we showed a transition from the homogeneous capillary network of early stages to an anarchic angioarchitecture of advanced ENU-glioma stages (Figure 3). It was found that the vessel density decreased and the vascular size increased in order to glioma malignity (Bulnes et al., 2009). The initial stage of ENU-glioma was constituted by microvessels similar to the brain capillaries, the intermediate stage by tortuous, disorganized and dilated vessels and the advanced stage by anarchic and aberrant vessels such as: multilayered "glomeruloid tuft"; "garland" of proliferated vessels and huge dilated vessels (Klehues et al., 2007).

One result to take in consideration was the gradient from the well-oxygenated tumour periphery to the central hypoxic core of ENU-glioblastoma. Dilated intratumour vessels, expressing VEGF (Lafuente et al., 1999) increase their lumen on account of endothelial elongation but not of cell proliferation (Helmlinger et al., 2000). The intratumour area displays irregularly branching vessels, variable intravascular spaces and large avascular areas. It is also worth mentioning that perivascular cells of aberrant vessels of ENU-GBM often displayed a high activity for BChE, depicted by a strong brown staining (Bulnes et al., 2009). BChE activity is strongly related to neurogenesis and cellular proliferation (Mack & Robitzki, 2000), having a great role in tumourigenesis. These findings have led us to postulate that these perivascular cells might be stem cells proliferating around intratumour vessels (Anderson et al., 2005; Brat et al., 2004) and migrating through the vascular extracellular matrix (Ruoslahti, 2002). This could corroborate the hypothesis that stem cells adapted to hypoxic stress use the vascular extracellular matrix for migration and invasion. In addition to this, in previous work we have shown that these cells co-expressed Ki-67 and VEGF (Bulnes & Lafuente, 2007).

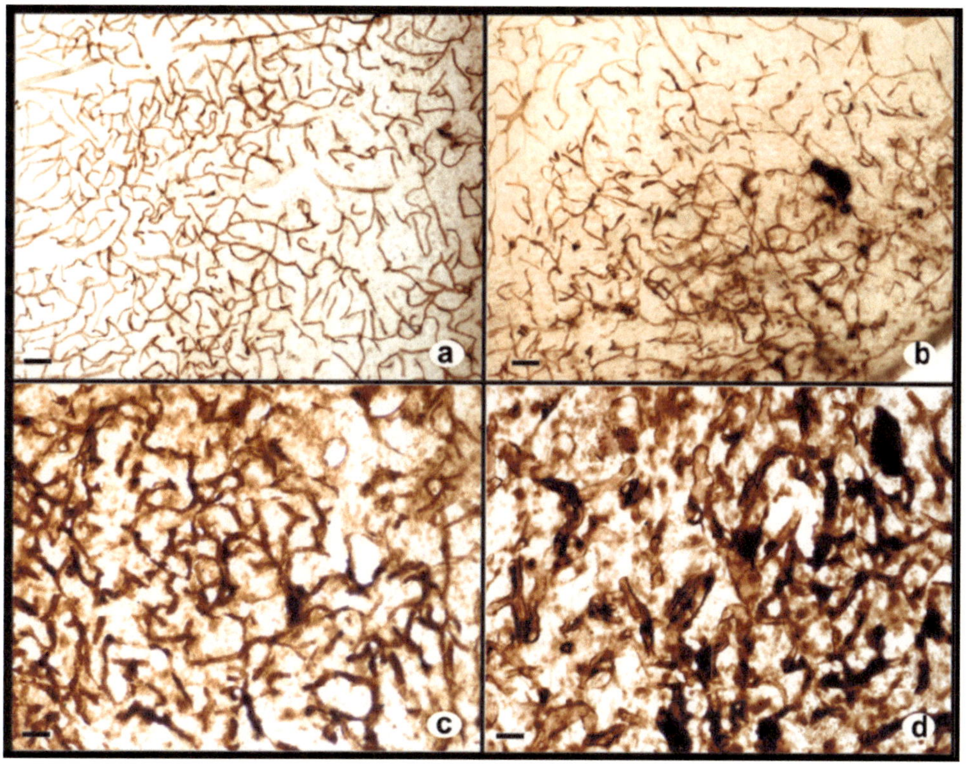

Fig. 3. Angioarchitecture study of gliomas shown by butyrylcholinesterase histochemistry. a) Angioarchitecture of the cerebral cortex of the rat brain. b) Periventricular small neoplastic mass (initial stage) showing some strongly-positive vessels for BChE. c) Intermediate ENU-glioma stage displaying a network of numerous tortuous capillaries of anarchic distribution. d) Malignant infiltrating macrotumour, with dilated vessels of the intratumour area with strongly BChE positive cells. (Scale bar of 50µm).

Glioma malignancy process is mediated by the vascular remodelling and the angiogenesis process where the blood brain barrier (BBB) function is implicated. The BBB is the set of mechanisms (physical and metabolic) that regulate the passage of elements from the blood plasma to neural tissue. This especial barrier is necessary for the cerebral homeostasis and it is associated with the hydrostatic and osmotic pressure gradients across the capillary (Hatashita & Hoff, 1986).

In pathological conditions, the increase of vascular permeability could be due to the blood brain barrier dysfunction, to a structural break-down or to its immaturity. Endothelial cells (ECs) of tumour vessels do not form a closed barrier, and pericytes are loosely attached (Baluk, et al., 2005). Defective tight junctions explain the tumour vessel leakiness which leads to blood brain barrier (BBB) breakdown and the oedema associated with brain tumours (Hashizume et al., 2000; Papadopoulos et al., 2004). Brain oedema in gliomas is an epiphenomenon related to BBB breakdown and is another cause of tumour mortality (Ballabh et al., 2004). The BBB distortion and permeability increase have been related to intravital dyes extravasation (Lafuente et al., 1994, 2004), Gd-DTPA contrast enhancement on T1-w images (Brasch & Turetschek, 2000; Cha et al., 2003; Claes et al., 2007) and to changes in the expression of BBB markers as glucose transporter-1 (GluT-1) (Dobrogowska & Vorbrodt, 1999) and structural rat specific antigen of BBB (EBA) (Argandona et al., 2005; Lafuente et al., 2006; Lin & Ginsberg, 2000; Krum et al., 2002; Sternberger et al., 1989; Zhu et al., 2001).

In our ENU model, vascular adaptations predominate over angiogenesis (Lafuente et al., 2000; Bian et al., 2006). Microvascular adaptations in early development stages are based on vasodilatation, endothelium elongation and permeability increase mediated by VEGF-A without BBB dysfunction. On the other hand, in malignant gliomas the microvascular adaptations vary according to blood flow perfusion. Permeability increase in intratumour vessels is not enough to supply the metabolic demand, and triggering of the angiogenesis process on the tumour border is necessary. When the blood flow inside and around the tumour becomes irregular and chaotic, partly due to the aberrant microvessels, the relative tissue hypoxia triggers the production of hypoxia inducible factor-1α (Chen et al., 2009; Jain et al., 2007), upregulating the expression of VEGF-A and endothelial nitric oxide synthase (eNOS). VEGF-A induces the synthesis of NO by phosphorylation of endothelial NO synthase via PI-3K/Akt kinase (Osuka et al., 2004, Ziche & Morbidelli, 2009), thus promoting BBB breakdown and increasing permeability. Although, the role of eNOS and VEGF-A in tumour induced brain oedema is still a matter of debate. Our previous studies demonstrates that eNOS overexpression in the microvasculature of intermediate and advanced ENU-gliomas correlates with the loss of immunostaining for primary BBB markers GluT-1 and EBA (Bulnes et al., 2010) (Figure 4).

Following the finding showed in human tissues, in ENU-malignant glioma astrocytic processes and pericytes were loosely attached to endothelial cells of tumour vessels without forming a continuous layer (Baluk et al., 2005) (result not published). In addition to this, defective tight junctions (TJs) without occludin protein expression, also lead to oedema associated with ENU induced brain tumours. We showed an intratumoural glioma oedema instead of peritumoural one by gadolinium contrast enhancement and intravital dyes extravasation (Bulnes et al., 2009, 2010).

6. Glioma stem cells and angiogenesis in ENU model

The moment named "angiogenenic switch", when the angiogenesis starts, is showed at ENU-glioma intermediate stage due to the presence of overexpression of VEGF and eNOS

(Bulnes et al., 2010). Because stem cells have been associated with the synthesis of VEGF (Bao et al., 2006), we focused on the identification of GSC using antibodies against the antigens CD133 and Nestin. We showed three distribution patterns of these cells (Figure 5): 1- isolated in the tumour periphery areas; 2- numerous small cells forming intratumour niches and 3- cells around the tortuous and aberrant vessel (intermediate-advanced stages).

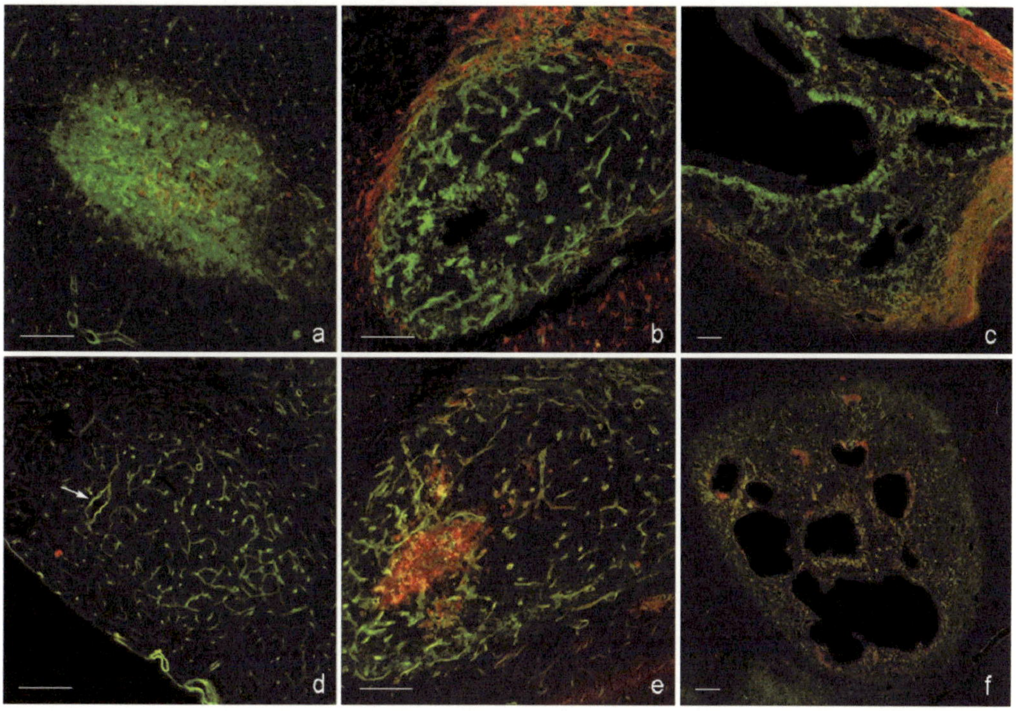

Fig. 4. Vascular endothelial growth factor and endothelial nitric oxide synthase expression during ENU-glioma development. Confocal microphotographs showing $VEGF_{165}$ (a-c, red) and eNOS (d-f, red) in different stages of glioma. Vascular network is showed by immunofluorescence for tomato lectin LEA (green). (a, d) Initial stages of gliomas display basal stain of $VEGF_{165}$ (a) and overexpression of eNOS only in dilated vessels (d, white arrow). (b, e) Anaplastic ENU-glioma corresponding with the intermediate tumour stage shows overexpression of $VEGF_{165}$ in the neoangiogenic tumour border (b) and overexpression of eNOS (e, yellow) in dilated and tortuous vessels from intratumour area. (c, f) ENU-induced glioblastomas show an heterogeneous pattern of expression for both markers. VEGF distribution is mainly showed in the peritumour neoangiogenic area (c) while eNOS overexpress as patching in vascular sections of intratumour aberrant microvessels (f). (Bar scale of 200 μm).

According to human astrocitomas, in ENU-glioma the number of positive cells for CD133 and Nestin antibodies increases with malignant grades of the tumour (Ma et al., 2008). Nestin+ cells were found in every stage of tumour development. It corroborated that the expression of Nestin is linked to the glioma grade, as stated in previous researches (Ehrmann et al., 2005).

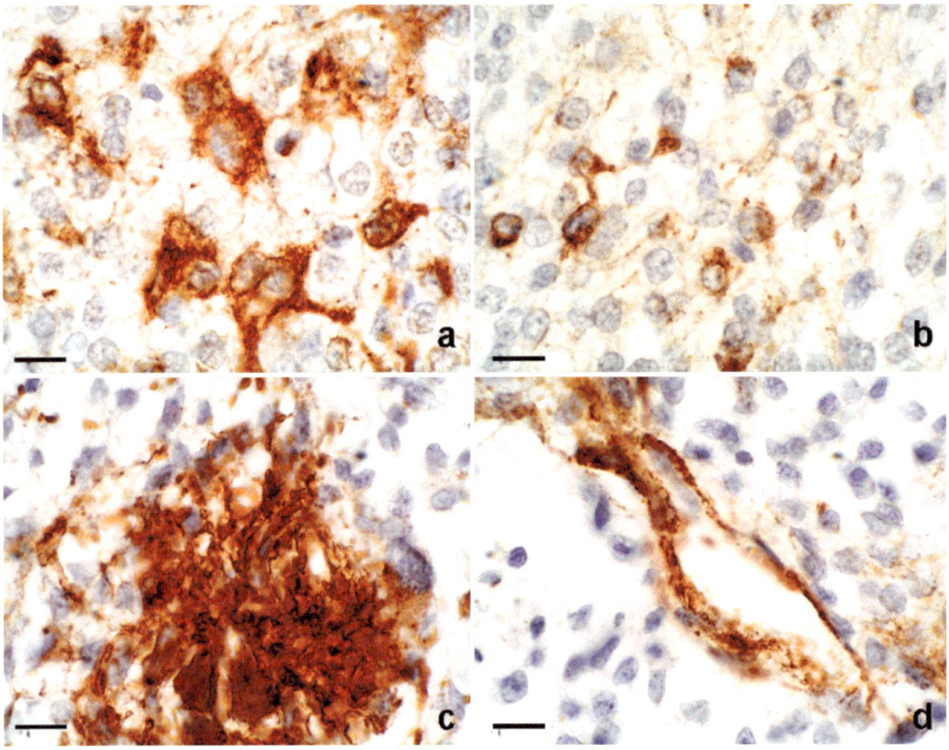

Fig. 5. Immunoexpression of Nestin antigen in 4 µm paraffin sections showed by DAB staining (Brown). a-b) Intratumour area of ENU-Glioma showing two kinds of isolated cells marked by Nestin antibody. a) Cells of big cytoplasm and nucleon distributed predominantly near the periphery of the tumour. They display an astrocyte shape and GFAP positivity. b) Small cells with scarce cytoplasm and prolongations. c-d) Two distribution of stem cells: Intratumour niches (c) and around the vascular endothelium of neoplastic microvessels (d). (Bar scale of 10µm).

By the other hand, CD133+ cells were only present since intermediate stages corresponding with "angiogenenic switch". The distribution of CD133+ cells corresponds mainly to overexpression of VEGF in neoangiogenic border and intratumour hypoxic areas of neoplasia (Bulnes & Lafuente, 2007). It has been reported that tumour stem cells over-express VEGF factor, so this cell population could be involved in the process of angiogenesis. Our results agree with the staining of CD133 described in the advanced and medium stage of human gliomas. Therefore, CD133 expression has been related to poor prognosis (Zeppernick et al., 2008).

We showed that some cells coexpress the antibodies Nestin, CD133 and $VEGF_{165}$. They were forming niches around microvessels or into hypoxic areas (Figure 6). Only cells distributed in the periphery of neoplasia were stained for GFAP and displayed astrocyte morphology.

The relationship between CD133+ cells and vessels wall was shown around the glomeruloid vessels, distributed in the neoangiogenic border of ENU-GBM, and delimiting huge dilated intratumour vessels (Figure 7). The presence of CD133+ cells near these aberrant vessels which display BBB disturbance may corroborate the pivotal role of stem cells in the neoplasia proliferation and invasion. These cells may be use extracellular matrix of vessel wall to migrate and infiltrate the brain parenchyma (Borovski et al., 2009).

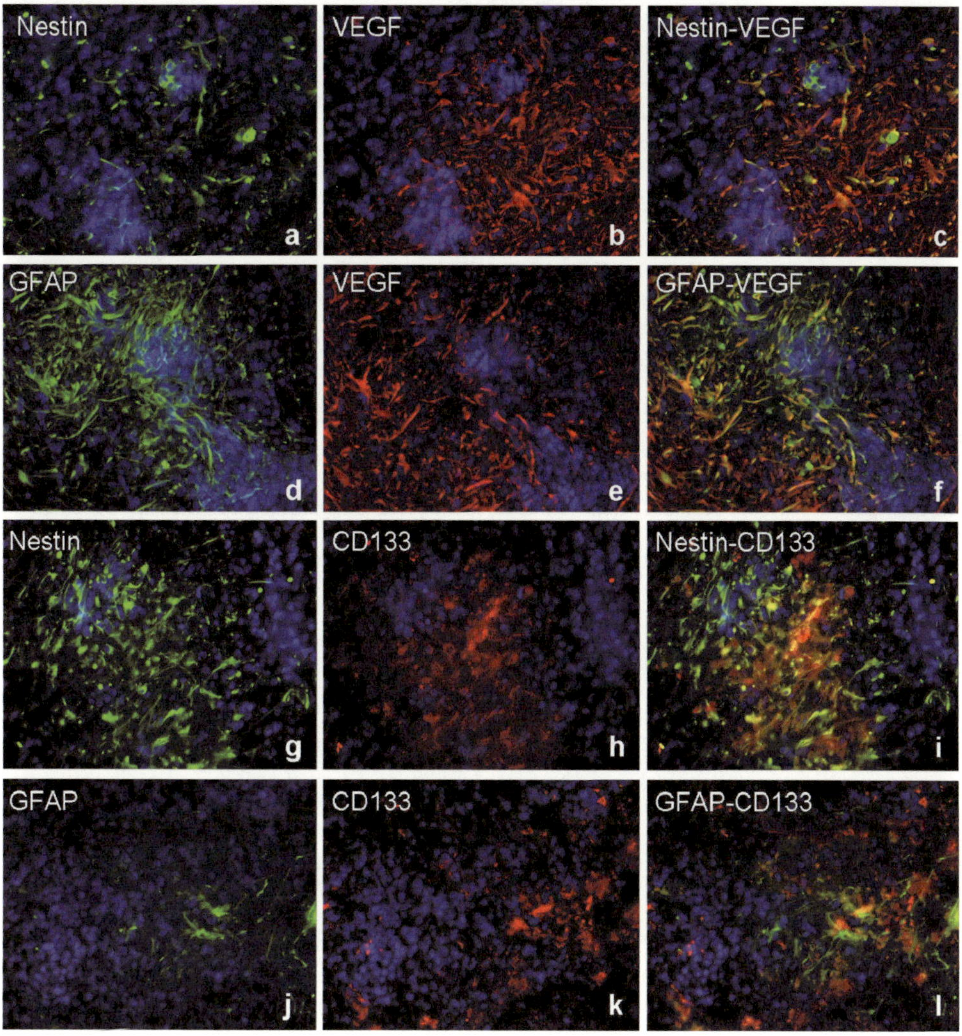

Fig. 6. Relationship between stem cell markers and proangiogenic factor VEGF in intratumour niches of advanced ENU-glioma stage. Study performed by double immunofluorescence, all tumours are counterstained with Hoechst. a-c) Microphotographs of Nestin+ cells (a, in green) and VEGF+ cells (b, in red) and colocalization (yellow, c). VEGF+ cells predominate over Nestin+ cells. Some cells with big cytoplasm are Nestin-VEGF+. Small Nestin+ cells form a cluster and lack the staining of VEGF (at the top). d-f) Colocalization (yellow) of glial fibrillary acidic protein (GFAP, green) and VEGF (red). All VEGF+ cells in this intratumour area are stained for GFAP and display the astrocyte shape. g-i) Relationship between the two markers of stem cells: Nestin (green) and CD133 (reed). This niche shows higher density of nestin+ cells (g) than CD133+ cells (h). Almost all of the CD133+ cells coexpress nestin antibody (i, yellow). j-l) Coexpression of GFAP (green) and CD133 (red). Some cells coexpress both antibodies (l, yellow). (x400 Amplification)

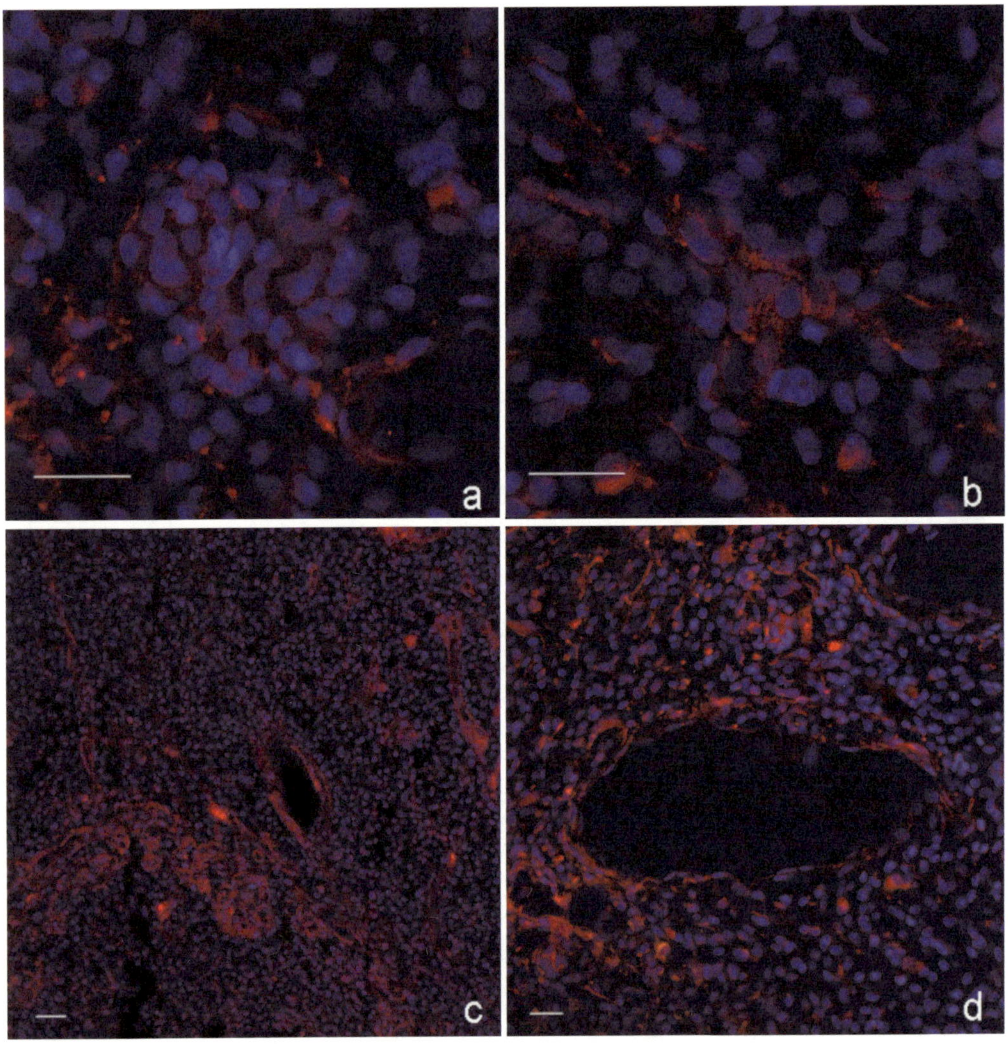

Fig. 7. Immunofluorescence confocal images of CD133 antibody (red) in ENU-glioblastoma. All sections are counterstained with Hoechst (blue). a) Intratumour niche displaying some CD133+ cells. b) Tortuous vessel of the periphery of the neoplasia with CD133+ structures attached to the vascular endothelium. c) Aberrant vessels sections demarcated by CD133+cells. d) Vessels with huge lumen display CD133+ cells around some vascular sections. (Scale bar of 20μm).

Although some authors proposed that CD133+ cells were selected cells with tumorigenic capacity (Schiffer et al., 2010), others postulated that a fraction of CD133+ cells might be related to the endothelial differentiation and could generate tumour vessels (Wang et al., 2010). Recently, Soda et al. (2011) reported that part of the vasculature of GBM was originated from tumour cells. Therefore, some researchers as Wang et al. (2010) and Ricci-Vitiani et al. (2010) were centred to describe the proportion of the stem cells that contributed to blood vessels in glioblastoma. After their results they postulated that glioblastoma microvessels were originated from tumour stem like cells.

7. Conclusion

Following evidences reported in the literature and our findings, the distribution of "glioma stem cells" close to microvascular wall during the glioma malignancy process suggests a synergistic role of both structures. Indeed, based on our results we corroborate the hypothesis that glioma stem cells may induce angiogenesis via VEGF synthesis or endothelial differentiation.

This knowledge will contribute to the generation of new antitumour therapy treatment against glioma stem cells. ENU experimental model would be considered as an useful option to check a design of treatment strategies against these cells.

8. Acknowledgment

This work has been partially supported by Gangoiti Foundation, SAIOTEK and GIC 491/10 Basque Government.

9. References

Al-Hajj, M.; Wicha, M.S.; Benito-Hernandez, A.; Morrison, SJ. & Clarke, M.F. (2003). Prospective identification of tumorigenic breast cancer cells. *Proceedings of the National academy of sciences of the United States of America*, Vol.100, No.7, (April 2003), pp. 3983-8, ISSN 0027-8424

Altman, J. & Das, G.D. (1966). Autoradiographic and histological studies of postnatal neurogenesis. I. A longitudinal investigation of the kinetics, migration and transformation of cells incorporating tritiated thymidine in neonate rats, with special reference to postnatal neurogenesis in some brain regions. *Journal of Comparaty Neurology*, Vol.126, No.3, (March 1966), pp. 337-89, ISSN 0021-9967

Alvarez-Buylla, A. & García-Verdugo, J.M. (2002). Neurogenesis in Adult Subventricular Zone. *Journal of Neuroscience*, Vol.22, No.3, (February 2002), pp. 629-34. ISSN 0270-6474

Anderson, S.A.; Glod, J.; Arbab, A.S.; Noel, M.; Ashari, P.; Fine, H.A. & Frank, J.A.(2005). Noninvasive MR imaging of magnetically labeled stem cells to directly identify neovasculature in a glioma model. *Blood*, Vol.105, No.1, (January 2005), pp. 420-425, ISSN 0006-4971

Argandoña, E.G.; Bengoetxea, H. & Lafuente, J.V. (2005). Lack of experience-mediated differences in the immunohistochemical expression of blood-brain barrier markers (EBA and GluT-1) during the postnatal development of the rat visual cortex. *Brain Research. Developmental Brain Research*, Vol.156, No.2, (May 2005), pp. 158-166, ISSN 0006-8993

Ballabh, P.; Braun, A. & Nedergaard, M. (2004). The blood-brain barrier: an overview: structure, regulation, and clinical implications. *Neurobiology of Disease*, Vol.16, No.1, pp.1-13. ISSN 0969-9961

Baluk, P.; Hashizume, H. & McDonald, D.M. (2005). Cellular abnormalities of blood vessels as targets in cancer. *Current Opinion in Genetics & Development*, Vol.15, No.1, (June 2004), pp. 102-111, ISSN 0959-437X

Bao, S.; Wu, Q., McLendon, R.E.; Hao, Y; Shi, Q.; Hjelmeland, A.B.; Dewhirst, M.W.; Bigner, D.D. and Rich, J.N. (2006). Glioma stem cells promote radioresistance by preferential activation of the DNA damage response. *Nature*, Vol.444, No.7120, (December 2006), pp. 756-60, ISSN 0028-0836

Bengoetxea, H.; Argandoña, E.G. & Lafuente, J.V. (2008). Effects of visual experience on vascular endothelial growth factor expression during the postnatal development of the rat visual cortex. *Cerebral Cortex*, Vol.18, No.7, (July 2008), pp. 1630-1639, ISSN 10473211

Bergsagel, D.E., & Valeriote, F.A. (1968). Growth characteristics of a mouse plasma cell tumor. *Cancer Research*, Vol. 28, No. 11, (November 1968), pp. 2187-2196, ISSN 00085472

Bergers, G. & Benjamin, L.E. (2003). Tumorigenesis and the angiogenic switch. *Nature Reviews Cancer*, Vol. 3, No.6, pp. 401-10, ISSN 1474175X

Bian, X.W.; Jiang X.F.; Chen, J.H.; Bai, J.S.; Dai, C.; Wang, Q.L.; Lu, J.Y.; Zhao, W.; Xin, R.; Liu, M.Y.; Shi, J.Q. & Wang, J.M. (2006). Increased angiogenic capabilities of endothelial cells from microvessels of malignant human gliomas. *International Immunopharmacology*, Vol.6, No.1, (January 2006), pp. 90-99, ISSN 15675769

Bielas, J.H. & Heddle, J.A. (2000). Proliferation is necessary for both repair and mutation in transgenic mouse cells. *Proceedings of the National Academy of Sciences of the United States of America*, Vol.97, No.21, (October 2000), pp. 11391-11396, ISSN 00278424

Bigner, D.D.; McLendon R.E. & Bruner, J.M. (1998) Russell & Rubinstenin´s. Pathology of tumors of the nervous system, 6th ed ., Arnold, London.

Blouw, B.; Song, H.; Tihan, T.; Bosze, J.; Ferrara, N.; Gerber, H.P.; Johnson, R.S. & Bergers, G. (2003). The hypoxic response of tumors is dependent on their microenvironment. *Cancer Cell*, Vol.4, No.2, (August 2003), pp. 133-146, ISSN 15356108

Bonnet, D. & Dick, J.E. (1977). Human acute myeloid leukemia is organized as a hierarchy that originates from a primitive hematopoietic cell. *Nature Medicine*, Vol.3, No.7, (July 1997), pp. 730-7, ISSN: 10788956

Borovski, T.; Verhoeff, J.J.; ten Cate, R.; Cameron, K.; de Vries, N.A.; van Tellingen, O.; Richel, D.J.; Van Furth, W.R.; Medema, J.P. & Sprick, M.R. (2009). Tumor microvasculature supports proliferation and expansion of glioma-propagating cells. *International Journal of Cancer*, Vol.125, No.5, (September 2009), pp. 1222-1230, ISSN 00207136

Brasch, R. & Turetschek K. (2000). MRI characterization of tumors and grading angiogenesis using macromolecular contrast media: status report. *European Journal of Radiology*, Vol.34, No.3, (June 2000), pp 148-155, ISSN 0720048X

Brat, D.J.; Castellano-Sanchez, A.A.; Hunter, S.B; Pecot, M.; Cohen, C.; Hammond, E.H.; Devi, S.N.; Kaur, B. & Van Meir, E.G. (2004). Pseudopalisades in glioblastoma are hypoxic, express extracellular matrix proteases, and are formed by an actively migrating cell population. *Cancer Research*, Vol.64, No.3, (February 2004), pp 920-927, ISSN 00085472

Bulnes, S. & Lafuente, J.V. (2007). VEGF immunopositivity related to malignancy degree, proliferative activity and angiogenesis in ENU-induced gliomas. *Journal of Molecular Neuroscience*, Vo.33, No.2, (October 2007), pp. 163-172, ISSN 08958696

Bulnes, S.; Argandona, E.G.; Bengoetxea, H.; Leis, O.; Ortuzar, N. & Lafuente, J.V. (2010). The role of eNOS in vascular permeability in ENU-induced gliomas. *Acta Neurochirgica. Supplement*, Vo.106, pp. 277-282, ISSN 00651419

Bulnes, S.; Bilbao, J. & Lafuente, J.V. (2009). Microvascular adaptive changes in experimental endogenous brain gliomas. *Histology and Histopathology*, Vo.24, No.6, (June 2009), pp. 693-706, ISSN 16995848

Bulnes-Sesma, S.; Ullibarri-Ortiz de, Z.N. & Lafuente-Sanchez, J.V. (2006). Tumour induction by ethylnitrosourea in the central nervous system. *Revista de Neurologia*, Vo.43, No.12, (December 2006), pp. 733-738, ISSN 02100010

Burger, P.C.; Shibata, T.; Aguzzi, A. & Kleihues, P. (1988). Selective induction by N-nitrosoethylurea of oligodendrogliomas in fetal forebrain transplants. *Cancer Research*, Vol.48, No.10, pp. 2871-2875, ISSN 00085472

Capilla-Gonzalez, V.; Gil-Perotin, S. & Garcia-Verdugo, J.M. (2010). Postnatal exposure to N-ethyl-N-nitrosurea disrupts the subventricular zone in adult rodents. *European Journal of Neuroscience*, Vol. 32, No.11, (December 2010), pp. 1789-1799, ISSN 0953816X

Carmeliet, P. & Jain, R.K. (2000). Angiogenesis in cancer and other diseases. *Nature*, Vol.407, No.6801, (September 2000), pp. 249-257, ISSN 00280836

Carmeliet, P. (2003). Angiogenesis in health and disease. *Nature Medicine*, Vol.9, No.6, (June 2003), pp. 653-660, ISSN 10788956

Cha, S.; Johnson, G.; Wadghiri, Y.Z.; Jin, O.; Babb, J.; Zagzag, D. & Turnbull, D.H. (2003). Dynamic, contrast-enhanced perfusion MRI in mouse gliomas: correlation with histopathology. *Magnetic Resonance in Medicine*, Vol. 49, No. 5, (May 2003), pp. 848-855, ISSN 07403194

Chen, L.; Endler, A.; & Shibasaki, F. (2009). Hypoxia and angiogenesis: regulation of hypoxia-inducible factors via novel binding factors. *Experimental and Molecular Medicine*, Vol. 41, No. 12, (December 2009), pp. 849-857, ISSN 12263613

Cheng, JX.; Liu, B.L. & Zhang, X. (2009). How powerful is CD133 as a cancer stem cell marker in brain tumors?. *Cancer Treatment Reviews*, Vol.35, No.5, (August 2009), pp. 403-8, ISSN 0305-7372

Claes, A.; Gambarota, G.; Hamans, B.; Van, T.O.; Wesseling, P.; Maass, C.; Heerschap, A. & Leenders, W. (2007). Magnetic resonance imaging-based detection of glial brain tumors in mice after antiangiogenic treatment. *International Journal of Cancer, Vol.* 122, No.9, (May 2008), pp. 1981-1986, ISSN 00207136

Collins, A.T.; Berry, P.A.; Hyde, C.; Stower, M.J. & Maitland, N.J. (2005). Prospective identification of tumorigenic prostate cancer stem cells. *Cancer Research*, Vol. 65, No.23, (December 2005), pp. 10946-10951, ISSN 00085472

Corbeil, D.; Röper, K.; Hellwig, A.; Tavian, M.; Miraglia, S.; Watt, S.M.; Simmons, P.J.; Peault, B.; Buck, D.W. & Huttner, W.B. (2000). The human AC133 hematopoietic stem cell antigen is also expressed in epithelial cells and targeted to plasma membrane protrusions. *Journal of Biological Chemistry*, Vol.275, No.8, (February 2000), pp. 5512-5520, ISSN 00219258

Dahlstrand, J.; Collins, V.P. & Lendahl, U. (1992). Expression of the class VI intermediate filament nestin in human central nervous system tumors. *Cancer Research*, Vol.52, No.19, pp. 5334-5341, ISSN 00085472

Dell'Albani, P. (2008). Stem cell markers in gliomas. *Neurochemical Research*, Vol. 33, No.12, (December 2008), pp. 2407-2415, ISSN 03643190

Dobrogowska, D.H. & Vorbrodt, A.W. (1999). Quantitative immunocytochemical study of blood-brain barrier glucose transporter (GLUT-1) in four regions of mouse brain.

Journal of Histochemistry and Cytochemistry, Vol. 47, No. 8, (August 1999), pp. 1021-1029, ISSN 00221554

Doetsch, F.; Caillé, I.; Lim, D.A.; García-Verdugo, J.M. & Alvarez-Buylla, A. (1999). Subventricular zone astrocytes are neural stem cells in the adult mammalian brain. *Cell*, Vol,97, No.6, pp. 703-716, ISSN 00928674

Donnenberg, V.S. & Donnenberg, A.D. (2005). Multiple drug resistance in cancer revisited: the cancer stem cell hypothesis. *Journal of Clinical Pharmacology*, Vol. 45, No.8, (August 2005), pp. 872-877, ISSN 00912700

Dvorak, H.F. (2006). Discovery of vascular permeability factor (VPF). *Experimental Cell Research*, Vol. 312, No. 5, (March 2006), pp. 522-526, ISSN 00144827

Ehrmann, J.; Kolar, Z. & Mokry, J. (2005). Nestin as a diagnostic and prognostic marker: immunohistochemical analysis of its expression in different tumours. *Journal of Clinical Pathology*, Vol.58, No. 2, (February 2005), pp.222-223, ISSN 00219746

Eriksson, P.S.; Perfilieva, E.; Bjork-Eriksson, T.; Alborn, A.M.; Nordborg, C.; Peterson, D.A. & Gage, F.H. (1998). Neurogenesis in the adult human hippocampus. *Nature Medicine*, Vol.4, No.11, (November 1998), pp. 1313-1317, ISSN 10788956

Esposito, I.; Kleeff, J.; Bischoff, S.C.; Fischer, L.; Collecchi, P.; Iorio, M.; Bevilacqua, G., Büchler, M.W. & Friess, H. (2002). The stem cell factor-c-kit system and mast cells in human pancreatic cancer. *Laboratory Investigation*, Vol.82, No.11, (November 2002), pp. 1481-1492, ISSN 00236837

Fan, X.; Salford, L.G. & Widegren, B. (2007). Glioma stem cells: Evidence and limitation. *Seminars in Cancer Biology*, Vol. 17, No. 3, (June 2007), pp. 214-218, ISSN 1044579X

Ferrara, N. (2001). Role of vascular endothelial growth factor in regulation of physiological angiogenesis. *American Journal of Physiology - Cell Physiology*, Vol. 280, No.6, pp. C1358-C1366, ISSN 03636143

Ferrara, N.; Gerber, H.P. & LeCouter, J. (2003). The biology of VEGF and its receptors. *Nature Medicine*, Vol. 9, No. 6, (June 2003), pp.669-676, ISSN 10788956

Fidler, I.J. & Kripke, M.L. (1997). Metastasis results from preexisting variant cells within a malignant tumor. *Science*, Vol. 197, No. 4306, pp. 893-895, ISSN 00368075

Folkman, J. (2006). Angiogenesis. *Annual Review of Medicine*, Volume 57, 2006, pp. 1-18, ISSN 00664219

Folkman, J. (2000). *Tumour angiogenesis*, Cancer Medicine. Hamilton, Ontario

Fong, G.H. (2008). Mechanisms of adaptive angiogenesis to tissue hypoxia. *Angiogenesis*, Vol. 11, No. 2, (June 2008), pp. 121-140, ISSN 09696970

Gangemi, R.M.; Griffero, F.; Marubbi, D.; Perera, M.; Capra, M.C.; Malatesta, P.; Ravetti, G.L.; Zona, G.L.; Daga, A. & Corte, G. (2009). SOX2 silencing in glioblastoma tumor-initiating cells causes stop of proliferation and loss of tumorigenicity. *Stem Cells*, Vol. 27, No.1, (January 2009), pp. 40-48,ISSN 10665099

Germano, I.; Swiss, V. & Casaccia, P. (2010). Primary brain tumors, neural stem cell, and brain tumor cancer cells: Where is the link?. *Neuropharmacology*, Vol. 58, No.6, (May 2010), pp. 903-910, ISSN 00283908

Götz, M. & Huttner, W.B. (2005). The cell biology of neurogenesis. *Nature Reviews Molecular Cell Biology*, Vol. 6, No.10, (November 2005), pp. 777-788, ISSN 14710072

Griguer, C.E.; Oliva, C.R.; Gobin, E.; Marcorelles, P.; Benos, D.J.; Lancaster, J.R. Jr, & Gillespie, G.Y. (2008). CD133 is a marker of bioenergetic stress in human glioma. *PLoS ONE*, Vol. 3, No. 11, (November 2008), Article number e3655, ISSN 19326203

Hadjipanayis, C.G. & Van Meir, E.G. (2009). Brain cancer propagating cells: biology, genetics and targeted therapies. *Trends in Molecular Medicine,* Vol. 15, No.11, (November 2009), pp.519-530, ISSN 14714914.

Hashizume, H.; Baluk, P.; Morikawa, S.; McLean, J.W.; Thurston, G.; Roberge, S.; Jain, R.K. & McDonald, D.M. (2000). Openings between defective endothelial cells explain tumor vessel leakiness. *American Journal of Pathology,* Vol. 156, No. 4, pp. 1363-1380, ISSN 00029440

Hatashita, S. & Hoff, J.T. (1986). Cortical tissue pressure gradients in early ischemic brain edema. *Journal of Cerebral Blood Flow and Metabolism,* Vol.6, No.1, 1, pp.1-7, ISSN 0271678X

Heddleston, J.M.; Li, Z.; McLendon, R.E.; Hjelmeland, A.B. & Rich, J.N. (2009). The hypoxic microenvironment maintains glioblastoma stem cells and promotes reprogramming towards a cancer stem cell phenotype. *Cell Cycle,* Vol. 8, No.20, (October 2009), pp. 3274-3284, ISSN 15384101.

Helmlinger, G.; Endo, M.; Ferrara, N.; Hlatky, L. & Jain, R.K. (2000). Growth factors: Formation of endothelial cell networks. *Nature,* Vol. 405, No. 6783, (May 2000), pp. 139-141, ISSN 00280836

Holland, E.C.; Li, Y.; Celestino, J.; Dai, C.; Schaefer, L.; Sawaya, R.A.; & Fuller, G.N. (2000). Astrocytes give rise to oligodendrogliomas and astrocytomas after gene transfer of polyoma virus middle T antigen in vivo. *American Journal of Pathology,* Vol. 157, No.3, pp. 1031-1037, ISSN 00029440

Holmin, S.; Almqvist, P.; Lendahl, U. & Mathiesen, T. (1997). Adult nestin-expressing subependymal cells differentiate to astrocytes in response to brain injury. *European Journal of Neuroscience,* Vol.9, No. 1, pp. 65-75, ISSN 0953816X

Ignatova, T.N.; Kukekov, V.G.; Laywell, E.D.; Suslov, O.N.; Vrionis, F.D. & Steindler, D.A. (2002). Human cortical glial tumors contain neural stem-like cells expressing astroglial and neuronal markers in vitro. *GLIA,* Vol.39, No. 3, (September 2002), pp. 193-206, ISSN 08941491

Jain, R.K.; di TE, Duda, D.G.; Loeffler, J.S.; Sorensen, A.G. & Batchelor, T.T. (2007) Angiogenesis in brain tumours. *Nature Reviews Neuroscience,* Vol.8, No.8, (August 2007), pp. 610-622, ISSN 1471003X

Jang, T.; Litofsky, N.S.; Smith, T.W.; Ross, A.H. & Recht, L.D. (2004). Aberrant nestin expression during ethylnitrosourea- (ENU)-induced neurocarcinogenesis. *Neurobiology of Disease,* Vol. 15, No. 3, (April 2004), pp. 544-552, ISSN 09699961

Jensen, R.L. (2006). Hypoxia in the tumorigenesis of gliomas and as a potential target for therapeutic measures. *Neurosurgical focus,* Vol. 20, No. 4, pp. E24, ISSN 10920684

Jin, K.; Zhu, Y.; Sun, Y.; Mao, X.O.; Xie, L. & Greenberg, D.A. (2002). Vascular endothelial growth factor (VEGF) stimulates neurogenesis in vitro and in vivo. *Proceedings of the National Academy of Sciences of the United States of America,* Vol. 99, No.18, (September 2002), pp. 11946-11950, ISSN 00278424

Jin, K.L.; Mao, X.O.; Nagayama, T.; Goldsmith, P.C. & Greenberg, D.A. (2000). Induction of vascular endothelial growth factor and hypoxia-inducible factor-1alpha by global ischemia in rat brain. *Neuroscience,* Vol.99, No.3, (August 2000), pp. 577-585, ISSN 03064522

Ke, L.D.; Shi, Y.X.; Im, S.A.; Chen, X. &Yung,W.K. (2000). The relevance of cell proliferation, vascular endothelial growth factor, and basic fibroblast growth factor production to angiogenesis and tumorigenicity in human glioma cell lines. *Clinical Cancer Research*, Vol. 6, Issue 6, (June 2000), pp. 2562-2572, ISSN 10780432

Kish, P.E.; Blaivas, M.; Strawderman, M.; Muraszko, K.M.; Ross, D.A.; Ross, B.D. & McMahon, G. (2001). Magnetic resonance imaging of ethyl-nitrosourea-induced rat gliomas: a model for experimental therapeutics of low-grade gliomas. *Journal of Neuro-Oncology*, Vol. 53, No.3, pp. 243-257, ISSN 0167594X

Kleihues, P.; Burger, P.C.; Aldape, K.D.; Brat, D.J.; Biernat, W.; Bigner, D.D.; Makazato, Y.; Plate, K.H.; Giangaspero,F.; von Deimling, A. & Ohgaki,H. (2007). Glioblastoma, In: *WHO Classification of tumours of the Central Nervous System*, Louis, D.N.; Ohgaki, H.; Wiestler, O.D. & Cavenee, W.K., (Ed.), 33-49. Agency for Research on Cancer (IARC), Lyon

Kokkinakis, D.M.; Rushing, E.J.; Shareef, M.M.; Ahmed, M.M.; Yang, S.; Singha, U.K. & Luo, J. (2004). Physiology and gene expression characteristics of carcinogen-initiated and tumor-transformed glial progenitor cells derived from the CNS of methylnitrosourea (MNU)-treated Sprague-Dawley rats. *Journal of Neuropathology and Experimental Neurology*, Vol. 63, Issue 11, (November 2004), pp. 1182-1199, ISSN 00223069

Krum, J.M.; Mani, N. & Rosenstein, J.M. (2002). Angiogenic and astroglial responses to vascular endothelial growth factor administration in adult rat brain. *Neuroscience*. Volume 110, Issue 4,(April 2002), pp. 589-604, ISSN 03064522

Lafuente, J.V. (2004). Involvement and consequences of Blood Brain Barrier permeability after minimal injury in rat cerebral cortex. In: *Blood-spinal cord and brain barriers in health and disease*. Sharma H.S. (eds)., 533-545 , Elsevier Academic Press. San Diego, California.

Lafuente, J.V.; Adán, B.; Alkiza, K.; Garibi, J.M.; Rossi, M. & Cruz-Sánchez, F.F. (1999). Expression of vascular endothelial growth factor (VEGF) and platelet-derived growth factor receptor-beta (PDGFR-beta) in human gliomas. *Journal of Molecular Neuroscience*, Volume 13, Issue 1-2, 1999, pp. 177-185, ISSN 08958696

Lafuente, J.V.; Alkiza, K.; Garibi, J.M.; Alvarez, A.; Bilbao, J.; Figols, J. & Cruz-Sanchez, F.F. (2000). Biologic parameters that correlate with the prognosis of human gliomas. *Neuropathology*, Vol. 20, No. 3, pp. 176-183, ISSN 09196544

Lafuente, J.V.; Argandona, E.G. & Mitre, B. (2006). VEGFR-2 expression in brain injury: its distribution related to brain-blood barrier markers. *Journal of Neural Transmission*, Vol. 113, No. 4, (April 2006), pp. 487-496, ISSN 03009564

Lafuente, J.V.; Bulnes, S.; Mitre, B. & Riese, H.H. (2002). Role of VEGF in an experimental model of cortical micronecrosis. *Amino Acids*, Vol. 23, No. 1-3, 2002, pp. 241-245, ISSN 09394451

Lafuente, J.V.; Cervos-Navarro, J. & Gutierrez Argandona, E. (1994). Evaluation of BBB damage in an UV irradiation model by endogenous protein tracers. *Acta Neurochirurgica, Supplement*, Vol. 60, pp. 139-141, ISSN 00651419

Lee, A.; Kessler, J.D.; Read, T.A.; Kaiser, C.; Corbeil, D.; Huttner, W.B.; Johnson, J.E. & Wechsler-Reya, R.J. (2005). Isolation of neural stem cells from the postnatal cerebellum. *Nature Neuroscience*, Vol.8, No.6, (June 2005), pp. 723-729, ISSN 10976256

Li, Z.; Bao, S.; Wu, Q.; Wang, H.; Eyler, C.; Sathornsumetee, S.; Shi, Q., Cao, Y. , Lathia, J., McLendon, R.E., Hjelmeland, A.B. & Rich, J.N. (2009). Hypoxia-inducible factors regulate tumorigenic capacity of glioma stem cells. *Cancer Cell,* Vol. 15, No.6, (June 2009), pp. 501-513, ISSN 15356108

Li, Z.; Wang, H.; Eyler, C.E.; Hjelmeland, A.B. & Rich, J.N. (2009). Turning cancer stem cells inside out: An exploration of glioma stem cell signaling pathways. *Journal of Biological Chemistry,* Vol. 284, No.25, 19 (June 2009), pp.16705-16709, ISSN 00219258

Lin, B. & Ginsberg, M.D. (2000). Quantitative assessment of the normal cerebral microvasculature by endothelial barrier antigen (EBA) immunohistochemistry: application to focal cerebral ischemia. *Brain Research,* Vol. 865, No. 2, (May 2000), pp. 237-244, ISSN 00068993

Lois, C. & Alvarez-Buylla, A. (1994). Long-distance neuronal migration in the adult mammalian brain. *Science,* Vol. 264, No.5162, (May 1994), pp. 1145-1148, ISSN 00368075

Ma, W.; Tavakoli, T.; Chen, S.; Maric, D.; Liu, J.L.; O'Shaughnessy, T.J. & Barker, J.L. (2008). Reconstruction of functional cortical-like tissues from neural stem and progenitor cells. *Tissue Engineering - Part A.* Vol. 14, No.10, (October 2008), pp. 1673-1686, ISSN 19373341

Machein, M.R. & Plate, K.H. (2004). Role of VEGF in developmental angiogenesis and in tumor angiogenesis in the brain. *Cancer treatment and research,* Vol. 117, 2004, pp. 191-218, ISSN 09273042

Mack, A. & Robitzki, A. (2000). The key role of butyrylcholinesterase during neurogenesis and neural disorders: An antisense-5'butyrylcholinesterase-DNA study. *Progress in Neurobiology,* Vol. 60, No. 6, (April 2000), pp. 607-628, ISSN

Marti, H.J.; Bernaudin, M.; Bellail, A.; Schoch, H.; Euler, M.; Petit, E. & Risau, W. (2000). Hypoxia-induced vascular endothelial growth factor expression precedes neovascularization after cerebral ischemia. *American Journal of Pathology,* Vol. 156, No.3, pp. 965-976, ISSN 00029440

Ment, L.R.; Stewart, W.B.; Fronc, R.; Seashore, C.; Mahooti, S.; Scaramuzzino, D. & Madri, J.A. (1997). Vascular endothelial growth factor mediates reactive angiogenesis in the postnatal developing brain. *Developmental Brain Research,* Vol. 100, No.1, (May 1997), pp. 52-61, ISSN 01653806

Millauer, B.; Wizigmann-Voos, S.; Schnurch, H.; Martinez, R.; Moller, N.P.; Risau, W. & Ullrich, A. (1993). High affinity VEGF binding and developmental expression suggest Flk-1 as a major regulator of vasculogenesis and angiogenesis. *Cell,* Vol. 72, No.6, pp. 835-846, ISSN 00928674

Mizrak, D.; Brittan, M. & Alison, M.R. (2008). CD133: molecule of the moment. *Journal of Pathology,* Vol. 214, No.1, (January 2008), pp. 3-9, ISSN 00223417

Müller, F.J; Snyder, E.Y & Loring, J.F. (2006). Gene therapy: Can neural stem cells deliver?. *Nature Reviews Neuroscience,* Vol.7, No.1, (January 2006), pp. 75-84, ISSN 1471003X

Nadig, R.R. (2009). Stem cell therapy-Hype or hope? A review. *Journal of Conservative Dentistry,* Vol.12, No.4, pp. 131-8, ISSN 0972-0707

Neufeld, G.; Cohen, T.; Gengrinovitch, S. & Poltorak, Z. (1999). Vascular endothelial growth factor (VEGF) and its receptors. *FASEB Journal,* (January 1999);Vol.13, No.1, pp. 9-22, ISSN 0892-6638

Nunes, M.C.; Roy, N.S.; Keyoung, H.M.; Goodman, R.R.; McKhann, G.; Jiang, L.; Kang, J.; Nedergaard, M. & Goldman, S.A. (2003). Identification and isolation of multipotential neural progenitor cells from the subcortical white matter of the adult human brain. *Nature Medicine*, Vol. 9, No.4, (April 2003), pp. 439-447, ISSN 10788956

O'Brien, C.A.; Pollett, A.; Gallinger, S. & Dick, J.E. (2007). A human colon cancer cell capable of initiating tumour growth in immunodeficient mice. *Nature*, Vol. 445, No.7123, (January 2007), pp. 106-110, ISSN 00280836

Ohgaki, H. & Kleihues, P. (2009). Genetic alterations and signaling pathways in the evolution of gliomas. *Cancer Science*, Vol. 100, No.12, December 2009, pp. 2235-2241, ISSN 13479032

O'Neill, J.P. (2000). DNA damage, DNA repair, cell proliferation, and DNA replication: how do gene mutations result?. *Proceedings of the National Academy of Sciences of the United States of America*, Vol. 97, No.21, (October 2000) , pp. 11137-11139. ISSN

Ortuzar, N.; Argandoña, E.G.; Bengoetxea, H. & Lafuente, J.V. (2011). Combination of intracortically administered VEGF and environmental enrichment enhances brain protection in developing rats. *Journal of Neural Transmission*, Vol.118, No.1, (January 2011), pp. 135-144, ISSN 03009564

Osuka, K.; Watanabe, Y.; Usuda, N.; Nakazawa, A.; Tokuda, M.; Yoshida, J. (2004). Modification of endothelial NO synthase through protein phosphorylation after forebrain cerebral ischemia/reperfusion. *Stroke*, Vol. 35, No.11, (November 2004), pp. 2582-2586, ISSN 00392499

Papadopoulos, M.C.; Saadoun, S.; Binder, D.K.; Manley, G.T.; Krishna, S. & Verkman, A.S. (2004). Molecular mechanisms of brain tumor edema. *Neuroscience*, Vol. 129, No.4, pp. 1011-1020, ISSN 03064522

Pistollato, F.; Abbadi, S.; Rampazzo, E.; Persano, L.; Della Puppa, A.; Frasson, C.; Sarto, E.; Scienza, R.; D'Avella, D. & Basso, G. (2010). Intratumoral hypoxic gradient drives stem cells distribution and MGMT expression in glioblastoma. *Stem Cells*, Vol. 28, No.6, (June 2010), pp. 851-862, ISSN 10665099

Plate, K.H. (1999). Mechanisms of angiogenesis in the brain. *Journal of Neuropathology and Experimental Neurology*, Vol. 58, No.4, (April 1999), pp. 313-320, ISSN 00223069

Reya, T.; Morrison, S.J.; Clarke, M.F. & Weissman, I.L. (2001). Stem cells, cancer, and cancer stem cells. *Nature*, Vol. 414, No.6859, (November 2001), pp. 105-111, ISSN 00280836

Reynolds, B.A., Weiss, S. (1992). Generation of neurons and astrocytes from isolated cells of the adult mammalian central nervous system. *Science*, Vol. 255, No.5052, 1992, pp. 1707-1710, ISSN 00368075

Ricci-Vitiani, L.; Pallini, R.; Biffoni, M.; Todaro, M.; Invernici, G.; Cenci, T.; Maira, G.; Parati, E.A.; Stassi, G.; Larocca, L.M. & De Maria, R. (2010). Tumour vascularization via endothelial differentiation of glioblastoma stem-like cells. *Nature*, Vol. 468, No.7325, (December 2010), pp. 824-830, ISSN 00280836

Rich, J.N. (2007). Cancer stem cells in radiation resistance. *Cancer Research*, Vol. 67, No.19, (October 2007), pp. 8980-8984, ISSN 00085472

Risau, W. & Flamme, I. (1995). Vasculogenesis. *Annual Review of Cell and Developmental Biology*, Vol. 11, 1995, pp. 73-91, ISSN 10810706

Risau, W. (1997). Mechanisms of angiogenesis. *Nature*, Vol. 386, No.6626, pp. 671-674, ISSN 00280836

Rosenstein, J.M. & Krum, J.M. (2004). New roles for VEGF in nervous tissue-beyond blood vessels. *Exp Experimental Neurology*, Vol. 187, No.2, (June 2004), pp. 246-253, ISSN 00144886

Ruoslahti, E. (2002). Specialization of tumour vasculature. *Nature Reviews Cancer,* Vol. 2, No.2, (February 2002), pp. 83-90, ISSN 1474175X

Schiffer, D.; Annovazzi, L.; Caldera, V. & Mellai, M. (2010). On the origin and growth of gliomas. *Anticancer Research,* Vol. 30, No.6, (June 2010), pp. 1977-1998, ISSN 02507005

Schlageter, K.E.; Molnar, P.; Lapin, G.D. & Groothuis D.R. (1999). Microvessel organization and structure in experimental brain tumors: microvessel populations with distinctive structural and functional properties. *Microvascular Research,* Vol. 58, No.3, (November 1999), pp. 312-328, ISSN 00262862

Semenza, G.L. (2003). Targeting HIF-1 for cancer therapy. *Nature Reviews Cancer,* Vol. 3, No.10, (October 2003), pp. 721-732, ISSN 1474175X

Shen, G.; Shen, F.; Shi, Z.; Liu, W.; Hu, W.; Zheng, X.; Wen, L. & Yang, X. (2008). Identification of cancer stem-like cells in the C6 glioma cell line and the limitation of current identification methods. *In Vitro Cellular and Developmental Biology – Animal,* Vol. 44, No.7, (August 2008), pp. 280-289, ISSN 10712690

Singh, S.K.; Clarke, I.D.; Terasaki, M.; Bonn, V.E.; Hawkins, C.; Squire, J. & Dirks, P.B. (2003). Identification of a cancer stem cell in human brain tumors. *Cancer Research,* Vol. 63, No.18, (September 2003), pp. 5821-5828, ISSN 00085472

Soda, Y.; Marumoto, T.; Friedmann-Morvinski, D.; Soda, M.; Liu, F.; Michiue, H.; Pastorino, S.; Yang, M.; Hoffman, R.M.; Kesari, S. & Verma, I.M. (2011). Transdifferentiation of glioblastoma cells into vascular endothelial cells. *Proceedings of the National Academy of Sciences of the United States of America,* Vol. 108, Issue 11, (March 2011), pp. 4274-4280, ISSN 00278424

Sternberger, N.H.; Sternberger, L.A.; Kies, M.W. & Shear, C.R. (1989). Cell surface endothelial proteins altered in experimental allergic encephalomyelitis. *Journal of Neuroimmunology,* Vol. 21, No.2-3, pp. 241-248, ISSN 01655728

Storkebaum, E.; Lambrechts, D. & Carmeliet, P. (2004). VEGF: once regarded as a specific angiogenic factor, now implicated in neuroprotection. *BioEssays,* Vol. 26, No.9, (September 2004), pp. 943-954, ISSN

Takebe, N. & Ivy, S.P. (2010). Controversies in cancer stem cells: targeting embryonic signaling pathways. *Clinical Cancer Research,* Vol. 16, No.12, (June 2010), pp. 3106-3112, ISSN 10780432

Tamaki, S.; Eckert, K.; He, D.; Sutton, R.; Doshe, M.; Jain, G.; Tushinski, R.; Reitsma, M.; Harris, B.; Tsukamoto, A.; Gage, F.; Weissman, I. & Uchida, N. (2002). Engraftment of sorted/expanded human central nervous system stem cells from fetal brain. *Journal of Neuroscience Research.* Vol. 69, No.6, (September 2002), pp. 976-986, ISSN 03604012

Till, J.E. & McCulloch, E.A. (2011). A direct measurement of radiation sensitivity of normal mouse bone marrow cells. 1961. *Radiation research,* Vol. 175, No.2, (February 2011), pp. 145-149, ISSN 19385404

Tonini, T.; Rossi, F. & Claudio, P.P. (2003) Molecular basis of angiogenesis and cancer. *Oncogene,* Vol. 22, No.43, (October 2003), pp. 6549-6556, ISSN 09509232

Vajkoczy, P. & Menger, M.D. (2004). Vascular microenvironment in gliomas. *Cancer treatment and research,* Vol. 117, pp. 249-262, ISSN 09273042

Vaquero, J.; Oya, S.; Coca, S. & Zurita, M. (1994). Experimental induction of primitive neuro-ectodermal tumours in rats: a re-appraisement of the ENU-model of neurocarcinogenesis. *Acta Neurochirurgica,* Vol. 131, No.3-4, pp. 294-301, ISSN 00016268

Wang, R.; Chadalavada, K.; Wilshire, J.; Kowalik, U.; Hovinga, K.E.; Geber, A.; Fligelman, B.; Leversha, M.; Brennan, C. & Tabar, V. (2010). Glioblastoma stem-like cells give rise to tumour endothelium. *Nature,* Vol. 468, No.7325, (December 2010), pp. 829-835, ISSN 00280836

Whitman, M.C. & Greer, C.A. (2009). Adult neurogenesis and the olfactory system. *Progress in Neurobiology,* Vol. 89, No.2, (October 2009), pp. 162-175, ISSN 03010082

Yancopoulos, G.D.; Davis, S.; Gale, N.W.; Rudge, J.S.; Wiegand, S.J. & Holash, J. (2000). Vascular-specific growth factors and blood vessel formation. *Nature,* Vol. 407, No.6801, (September 2000), pp. 242-248, ISSN 00280836

Yoshimura, F.; Kaidoh, T.; Inokuchi, T. & Shigemori, M. (1998). Changes in VEGF expression and in the vasculature during the growth of early-stage ethylnitrosourea-induced malignant astrocytomas in rats. *Virchows Archiv,* Vol.433, No.5, pp. 457-463, ISSN 09456317

Zagzag, D.; Friedlander, D.R.; Margolis, B.; Grumet, M.; Semenza, G.L.; Zhong, H.; Simons, J.W.; Holash, J.; Wiegand, S.J. & Yancopoulos, G.D. (2000). Molecular events implicated in brain tumor angiogenesis and invasion. *Pediatric Neurosurgery,* Vol. 33, No.1, pp. 49-55, ISSN 10162291

Zeppernick, F.; Ahmadi, R.; Campos, B.; Dictus, C.; Helmke, B.M.; Becker, N.; Lichter, P.; Unterberg, A.; Radlwimmer, B. & Herold-Mende, C.C. (2008). Stem cell marker CD133 affects clinical outcome in glioma patients. *Clinical Cancer Research,* Vol.14, No.1, (January 2008), pp. 123-129, ISSN 10780432

Zhu, C.; Ghabriel, M.N.; Blumbergs, P.C.; Reilly, P.L.; Manavis, J.; Youssef, J.; Hatami, S. & Finnie, J.W. (2001). Clostridium perfringens prototoxin-induced alteration of endothelial barrier antigen (EBA) immunoreactivity at the blood-brain barrier (BBB). *Experimental Neurology,* Vol.169, No. 1, pp. 72-82, ISSN 00144886

Ziche, M. & Morbidelli, L. (2009). Molecular regulation of tumour angiogenesis by nitric oxide. *European Cytokine Network,* Vol.20, No.4, (December 2009), pp. 164-170, ISSN 11485493

Zook, B.C.; Simmens, S.J. & Jones, R.V. (2000). Evaluation of ENU-induced gliomas in rats: nomenclature, immunochemistry, and malignancy. *Toxicologic Pathology,* Vol.28, No. 1, 2000, pp. 193-201, ISSN 01926233

19

Copy Number Alterations in Glioma Cell Lines

Bárbara Meléndez et al.*
Virgen de la Salud Hospital, Toledo, Spain

1. Introduction

Established tumor-derived cell lines are widely and routinely used as *in vitro* cancer models for various kinds of biomedical research. The easy management of these cell cultures, in contrast to the inherent difficulty in establishing and mantaining primary tumoral cultures, has contributed to the wide use of these inmortalized cell lines in order to characterize the biological significance of specific genomic aberrations identified in primary tumors. Therefore, it has been assumed that the genomic and expression aberrations of long-term established cell lines resemble, and are representative, of the primary tumor from which the cell line was derived. Indeed, the cell line-based research has been performed, not only for the definition of the molecular biology of several cancer models, but also for the investigation of new targeted therapeutic agents in a prior step to clinical practice. The use of tumor-derived cell lines has been highly relevant for the testing and development of new therapeutical agents, with several cancer cell-line panels having been developed for drug sensitivity screening and new agents' discovery (Sharma et al, 2010).

Controversial concerning the ability of tumor-derived cell lines to accurately reflect the phenotype and genotype of the parental histology has been documented. A previous report of Greshock and coworkers using array-based Comparative Genomic Hybridization (aCGH) data of seven diagnosis-specific matched tumors and cell lines showed that, on average, cell lines preserve *in vitro* the genetic aberrations that are unique to the parent histology from which they were derived, while acquiring additional locus-specific alterations in long-term cultures (Greshock et al, 2007). In contrast, a study on breast cancer cell lines and primary tumors highlight that cell lines do not always represent the genotypes of parental tumor tissues (Tsuji et al, 2010). Furthermore, a parallel genomic and expression study on glioma cell lines and primary tumors states that in this specific cancer type, cell lines are poor representative of the primary tumors (Li et al, 2008). Given the importance of the use of cell lines as models for the study of the biology and development of tumors, and for the testing of the mode of action of new therapeutical agents, the knowledge of which genomic alterations are tumor-specific or which are necessary for the maintenance of the cell line in culture, becomes essential.

---

* Ainoha García-Claver[1], Yolanda Ruano[1], Yolanda Campos-Martín[1], Ángel Rodríguez de Lope[1], Elisa Pérez-Magán[1], Pilar Mur[1], Sofía Torres[2], Mar Lorente[2], Guillermo Velasco[2] and Manuela Mollejo[1]
[1] *Virgen de la Salud Hospital, Toledo, Spain*
[2] *Universidad Complutense, Madrid, Spain*

Sometimes cell line studies are interpreted in the context of artifacts introduced by selection and establishment of cell lines in vitro, given the prevalence of documented cell line-specific cytogenetic changes acquired with multiple growth passages which is associated with random genomic instability. Therefore, the ability of glioma cell-line models to accurately reflect the phenotype and genotype of the parental glioma tumors remains unstudied. The aim of this study is to compare the genomic aberrations of the most commonly used glioma cell lines for *in vitro* analysis with those alterations more prevalent in primary glioma tumors.

2. Copy number alterations in glioma cell lines

2.1 High-level DNA copy number alterations in glioma cell lines

2.1.1 Amplifications

Genomic high-level DNA copy number gains (regions of amplification, or amplicons, i.e. chromosome regions that show more than 5- to 10-fold copy number increases) were detected at 4q, 10q and 19q in two of the cell lines: SW1783 (4q12) and SF767 (10q21.2-q23.1 and 19p12) (table 1, figure 1). The MLPA analysis confirmed some of the genomic alterations observed by aCGH, such as the amplification of *PDGFRA* (4q12) which was observed in SW1783 cell line (see below table 3).

CHROMOSOME	GENES	CELL LINE (Region Size Mb)
4q12	CHIC2, GSH2, PDGFRA, KIT, KDR, SRD5A2L, TMEM165, CLOCK, PDCL2, NMU, EXOC1, CEP135, AASDH, PPAT, PAICS, SRP72, HOP, SPINK2, REST, OLR2B, IGFBP7	SW1783 (3.57)
10q21.2 - q23.1	COL13A1, H2AFY2, AIFM2, TYSND1, SAR1A, PPA1, NPFFR1, LRRC20, EIF4EBP2, NODAL, PRF1, ADAMTS14, SGPL1, PCBD1, UNC5B, SLC29A3, CDH23, PSAP, CHST3, SPOCK2, ASCC1, DNAJB12, CBARA1, CCDC109A, OIT3, PLA2G12B, P4HA1, NUDT13, ECD, DNAJC9, MRPS16, TTC18, ANXA7, ZMYND17, PPP3CB, , USP54, MYOZ1, SYNPO2L, SEC24C, FUT11, NDST2, CAMK2G, PLAU, VCL, AP3M1, ADK, MYST4, DUSP13, SAMD8, VDAC2, KCNMA1, DLG5, NAG13, POLR3A, RPS24, ZMIZ1, PPIF, SFTPD, ANXA11, MAT1A, DYDC1, DYDC2, TSPAN14, NRG3	SF767 (13.37)
19p12	ZNF43,SINE-R ,ZNF208,ZNF257	SF767 (0.28)

Table 1. Summary of high-level gains (amplifications) detected by aCGH

Amplification of the EGFR gene, located on chromosome 7, and subsequent over-expression of EGFR protein, is the most common genetic alteration found in primary glioblastoma (GBM), the most aggressive high-grade glioma. This amplification is detected in about 40% of these tumors, and is present as double-minute extrachromosomal elements (Louis et al, 2007). Amplification of the EGFR gene is often associated with structural rearrangements, resulting in tumors expressing both wild-type EGFR as well as the mutated EGFR. The most common truncated EGFR variant is the EGFRvIII one, consisting of 801-bp in-frame deletion comprising exons 2-7 of the gene.

Among the cell lines analyzed in this study, some of them derived from primary GBMs, none of them carried either amplification of the EGFR gene, nor the EGFRvIII mutant form of the receptor (Figure 2). Besides, EGFR sequence analysis of exons 18-21, coding for the tyrosine kinase domain, revealed not a mutation in this region, unlike what is found in non-small lung cancer tumors.

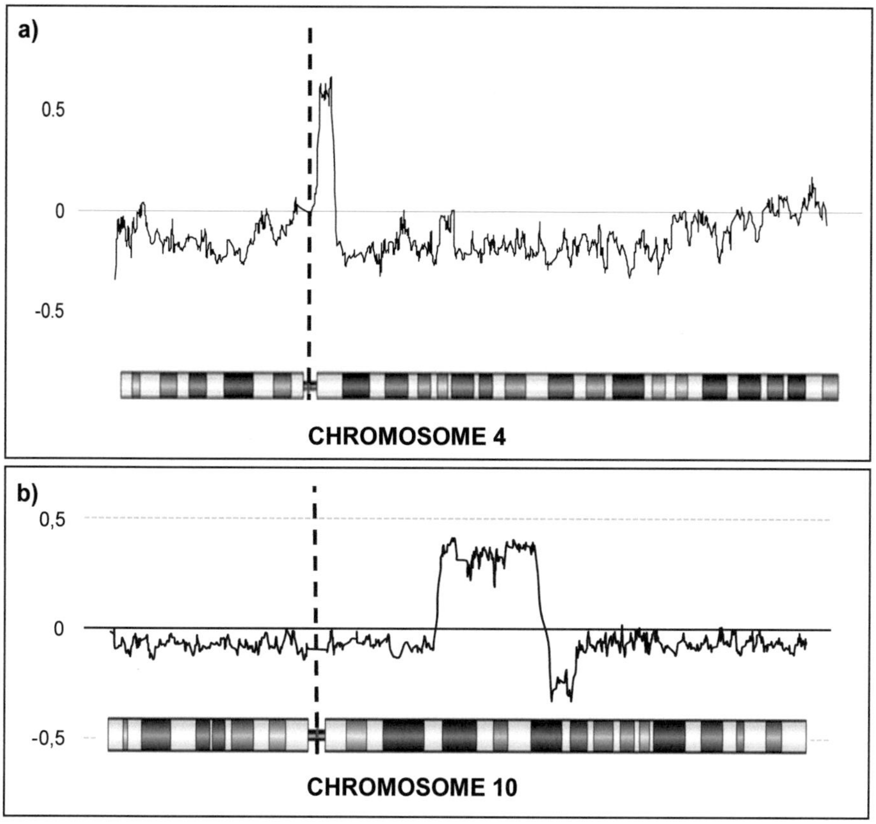

Fig. 1. aCGH results of chromosomes 4 (a) and 10 (b) in SW1783 and SF767 cell lines, respectively. Moving average of log_2-genomic ratios over five neighbouring genes are plotted.

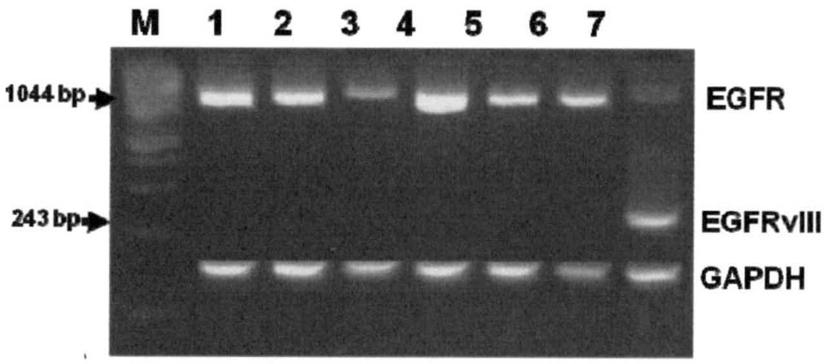

Fig. 2. RT-PCR analysis for the detection of EGFR wild-type (EGFRwt) and EGFRvIII mutant receptor. The inset shows control gene GAPDH results. Line 1: GOS3, 2: A172, 3: U118, 4: SF767, 5: T98, 6: wt EGFR control, 7: EGFRvIII control; M: molecular marker.

2.1.2 Homozygous deletions

Analysis of the high-level copy number changes detected by aCGH in the eleven glioma cell lines revealed higher frequency of genomic losses than gains. A stringent filter was applied in order to detect homozygous deletions.

Genomic homozygous losses were detected at 1p, 1q, 2q, 3p, 4q, 5q, 6q, 7p, 9p, 10p, 10q and 21p (Table 2).
Homozygous losses affecting two or more cell lines were detected at 1p33, 9p21.3-21.1, 10q23.2-23.3 and 21p11.1 (Table 2). Main target genes of these regions were: *CDKN2C* ($p18^{INK4c}$) on chromosome 1, *CDKN2A* ($p16^{INK4a}$) and CDKN2B ($p15^{INK4b}$) on chromosome 9, and *PTEN* on chromosome 10. The most frequent homozygous gene loss was the loss of *CDKN2A* ($p16^{INK4a}$) and *CDKN2B* ($p15^{INK4b}$), affecting nine (82%) and eight (73%) of 11 glioma cell lines, respectively.

2.1.2.1 Loss of *CDKN2C*

The Cancer Cell Line project (CCL) database from the Genome Cancer Project of the Sanger Institute (http://www.sanger.ac.uk/genetics/CGP/CellLines/) was used to confirm these alterations when possible. Homozygous deletion of CDKN2C (1p33) was described in this project for T98 and U87 cell lines. Homozygous deletion of CDKN2C on U373 cell line was not reported in this project. By contrast, this deletion was not reported in the study of Li and coworkers for T98 and U87 cell lines (Li et al, 2008).

2.1.2.2 Loss of *CDKN2A* and *CDKN2B*

CDKN2A (9p21.3) loss of cell lines A172, H4, SW1088, T98, U118 and U87 was reported by the CCL project. Similarly, this gene was described as not mutated in SW1783, therefore confirming our results. Data from GOS3, LN18 and U373 were not provided in this database. Deletion of the 9p21 region was also reported in A172 and U87 cell lines by Li and coworkers, again validating our findings. Strikingly, T98 cell line was not deleted in that study (Li et al, 2008). Furthermore, the MLPA analyses performed on the cell lines confirmed the homozygous deletions observed by aCGH (Table 2). Therefore homozygous deletion of the *CDKN2A* gene was present in 9 of the 11 glioma cell lines (Table 2, Figure 3).
Remarkably, there were two cell lines that lack any alteration at the *CDNK2A* locus, either by homozygous or hemizygous loss of the region.

2.1.2.3 Loss of *PTEN*

The aCGH analysis revealed homozygous deletion of PTEN in SW1088 and H4 cell lines (Table 2), which was confirmed by the MLPA assay (Figure 4). In addition, homozygous deletion of PTEN in these cell lines was also reported by the CCL project. PTEN hemizygous deletion was detected in SF767 and GOS3 cell lines by aCGH and MLPA. Surprisingly, A172 cell line had homozygous deletion of all the PTEN probes of the MLPA assay except those of exons 1 and 2. This loss could not be detected by the aCGH analysis, probably because only two of the three probes included in the microarray were in the deleted part of PTEN (homozygous losses were considered as present when three consecutive clones were under the threshold 1.0) (Figure 4).
Further analyses of PTEN sequence were performed attending to PTEN expression (see Table 5 in section 3). Western-blot analysis showed PTEN expression in T98, LN18, GOS3 and SF767 (the two latter carring hemizygous deletion of the gene). Lack of protein expression was found in 7 of the eleven cell lines, three of them having homozygous deletion of PTEN. Therefore, we carried out exon-sequencing analysis of the other four PTEN deficient cell lines (U118, U87, U373 and SW1783) in order to detect putative mutations of the genomic sequence that could explain the observed suppression of protein expression. U118 and U87 presented a substitution mutation (G>T) in the splicing site of exons 8 (c.1026+1G>T) and 3 (c.209+1G>T), respectively; U373 showed an homozygous TT insertion in exon 7 causing a shift in the reading frame (c.723_724insTT); and SW1783

showed a substitution in exon 7 (c.691C>T) which results in a stop codon (CGA>TGA). The latter mutation was confirmed with the database from the Cancer Genome Project (CGP, Sanger Institute). The CGP report the same mutation that we found in cell line U373, for the U251 glioma cell line, which is derived from the same tumour as U373, and thus contains the same TT insertion mutation in PTEN.

CHROMOSOME	GENES	CELL LINE (Mb lost)
1p33	FAF1, CDKN2C	U87 (0.17), T98 (0.07), U373 (0.23)
1p31.1	LRRC44, FPGT, TNNI3K, CRYZ, TYW3	U118
1q42.2	DISC1,SIPA1L2,PCNXL2	GOS3 (1.33)
2q42.2	BAZ2B	GOS3 (0.12)
3p24.3	TBC1D5,SATB1,KCNH8, EFHB,RAB5A, SGOL1, PCAF	H4 (4.63)
3p24.1	TGFBR2	SF767 (0.23)
3p12.2-p11.2	IGSF4D,VGLL3,CHMP2B, POU1F1,HTR1F, CGGBP1	LN18 (6.32)
4q34.1	FBXO8,HPGD,GLRA3	U118 (0.40)
5q14.1	THBS4, SERINC5	SF767 (0.13)
6q22.2	ROS1,DCBLD1	U118 (0.17)
7p21.2-p21.1	ETV1, DGKB, MEOX2, OSTDC1, ANKMY2, BZW2, TSPAN13, AGR2, BCMP11, AHR, SNX13, HDAC9	SF767 (5.09)
9p22.1-p21.1	SLC24A2	LN18 (6.37)
9p21.3-p21.1	MLLT3, IFNB1	U118 (10.86), U87 (3.52), LN18
	IFNW1	U118, U87,LN18, H4 (1.22)
	KLHL9,IFNA2,IFNA8	U118, U87,LN18, H4, SW1088 (7.22)
	IFNE1,MTAP	U118, U87,LN18, H4, SW1088,A172 (0.71)
	CDKN2A	U118,U87,LN18,H4,SW1088,T98,U373,A172,GOS3 (0.18)
	CDKN2B	U118, U87,LN18, H4, SW1088, U373, A172, GOS3
	ELAVL2	U118, LN18, SW1088
	hel-N1	U118, LN18
	PLAA, IFT74, LNG01784, TEK, MOBKL2B, LRRN6C	U118, SW1088
	LINGO2	U118
10p11.21	PARD3	T98 (0.11)
10q23.2 - q23.31	MINPP1	H4 (0.73)
	PAPSS2,ATAD1,PTEN	H4,SW1088
	LIPF,ANKRD22,STAMBPL1, ACTA2, FAS,CH25H,LIPA	SW1088 (1.50)
10q25.2	TCF7L2	T98 (0.16)
12q21.2	PAWR	GOS3 (0.14)
21p11.1	BAGE4,BAGE5,BAGE3,BAGE2, BAGE	H4 A172, U118, GOS3 (0.04)

Table 2. Homozygous losses detected in glioma cell lines by aCGH

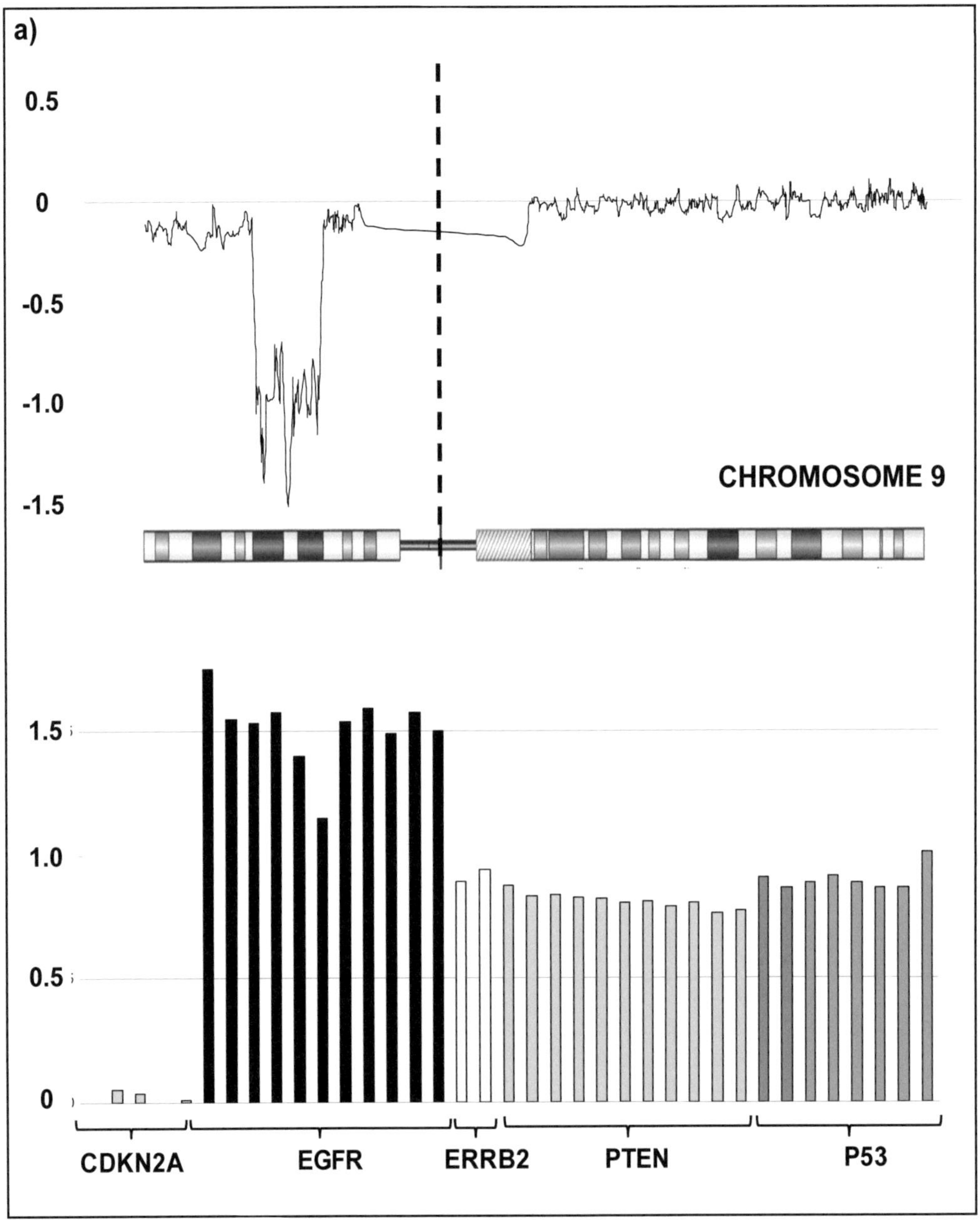
a)
0.5
0
-0.5
-1.0
-1.5
CHROMOSOME 9
1.5
1.0
0.5
0
CDKN2A
EGFR
ERRB2
PTEN
P53

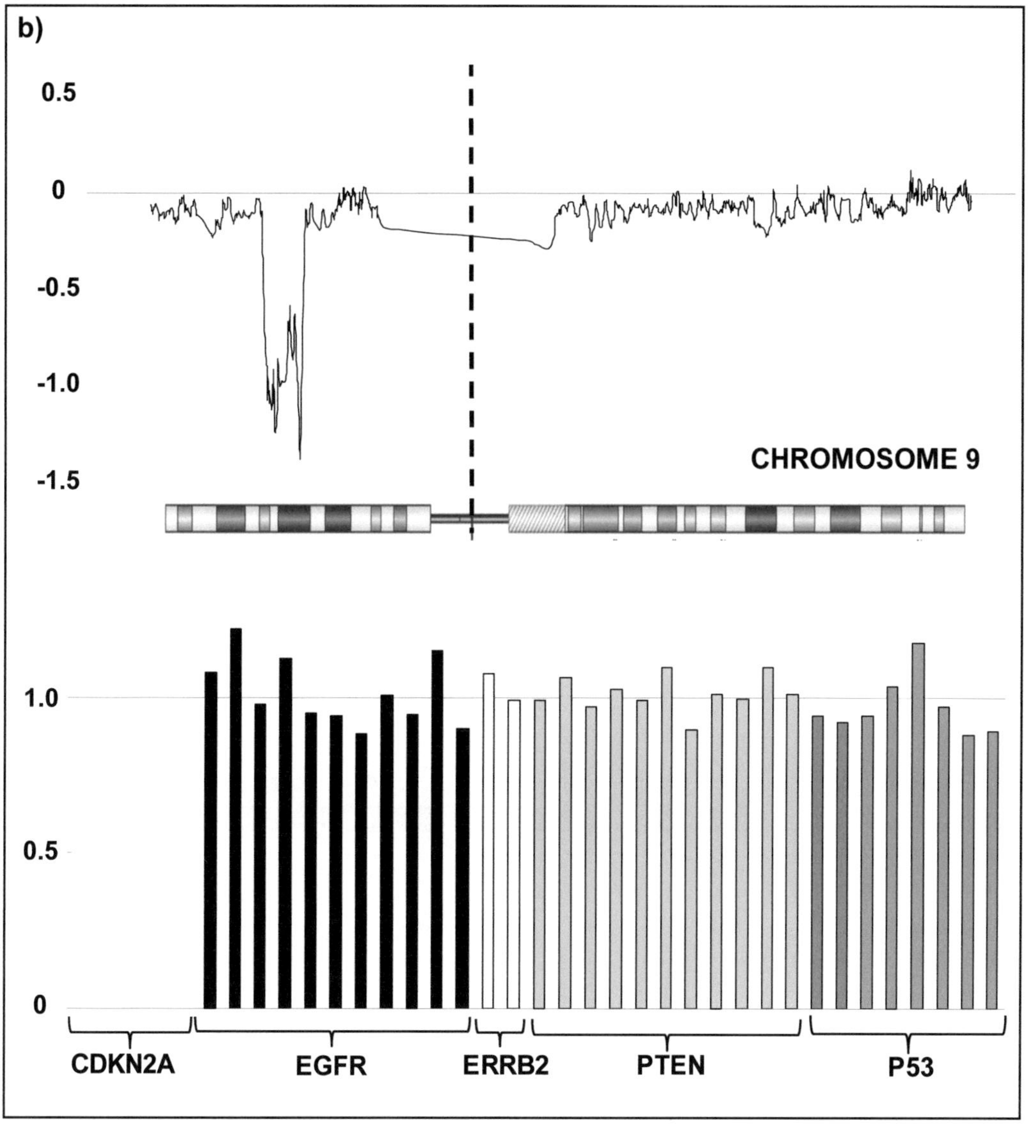

Fig. 3. Homozygous loss detected on chromosome 9 (including *CDKN2A*locus) in two representative cell lines: U118 (a) and LN18 (b). Upper panel: aCGH plot (moving average of log_2-genomic ratios over five neighbouring genes); Lower panel: MLPA graph (each bar represents a probe of the MLPA assay).

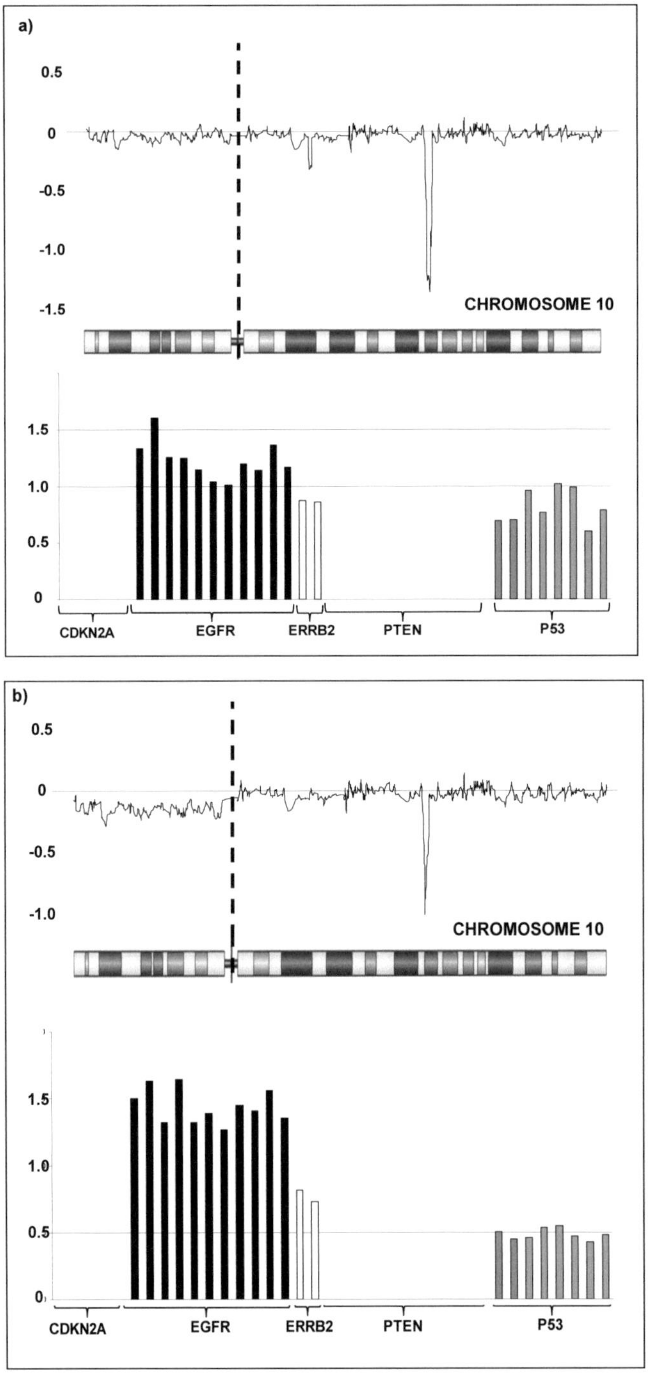

Fig. 4. Homozygous loss detected on chromosome 10 (including *PTEN*) in two representative cell lines: SW1088 (a) and H4 (b). Upper panel: aCGH plot (moving average of log_2-genomic ratios over five neighbouring genes); Lower panel: MLPA graph (each bar represents a probe of the MLPA assay).

2.2 Low-level DNA copy number alterations in glioma cell lines

Analyses of the DNA copy number changes in 11 of the most commonly used glioma cell lines revealed higher frecquency of genomic losses than gains. While 22.15% of the analyzed probes were lost, only 12.35% of them presented gains. Chromosomes containing frequently gained probes among all the cell lines included chromosomes 7, 16, 17, 19 and 20. Similarly, chromosomes containing frequently lost probes included chromosomes 4, 6, 10, 13, 14 and 18 (Figure 5). Surprisingly, chromosome 9, presenting loss of the *CDKN2A/CDKN2B* locus in most of the cell lines (9 out of 11 cell lines) presented a similar percentage of gained and loss probes. This result may be explained due to this loss is relatively small in most of the cell lines, and to the low-level DNA copy number gain of most of chromosome 9 in SF767 cell line (data not shown).

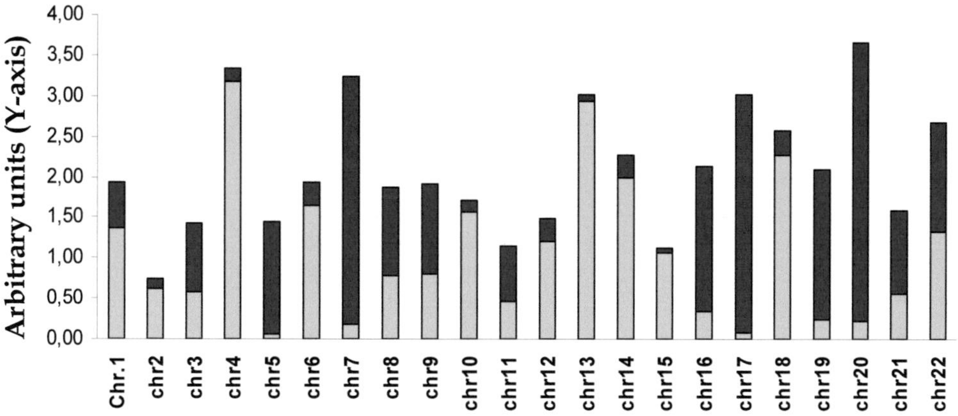

Fig. 5. Percentage of low-level DNA copy number gains (black) and losses (grey) relative to the analyzed probes in the microarray per chromosome.

Chromosome 7 was one of the most gained chromosomes, with complete or almost complete chromosome 7 gain in SW1088 and GOS3 cell lines, or with relative wide regions of gain in H4, U373, U118 or A172 cell lines. Gain of the *EGFR* gene (located at 7p12) was evaluated by MLPA assays, showing EGFR low-level copy number gain in 8 out of the 11 cell lines (table 3).

Other gains detected by MLPA analysis were *PI3KCA, BRAF* and *BIRC5*. Three of the cell lines presented a *PI3KCA* gain (3q). *PIK3CA* is one of the three genes encoding components of PI3K which is involved in activation of AKT signaling. Amplification of *PIK3CA* has been observed in various types of cancer, including gliomas (Karakas, 2006; Kita, 2007; Vogt, 2006). *BRAF* oncogene (7q34) was gained in five of the cell lines. BRAF is a serine/threonine kinase that is frequently activated in many types of cancer by a specific mutation (V600E). In pilocytic astrocytomas, BRAF is frequently activated by tandem duplication and rearrangement of part of the gene, resulting in fusion proteins containing the kinase domain (exons 9-18). Activation of BRAF through these mechanisms of duplication or fusion is infrequent in diffusely infiltrating astrocytic gliomas (Bar et al, 2008; Riemenscheneider et al, 2010). All the cell lines analyzed in this study were obtained from adult patients with high grade gliomas.

BIRC5 or survivin (17q) was gained in five of the cell lines. Survivin, which promotes cell proliferation, angiogenes and inhibits apoptosis, is frequently overexpressed in proliferating tissues and tumors (Zhen et al, 2005). In gliomas, survivin overexpression is significantly associated with tumorigenesis and progression, and with a worse prognosis of patients (Shirai et al, 2009). Previous studies revealed, as well, BIRC5 gain and overexpression in oligodendroglial tumors (Blesa et al, 2009). High expression of BIRC5 in nervous system tumors have been already reported (Das, 2002; Hogdson, 2009; Sasaki, 2002).
As a summary, at the gene-level, the most represented gains and losses in the 11 analyzed cell lines are shown in table 4.

	CHROMOSOME	GENE NAME	CELL LINE
HOM LOSS	9p21	*CDKN2A*	U373, U118, SW1088, GOS3, A172, H4, T98, U87, LN18
	10q23	*PTEN*	A172, SW1088, H4
HEMI LOSS	1p13.2	*NRAS*	A172, H4
	10q23	*PTEN*	SF767, GOS3
GAIN	1p13.2	*NRAS*	U373
	1q32	*PI3KC2B*	A172
	2q35	*IGFBP2*	SW1088
	3q26.3	*PIK3CA*	A172, SW1783, H4
	7p12	*EGFR*	U373, U118, SW1088, GOS3, A172, H4, T98, SF767
	7q34	*BRAF*	U87, U373, SW1088, GOS3, T98
	17p11.2	*TOM1L2*	LN18
	17q25	*BIRC5*	H4, LN18, T98, U373, SW1783
	21q22.3	*RUNX1*	H4, A172, T98
A	4q11	*PDGFRA*	SW1783

Table 3. Summary of gene-specific MLPA-validated copy number alterations (HOM LOSS: homozygous loss; HEMI LOSS: one copy loss; GAIN: low-level copy number gains; A: amplifications).

GAIN		HOMOZYGOUS DELETION	
Gene (location)	Total	Gene (location)	Total
EGFR (7p12)	8	CDKN2A (9p21)	9
BRAF (7q34)	5	CDKN2B (9p21)	8
BIRC5 (17q25)	5	MTAP (& others; 9p21)	6
PI3KCA (3q26.3)	3	BAGE (21p11.1)	4
		PTEN (10q23)	3
		CDKN2C (1p33)	3

Table 4. Summary of the alterations most represented on the eleven glioma cell lines studied. (Total: number of cell lines presenting the alteration described)

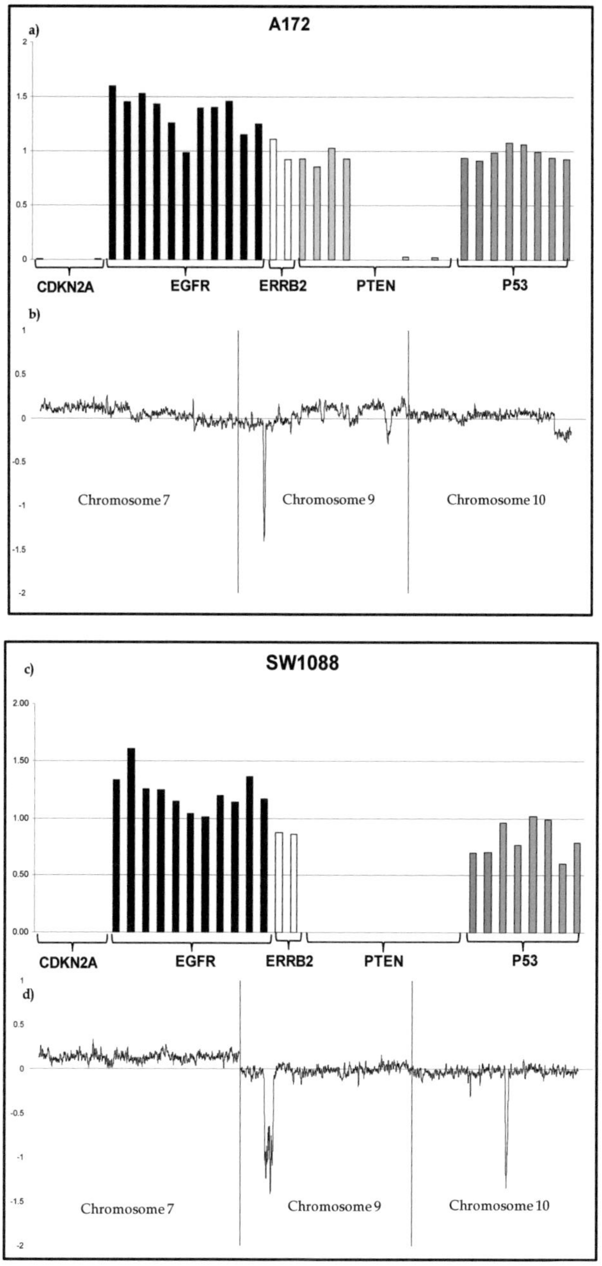

Fig. 6. Genomic analysis of A172 (a, b) and SW1088 cell lines (c, d). a) MLPA analysis (each bar represents a probe of the MLPA assay) showing *EGFR* gain, *CDKN2A* homozygous deletion, and *PTEN* homozygous deletions except for exons 1 and 2. b) aCGH analysis (moving average of log_2-genomic ratios over five neighbouring genes) of chromosomes 7, 9 and 10. c) MLPA analysis showing *EGFR* gain, and homozygous deletions of *CDKN2A* and *PTEN* d) aCGH analysis of chromosomes 7, 9 and 10. Observe that no *PTEN* deletions (10q23.2) were detected in A172 cell line compared to SW1088.

3. Comparison between copy number alterations in glioma cell lines and primary tumors

Gliomas are the most frequent primary brain tumors, and include a variety of different histological tumor types and malignancy grades. High-grade gliomas are those graded as III or IV according to the criteria of the World Health Organization (WHO) classification system (Louis et al, 2007), including anaplasic astrocytoma (WHO grade III) and GBM (WHO grade IV). High-grade gliomas may arise from diffuse astrocytoma WHO grade II or III, or *de novo,* i.e. without evidence of a less malignant precursor lesion. GBM is the most frequent primary brain tumor. Primary GBM manifest rapidly de novo, while secondary GBM develops slowly from diffuse or anaplastic astrocytomas.

It is important to note that most of the cell lines used in this study derived from astrocytoma tumors of high-grade (8 cell lines: T98, LN18, U373, SW1088, H4, SW1783, U118, and A172), with the exception of GOS3 cell line that was derived from a high-grade mixed tumor with oligodendroglial component.

From a genetic point of view, progression to malignancy in gliomas is a multistep process, driven by the sequential acquisition and accumulation of genetic alterations. Distinctions between the genetic alterations identified in primary and secondary GBM have been made, with *TP53* mutations occurring more commonly in secondary GBMs and *EGFR* amplifications, and *PTEN* mutations occurring more frequently in primary GBMs. However, none of these alterations sufficiently distinguishes between primary and secondary GBM.

Recently, a comprehensive sequencing and genomic copy number analysis of GBM tumors showed that the majority of the tumors analyzed had alterations in genes encoding components of each of the *TP53, RB1,* and *PI3K* pathways, previously known to be altered in GBMs (Parsons et al, 2008). In these tumors, all but one of the cancers with mutations in members of a pathway did not have alterations in other members of the same family, suggesting that such alterations are functionally equivalent in tumorigenesis. Opposite to what is found in primary and secondary GBMs, glioma cell lines usually harbor functional alterations of the three pathways simultaneously (e.g. SW1088, SW1783 or U118, table 5).

Alteration mutations of the tumor suppressor gene *TP53* (located at 17p13.1) and loss of heterozygosity on chromosome arm 17p are frequent in secondary GBM. While *TP53* copy number analysis showed nor gains or losses in the cell lines tested, neither by CGH nor by MLPA, point mutations have been reported by the Sanger database in some of the analyzed cell lines (Table 5).

Primary GBM, on another hand, characterises by *EGFR* amplification or overexpression, *PTEN* mutation, trisomy of chromosome 7, monosomy of 10 and genomic gains of 12p, 19q and 20q (Riemenschneider et al, 2010).

Regarding alterations of *PTEN* gen (*PI3K* pathway), loss of chromosome 10 is one of the most frequent alteration in primary GBM tumors (60-80% of cases). While many tumors show loss of one entire copy of chromosome 10, loss of heterozygosity (LOH) studies have reported the involvement of several regions of LOH, suggesting several potential tumor suppressor genes in addition to *PTEN.* The cell lines analyzed in our study frequently presented alteration of *PTEN* gene (nine out of 11 cell lines), either by mutation or genomic loss. Absence of PTEN protein expression in these cell lines was confirmed in seven of these cell lines by western blot (data not shown).

Concerning amplifications, EGFR high-level copy number gain is the most frequent alteration found in primary GBM. As mentioned before, this alteration is present as double-minutes, i.e. small and circular fragments of extrachromosomal DNA that are replicated in the nucleus of the cell during cell division but that, unlike actual chromosomes, lack centromere or telomere. This EGFR amplification has not been detected in any of the analyzed glioma cell lines, probably due to the difficulty in maintaining a highly unstable extrachromosomal fragment that lacks centromere, in long-term cultures. A recent report, however, describes another type of EGFR gain in which extra copies (in small numbers) of EGFR are inserted in different loci of chromosome 7 (Lopez-Gines et al, 2010). The presence of this type of gain in glioma cell lines remains to be studied.

	RB pathway	*PI3K* pathway				*TP53* pathway	
	CDKN2A	***PTEN***	***PTEN seq***	***EGFR***	***EGFRvIII***	***Tp53***	***p53 mut***
T98G	del HOMO	N	-	G	No	N	p.M237I
LN18	del HOMO	N	-	N	No	N*	nd
SF767	N	del HEMI	-	G	No	N*	nd
U373	del HOMO	N*	c.723_724insTT	G	No	N	nd
U87MG	del HOMO	N*	c.209+1G>T	N	No	N*	nd
SW1088	del HOMO	del HOMO*	-	G	No	N	p.R273C
H4	del HOMO	del HOMO*	-	G	No	N*	nd
SW1783	N	N*	c.691C>T	N	No	N	p.R273C
U118	del HOMO	N*	c.1026+1G>T	G	No	N	p.R213Q
GOS3	del HOMO	del HEMI	-	G	No	N	nd
A172	del HOMO	del HOMO*,#	-	G	No	N*	nd

*Protein expression not detected (Western-blot or Immunohistochemistry, data not shown) #deletion except for exons 1 and 2. del HOMO: homozygous deletion; del Hemi: hemizygous deletion; G: Gain; N: No copy number change; No: EGFRvIII mutation not detected; p53 mut: data from the Sanger database; nd: no data from available.

Table 5. Alterations of the RB, TP53 and PI3K pathways.

Thus, at least for what concerns to the EGFR amplification, glioma cell lines seem not to resemble primary tumors. This result contrast to what is found in breast cancer cell lines, where amplification of *ERBB2* (17q12) is detected indeed more frequently in cell lines that in primary tumors (Tsuji et al, 2010). Of note, amplification of *ERBB2* takes place within homogeneously staining regions, where the extra copies of the gene are integrated within the chromosome, thus allowing its maintenance in established cell lines.

Similarly, other amplifications reported in primary GBM tumors have not been found in these cell lines, such as those of 1q (*MDM4, PIK3C2B*), 7q (*MET, PEX1, CDK6*), 12p (*CCDN2*) 12q (*MDM2, GLI, CDK4*) or 13q (Rao et al, 2010; Ruano et al, 2006). The only common amplification detected in glioma cell lines and tumors was that of 4q (*PDGFRA*) which was detected in SW1783 cell line. *PDGFRA* encodes for a cell surface tyrosine kinase receptor of the members of the platelet-derived growth factor family. These growth factors are mitogens for cells of mesenchymal origin and activate intracellular signaling through the MAPK, PI3K and PKCgamma pathways with roles in the regulation of many biological processes including embryonic development, angiogenesis, cell proliferation and differentiation. On the other hand, to our knowledge, amplifications of 10q and 19p detected in SF767 cell line have not been reported before in glioma tumors.

Digital karyotyping for eight tumor-derived cultured samples and one bulk tumor was used by Rao and coworkers (2010) to describe genomic alterations in GBM. This group described amplifications in 1q, 7p, 8q and 12q, and homozygous deletions in 1p, 9p and 9q. However 7p11.2-12.1 (*EGFR*), 8q24.21 (*MYC*) and 12q15 (*MDM2*) amplifications were found just in case of the tumor sample, consistent with previous observations that adherent GBM cells tend to lose EGFR amplification during culturing. The most frequent amplifications found by this group was 12q13.3-q14.1, which targeted *GLI1* and *CDK4* oncogenes, affecting 3 samples. Two of the samples showed amplification of *PI3KC2B* and *MDM4* in 1q32.1. Table 6 shows comparison of our results with those published by Rao and coworkers (2010). Low-level copy number gains (e.g. *PI3KC2B*: A172 cell lines; *EGFR:* 8/11 cell lines) but not amplifications were detected in the cell lines.

The p16ink4a/CDK4/RB1 pathway is important for the control of progression through G1 into the S phase of the cell cycle. In GBM tumors, alterations affecting this pathway are found at an overall frequency of 40-50% (Louis et al, 2007). Homozygous deletions affecting *CDKN2A* locus (9p21) were described by digital karyotyping in 44% of cultured samples (four out of nine) (Rao et al, 2010). Our study reveals 82% (9/11) and 73% (8/11) of cell lines carrying homozygous deletions for *CDKN2A* and *CDKN2B* genes, respectively (Table 6).

Chromosome band	**Target oncogene**	**Rao % (n=9)**	**Our group % (n=11)**
Amplifications/Gains (G)			
1q32.1	PIK3C2B	22	9 (G)
1q32.1	MDM4	22	0
7p11.2-12.1	EGFR	11	73 (G)
8q24.21	MYC	11	45 (G)
12q13.3-q14.1	GLI1,CD4	33	18 (G)
12q14.1	Unknown	22	9 (G)
12q15	MDM2	11	0
Homozygous deletions			
1p36.31-p36.23	TP73, LRRC47, DFFB	33	18
9p21.3-22.3	CDKN2A, CDKN2B	44	82, 73
9q34.3	CACNA1B	44	0

Table 6. Comparison of results obtained by Digital Karyotyping (Rao et al, 2010) with aCGH alterations observed in glioma cell lines. Only amplification data from Rao´s study was available.

Finally, regarding the number of DNA copy number alterations in cell lines, the lost probes almost doubled the gained ones, with an average of losses and gains per cell line of 9,908 and 5,072 probes, respectively. This result contrast to what is observed in primary GBM tumors, having similar numbers of gains and losses (Ruano et al, 2006). Accordingly, similar results were obtained in tumor-derived cell lines from other histologies (Greshock et al, 2007) and specifically in breast cancer cell lines (Tsuji et al, 2010; Naylor et al, 2005), with more alterations found in cell lines than in tissue specimens, as a general trend. In fact, genomic losses in breast cancer cell lines almost doubled the gains (Tsuji et al, 2010). These observations may suggest the accumulation of genomic alterations in long-term cultures that are not present in primary tissues.

4. Cell culture specific aberrations

Several of the frequent genomic alterations detected in glioma cell lines are not found in primary tumors, suggesting that some of the commonly seen alterations *in vitro* could be artifacts secondary to the selection pressure for optimal cell growth *in vitro* following years of passage. This observation has been reported previously in gliomas (Li et al, 2008), but the presence of acquired locus-specific alterations in culture has also been recognized in tumors and cell lines of other histologies (Greshock et al, 2007). For example, genome-specific copy number alterations of chromosomes 5 (gained), 8, 11 and 18 (lost) in glioma cell lines have been attributed exclusively to the phenotype of established cell lines. Furthermore, other copy number alterations not commonly found in cell lines, such as those of specific areas of chromosomes 2, 3, 6 and 8 have been rarely observed in primary tumors.

Our findings (Figure 5) have identified areas of low-level gain on chromosomes 5, 16 and 17 affecting between 5 and 7 cell lines, which do not feature GBM tumors. In addition, areas of loss of chromosomes 6, 8, 11, and, most importantly, loss of chromosome 18 have been identified in most of cell lines. These alterations seem to be culture-associated changes present in cell lines and suggest a genomic instability phenotype in established cell lines that is not present in primary tumor tissues.

Absence of chromosome 13 deletions in glioma cell lines, which were commonly found in primary GBMs, was reported by Li and coworkers (2008) as a striking discrepancy between cell lines and tumors. Our study, however, did detected chromosome 13 losses (Figure 5). In the present study, complete loss of chromosome 13 was identified by aCGH in H4, LN18, U373, SW1088 and U118 cell lines, while partial loss was detected in U87, SF767, SW1783 and A172 cell lines. No loss was observed in T98 and GOS3 cell lines. Curiously, cell lines analyzed in common by our study and that of Li, had partial chromosome 13 loss in our study and partial chromosome 13 LOH in the study of Li and coworkers (U87 and A172), or no chosmosome 13 loss in both studies (T98).

5. Material and methods

5.1 Cell lines and cell culture

The human glioma cell lines GOS3, U87MG (U87), A172, SW1783, U118 MG (U118), T98G (T98), SW1088, H4, LN18, U373MG (U373) and SF767WL (SF767) were kindly provided by Dr. Velasco (Complutense University of Madrid, Spain) or Dr. Setién (Catalan Institute of Oncology, Spain). These cell lines were maintained in RPMI medium containing 10% FBS (Gibco, Grand Island, NY) in standard culture conditions. Total DNA and RNA were extracted from cell cultures according to standard phenol-chloroform and Trizol (Invitrogen, Carlsbad, CA) techniques, respectively. Nucleic acids obtained were quantified using NanoDrop-1000 (NanoDrop Technologies, Inc., Wilmington, DE).

5.2 Comparative genomic hybridization

Copy number analyses of the 11 glioma cell lines were screened by array-based Comparative Genomic Hybridization (aCGH) in the Microarrays Analysis Service of the CIPF (Centro de Investigación Principe Felipe, Valencia). "Agilent Oligonucleotide Array-Based CGH for Genomic DNA Analysis" protocol Version 4.0 (Agilent Technologies, Palo Alto, California USA. p/n G4410-90010) was followed to obtain labeled DNA. 2000 ng of DNA from samples and reference DNA (pool of sex-matched normal brain DNA) was fragmented and labeled (Cyanine 3-dUTP for the cell lines DNA and cyanine 5-dUTP for the reference DNA) according to the "Agilent Genomic DNA labeling kit plus" protocol. Labeled DNA was hybridized with Human Genome CGH Microarray 44 k (Agilent p/n G4426B-014950) containing 45,214 probes with 42,494 distinct biological features. Arrays were scanned in an Agilent Microarray Scanner (Agilent G2565BA). Data was analyzed using DNA Analytics 4.0 CGH Module (Agilent Technologies). Genomic alterations were detected using an ADM-2 algorithm with two different filters: one, used to detect low level alterations, , detects those alterations affecting to three consecutive probes with a ratio above or below to 0.25; the other, used to obtain amplifications or homozygous deletion, included in 2.1 section, detects only three consecutive probes above or below a ratio of 1.0.

5.3 MLPA analysis

Specific gene alterations were validated by Multiple ligation probe assay experiments (MLPA®, Mrc-Holland, The Netherlands) with SALSA MLPA kit P105 Glioma-2 for EGFR, PTEN, CDKN2A and p53. Besides, SALSA® MLPA® kit P173 was used to detect copy number alteration of several genes which are frequently altered in several tumors, such as: BCL2L11, BIRC5, BRAF, ERBB4, JAK2, NRAS, PDGFRA, PIK3C2B, PIK3CA. MLPA assays were carried in total DNA from the eleven cell lines, obtained by standard methods, following manufacturers' conditions. Polymerase chain reaction products were separated and quantified on an ABI PRISM 310 DNA sequencer (Applied Biosystems), and electropherograms were analyzed using GeneMapper v.3.7 software (Applied Biosystems). Three nontumor reference samples were included in each run.

5.4 EGFRvIII analysis

Presence of EGFR vIII variant was determined by RT-PCR from total RNA of the cell cultures. cDNA was obtained from 1μg of total RNA using the Superscript System (Gibco®). Primers and PCR conditions used were previously described (Lee et al, 2006). Amplifications products were visualized in bromure ethydium 2% agarose gel.

5.5 EGFR and PTEN sequence analysis

Mutations in exons 1 to 9 of PTEN gene and 18 to 21 of the EGFR gene were screened by direct sequencing in an ABI PRISM 310 DNA Analyser (Applied Biosystems) according to the manufacturer's instructions. PCR primers and conditions for EGFR amplification were previously described (Hsieh et al, 2006).

Exon	Upstream primer 5'-3'	Downstream primer 5'-3'	Annealing T (°C)
1	TCCTCCTTTTTCTTCAGCCAC	GAAAGGTAAAGAGGAGCAGCC	56
2	GCTGCATATTTCAATCAAACTAA	ACATCAATATTTGAAATAGAAAATC	54
3	TGTTAATGGTGGCTTTTTG	GCAAGCATACAAATAAGAAAAC	56
4	TTCCTAAGTGCAAAAGATAAC	TACAGTCTATCGGGTTTAAGT	56
5	TTTTTTTTTCTTATTCTGAGGTTAT	GAAGAGGAAAGGAAAAACATC	51
6	AGTGAAATAACTATAATGGAACA	GAAGGATGAGAATTTCAAGC	54
7	AATACTGGTATGTATTTAACCAT	TCTCCCAATGAAAGTAAAGTA	56
8	TTTTTAGGACAAAATGTTTCAC	CCCACAAAATGTTTAATTTAAC	54
9	GTTTTCATTTTAAATTTTCTTTC	TGGTGTTTTATCCCTCTTG	54

Table 7. PTEN sequence and annealing temperature used for PCR reactions of nine exon primers

6. Conclusion

High-level copy number alterations have been observed in cell lines of different sources such as breast, melanoma or lung tumors. Some authors suggest that some of the commonly seen alterations in the glioma cell lines can be due to the *in vitro* cell growth process following long term passage cultures. These observations are based on (i) the comparison of the genomic alterations of glioma and other non glioma cancer cell lines: some of these alterations are common between established cancer cell lines from different origin and uncommon in glioma tumors (Li et al, 2008). ii) Differential expression analyses suggest that established cancer cell lines share an underlying molecular similarity more closely related to their *in vitro* culture conditions than to their original tumor type of origin. Although some functional signalling pathways are up-regulated both in glioma tumors and glioma cell lines (epidermal growth factor receptor, vascular endothelial growth factor receptor, p53, PI3K pathway), there are some others gene expression sets whose up-regulation is just seen in cancer cell lines (cell cycle, proteasome activity, purine metabolism, mitochondrial activity).
Our findings show that established glioma cell lines and glioma tumours have differences in genomic alterations, concluding that glioma cell lines may not be such an accurate representation or model system for primary gliomas as would be desirable. As opposed to primary tumors, glioma cell lines did not present either *EGFR* amplification, or presence of EGFRvIII variant, events that are frequent in high-grade gliomas. Homozygous *CDKN2A* deletion was frequently observed in glioma cell lines, as occur in cell lines derived from other histologies and in glioma tumors. Chromosome 7 gain and *PTEN* deletions represent the most specific glioma alterations present in these cell lines.
The easy of management of glioma cell lines make these cell lines as good candidate models for exploring basic glioma biology and for the use and discovery of therapeutic agents in preclinical screens. However, it is of interest that cell clycle-related alterations of gene expression are importantly affected in these cell lines, and that most drugs have been tested for cytotoxicity against rapidly dividing cells. Therefore, selection bias toward the identification of therapeutic agents involved in molecular functions more related to the long term culture than to glioma biology could occur.
On the other hand, many efforts are being done to create adequate culture conditions that allow the maintenance of the genomic profiles of the original tumor, such as glioma stem-like cell cultures, which may be more representative of their parent tumors. Several reports have demonstrated that glioma cultures under serum free conditions and stimulated with mitogens, epidermal growth factor and fibroblast growth factor, grow as neurospheres and maintain a phenotype and genotype closer to that typical of primary tumours compared to traditional serum-derived cell lines and culture techniques (Fael Al-Mayhani et al, 2009; Ernst et al, 2009). Perhaps, the standardization of this culture method could enhance and improve the research with cell lines in brain tumors.

7. Acknowledgment

We gratefully acknowledge Drs. G. Velasco and F. Setien for kindly provinding cell lines. This work was partially supported by grants G-2009_E/04 from Fundación Sociosanitaria de Castilla-La Mancha and the Consejería de Salud y Bienestar Social, Junta de Comunidades de Castilla-La Mancha; and FIS PI07/0662, FIS10/01974 from the Fondo de Investigaciones Sanitarias (FIS) of the Instituto de Salud Carlos III (Spain).

8. References

Bar, E.E, Lin, A., Tihan, T., Burger, P.C. & Eberhart C.G. (2008) Frequent gains at chromosome 7q34 involving BRAF in pilocytic astrocytoma. Journal of Neuropathology and Experimental Neurology (September 2008) Vol. 67, No. 9, pp 878-887. ISSN 0022-3069

Blesa, D., Mollejo, M., Ruano, Y, Rodriguez de Lope, A., Fiaño, F., Ribalta, T., García, J., Campos-Martin, Y., Hernandez-Moneo, J., Cigudosa, J., Melendez, B. (2009) Novel genomic alterations and mechanisms associated with tumor progression in oligodendroglioma and mixed oligoastrocytoma. *Journal of Neuropathology and Experimental Neurology*. Vol.68, No.3, (March 2009), pp 274-285 ISSN ISSN 0022-3069

Das, A., Tan, W.L., Teo, J. & Smith, D.R.(2002) Expression of survivin in primary glioblastomas. *Journal of Cancer Research and Clinical Oncology*, (June 2002), Vol. 128, No. 6, pp 302-306. ISSN: 1432-1335

Ernst, A., Hofmann, S., Ahmadi, R., Becker, N., Korshunov, A., Engel, F., et al. (2009). Genomic and expression profiling of glioblastoma stem cell-like spheroid cultures identifies novel tumor-relevant genes associated with survival. *Clinical Cancer Research*. Vol. 15, No. 21, (November 2009), pp 6541-6550, ISSN 1078-0432

Fael Al-Mayhania, T., Balla, S., Zhaoa, J., Fawcetta, J., Ichimurab, K., Collins, P. & Watts, C. (2009) An efficient method for derivation and propagation of glioblastoma cell lines that conserves the molecular profile of their original tumours . *Journal of Neuroscience Methods* (July 2008), Vol.176, pp 192-199. ISSN 0165- 0270

Greshock, J., Nathanson, K., Martin, AM, Zhang, L., Coukos, G., Weber, BL. & Zaks, Z. (2007) Cancer Cell Lines as Genetic Models of Their Parent Histology: Analyses Based on Array Comparative Genomic Hybridization. *Cancer Research. Vol.* 67, No. 8, (April 2007), pp. 3594-3600, ISSN 0008-5472

Hsieh, MH., Fang, YF., Chang, WC., Kuo, H., Lin, S.Y., Liu, H., Liu, C., Chen, HC., Ku, Y., Chen, Y.T., Chang, Y.H., Chen, Y.T., His, B., Tsai, S., Huang, S.F. (2006) Complex mutation patterns of epidermal growth factor receptor gene associated with variable responses to gefitinib treatment in patients with non-small cell lung cancer. *Lung Cancer (*September 2006), Vol.53, No.3, pp 311-322. ISSN 0169-5002

Karakas, B., Bachman, K.E. & Park, B.h. (2006) Mutation of the PI3KCA oncogene in human cancers British Journal of Cancer (January 2006), Vol. 94, pp 455-459, ISSN 1532-1827

Kita, D., Yonekawa, Y., Weller, M. & Ohgaki, H. (2007) PI3KCA alterations in primary (de novo) and secondary glioblastomas. *Acta Neuropathologica* (January 2007), Vol. 113, pp 295–302. ISSN 1432-0533

Lee, J., Vivanco, I., Beroukhim, R., Huang, J., Feng, W., DeBiasil, R. et al. (2006) Epidermal growth factor receptor activation in glioblastoma through novel missense mutations in the extracellular domain. PLOS Medicine (December 2006), Vol. 3, No.12. pp 2264-2273. ISSN 15491676

Li, A., Walling, J., Kotliarow, Y., Center, A., et al. (2008) Genomic changes and gene expression profiles reveal that established glioma cell lines are poorly representative of primary human gliomas. *Molecular Cancer Research* (January 2008), Vol. 6, No.1, pp 21–30. ISSN 1541-7786

Lopez-Gines, C., Gil-Benso, R., Ferrer-Luna, R., Benito, R. , Serna, E., Gonzalez-Darder, J., Quilis, V., Monleon, D., Celda, B., Cerdá-Nicolas, M. (2010) New pattern of EGFR amplification in glioblastoma and the relationship of gene copy number with gene expression profile. *Modern Pathology* (June 2010), Vol.23, No.6, pp 856-865. ISSN 0893-3952

Louis, DN., Ohgaki, H. Wiestler, OD., Cavenee, WKK. (2007). *WHO classification of tumours of the central nervous system,* (3rd edition), IARC Press, ISBN 9789283224303, Lyon, France.

Naylor, T.L., Greshock, J., Wang, Y., Colligon, T., Yu, Q.C., Clemmer, V., Zaks, T.Z., Weber, B.L. (2005) High resolution genomic analysis of sporadic breast cancer using array-based comparative genomic hybridization. *Breast Cancer Research* (October 2005), Vol. 7, No.6, pp 1186-1198, ISSN 1465-5411

Parsons, D.W., Jones, S., Zhang, X., Lin, J.C., Leary, R.J., Angenendt, P., Mankoo, P., Carter H., Siu, I.M., Gallia, G.L., Olivi, A., McLendon, R., Rasheed, B.A., Keir, S., Nikolskaya, T., Nikolsky, Y., Busam, D.A., Tekleab, H., Diaz, LA., Hartigan, J., Smith, D.R., Strausberg, R., Marie, S., Shinjo, S.M., Yan, H., Riggins, G., Bigner, D., Karchin, R., Papadopoulos, N., Parmigiani, G., Vogelstein, B., Velculescu, V.E., Kinzler, K.W. (2008) An integrated genomic analysis of human glioblastoma multiforme. *Science* (September 2008) Vol.26, No.321, pp 1807-1812. ISSN 1095-9203

Rao, S., Edwards, J., Joshi, A., Siu, M., Riggins, G (2009) A survey of glioblastoma genomic amplifications and deletions. *Journal of Neuro-oncology* (July 2009) Vol. 93, pp 169-179. ISSN: 1573-7373

Riemenschneider, MJ., Jeuken, JWM., Wesseling, P., Reifenberger, G. (2010) Molecular diagnostics of gliomas: state of the art. *Acta Neuropathologica,* (July 2010) Vol. 120, No. 5 , pp 567-584, ISSN 1432-0533

Ruano, Y., Mollejo, M., Ribalta T., et al. (2006) Identification of novel candidate target genes in amplicons of Glioblastoma multiforme tumors detected by expression and CGH microarray profiling. *Molecular Cancer.* (September 2006), Vol. 5, No.39, pp 44-55, ISSN 1476-4598

Sasaki, T., Lopes. M.B., Hankins, G.R. & Helm, G.A. (2002) Expression of surviving, an inhibitor of apoptosis protein, in tumors of the nervous system. *Acta Neuropathologica* (July 2002), Vol. 104, No.1, pp 105-109, ISSN 1432-0533

Sharma, SV., Haber DA. & Settleman, J.(2010) Cell line-based platforms to evaluatethe therapeutic efficacy of candidate anticancer agents. *Nature Reviews Cancer,* (April 2010), Vol. 10, No. 4, pp.241-253. ISSN:1474-1768

Shirai, K., Suzuki, Y., Oka, K., Noda, S., Katoh, H., Suzuki, Y., Itoh, J., Itoh, H., Ishiuchi, S., Sakurai, H., Hasegawa, M., Nakano, T. (2009) Nuclear survivin expression predicts poorer prognosis in glioblastoma. *Journal of Neuro-Oncology,* Vol. 91, No.3, (February 2009) pp 353-358. ISSN: 1573-7373

Vogt, P.K., Bader, A.G. & Kang, S. (2006) PI3-Kinases, Hidden Potentials Revealed. *Cell cycle* (May 2006), Vol. 5, No.9 pp 946-949, ISSN: 1551-4005

Zhen, H., Zhang, X., Hu, P., Yang, T., Fei, Z. et al. (2005) Survivin expression and its relation with proliferation, apoptosis, and angiogenesis in brain gliomas. *Cancer* (April 2005) Vol. 104, pp 2775-2783, ISSN: 1097-0142

Part 6

Miscellaneous

20

Oxidative Stress and Glutamate Release in Glioma

Robert Ungard and Gurmit Singh
McMaster University
Canada

1. Introduction

Glioma are a family of glial cell tumours of the central nervous system (CNS) well-characterized as aggressive cancers with dismally limited treatment options. The relatively recent discoveries of mechanisms surrounding glioma cell antioxidant protection and neuronal and glial cell destruction have opened the gates to a new therapeutic avenue whose implications to the field of cancer biology extend far beyond the treatment of glioma alone. Stemming from the discovery of significant glutamate release and glutathione production by glioma cells, the mechanisms through which glioma mediate oxidative stress and influence their extracellular microenvironment are now being unravelled.

This chapter will discuss the upregulation of the cystine/glutamate antiporter, system x_c^-, in glioma and the far ranging consequences that stem from this compensatory action. Specifically, a characteristic shift of cancer cell metabolism away from the tricarboxylic acid (TCA) cycle and towards increased rates of glycolysis, a process termed the Warburg effect, produces a high amount of reactive oxygen species (ROS) that would prove cytotoxic without adequate cellular antioxidant defences. In response to this metabolic abnormality, glioma have demonstrated increased synthesis of the primary cellular antioxidant glutathione and an increased circulation of the cystine/cysteine redox cycle. These antioxidant increases are driven by an upregulation of system x_c^-, which supplies the cell with the rate limiting substrate for glutathione synthesis, cysteine, and acts as one half of the transport machinery for the cystine/cysteine cycle. The increased tolerance to oxidative stress that is conferred by these mechanisms allows glioma survival and growth advantages and mediate chemo- and radiation-resistance to treatment. The corollary effect of cystine import *via* system x_c^- is the export of the neurotransmitter and ubiquitous cell-signalling molecule, glutamate. This release has destructive consequences for the peritumoral brain. Glutamate induces neuronal and glial excitotoxic cell death, and acts in an autocrine and paracrine signalling manner to stimulate glioma cell growth and migration. Treatments based on these mechanisms are currently under development and some have progressed as far as clinical trials. Glutamate receptor antagonists and system x_c^- inhibitors are as of yet the primary avenues of investigation. The potential treatment benefits of targeting these pathways are great, and the discovery of system x_c^- prevalence in other cancers beyond glioma suggests that study of this pathway may produce wide-ranging cancer treatment options.

2. Glioma metabolism and oxidative stress

Cancer cells exist under self-induced conditions of abnormally elevated oxidative stress resulting from a characteristic shift in glucose metabolism away from the TCA cycle and towards a high rate of aerobic glycolysis (Kroemer & Pouyssegur, 2008). This metabolic shift results in less efficient ATP production from glucose by the cell, but serves to confer unique benefits upon the cancer cell allowing survival in conditions of high proliferation, high oxidative stress, and varying access to blood vasculature. One adaptive characteristic of cancer cells is the upregulation of antioxidant defence mechanisms, necessary for protection from the high level of ROS generated by escalated glycolysis.

2.1 Cancer cell metabolism

In normal cells, the metabolism of glucose generates ATP through glycolysis followed by a high rate of pyruvate metabolism through the TCA cycle. The final electron acceptor in the TCA cycle is oxygen, without which, the cycle ceases to function, and pyruvate is converted to lactate *via* anaerobic glycolysis (Kim & Dang, 2006). Anaerobic glycolysis is prevalent in hypoxic environments when the TCA cycle has no access to oxygen, however, glycolysis is also predominant in cancer cells even during aerobic conditions (Kim & Dang, 2006). This phenomenon of cancer cell metabolism was first described in the 1920s by Nobel laureate Otto Warburg and is to this day termed the Warburg effect, or aerobic glycolysis (Warburg et al., 1927). Most cancer cells, limited with regards to energy production by their shift away from the efficiency of the TCA cycle, rely upon an increased rate of glucose uptake for glycolytic ATP production. This allows the cell a number of advantages including the use of glycolytic intermediates for anabolic reactions, without which, rapidly proliferating cells in conditions of fluctuating oxygen availability could not survive (See review by Kroemer & Pouyssegur, 2008). All aerobic respiration generates ROS which induces oxidative damage within the cell (Balendiran et al., 2004). The enhanced metabolic activity of cancer cells raises ROS production to a level that demands adaptation by the cell to survive and proliferate despite the resulting high level of oxidative stress (Halliwell, 2007). The Warburg effect has been identified as a key factor in the increased oxidative stress that cancer cells face, and has also been directly implicated in the activation of oncogenes and the loss of tumour suppressor genes (Le et al., 2010).

2.2 Glutathione synthesis response

Glutathione (GSH) is a tripeptide thiol synthesized intracellularly from the amino acids glutamate, cysteine and glycine. In the cell it performs a number of functions, one of which is as the predominant cellular antioxidant in the body (Meister, 1995). GSH fulfils this role by acting as a substrate for several antioxidant enzymes as well as by acting directly upon free radicals in its reduced form, GSH, or in its oxidized form, glutathione disulfide (Meister, 1995). The rate-limiting step in GSH biosynthesis is the availability of cysteine, which in glioma cannot be synthesized intracellularly (Ishii et al., 1992). In glioma, increased oxidation of intracellular GSH and elevated oxidative stress induce the upregulation of cystine transport into the cell, allowing the dual processes of increased GSH biosynthesis, and increased cycling of the cystine/cysteine redox cycle, both of which counter the effects of ROS mediated damage (Banjac et al., 2008; Chung et al., 2005).

3. The System x_c^- antiporter and glioma

In several cancers including glioma, cysteine must be obtained through the import of cystine from the extracellular environment. Cystine is imported into the cell *via* the system x_c^- cystine/glutamate antiporter; a transporter that is a feature of many cancer cell lines and endogenous to many tissues in the body. Cystine is the oxidized form of the amino acid, comprised of two cysteine molecules joined by a covalent double bond, and more prevalent in the oxidizing extracellular space. In the reducing environment of the cell, imported cystine is rapidly reduced to cysteine which is then incorporated as a substrate in GSH biosynthesis or serves to propel the cystine/cysteine redox cycle that plays a large role in maintaining extracellular redox balance (Ishii et al., 1992). The exported glutamate can have a number of deleterious effects upon the surrounding host tissue, many of which favour cancer cell survival and progression (Ishii et al., 1992).

3.1 System x_c^-

System x_c^- is the name given to the Na^+ independent electroneutral exchanger of cystine and glutamate first described in human fibroblasts by Bannai & Kitamura (1980), and later named by Makowske & Christensen (1982). It is classified within the family of heteromeric amino acid transporters, all of which are comprised of a single heavy polypeptide subunit (SLC3 family) and a single light subunit (SLC7 family) coupled *via* a disulfide bridge (Chillarón et al., 2001). These transporters are essential for the import of amino acids to the cell that cannot be intracellularly synthesized. In system x_c^- the heavy subunit is 4F2hc (SLC3A2), a type II membrane glycoprotein common to many amino acid transporters (Verrey et al., 2004). It plays a regulatory role, functioning to traffic and adhere the transporter complex to the cell membrane. It features one transmembrane domain, and has a molecular weight of ~85 kDa (Lim & Donaldson, 2010). 4F2hc is not essential to the transport action of system x_c^-, and can be supplanted with another heavy chain polypeptide with similar transport and adherence capabilities, (ex. rBAT) without losing antiporter function (Wang et al., 2003). The light subunit of system x_c^- is xCT (SLC7A11), which is entirely responsible for the amino acid exchange function of the transporter and unique to system x_c^-. It features 12 transmembrane domains, and has a molecular weight of ~55 kDa (Lim & Donaldson, 2010). Cystine and glutamate are exchanged with a 1:1 stoichiometry that does not require an ionic gradient, rather it is thought that glutamate, which must be eliminated from the cytosol to prevent toxicity, provides the concentration gradient necessary for transporter function (Bannai & Ishii, 1988).

3.1.1 System x_c^- in glia

System x_c^- is expressed endogenously in a number of tissues in the body. In the human brain, it is a feature of both neurons and glial cells. Specifically, xCT was found to be expressed in neurons of the cerebral cortex, GFAP positive glial cells, vascular endothelial cells and the leptomeninges (Burdo et al., 2006). The prominence of system x_c^- in the brain is thought to be related to the organ's relatively high rate of glucose metabolism and the need for antioxidants to protect highly sensitive neurons from the resulting ROS production (Conrad & Sato, 2011). The expression of xCT fluctuates greatly, and can be readily induced under a number of stimuli including low levels of extracellular cystine (Bannai & Kitamura, 1982), and oxidative stress (Bannai et al., 1991). In astrocytes, the induced upregulation of xCT increased GSH synthesis and release and conferred antioxidant protection on immature neurons in an *in vitro* co-culture model (Shih et al., 2006). Due to its critical role in maintaining antioxidant and glutamate balance, the misregulation of system x_c^- has the potential for great damage, and the transporter has been implicated in a number of CNS pathologies, including some characteristic features of morbidity in glioma.

3.1.2 System x_c^- in glioma

The ability of xCT to be readily induced upon exposure to oxidative stress or cysteine deficit is thought to be responsible for the presence of system x_c^- as a cell-culture induced artifact in some cell lines. In glioma cell lines this is not the case; system x_c^- has not only been demonstrated in established cell lines (Chung et al., 2005), but also in normal glia (Burdo et al., 2006), and in glioma tumour samples from patients (Lyons et al., 2007).

In glioma, glucose metabolism is significantly escalated, as is characteristic of cancer cell metabolism. The resulting increase in the production of ROS from aerobic glycolysis induces the upregulation of xCT expression (Kim et al., 2001). With 4F2hc present in abundance, this xCT increase is sufficient to initiate an upregulation of system x_c^- characteristic of glioma (Sontheimer, 2008). The consequences of this system x_c^- upregulation are immensely detrimental to the patient as a result of both of the substrate actions of the antiporter. The greater import of cystine by system x_c^- allows the cell to survive and proliferate in conditions of oxidative stress that would be lethal to other cells. This increased resistance has a destructive outcome for the patient, allowing the glioma to survive and progress to a greater extent, and endowing the cell with resistance to cancer treatments, many of which attack cancer cells through increased oxidative stress. The simultaneous export of high levels of glutamate into the microenvironment of glutamate-sensitive brain tissues induces neuron and glial cell death and promotes the growth and migration of the tumour. These uniquely destructive outcomes from the action of system x_c^- ultimately aid the progression of the cancer. (See Fig. 1 concept model).

4. System x_c^- and oxidative stress in glioma

The upregulation of xCT readily occurs in response to oxidative stress. To mediate oxidative damage, the system x_c^- antiporter acts in two cystine-dependent manners to provide antioxidant capabilities to the cell and surrounding microenvironment. By increasing the availability of intracellular cysteine, this rate-limiting substrate is provided for both the synthesis of GSH, and for the completion of one half of the cystine/cysteine redox cycle.

4.1 System x_c^- drives glutathione synthesis

Within the cell, the tripeptide GSH is synthesized from its constituent amino acids, glycine, glutamate and cysteine *via* the enzymes γ-glutamylcysteine synthetase, adding glutamate; and glutathione synthetase, adding glycine in two steps (See Fig. 2). Oxidized GSH can be reduced back to its active form *via* glutathione reductase (Conrad & Sato, 2011). The rate-limiting factor in this pathway is the availability of intracellular cysteine (Ishii et al., 1987). Most mammalian cells have the ability to directly import cysteine with a number of transporters (Lo et al., 2008), however cysteine is not prevalent in the extracellular space to the degree of cystine. Upon export from the cell, cysteine, the reduced and more prominent intracellular form of the amino acid, is rapidly oxidized to cystine, which is vastly more

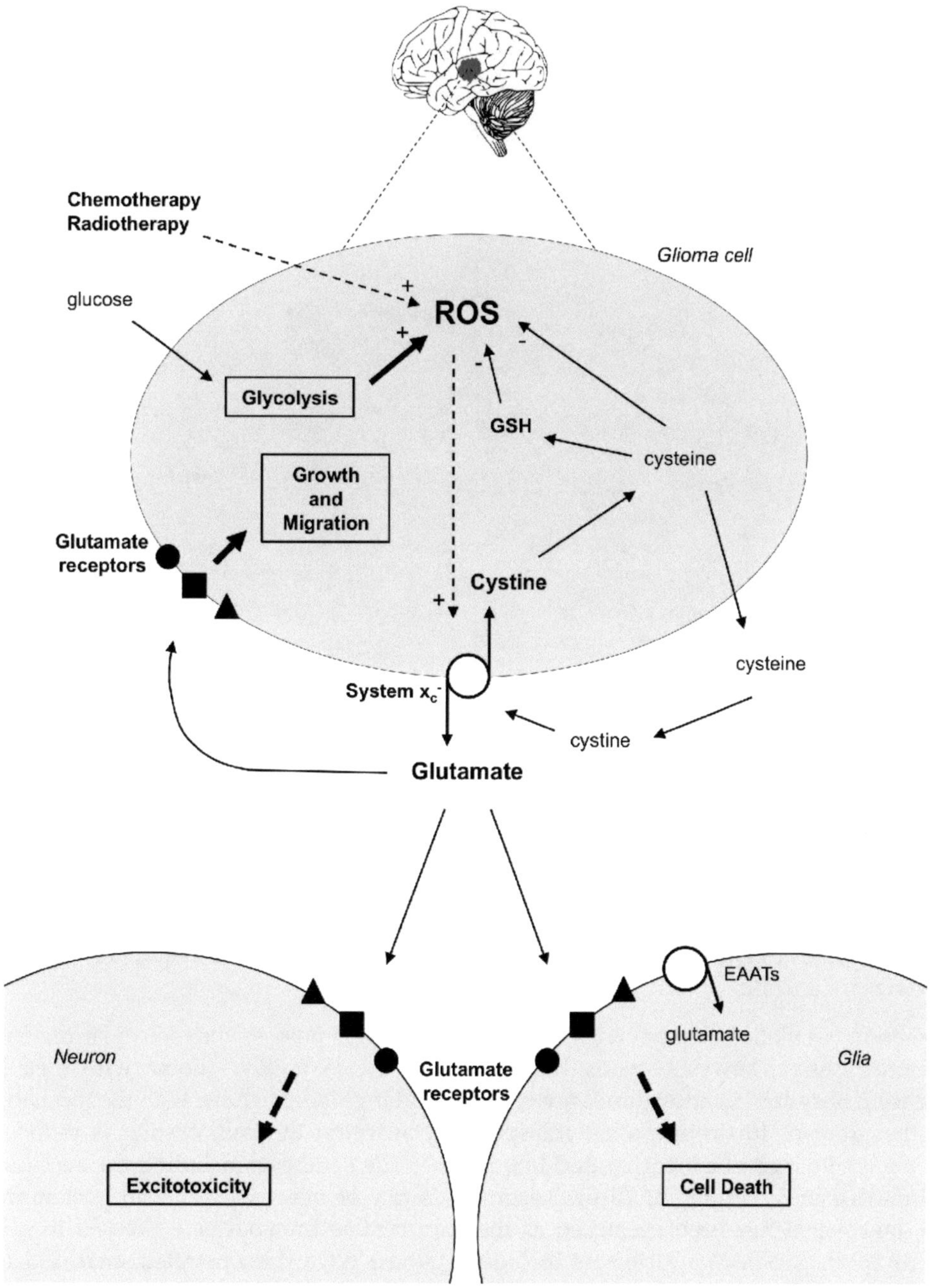

Fig. 1. Summary concept model demonstrating the impact of altered cancer cell metabolism and cytotoxic treatments on cellular ROS, the upregulation of system x_c^-, and the consequent import of cystine and export of glutamate. Cystine import allows the synthesis of GSH and the cycling of the cystine/cysteine redox cycle. The export of glutamate has cytotoxic effects on brain cells within the tumour microenvironment, and autocrine and paracrine effects on the glioma initiating growth and increased migration.

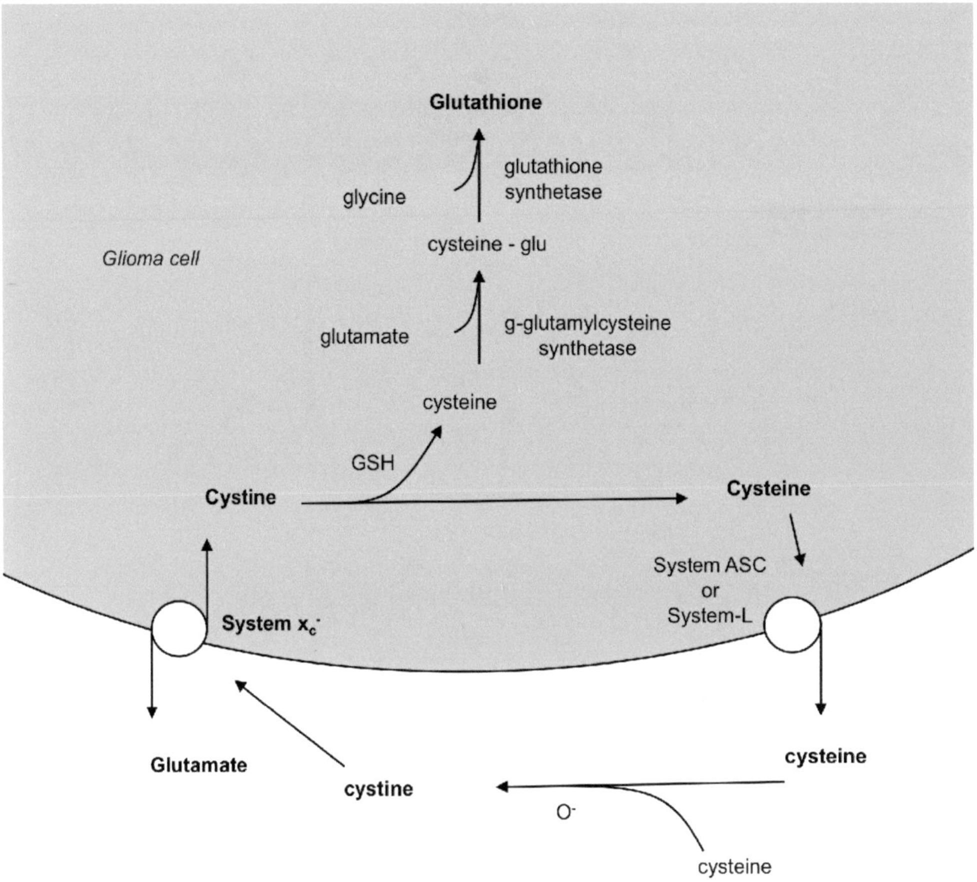

Fig. 2. Glutathione biosynthesis and the cystine/cysteine redox cycle as driven by amino acid transporters in glioma. Glutamate is secreted by system x_c^- which requires both substrates to function.

common in circulation (Bannai & Ishii, 1988). Not all cells possess the molecular machinery to import cystine, however, many brain cells and consequently, glioma with their high expression of system x_c^- and abundance of intracellular glutamate have both the mechanisms and the gradient to drive cystine transport. Once inside the cell, cystine is reduced to cysteine where it can be incorporated into polypeptide synthesis including the synthesis of GSH (Savaskan & Eyüpoglu, 2010). System x_c^- is one of many cystine transporters in the CNS, however it has been identified as the only cystine transporter expressed in glioma (Chung et al., 2005). Many cancers including glioma have demonstrated increased basal levels of intracellular GSH (Louw et al., 1997). Pharmacological inhibition of system x_c^-, and therefore limitation or elimination of available intracellular cysteine is able to deplete intracellular GSH almost entirely in a dose and time-dependent manner in glioma cell lines (Chung et al., 2005; Chung & Sontheimer, 2009; Pham et al., 2010). The negative effects of this GSH limitation on cell growth can be rescued entirely by the introduction of membrane permeable exogenous GSH, suggesting that cysteine availability for GSH production is critical for glioma cell growth (Chung & Sontheimer, 2009).

4.2 System x_c^- drives the cystine/cysteine redox cycle

As cysteine is rate-limiting in GSH synthesis, it is well expected that increased availability of the amino acid from system x_c^- upregulation would have the observed positive impact on GSH levels. Increased cystine import in glioma has also been demonstrated to drive the cystine/cysteine redox cycle across the cell membrane, which acts independently of GSH to counter ROS. To cycle the amino acid , cystine is imported by system x_c^-, where it is promptly reduced in the cytoplasm, likely by GSH, and conversely cysteine is exported by the amino acid transporters system-L or system ASC to the extracellular environment where it is promptly oxidized (Conrad & Sato, 2011). It was discovered in xCT induced lymphoma cells that the cystine/cysteine cycle raised concentrations of extracellular cysteine and acted as an effective antioxidant even in cases of GSH depletion (Banjac et al., 2008). A subsequent study found that in cells negative for γ-glutamylcysteine synthetase and therefore unable to produce GSH, the cystine/cysteine cycle was sufficient to maintain oxidative stress protection (Mandal et al., 2010). This suggests that alternative redox systems can compensate for each other to the point of redundancy, and in this case, both cycles are driven by the import of cystine (Mandal et al., 2010). Both this redox cycle and GSH synthesis are enabled by the actions of system x_c^- and in glioma, both confer protection from oxidative stress to the cell.

4.3 Consequences of ROS resistance

The upregulation of antioxidant defences in glioma cells confers proliferation and survival benefits to glioma above those of normal cells without which, glioma could not thrive in their self-induced oxidative environment. The ability of glioma to upregulate antioxidant production in the face of ROS has long been suspected to contribute to the chemotherapy and radiation-resistance that is devastatingly common in the treatment of glioma, a condition already characterized by poor prognoses (Sontheimer, 2008). A large scale microarray to coordinate transporter gene expression in 60 cancer cell lines with the activity of 1400 anticancer drugs revealed 39 drugs that positively correlate with SLC7a11 (xCT) expression and 296 that negatively correlate (Huang & Sadée, 2006). An example of a positively correlating drug is L-alanosine, an amino acid analogue whose uptake is mediated by system x_c^-. The authors demonstrated that pharmacologic system x_c^- inhibition reduced the efficacy of L-alanosine by impeding its system x_c^- mediated uptake. A negatively correlating drug is geldanamycin, an antibiotic that targets heat shock protein 90 (Hsp90). System x_c^- inhibition increased the efficacy of geldanamycin through a reduction of intracellular GSH which reduced cellular resistance to the drug's cytotoxicity (Huang et al., 2005). Celastrol is another Hsp90 targeting drug that has demonstrated antitumoral properties specifically in glioma, and is also very negatively correlated with SLC7a11 expression (Huang et al., 2008). Inhibition of system x_c^- in celastrol-resistant glioma cells reduced chemoresistance to celastrol treatment, as did other negative modulators of GSH synthesis, indicating that celastrol resistance in glioma is at least in part mediated through the availability of GSH (Pham et al., 2010).

5. System x_c^- and glutamate

The corollary effect of system x_c^- mediated cystine uptake is the necessary secretion of glutamate into the extracellular space, without which system x_c^- cannot function. It has been demonstrated that glioma cells secrete amounts of glutamate *via* this mechanism that are significant enough to mediate excitotoxic cell death in the brain (Sontheimer, 2003; Takano et al., 2001; Ye & Sontheimer, 1999). The amino acid glutamate is most well known as the primary excitatory neurotransmitter in the CNS, however it also functions as a growth factor and motogen to different cell types in the brain (de Groot & Sontheimer, 2010), and mediates critical cell signalling in many non-neuronal tissues (Hinoi et al., 2004).

5.1 Glutamate release

The normal brain usually does not harbour extracellular glutamate in excess of 1-3μM, likely due to the glutamate reuptake mechanisms of glia (de Groot & Sontheimer, 2010). *In vitro*, astrocyte cultures demonstrate the ability to reduce extracellular glutamate concentrations to near 1μM from 92μM within 3 hours, while conversely several glioma cell lines raised extracellular glutamate to 400-500μM in a 12-hour period (Ye & Sontheimer, 1999). When neurons were grown in co-culture or treated with media from independent glioma cultures, neurons died from glutamate-mediated excitotoxicity (Ye & Sontheimer, 1999). In normal brain, glutamate released into the extracellular space is rapidly removed, either back into the presynaptic nerve terminal, or, more commonly, by glial cells *via* one of the excitatory amino acid transporters (EAAT1 or EAAT2) (Danbolt, 2001). Glutamate reuptake is a key feature of normal glial cells that surround the synaptic cleft, a mechanism that contributes to neuron protection and signal consistency (de Groot & Sontheimer, 2010). It has been demonstrated by microarray that EAAT2 expression in glioma is negatively correlated with tumour progression, and that induction of glioma with EAAT2 expression dose-dependently limits cell growth, suggesting that the loss of EAAT function in glioma cells may play a role in the accumulation of extracellular glutamate (de Groot et al., 2005). Glutamate release from glioma was confirmed *in vivo* through glioma cells implanted into rat brain. Glutamate was measured to be highest in peritumoral regions, significantly higher than in the normal brain and the tumour itself (Behrens et al., 2000; Takano et al., 2001). Cells of the same type cloned as to not release glutamate grew significantly smaller tumours than their glutamate-releasing counterparts (Takano et al., 2001). In glioma patients, despite conflicting reports, it appears that glutamate concentrations are significantly elevated in glioma in both the tumour (Behrens et al., 2000) and the peritumoural region (Roslin et al., 2003).

5.2 Consequences of glutamate release

Glutamate release into the peritumoral environment has a number of cytotoxic and cell signalling effects whose results are advantageous to glioma and seriously deleterious to the host. It has been suggested that glutamate release confers an adaptive advantage upon glioma (Sontheimer, 2003), but it is also possible that the release in great quantities of such a ubiquitous signalling molecule into a tissue that is highly sensitive to such molecules exerts a disruptive influence simply as a side-effect. This has also been demonstrated as a feature of glutamate-releasing cancers metastasized to bone, a tissue where glutamate is an important intercellular communication molecule (Seidlitz et al., 2010).

Glioma exist in an environment physically constrained to the cavity of the cranium, a space consumed by 85% tissue and 15% cerebrospinal fluid (CSF). To grow, glioma must create space to occupy, as compression cannot occur in a vessel filled with fluid. Glutamate-induced excitotoxic cell death is thought to be principally responsible for the clearance of brain cells along the tumour borders that allows glioma progression. Indicating the succeptability of brain tissues to glutamatergic disruption is that no cell type in the brain is without receptors for glutamate. The inhibition of system x_c^- in glioma significantly reduces extracellular glutamate levels, as well as neurodegeneration and cellular edema both *in vitro* and *in vivo,* indicating the role of system x_c^- in the induction of these morbidities (Savaskan et al., 2008). Excitotoxicity is thought to be initiated as a result of excessive activation of glutamate receptors resulting in the uncontrolled increase of intracellular Ca^{2+} which stimulates the activation of cytotoxic enzymes (Choi, 1988). Neurons possess both the ionotropic α-amino-3-hydroxy-5-methyl-4-isoaxazolepropionate acid (AMPA) glutamate receptors, and N-methyl-D-aspartate (NMDA) glutamate receptors for excitatory glutamate signal transmission. Neurons in coculture and *in vivo* were shown to be highly sensitive to excitotoxic cell death when exposed to glutamate release from glioma (Takano et al., 2001). Treatment with the NMDA receptor antagonist MK801 reduced but did not entirely eliminate this excitotoxicity (Takano et al., 2001).

Normal glial cells are also highly receptive to glutamate. Oligodendrocytes demonstrate a similar low tolerance to glutamate exposure as neurons, while astrocytes can tolerate much higher concentrations (Oka et al., 1993). Astrocytes normally function to remove glutamate from the extracellular space, so their tolerance to high glutamate concentrations is not surprising; however they too are eventually killed by an expanding glioma. Whether this cell death is also mediated by exposure to glutamate is not yet understood (de Groot & Sontheimer, 2010).

It has also been reported that glutamate may have an autocrine or paracrine signalling effect on glioma cells. AMPA, NMDA, Kainate, and the metabotropic glutamate receptors mGluR3 and mGLuR5 have all been identified in glioma, and growth-effects have been demonstrated through manipulation of both AMPA and NMDA receptors. Most glioma express AMPA receptors that are permeable to Ca^{2+} upon activation by glutamate (Ishiuchi et al., 2007). Induced expression of the GluR2 receptor subunit which renders AMPA receptors Ca^{2+} impermeable sensitized glioma cells to apoptosis and reduced tumour growth *in vivo,* suggesting the ability of glioma-derived glutamate signalling through AMPA receptors to act in an autocrine/paracrine manner to stimulate cell growth (Ishiuchi et al., 2007).

Exogenous glutamate has a stimulatory effect on growth when applied to glioma cells, and conversely, antiproliferative effects on glioma have been demonstrated individually with several AMPA receptor antagonists and several NMDA receptor antagonists (Rzeski et al., 2001). Inhibition of mGlu2/3 receptors with the antagonist LY341495 in glioma cells positive for both receptors also was able to reduce glioma cell growth both *in vitro* and *in vivo* (Arcella et al., 2005). Taken together, these results obtained through the blockade of nearly all glutamate receptors expressed in glioma suggest a significant autocrine/paracrine effect on growth of glioma-derived glutamate.

6. Experimental therapeutics

The myriad consequences originating from the upregulation of xCT in glioma have uncovered several novel possibilities for treatment of glioma. Any therapeutic targeting of the mechanisms of antioxidant production and glutamate release could prove to be critical in the treatment of glioma, as current therapies are limited in efficacy and often become redundant through acquired cell-resistance (Sontheimer, 2008). Symptom management may also arise from treating glutamate release, as it is hypothesized that frequent seizures, a morbidity that affects over 80% of glioma sufferers could be related to glutamate-induced hyperexcitability in the CNS, possibly in advance of neuron excitotoxic death and possibly an early indication of the cancer (de Groot & Sontheimer, 2010).

6.1 Targeting glutamate receptors

AMPA receptor targeting has emerged as the most prolific avenue of interest for treatment from glioma glutamate-release work. An AMPA antagonist called talampanel is currently the most likely candidate for glioma treatment in this manner in large part because it does not exhibit the side-effects of most glutamate receptor antagonists in the CNS, and it has been shown to increase the lifespan of mice xenografted with human glioma (Goudar et al., 2004). Two clinical trials have developed from these findings. The first, begun in 2009, was a phase II trial designed to examine the efficacy of talampanel in conjunction with standard radiation and temozolomide treatments in improving survival in adults with newly diagnosed glioblastoma (Grossman et al., 2009). This trial concluded that patients treated with talampanel demonstrated significantly longer survival than those who received standard care alone (Grossman et al., 2010). While this is promising and certainly demands further investigation, this study alone cannot be deemed conclusive. The second trial, a smaller phase II trial, examined the effects of talampanel alone on 6-month survival of patients with recurrent malignant glioma (Iwamoto et al., 2010). This trial determined that talampanel alone conferred no obvious advantage on patient survival, but the drug was tolerated well with no severe side-effects (Iwamoto et al., 2010).

Inhibitors of other glutamate receptors have not yet been clinically evaluated, however the preliminary success of animal models of glioma treatment as mentioned above will certainly lead to trials of other glutamate receptor antagonists in the near future. Significant promise is held by these inhibitors as both candidate adjuvant therapies capable of supplementing treatment cytotoxicity or of mediating the effects of glutamate on the brain.

6.2 System x_c^- Inhibition

While the above-mentioned therapies for mediating the excess glutamate released by glioma are promising, certainly the most attractive potential therapies to arise from these studies are those that involve the inhibition of system x_c^-. Rather than mediate the consequences of destructive glutamate release and treatment-resistance, system x_c^- inhibition could eliminate the function of the transporter responsible for the excess glutamate, and consequently limit the multiple morbidities of glutamate release rather than manage its downstream effects. In addition, system x_c^- inhibition would limit cysteine availability to the glioma cell and therefore inhibit its antioxidative capabilities by way of both limiting glutathione synthesis and halting the drive of the cystine/cysteine redox cycle. There are many chemical inhibitors of system x_c^-; of these, the cyclic glutamate analogue S-(4)-carboxyphenylglycine has emerged as the most potent inhibitor (Patel et al., 2004), and the FDA approved anti-inflammatory drug sulfasalazine has garnered the most clinical interest. Sulfasalazine has been demonstrated in animal models to effectively slow the growth of glioma and reduce levels of both intracellular GSH and extracellular glutamate (Chung et al., 2005; Chung & Sontheimer, 2009). A phase I clinical trial of sulfasalazine to evaluate drug safety and effects on tumour growth in the treatment of grade 3 glioma in a small number of patients was prematurely terminated due to several adverse effects during treatment (Robe et al., 2009; 2006). This study was initiated on the basis on sulfasalazine acting as an inhibitor of NFkB, however treatment did not differ from that required for system x_c^- inhibition. Although the poor outcomes from this trial are unfortunate, they do little to dampen the potential of sulfasalazine for glioma treatment or system x_c^- as a therapeutic target. Another phase I clinical trial has just recently been initiated with the intent to examine the effects of sulfasalazine on glutamate release in the brain, and on seizures in low-grade, newly-diagnosed glioma patients (de Groot & Sontheimer, 2010). The upcoming results of this trial will be the first clinical evidence of treatments directed at system x_c^- inhibition, and will contribute greatly to the establishment of the role of this critical transporter in glioma morbidity and treatment.

7. Conclusion

Glioma exist in conditions of high oxidative stress as a result of the metabolic shift away from the TCA cycle and towards increased rates of glycolysis. This metabolic shift, the Warburg effect, is characteristic of cancer cells and confers unique benefits to the cell which allow survival and proliferation in conditions of rapid growth, division and variable access to blood vasculature. However, a result of this reliance on glycolysis is the increased prevalence of ROS in the cancer cell. To survive these conditions, cancer cells must possess upregulated mechanisms of antioxidation. Glioma exhibit an oxidative stress-mediated upregulation of the xCT coding gene SLC7a11, which, along with the membrane-anchoring protein 4F2hc comprise the two subunits of the Na^+ independent electroneutral cystine/glutamate antiporter called system x_c^-. This antiporter drives the molecular turnover that is ultimately responsible for several of the features of morbidity in glioma, as well as its characteristic chemo- and radiation-resistance. The import of cystine into the cell increases the availability of cysteine for the GSH synthesis pathway and for the cystine/cysteine redox cycle. These two antioxidant pathways function to relieve the glioma cell of significant oxidative stress, allowing increased proliferation and survival of the cancer cells. This also allows resistance of glioma to oxidative stress-inducing radiation and chemotherapies. Conversely, the export of glutamate results in the neurotoxic death of neurons and glial cells in the vicinity of the tumour, and acts in an autocrine/paracrine manner to stimulate glioma proliferation and migration. Therapies are currently under development with these mechanisms in mind. Glutamate receptor antagonists have been demonstrated to limit brain cell death and to inhibit tumour growth *in vitro* and in xenograft animal models of glioma. System x_c^- inhibitors that prevent the import of cystine for antioxidant purposes and also prevent the release of glutamate into the extracellular environment have also demonstrated success *in vitro* and *in vivo*, and a clinical trial is currently underway with the inhibitor sulfasalazine. This work opens new pathways for investigation in a condition well known for poor prognoses and limited treatment options. The evidence of system x_c^- in other cancers in addition to glioma suggests that this mechanism may soon become of great importance to cancer treatment.

8. References

Arcella, A., Carpinelli, G., Battaglia, G., D'Onofrio, M., Santoro, F., Ngomba, R. T., et al. (2005). Pharmacological blockade of group II metabotropic glutamate receptors reduces the growth of glioma cells in vivo. *Neuro-oncology*, *7*(3), 236-45.

Balendiran, G. K., Dabur, R., & Fraser, D. (2004). The role of glutathione in cancer. *Cell biochemistry and function*, *22*(6), 343-52.

Banjac, A., Perisic, T, Sato, H, Seiler, A, Bannai, S, Weiss, N, et al. (2008). The cystine/cysteine cycle: a redox cycle regulating susceptibility versus resistance to cell death. *Oncogene*, *27*, 1618-1628.

Bannai, S, & Ishii, T. (1988). A novel function of glutamine in cell culture: utilization of glutamine for the uptake of cystine in human fibroblasts. *Journal of cellular physiology, 137*(2), 360-6.

Bannai, S, & Kitamura, E. (1980). Transport interaction of L-cystine and L-glutamate in human diploid fibroblasts in culture. *The Journal of biological chemistry, 255*(6), 2372-6.

Bannai, S, & Kitamura, E. (1982). Adaptive enhancement of cystine and glutamate uptake in human diploid fibroblasts in culture. *Biochimica et biophysica acta, 721*(1), 1-10.

Bannai, S, Sato, H, Ishii, T., & Taketani, S. (1991). Enhancement of glutathione levels in mouse peritoneal macrophages by sodium arsenite, cadmium chloride and glucose/glucose oxidase. *Biochimica et biophysica acta, 1092*(2), 175-9.

Behrens, P. F., Langemann, H., Strohschein, R., Draeger, J., & Hennig, J. (2000). Extracellular glutamate and other metabolites in and around RG2 rat glioma: an intracerebral microdialysis study. *Journal of neuro-oncology, 47*(1), 11-22.

Burdo, J., Dargusch, R., & Schubert, D. (2006). Distribution of the cystine/glutamate antiporter system xc- in the brain, kidney, and duodenum. *Journal of Histochemistry and Cytochemistry, 54*(5), 549-557.

Chillarón, J., Roca, R., Valencia, A., Zorzano, A., & Palacín, M. (2001). Heteromeric amino acid transporters: biochemistry, genetics, and physiology. *American journal of physiology. Renal physiology, 281*(6), 995-1018.

Choi, D. W. (1988). Glutamate neurotoxicity and diseases of the nervous system. *Neuron, 1*(8), 623-34.

Chung, W J, Lyons, S A, Nelson, G. M., Hamza, H., Gladson, C. L., Gillespie, G. Y., et al. (2005). Inhibition of cystine uptake disrupts the growth of primary brain tumors. *Journal of Neuroscience, 25(31),* 7101-7110.

Chung, W J, & Sontheimer, H. (2009). Sulfasalazine inhibits the growth of primary brain tumors independent of Nuclear factor-kappaB. *Journal of Neurochemistry, 110,* 182-193.

Conrad, Marcus, & Sato, Hideyo. (2011). The oxidative stress-inducible cystine/glutamate antiporter, system x (c) (-) : cystine supplier and beyond. *Amino acids.* Electronic Advance Copy.

deGroot, J., & Sontheimer, Harald. (2010). Glutamate and the biology of gliomas. *Glia.* Electronic Advance Copy.

Goudar, R. K., Keir, S. T., Bigner, D. D., & Friedman, H. S. (2004). NMDA and AMPA glutamate receptor antagonists in the treatment of human malignant glioma xenografts. *AACR Meeting Abstracts, 2004*(1), 1053.

Grossman, S. A., Ye, X., Chamberlain, M., Mikkelsen, T., Batchelor, T., Desideri, S., et al. (2009). Talampanel with standard radiation and temozolomide in patients with newly diagnosed glioblastoma: a multicenter phase II trial. *Journal of clinical oncology : official journal of the American Society of Clinical Oncology, 27*(25), 4155-61.

Grossman, S. A., Ye, X., Piantadosi, S., Desideri, S., Nabors, L. B., Rosenfeld, M., et al. (2010). Survival of patients with newly diagnosed glioblastoma treated with radiation and temozolomide in research studies in the United States. *Clinical cancer research : an official journal of the American Association for Cancer Research, 16*(8), 2443-9.

Halliwell, B. (2007). Oxidative stress and cancer: have we moved forward? *The Biochemical journal, 401*(1), 1-11.

Hinoi, E., Takarada, T., Ueshima, T., Tsuchihashi, Y., & Yoneda, Y. (2004). Glutamate signaling in peripheral tissues. *European Journal of Biochemistry, 271,* 1-13.

Huang, Ying, Dai, Z., Barbacioru, C., & Sadée, W. (2005). Cystine-glutamate transporter SLC7A11 in cancer chemosensitivity and chemoresistance. *Cancer research, 65*(16), 7446-54.

Huang, Ying, & Sadée, W. (2006). Membrane transporters and channels in chemoresistance and -sensitivity of tumor cells. *Cancer letters, 239*(2), 168-82.

Huang, Yulun, Zhou, Y., Fan, Y., & Zhou, D. (2008). Celastrol inhibits the growth of human glioma xenografts in nude mice through suppressing VEGFR expression. *Cancer letters, 264*(1), 101-6.

Ishii, T., Sato, H, Miura, K., Sagara, J., & Bannai, S. (1992). Induction of cystine transport activity by stress. *Annals of the New York Academy of Sciences, 663*, 497-8.

Ishii, T., Sugita, Y., & Bannai, S. (1987). Regulation of glutathione levels in mouse spleen lymphocytes by transport of cysteine. *Journal of cellular physiology, 133*(2), 330-6.

Ishiuchi, S., Yoshida, Y., Sugawara, K., Aihara, M., Ohtani, T., Watanabe, T., et al. (2007). Ca2+-permeable AMPA receptors regulate growth of human glioblastoma via Akt activation. *The Journal of neuroscience : the official journal of the Society for Neuroscience, 27*(30), 7987-8001.

Iwamoto, F. M., Kreisl, T. N., Kim, L., Duic, J. P., Butman, J. A., Albert, P. S., et al. (2010). Phase 2 trial of talampanel, a glutamate receptor inhibitor, for adults with recurrent malignant gliomas. *Cancer, 116*(7), 1776-82.

Kim, J. Y., Kanai, Y, Chairoungdua, A., Cha, S. H., Matsuo, H., Kim, D. K., et al. (2001). Human cystine/glutamate transporter: cDNA cloning and upregulation by oxidative stress in glioma cells. *Biochimica et biophysica acta, 1512*(2), 335-44.

Kim, J.-whan, & Dang, C. V. (2006). Cancer's molecular sweet tooth and the Warburg effect. *Cancer research, 66*(18), 8927-30.

Kroemer, G., & Pouyssegur, J. (2008). Tumor cell metabolism: cancer's Achilles' heel. *Cancer cell, 13*(6), 472-82.

Le, A., Cooper, C. R., Gouw, A. M., Dinavahi, R., Maitra, A., Deck, L. M., et al. (2010). Inhibition of lactate dehydrogenase A induces oxidative stress and inhibits tumor progression. *Proceedings of the National Academy of Sciences of the United States of America, 107*(5), 2037-42.

Lim, J. C., & Donaldson, P. J. (2010). Focus On Molecules: The cystine/glutamate exchanger (System x(c)(-)). *Experimental eye research. 92*(3),162-3

Lo, M., Wang, Y. Z., & Gout, P W. (2008). The x(c) (-) cystine/glutamate antiporter: A potential target for therapy of cancer and other diseases. *Journal of Cellular Physiology, 215*(1097-4652).

Louw, D. F., Bose, R., Sima, A. A., & Sutherland, G. R. (1997). Evidence for a high free radical state in low-grade astrocytomas. *Neurosurgery, 41*(5), 1146-50.

Lyons, Susan A, Chung, W Joon, Weaver, A. K., Ogunrinu, T., & Sontheimer, Harald. (2007). Autocrine glutamate signaling promotes glioma cell invasion. *Cancer research, 67*(19), 9463-71.

Makowske, M., & Christensen, H. N. (1982). Contrasts in transport systems for anionic amino acids in hepatocytes and a hepatoma cell line HTC. *The Journal of biological chemistry, 257*(10), 5663-70.

Mandal, P. K., Seiler, Alexander, Perisic, Tamara, Koelle, P., Banjac Canak, A., Foester, H., et al. (2010). System xC- and thioredoxin reductase 1 cooperatively rescue glutathione deficiency. *The Journal of biological chemistry.*

Meister, A. (1995). Glutathione metabolism. *Methods in enzymology, 251*, 3-7.

Oka, A., Belliveau, M. J., Rosenberg, P. A., & Volpe, J. J. (1993). Vulnerability of oligodendroglia to glutamate: pharmacology, mechanisms, and prevention. *The Journal of neuroscience : the official journal of the Society for Neuroscience, 13*(4), 1441-53.

Patel, S. A., Warren, B. A., Rhoderick, J. F., & Bridges, R. J. (2004). Differentiation of substrate and non-substrate inhibitors of transport system xc(-): an obligate exchanger of L-glutamate and L-cystine. *Neuropharmacology*, *46*(2), 273-84.

Pham, A.-N., Blower, P. E., Alvarado, O., Ravula, R., Gout, Peter W, & Huang, Ying. (2010). Pharmacogenomic approach reveals a role for the x(c)- cystine/glutamate antiporter in growth and celastrol resistance of glioma cell lines. *The Journal of pharmacology and experimental therapeutics*, *332*(3), 949-58.

Robe, P. A., Martin, D. H., Nguyen-Khac, M. T., Artesi, M., Deprez, M., Albert, A., et al. (2009). Early termination of ISRCTN45828668, a phase 1/2 prospective, randomized study of sulfasalazine for the treatment of progressing malignant gliomas in adults. *BMC cancer*, *9*, 372.

Robe, P. A., Martin, D., Albert, A., Deprez, M., Chariot, A., & Bours, V. (2006). A phase 1-2, prospective, double blind, randomized study of the safety and efficacy of Sulfasalazine for the treatment of progressing malignant gliomas: study protocol of [ISRCTN45828668]. *BMC cancer*, *6*, 29.

Roslin, M., Henriksson, R., Bergström, P., Ungerstedt, U., & Bergenheim, A. T. (2003). Baseline levels of glucose metabolites, glutamate and glycerol in malignant glioma assessed by stereotactic microdialysis. *Journal of neuro-oncology*, *61*(2), 151-60.

Rzeski, W., Turski, L., & Ikonomidou, C. (2001). Glutamate antagonists limit tumor growth. *Proceedings of the National Academy of Sciences of the United States of America*, *98*(11), 6372-7.

Savaskan, Nic E, & Eyüpoglu, I. Y. (2010). xCT modulation in gliomas: Relevance to energy metabolism and tumor microenvironment normalization. *Annals of anatomy = Anatomischer Anzeiger : official organ of the Anatomische Gesellschaft*.

Savaskan, Nicolai E, Heckel, A., Hahnen, E., Engelhorn, T., Doerfler, A., Ganslandt, O., et al. (2008). Small interfering RNA-mediated xCT silencing in gliomas inhibits neurodegeneration and alleviates brain edema. *Nature medicine*, *14*(6), 629-32.

Seidlitz, E. P., Sharma, M. K., & Singh, G. (2010). Extracellular glutamate alters mature osteoclast and osteoblast functions. *Canadian journal of physiology and pharmacology*, *88*(9), 929-36.

Shih, A. Y., Erb, H., Sun, X., Toda, S., Kalivas, P. W., & Murphy, T. H. (2006). Cystine/glutamate exchange modulates glutathione supply for neuroprotection from oxidative stress and cell proliferation. *The Journal of neuroscience : the official journal of the Society for Neuroscience*, *26*(41), 10514-23.

Sontheimer, Harald. (2003). Malignant gliomas: perverting glutamate and ion homeostasis for selective advantage. *Trends in neurosciences*, *26*(10), 543-9.

Sontheimer, Harald. (2008). A role for glutamate in growth and invasion of primary brain tumors. *Journal of neurochemistry*, *105*(2), 287-95.

Takano, T., Lin, J. H., Arcuino, G., Gao, Q., Yang, J., & Nedergaard, M. (2001). Glutamate release promotes growth of malignant gliomas. *Nature medicine*, *7*(9), 1010-5.

Verrey, F., Closs, E. I., Wagner, C. A., Palacin, M., Endou, Hitoshi, & Kanai, Yoshikatsu. (2004). CATs and HATs: the SLC7 family of amino acid transporters. *Pflügers Archiv : European journal of physiology*, *447*(5), 532-42.

Wang, H., Tamba, M., Kimata, M., Sakamoto, K., Bannai, Shiro, & Sato, Hideyo. (2003). Expression of the activity of cystine/glutamate exchange transporter, system x(c)(-), by xCT and rBAT. *Biochemical and biophysical research communications*, *305*(3), 611-8.

Warburg, O., Wind, F., & Negelein, E. (1927). The metabolism of tumours in the body. *The Journal of general physiology*, *8*(6), 519-30.

Ye, Z. C., & Sontheimer, H. (1999). Glioma cells release excitotoxic concentrations of glutamate. *Cancer research*, *59*(17), 4383-91.

21

Improving the Efficiency of Chemotherapeutic Drugs by the Action on Neuroepithelial Tumors

Vladimir A. Kulchitsky et al.*
Institute of Physiology, National Academy of Sciences of Belarus, Minsk Belarus

1. Introduction

The problem of cancer embraces a lot of unresolved issues, among which there dominates the problem of ascertainment of the mechanisms of uncontrolled growth and cellular spill of tumor neoplasm, composed of dividing cancer cells and cancer stem cells (Schatton & Frank MH, 2009; Schatton et al., 2009; Frank NY et al., 2010). It is impossible to answer the question about a complete removal of the tumor tissue and simultaneous minimizing the adverse effects of surgical and other manipulations while removing the tumor without solving this problem. This is a particularly relevant goal for physicians who are engaged in treatment of brain tumors. The destruction of nerve tissue nonaffected by tumor growth has a negative impact on the integrative brain activity and at least on the central control of all bodily functions and homeostasis maintenance. How is it possible to reduce by-effects of major therapeutic technologies in neurooncology (surgical, radiological, chemotherapeutic), having preserved or enhanced their selective tumor damaging action?

Since you choose chemotherapy as one of the ways to impact on tumor tissue, it is impossible not to mention the commonly known toxic effect of chemotherapeutic agents on all body tissues. Destroying the tumor cells, cytotoxic agents kill healthy cells and tissues. Thus, local or systemic applying the chemotherapy leads inevitably to the destruction of healthy brain cells in case of the tumor localization within the cranial cavity and the spinal canal. Thus, one of the objectives of this work was to develop methodic of leveling the general toxic effects of chemotherapy while strengthening their local destructive effect on tumor tissue. What ways have been chosen to solve this problem?

Tumors of the brain and spinal cord have extremely variety (set) of histological forms which are accounted for their origin from the elements of various tissues and for peculiarity of

---

*Michael V. Talabaev[2], Alexander N. Chernov[1], Dmitry G. Grigoriev[3], Yuri E. Demidchik[4], Dmitry G. Shcharbin[5], Nicholas M. Chekan[6], Vladimir V.Kazbanov[1], Tatiana A. Gurinovich[1], Anatoly I. Gordienko[6], Elena K. Sergeeva[6], Vladimir I. Potkin[7] and Vladimir N. Kalunov[1]
[1]*Institute of Physiology, National Academy of Sciences of Belarus, Minsk;Belarus*
[2] *Clinical Hospital of Emergency, Minsk;Belarus*
[3]*Belarusian State Medical University, Minsk;Belarus*
[4]*Belarusian Medical Academy of Post-Graduate Education, Minsk;Belarus*
[5]*Institute of Biophysics and Cell Engineering, National Academy of Sciences of Belarus, Minsk; Belarus*
[6]*Physical-Technical Institute, National Academy of Sciences of Belarus, Minsk; Belarus*
[7]*Institute of Physical Organic Chemistry, National Academy of Sciences of Belarus, Minsk, Belarus*

genesis not solved up to the end in respect to especially neuroepithelial tumors (Hirose & Yoshida, 2006; Nicholas et al., 2011; Van den Eynde et al., 2011). The nervous system tumors account for almost 10% of all human neoplasms, and up to 20% for children (Alomar, 2010; Davis et al., 2010; Myung et al., 2010). Neoplasms of brain and spinal cord are the most common solid tumors in childhood. They take the second place in frequency after leukemia of all child malignancies. In childhood (under 14 years) the vast majority of cases occur in neuroepithelial tumors. Of these, about 80% are of six histological forms: medulloblastoma, juvenile pilocytic astrocytoma, diffuse astrocytoma, ependymoma, craniopharyngioma, and neuroblastoma.

Among the tumors of neuroepithelial tissues 9 sub-groups are selected out: astrocytic, oligodendroglial, ependymal, oligoastrocytic tumors (mixed gliomas), tumors of vascular plexus, and other neuroepithelial tumors (glial tumors of unspecified origin), neuronal and neuronal-glial, pineal, and embryonal tumors. In most cases glial tumors (gliomas) such as astrocytic, oligodendroglial, and ependymal glioma ones are detected. Histological diagnosis was based on identifying the predominant cell type.

Combined treatment of the brain cancer (children including), which supposes surgery interference together with chemo- and radiotherapy, does not so far reach the desired impact. According to statistics concerning only medulloblastoma, the average disease-free and overall survival during 2-7 years for patients up to 4 years old is respectively 46% and 54%. So, tiny comforting is aggravated by data that uniquely ascertain the growth of intracerebral cancer. Thus, in the U.S. during 30 years from 1973 to 2003 it increased from 4.1 to 5.2 for women and from 5.9 to 7.0 for men per 100 000 population (Alomar, 2010). Similar dynamics were recorded by The Child Cancer Registry of the Belarusian Republic. The percentage of brain tumors rose from 2.5 to 3.3 per 100 000 children living in Belarus from 1989 to 2005.

A number of intractable causes is due to a low curability of brain tumors. The most productive radical method of removal of cancer neoplasm is often limited by the fact of their location near vital centers. Courses of medical and radiation treatment in accordance with approved protocols HIT`91, PO/02-PO/04 (Dunkel et al., 2010; Rosenfeld et al., 2010) along with known positive ones embrace recognizable negative aspects. To the negative ones there pertain as follows: i) a low permeability of the blood-brain barrier being created by tight contacts of micro vessel intracerebral network, which became completed with a set of proteins (Claudine 1,5, Occludin and others), which are impermeable to hydrophilic low soluble compounds exceeding a diameter of 18 Å and a molecular weight of 180 Da. The vast majority of cytotoxic drugs pertain to them (Erdlenbruch et al., 2000; Kemper et al., 2004; Xie et al., 2005); ii) a weak selectivity of the concentration of cytostatic in the place of neoplasm (Cragnolini & Friedman, 2008); iii) an insufficiently studied mechanism of the action of traditional and new pharmacological agents, as well as their clearance, which hinders a reasonable estimation of the amount of molecules that come in direct contact with tumor cells (Gerstner & Fine, 2007; Ta et al., 2009); iv) a lack of unified schemes of medical product application, taking into account the morphological structure of complex heterogeneous neoplasias, stages of their malignancy, and individual sensitivity of the tumor cells to them and patient age (Alomar, 2010; Myung, et al., 2010); v) a symptomatic toxic side effect, reduced to a violation of general tissue metabolism and endocrine function, to immunity suppression, involvement in a destructive reaction of abnormal elements along with intact (healthy) cell ones, as well as the development of complications (acute arachnoiditis, meningo encephalopathy, renal failure, passing deviation from the motor areas, speech, vision, hearing, stop of growth, and cognitive deficits with reduced intelligence), what in totality leads to disability (Kemper et al., 2004; Vega et al., 2003); vi) a limited range of available medications.

The postulates set forward underline the actuality of further improving of existing strategies and creating new ones for earlier diagnosis, prognosis and a more successful fight against cancer. One of the ways to the aim is a broad involvement in oncology of a very representative class of multifunctional endogenous biological regulators of peptide nature, generally called as growth factors. In own structure they number a series of families, among which are neurotrophins (Nerve Growth Factor (NGF), Brain-Derived Neurotrophic Factor (BDNF), Neurotrophins 3, 4, 5 (NT), Transforming Growth Factor (TGF), Fibroblast Growth Factor (FGF), Epidermal Growth Factor (EGF), Vascular Endothelial Growth Factor (VEGF), Insulin-Like Growth factor (IGF), and others, rating more than 50 different variants (Antonelli et al., 2007; Beebe et al., 2003). The key role belongs to growth factors in the capacity of epigenetic "directive" signals in the control of such fundamental morphogenetic processes in ontogenesis as growth, survival, proliferation, differentiation (i.e., the selection of the terminal tract of specialization by stem and progenitor cells), guided migration and elongation processes, synaptogenesis, regulation of cell homeostasis by apoptosis, regeneration, as well as maintaining a normal cyto-biochemical status of mature cells and their resistance to damaging factors (Alam et al., 2010; Charles et al., 2011; Vinores & Perez-Polo, 1983; Xie et al., 2005).

The interest to determine the significance of these compounds in tumor formation and in their reverse transforming potential has just relatively recently emerged, when it became vivid that virtually all types of neoplasias are synthesized not only by growth factors but actively expressize their receptors (Antonelli et al., 2007; Barnes et al., 2009; Blum & Konnerth, 2005; Brossard et al., 2009; Evangelopoulos et al, 2004; Krűttgen et al., 2006; Nakagawara, 2001). At the same time we point out a startling fact: NGF was purified for the first time from sarcoma secretions S180, and protooncogenes sites, which take it, were purified from high-affinity TrkA and low relational P75 from biopsies of colon carcinoma (*intestinum crassum*) and human melanoma. It is much more interesting that bio testing of growth factors on its activity is performed on rat pheochromocytoma PC12 (Krűttgen et al., 2006).

The experiments proved that *in vitro* the cell lines of neuroblastoma (IMR-32, SY-5Y, SK-N-SH, NB-GR) and medullary pheochromocytoma cease to divide in the presence of NGF and are transformed into neuron-like elements at braking formation of DNA, at the intensification of including labeled amino acids, at the appearance of sprouts, at the growth of size, substrate adhesion together with the formation of pseudoganglies and at the occurrence in membrane of electrical excitability (Krűttgen et al., 2006; Poluha et al., 1995). On the other hand, the ability of NGF *in vivo* to reduce the number of induced nitrosourea by neurinomas was revealed, as well as the speed of their development, and the ability to reduce the volume and to prolong animal survival after subcutaneous injection or intracerebral implantation of anaplastic glioma cell F98, T9, and neurinomas (Yaeger et al., 1992). The predictive value of identification of perceiving Neurotrophins receptors is overviewed. So thus the over expression of TrkA and C (for NT-3) in neuro-, medulla and glioblastomas promises a favorable outcome, due to a spontaneous regression (through differentiation), the inclusion of suicide programs or autophagy (Blum & Konnerth, 2005; Collins, 2004; Krűttgen et al., 2006; Yamaguchi et al., 2007). Patients with low or no detectable levels of these receptors in medulloblastoma exhibit 5-fold risk of death than with

a high level (Krűttgen et al., 2006). *Per contra*, the enhanced expression of TrkB (ligand BDNF), which takes place in aggressive tumors, where isoforms often truncated and lacked of intracellular domain, goes with the pessimistic ending.
In this light the aim of the research was to study individual and combined effects of some of cytostatic and growth factors (Liu et al., 2010), which are in circulation, on the survival of primary culture of cells. Alongside an attempt of the combined action of cytostatic, that is the factor of Nerve Growth and Dendrimers (or Heterocyclic Compounds) on primary culture cells of neuroepithelial tumors was undertaken. Dendrimers are the extended three-dimensional molecules which contain a large number of active functional groups on the outer surface (Morgan et al., 2006; Waite & Roth, 2009). We focused on one of the most common types of Dendrimers - Polyamidoamine, (PAMAM), containing ethylenediamine core and branching of methyl acrylate and ethylenediamine (Kang et al., 2010). We aimed at verifying the hypothesis about the possibility of dose reducing of cytostatic at combined application of chemotherapy with growth factors and nanoparticles, in particular Dendrimers in these experiments. The fifth generation of Dendrimer (PAMAM G5) was used. The effect of combinations of cytostatic, Nerve Growth Factor and Dendrimers or the cytostatic agent, Nerve Growth Factor and Heterocyclic Compounds was studied in separate series of experiments. Heterocycles of isoxazole series (Isoxazole) and isothiazolyl (Isothiazole) (typical representatives of 1,2-azoles) are structural fragments of a wide range molecules of active physiologically substances, what causes a growing interest in the research of the synthesis and in the study of the biological properties of these compounds. Isoxazole heterocycle is a compound part of molecules of the cytotoxic, antitubercular agents, anticonvulsants, and pesticides.
The compounds to be perspective for the treatment of Alzheimer's disease and inflammatory, antithrombosis and anticonvulsive drugs were identified among the derivatives of isothiazolyl. It was recently found that some isothiazolyls were inhibitors of kinases and could be used in the treatment of tumors. For example, isothiazolyl with urea function in position 3 is an inhibitor of tyrosine kinases and now it is under studying as an anticancer drug CP-547, 632 (Beebe et al., 2003). The fellow-colleagues of Institute of Physical Organic Chemistry NAS of Belarus developed methods for the synthesis of new 5-substituted 1,2-thiazol-3-ilcarbamids and their heteroanalogs - 1,2-oxazole-3-ilcarbamids - isosteres known as inhibitors of tyrosine kinases, which are of some interest for testing in our planned experiments. The goal of these experiments was to find ways of reducing the dose of cytotoxic drugs, under condition of preserving or increasing the toxic effects of chemotherapy on tumor tissue.

2. Methodic

The biopsy material was taken from 67 children aged from 1 to 15 years old who were treated at the children's neurosurgical department of Municipal Clinical Emergency Hospital in Minsk from November 2008 to December 2010.

2.1 The research protocol

The biopsy material taken during the fine-needle stereotactic or neurosurgical operation was transported in an hour to the Pathology Laboratory to determine the histology forms of the tumor and degrees of its malignancy, and was simultaneously delivered to the Laboratory of Cell Monitoring to assess individual sensitivity of tumor cells to chemotherapeutic drugs *in vitro*. After the mentioned period 0.5 ml of chemotherapy was added in doses approved by instructions and converted either to a square cup (10.0 cm^2) or to β-subunit of recombinant human NGF (Sigma-Aldrich, USA, 1.0 µg / ml) or to Dendrimers (PAMAM 0.1, 1.0, 10.0 µg / ml, Sigma-Aldrich, USA), or to heterocyclic compounds (0.1, 1.0, 10.0 µg / ml), or to these or others in various combinations. Each series of observations *in vitro* consisted of 30 applications (n = 30). Assessment of the viability of tumor cells was estimated in 24 hours after putting test compounds into the environment for their ability to incorporate trypan blue. For this matter the cell suspension was mixed with 2% dye solution in saline buffer pH = 7.2 at a ratio of 1:10 and transferred into Goryaev's chamber, where the number of dead (paint over) and living (light) elements was counted at a percentage. The obtained data were reported to neurosurgeons who together with other specialists developed the tactics of post-operative treatment and determined prognosis.

2.2 Cytoscopic study

Cytoscopic study of surgical specimens was carried out after using the methods of frozen sections, or the crushed drop. The final conclusion of the histological form of the tumor and its malignancy degree was made after alcohol treatment, filling material in paraffin, sectioning and staining by the following methodic: a method of staining with hematoxylin and eosin; histochemical methods for the detection of glial filaments, collagen and reticulin fibers; immunohistochemical studies for detection of acidic glial fibrillary protein, neurofilaments, synaptophysin, and neuron-specific enolase; a definition of PCNA, Ki-67, cyclins in order to clarify the nature of proliferative activity. The conducted cytoscopic research allowed to identify indications of malignancy and was a guide to neurosurgeons in case of choosing the treatment tactics.

2.3 Cultural studies

Pieces of biopsy material were washed from the blood and mechanically comminuted in Hank's solution (Sigma-Aldrich, USA) with Gentamicin sulfate added, and then for 30 min they were put in a mixture of 0.25% trypsin solution in Ethylenediaminetetraacetic acid (EDTA) (2 ml) at a ratio of 1:3. The effect of the enzyme was inhibited by adding 3 ml Fetal Calf Serum - FCS (Sigma-Aldrich, USA) for a period of 3-5 minutes. The material treated in such a way was crushed under a microscope with a sterile blade up to pasty consistency and then was taken to a sterile Petri dish with medium Dulbecco's Modified Eagle's Medium (DMEM) (Sigma-Aldrich, USA), with adding ETS at a ratio of 1:10 and 4% sulfate solution Gentamicin (10^{-4} g / l). The cells obtained from the substrate were grown in a medium of this composition for 2-7 days at 37°C, 95% humidity and 5% partial pressure of CO_2 (Chekan et al., 2009). Stay duration of the cells *in vitro* was dictated by the speed of the attachment to the substrate.

2.4 Clinical, laboratory and instrumental methods

Clinical, laboratory and instrumental methods of the study included a list of routine clinical examination methods and laboratory diagnostics, as well as computed tomography and nuclear magnetic resonance. The credibility of differences between the average values was set by a Mann-Whitney test for nonparametric samples using the computer program StatPlus 2005. Differences were estimated to be significant at $P < 0.05$.

3. Results

The following types of cancer were included according to the histological conclusions based on classification of brain tumors (WHO, 2007) into the observations: astrocytic, embryonic, and compiled under the title "other types" of neoplasm. In the group of cancers of astrocytic origin were present: pilocytic, pilomixoidnic, protoplasmic, pleomorphic, anaplastic neoplasm. Medulloblastoma, atypical teratoidnic/rabdoidnic tumor of posterior fossa, and malignant neuroectodermal tumor of the left temporal lobe were in the category of embryonic tumors. The category of "the other options" of neoplasm included: anaplastic oligodendrogliomas, oligoastrocytomas of a cerebellar vermis, ependymoma, gangliogliomas of a mixed neuroglial type, immature teratoma of a pineal region, which was attributable to germinocell tumors, glioma of an optic chiasm, and a gemangioblastoma to be regarded as an intramedullary tumor of a cervical spinal cord.

It was revealed in the experiments *in vitro* that Cisplatin (Merck, USA, 1.0 µg / ml) took priority in the samples of pilocytic astrocytoma, medulloblastoma, and malignant neuroectodermal tumors of the temporal lobe, where the percentage of dead cells reached respectively 61.9 ± 12.9, 40.9 ± 11.4, 41.6 ± 8.5, 68.6 ± 7.8 reliably exceeding the one in those experiments where the cells of a primary culture of neuroepithelial tissue devolved out of contact with chemotherapy (14.3 ± 5.0%). A similar position was taken by Carboplatin (Merck, USA, 4.0 µg / ml) in biopsies from pleyomorfic xanthoastrocytoma, anaplastic oligodendroglioma (Fig. 1), optic chiasm glioma and atypical teratoid / rhabdoid tumors (Fig. 2) with lethality according to the order of enumeration 57.9 ± 5.9, 68.4 ± 10.6, 78.9 ± 4.1 and 79.5 ± 1.0%.

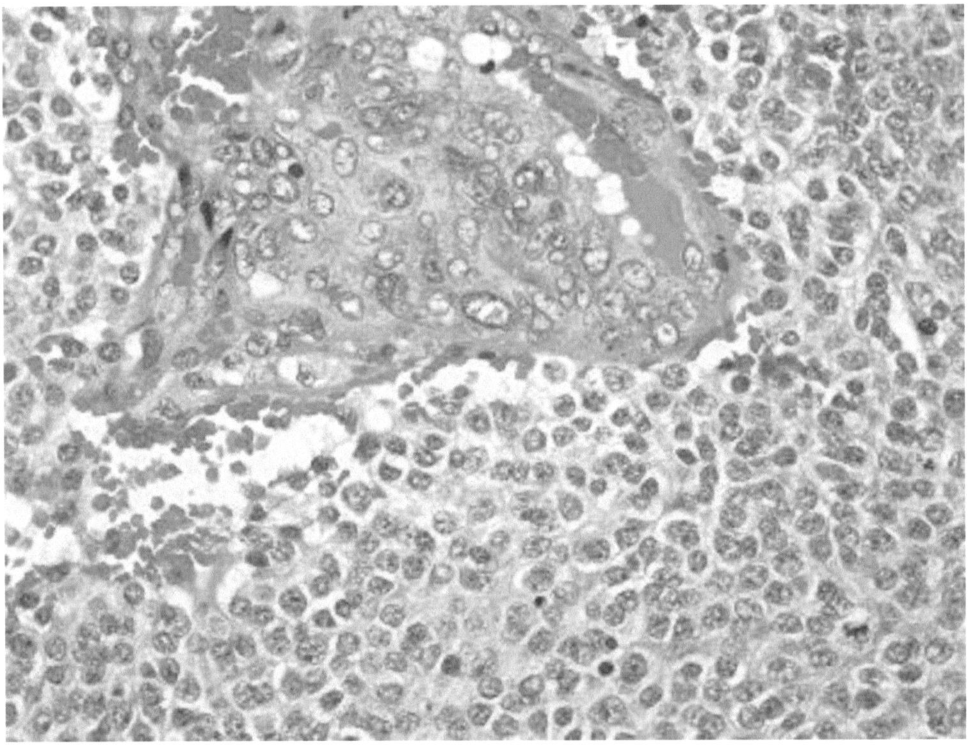

Fig. 1. Anaplastic oligodendroglioma

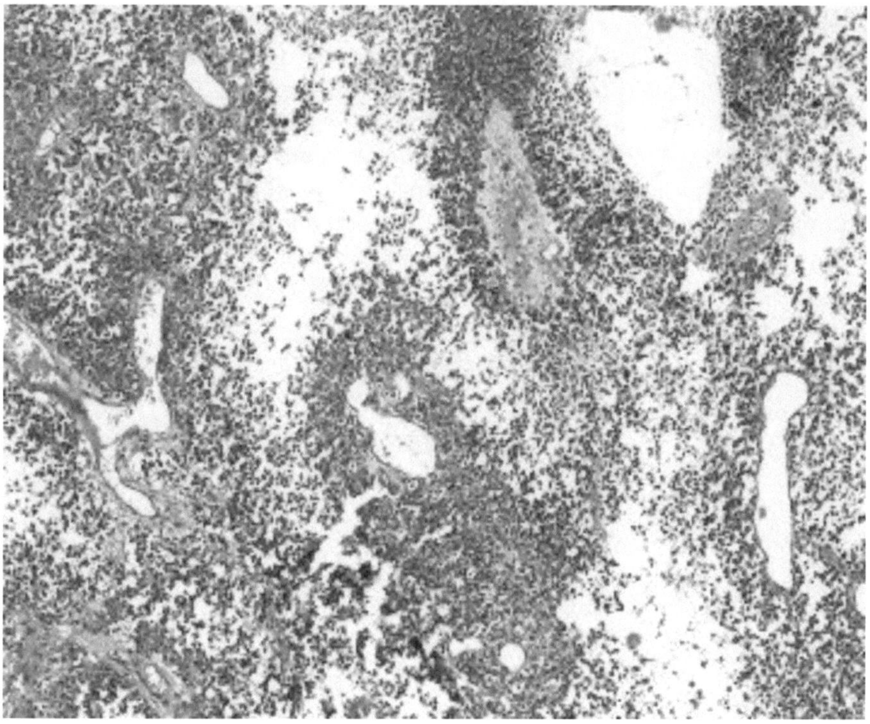

Fig. 2. Atypical teratoid / rhabdoid tumor

The same can be said about Etoposide (Ebewe Artsnaym., Austria, 1.0 µg / ml) in relation to the protoplasmic astrocytoma cells (61.0 ± 4.7%), oligoastrocytoma (55.1 ± 8.5%) (Fig. 3 a, b) and especially about hemangioblastoma (74.7 ± 3.9%).

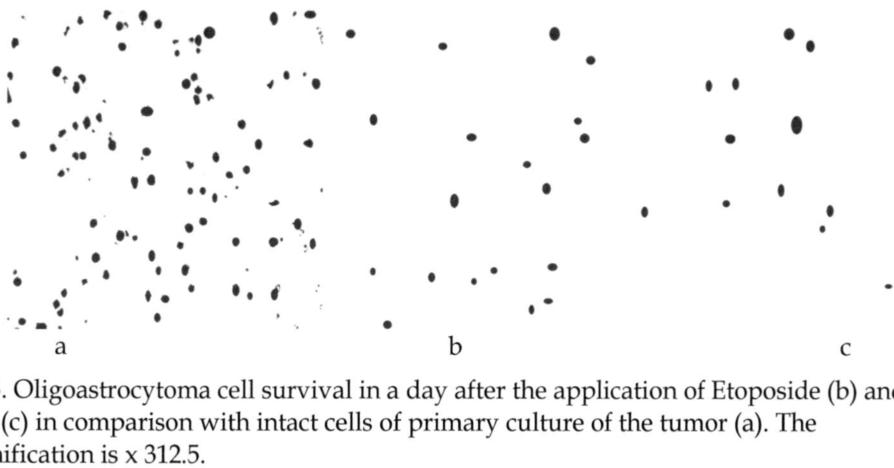

Fig. 3. Oligoastrocytoma cell survival in a day after the application of Etoposide (b) and β-NGF (c) in comparison with intact cells of primary culture of the tumor (a). The magnification is x 312.5.

Cytarabine (Belmedpreparaty, Belarus, 1.0 µg / ml) effectively suppressed the cell vitality in cultures of anaplastic astrocytoma (51.4 ± 5.9%) and immature teratoma (90.6 ± 5.0%). Other substances - Methotrexate (Ebewe Artsnaym., Austria, 50.0 µg / ml) and Gemcitabine (Wee-Em-Gee Pharmaceuticals Pvt. Ltd., India, 2.0 µg / ml) though were not included in the list of leading substances, often successfully shared with them the second or third position. However, in a case of anaplastic oligodendroglioma the latter was not effective. Moreover, in its presence the cells of pleomorphic xanthoastrocytoma like Etoposide ones demonstrated a paradoxical reaction - a statistically significant increase of survival potential. The same is with carboplatin. Maximum susceptibility to it is shown by document in the samples of four neoplasm, and first of all of atypical teratoid / rabdoid tumor and optic chiasm glioma to have lost 79.5 ± 1.0 and 78.9 ± 4.1% viable units. These compounds are followed by Etoposide, which predominant efficacy was also recorded in three types of tumor cells, especially in glioblastoma.

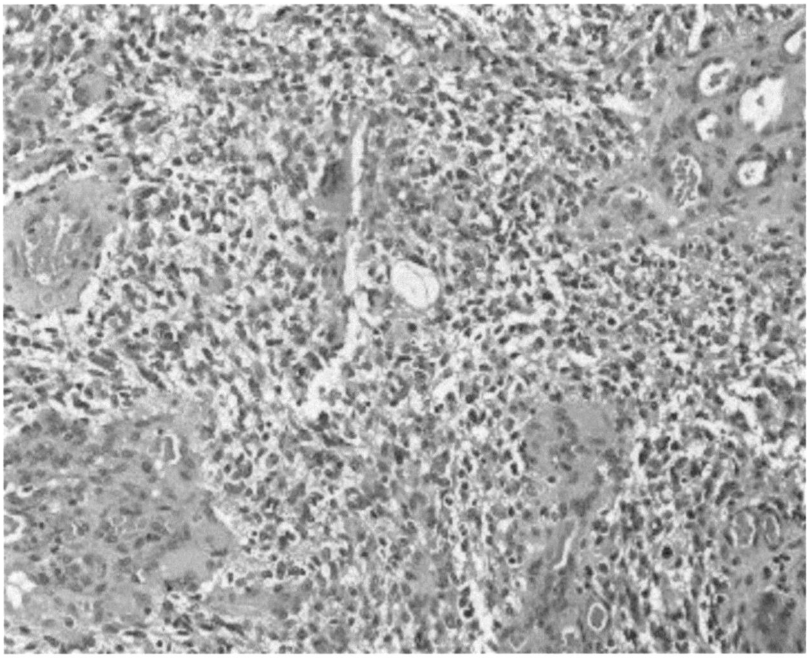

Fig. 4. Glioblastoma with marked vascular proliferation and the formation of glomerular structures.

It is right to note the following fact: culture objects manifested almost the same (competitive) sensitivity to two or more agents in virtually all cases, if one takes into consideration the closeness of a number of infected cells, differences of which were not included in the validation category. As for β-NGF, its superiority (although not statistically significant) over the cytostatic regarding a number of perished *in vitro* units occurred in biopsies of pilomixoid astrocytoma (47.6 ± 1.3% vs. 40.9 ± 11.4% of Cisplatin), medulloblastoma (Fig. 5) (44.9 ± 2.9 vs. 41.6 ± 8.5% from the same preparation), oligoastrocytoma (78.3 ± 0.9 vs. 55.1 ± 8.5% of Etoposide) (Fig. 3 a, b, c) and ependymoma (62.4 ± 6.0 vs. 58.6 ± 4.4% of Carboplatin).

The efficiency of β-NGF (68.2 ± 0.5%) almost coincided with that of Cytarabine (68.9 ± 11.9%), and under the contact with the cells of anaplastic astrocytomas (Fig. 6) (38.2 ± 2.3%) reached the 2nd position after for Cytarabine (54.4 ± 5.9%), pushing on the third place Carboplatin (35.9 ± 1.8%) when glioblastoma was applied to the cells the primary culture. In the contrast, the derivatives of pleomorphic xanthoastrocytoma responded to β-NGF by a significant increase in its resistance to the toxin (an increase of vitality). Their death was 13.6 ± 2.9% in relation to the fixed one in the tumor cells which were not subjected to any influence - 31.7 ± 0.5%, whereas the culture of ganglioglioma was generally indifferent to cytostatics.

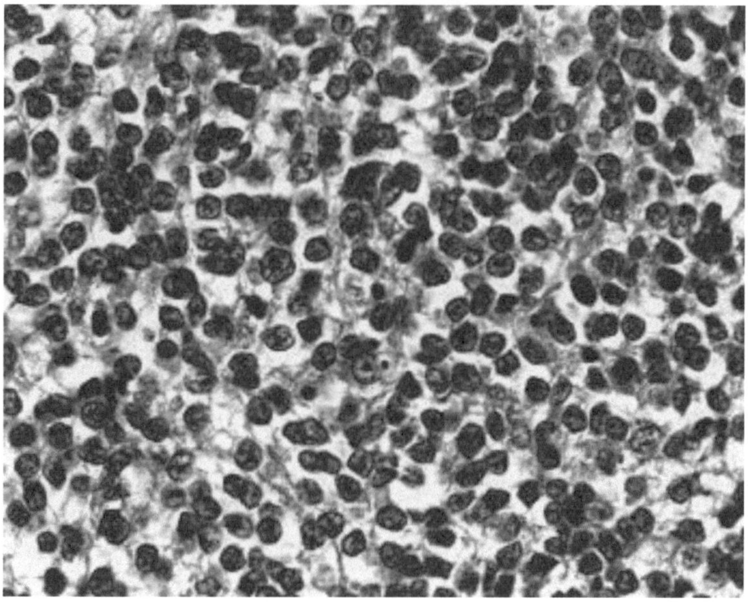

Fig. 5. Undifferentiated medulloblastoma

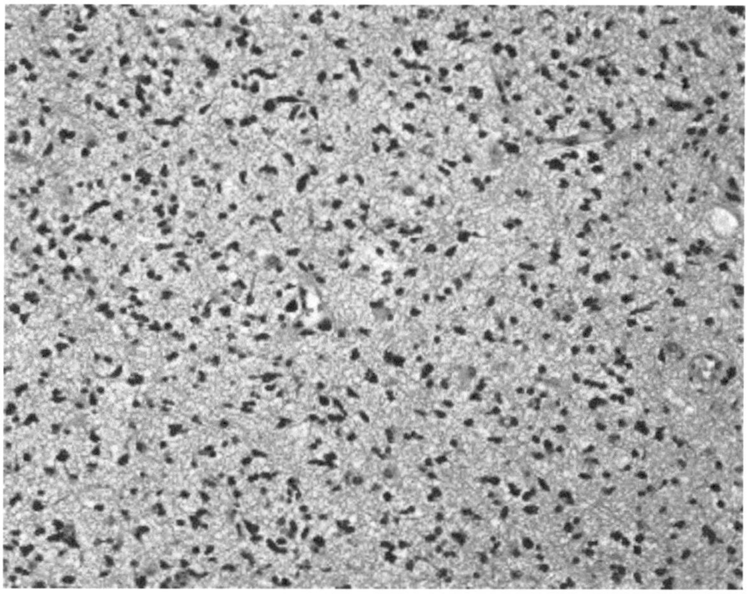

Fig. 6. Anaplastic astrocytoma. Moderate cellularity. Nuclear polymorphism

The access to the analysis of a destructive influence of combined test compounds application, while keeping in mind the possibility of potentiation of their individual effects was the logical corollary from an analysis of the brought materials. It turned out that in most combinations (excluding β-NGF + Methotrexate in the case of pilocytic astrocytoma), a marked tendency of a destructive cellular reactions increase in comparison with those described in the isolated introduction of preparation) was observed. A combination of Cisplatin + Etoposide (89.5 ± 0.8%), Carboplatin + Cytarabine (81.4 ± 2.0%), Carboplatin + Etoposide (69.2 ± 3.0%) and Cisplatin + Carboplatin (68.8 ± 7.3%) for cells oligoastrocytoma, and Cisplatin + Carboplatin (78.1 ± 1.9%) and β-NGF + Cisplatin (55.5 ± 3.2%) shown with an example of cells of ganglioglioma was especially attractive *in vitro* conditions. In these cases, the combined effect of cytotoxic drugs significantly exceeded observed ones under individual applications of each component from every pair of drugs. It's worth noting that β-NGF, despite the decline of its performance in a variant of samples from oligoastrocytoma, tends as a rule to significantly increasing toxic effects on the tumor cells survival in a combination with cytotoxic drugs. This raises a question of reasonableness of the further research in terms of the simultaneous application of these agents. For the sake of fairness it should be emphasized that in any case of their combination one failed to reveal signs of synergy, where the reaction to the combination would have excelled the arithmetic sum of the personal effects, included as components in its structure. This can be conditioned by complex polymorphism of brain tumors, including dividing tumor cells and stem tumor cells at that. The survival of an even single cancer stem cell could lead to a recurrence of tumor metastasis and uncontrolled process in other parts of the central nervous system.

It is important to point out that varying selective affinity touched not only biopsy samples belonging to different types of tumors, but also tumors taken away from an absolutely analogous composition accordingly to histological compounds and a measure of tumor progression. For example, the maximum destruction of cultured cells was recorded against a background application Cytarabine (68.3 ± 6.9%, $P < 0.05$), and to a lesser extent Cisplatin (49.4 ± 5.4%, P <0.05), and Methotrexate (39.7 ± 7.2%, $P < 0.05$) in three patients with medulloblastoma of the IV stage. The other chemotherapy drugs effect on cells of tumor had actually no difference in growth of cell culture without the application of cytostatic. This circumstance makes relevant carrying out a preliminary rapid assessment of individual susceptibility of patients to chemotherapeutic drugs with involvement of cultural systems.

Moreover, it was possible to show by a document a certain correlation between the effectiveness of test compounds and the degree of malignancy at the same astrocytic nature of the tumors. Let us demonstrate this by the following examples. Thus Cisplatin (61.9 ± 12.9%), Carboplatin (53.8 ± 7.9%) and Methotrexate (47.0 ± 7.2%) came into the triad of superior according to induction of cell lethality at the Ist stage. At the IInd stage Carboplatin (57.9 ± 5.9%), Methotrexate (51.1 ± 4.0%) and Cytarabine (50.2 ± 9.4%) occupied the dominant position. On the IIId - Cytarabine (54.4 ± 5.9%), Carboplatin (35.9 ± 1.8%) and Etoposide (34.5 ± 4.4%), and at the IVth - Cytarabine (68.9 ± 11.9%), Etoposide (63.1 ± 0.4%) and Gemcitabine (61.5 ± 1.7%). As a matter of fact the mentioned graduation should be viewed with a certain degree of conditionality, since statistically significant differences between the members of each triad could not be established. It's noteworthy, however, that β-NGF, occupying a relatively modest position in the first phase of malignancy acquired a tough competition (68.2 ± 0.5%) leading to the IVth stage of Cytarabine (68.9 ± 11.9%) and bunched over (38.2 ± 2.3%) from the 2nd stage (35.9 ± 1.8%) of Carboplatin (please, bear in mind: at isolated applications of β-NGF).

The dependence of the destructive action of cytostatic and β-NGF also correlated with the age of the patients. Differences in digital indicators which characterize the percentage of cell loss of primary tumor culture *in vitro* gave evidence of the complex mechanisms of interaction between tumor cells with cytotoxic drugs coming in the triad of the most active compounds. So, at the child age under 3 years old the tumor generating effect was observed in Carboplatin (59.7 ± 4.1%), Cisplatin (51.4 ± 4.5%) and Cytarabine (48.3 ± 2.4%), and at the age from 4 to 6 years old β-NGF (63.2 ± 4.8%), Cisplatin (62.3 ± 7.6%) and Methotrexate (49.4 ± 5.8%) were in the lead. At the age from 7 to 10 years old the toxic substances rating looked like follows: Carboplatin (38.1 ± 8.8), β-NGF (27.1 ± 6.1%) and Methotrexate (26.2 ± 3.1%). At the age from 11 to 15 years old Methotrexate moved to the first position (56.0 ± 3.8%), slightly ahead of Carboplatin (54.4 ± 2.9%) and Cisplatin (53.6 ± 3.7%). β-NGF, taking the first place in terms of suppression of cell survival in the intermediate age groups, showed in the fourth (most mature) group an inverted effect, which increased cell survival significantly (13.3 ± 2.9%) compared with control (32.9 ± 3.0%).
Experiments conducted *in vitro* demonstrated once again the well-known position of the highest individual sensitivity of glioma to cytostatics. No one has ever managed to fix the same sequence in the effectiveness of tumor destroying the action by the protocol approved cytostatic at absolutely identical histological diagnoses. Registered dependence of differences of effects from sex and age did not permit to explain the inner workings of such a high individual sensitivity of glioma to chemotherapy. It is obvious that one of explanations for this phenomenon can be a different degree of presence of stem tumor cells in tumor tissue. The high stability of stem tumor cells to damaging agents is well known.
We are therefore got interested in the effect of enhancing the anticancer effect of cytostatics and NGF presence. As a hypothesis we can suggest that a strengthening of an anticancer effect of a combination of chemotherapeutic drugs and NGF is determined by an influence of drugs not only on dividing tumor cells but also on stem tumor cells. If it is so, then it is advisable to try to test different combinations of chemotherapy with cytotoxic substances of a new generation. In particular, we talk about the heterocyclic compounds, many of which are capable of inhibiting the intracellular tyrosine kinas path and, thus, to initiate the mechanisms of apoptosis in tumor tissue. The use of nanoparticles, in particular, Fullerenes or Dendrimers seems making a promise for these tasks. More details will be discussed below. There are many more challenges in oncology on the way to more effective cancer therapy. The well known high toxicity of chemotherapeutic drugs for all organs and systems of a living organism stimulates scientists and oncologists to find ways of reducing the general toxic action of cytostatic, and maintaining their anti-tumor effect. The result in these experiments on primary culture oligoastrocytoma cerebellar vermis can be given as an example of such a design. The data are presented in Table 1.
The following fact draws attention at analyzing the data. In comparison with the natural death of cells the addition of Carboplatin, Methotrexate or Cisplatin was accompanied by an increase in the percentage of dead cells in a Petri dish from 35% to 47 % in the control (when cells of primary culture of oligoastrocytoma cerebellar vermis were developing in the culture medium without any contact with the chemotherapy). The combination of one of these three chemotherapy drugs with Nerve Growth Factor under decreasing doses of the cytostatic factor led in 10 times to the preservation or even an increase of the cytostatic effect (Table 1). The effect of two cytostatics - Carboplatin and Methotrexate increased especially

demonstratively. If you are not going to speculate on possible mechanisms of this phenomenon, then one is competent to conclude that the concentration of cytostatic can be significantly reduced in situations of combined use of chemotherapy with NGF. This reduction of dosage will be accompanied by a decline in general toxic action of chemotherapy drugs (which is critical for every cancer patient) and a persistence of the cytostatic action in relation to tumor cells (what is critical for a patient and a physician). A similar cytotoxic effect was observed earlier while applying diamond-like structures (Chekan et al., 2009). Experiments *in vitro* decreased survival of rat C6 glioma cells in the presence of implants made of titanium alloy VT-16. Putting diamond-like carbon coatings on the alloy VT-16 was accompanied with an increase in the percentage of cell death on the fifth day of cultivation, compared with the control: 39.9 ± 2.1% and 5.4 ± 0.3%, respectively. A more significant decrease in mitotic activity and cell viability was observed when C6 glioma cells contacted with diamond-like carbon coating, comprising silver nanoparticles. The number of cell destruction of glioma C6 at contact with the diamond-like carbon covering, including up to 3.5 % Silver nanoparticles, made 53.7 ± 2.1%, and at doping up to 6.7 % Silver the cell destruction reached 66.7 ± 3.2% ($P < 0.05$) in comparison with the control. Hence, the maximum toxic effect in regard to C6 glioma was detected in samples coated with diamond-like film, including silver nanoparticles. Similar results were obtained in the application of diamond coatings on the primary culture of human gliomas. If the surface of titanium samples with a diamond-like coatings included additional silver nanoparticles, the cytotoxic effect on the second day after exposure of cells of oligodendrogliomas with the surface of the samples would be disastrous for the viability of these cells. As it is shown in Fig. 7 A, processes of proliferation are continuing in tumor cells outside the titanium samples, while at the site location on a Petri dish of titanium sample almost all cells died (Fig. 7 B).

Title Series	Cell death, %
Control	12.5 ± 4.2
Carboplatin 4.0 µg / ml	35.3 ± 0.9*
Carboplatin 0.4 µg / ml + β NGF 0.1 µg / ml	57.1 ± 12.5*
Methotrexate 50.0 µg / ml	43.7 ± 8.6*
Methotrexate 5.0 µg / ml + β NGF 0.1 µg / ml	72.4 ± 2.5*
Cisplatin 1.0 µg / ml	47.4 ± 3.0*
Cisplatin 0.1 µg / ml + β NGF 0.1 µg / ml	50.0 ± 8.1*

Table 1. Percentage of cell death oligoastrocytoma cerebellar vermis at a combination of different doses of cytostatics with Nerve Growth Factor (NGF). (The asterisk * denotes the reliability of $P < 0.05$)

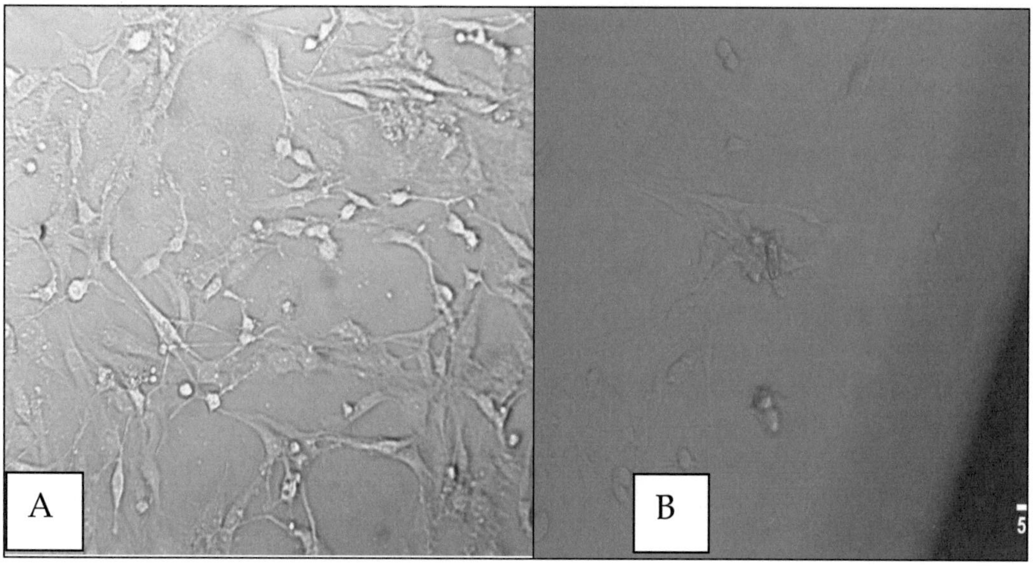

Fig. 7. Oligodendrogliomas cell distribution in twenty-four hours at 40 mm from the titanium sample with diamond-like coating containing silver nanoparticles (A), and at 1 mm from the edge of the sample (B)

It was established that if the titanium samples were coated with titanium dioxide (TiO_2), a cytotoxic effect of these samples (Fig. 8 A and B) would not differ from a cytotoxic effect of those which coating consisted of silver nanoparticles.

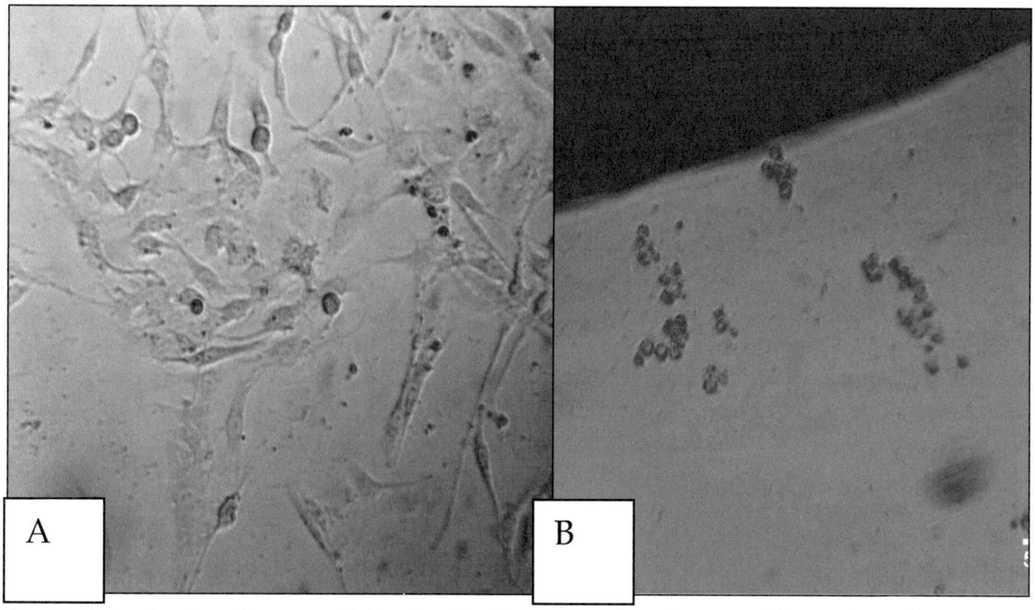

Fig. 8. Oligodendrogliomas cell distribution in twenty-four hours at 40 mm from the titanium sample with titanium dioxide (TiO_2) (A), and at 1 mm from the edge of the sample (B)

The highest potentiating effect of the combination of chemotherapy and nanoparticles was obtained by the application of Dendrimers. Series of experiments of a Cisplatin combination with PAMAM on the primary culture of medulloblastoma are in Table 2.

Title Series	**Cell death**, %
Control	20.7 ± 3.3
Cisplatin 1.0 µg / ml	67.6 ± 7.4*
Cisplatin 1.0 µg / ml + β NGF 0.1 µg / ml	49.2 ± 6.8*
PAMAM 30 mM (10.0 µl)	45.5 ± 6.7*
Cisplatin 1.0 µg / ml + PAMAM 30 mM (10.0 µl)	92.7 ± 4.9*
Cisplatin 0.1 µg / ml + PAMAM 30 mM (10.0 µl)	98.4 ± 1.5*

Table 2. Percentage of cell death medulloblastoma IV at a combination of different doses of Cisplatin with Polyamidoamine (PAMAM) Dendrimer (the asterisk * denotes the reliability of $P < 0.05$)

As it is seen in Table 2, the percentage of cell death of malignant medulloblastoma increased significantly in primary culture under the action of Cisplatin and paradoxically reduced by a combination of Cisplatin with NGF. This fact does illustrate once again the high specificity of each particular tumor in each patient, what determines the choice of individual treatment strategy in each case. This choice should be guided by research data and the sensitivity of cells in primary culture *in vitro*.

Application of PAMAM 30 mM (10.0 µl) in a Petri dish was accompanied by increased cell death in comparison with control ones. In principle, the anticancer effect of Dendrimer is described in literature but has not been studied in detail (Bei et al., 2010). At this stage we have only stated such an action of PAMAM. Surprisingly a stable toxic effect of a combination Cisplatin with PAMAM was demonstrated at using two different concentrations of chemotherapeutic drugs (Table 2). The anticancer effect of this drug combination ranged from 92% to 98% (Fig. 9, and Fig. 10). Therefore it is very important to find such a combination chemotherapy with growth factors and nanoparticles, which would reduce the dose of cytostatics, when we tried to determine the sensitivity of individual tumor *in vitro* to cytostatic in the next phase of the research. At the same cytotoxic effect of substances used must be maintained at maximum levels. Dendrimers belong to a class of polymeric compounds whose molecules have a large number of branches. At their acquisition a number of branches of the molecule increase with every elementary act of growth. As a result, the shape and rigidity of the molecules change with increasing molecular weight of these compounds, what is usually accompanied with changes in physical and chemical properties of Dendrimers. Inside Dendrimers cavities are formed which can be filled in with a variety of substances, such as cytostatic. This ability of Dendrimers was one of the factors to determine the decision to use them for enhancement of their anticancer effect of chemotherapy.

The paper drew attention also to other compounds that might be effective against tumor growth. The input material for the synthesis of heterocyclic compounds was 1,2-azole-3-carboxylic acids, which were consistently converted into azides or carbamide. Implemented computer modeling of ligand-protein complexes of carbamide was carried out in the framework of the methods of molecular mechanics using the program Dock 6.4 and USF

Chimera. Evaluation of energy characteristics of the van der Waals and electrostatic interaction suggests the possibility of efficient binding of 1,2-azole ligand protein. These studies helped to choose the best version of heterocyclic compounds (Carbamide), which application in a combination with cytostatic agents and Nerve Growth Factor allowed reducing the dose of the cytostatic factor in 10 times at maintaining *in vitro* the tumor generating effect on primary cell cultures. There are the above listed drawings as a demonstration.

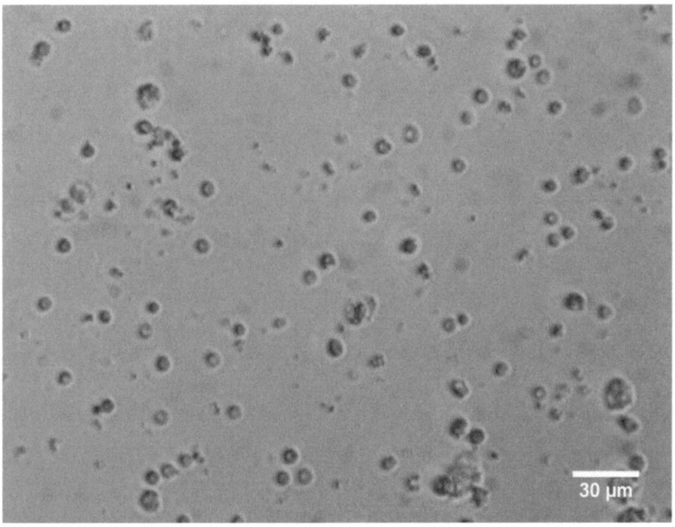

Fig. 9. Atypical teratoid / rhabdoid tumor cells remaining in a day after the application of Cisplatin (1.0 µg / ml), β-NGF (0.1 µg / ml), Polyamidoamine Dendrimer (30 mM, 10.0 µl)

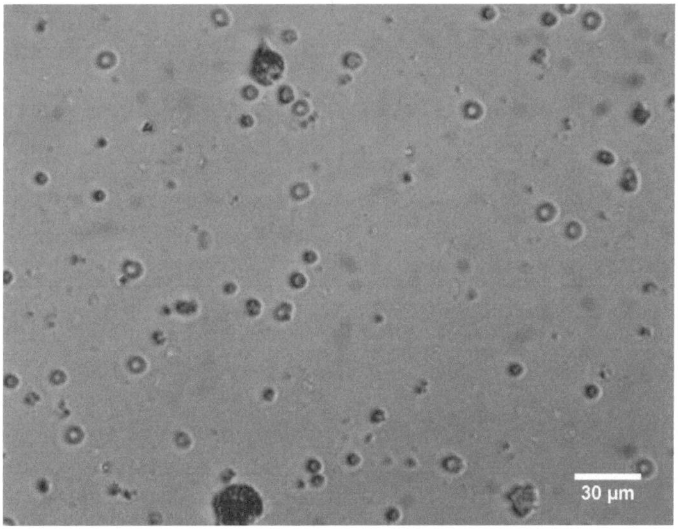

Fig. 10. Atypical teratoid / rhabdoid tumor cells remaining in a day after the application of Cisplatin (0.1 µg / ml), β-NGF (0.1 µg / ml), Polyamidoamine Dendrimer (30 mM, 10.0 µl)

Anticancer effects of heterocyclic compounds in one more series of experiments were approved (Figs. 11-13). The Fig. 11 shows the primary tumor cells of pilocytic astrocytoma in two days after passage. Figure 12 shows primary tumor cells pilocytic astrocytoma in two days after the addition of Azide at a concentration of 1.0 mg / ml. Figure 13 shows primary tumor cells pilocytic astrocytoma in two days after the addition of Carbamide at a concentration of 1.0 mg / ml. Toxic properties of Azides and Carbamide can be explained by their ability to inhibit the tyrosine kinase pathway. This mechanism can be implemented in the subsequent initiation of apoptosis in tumor cells.

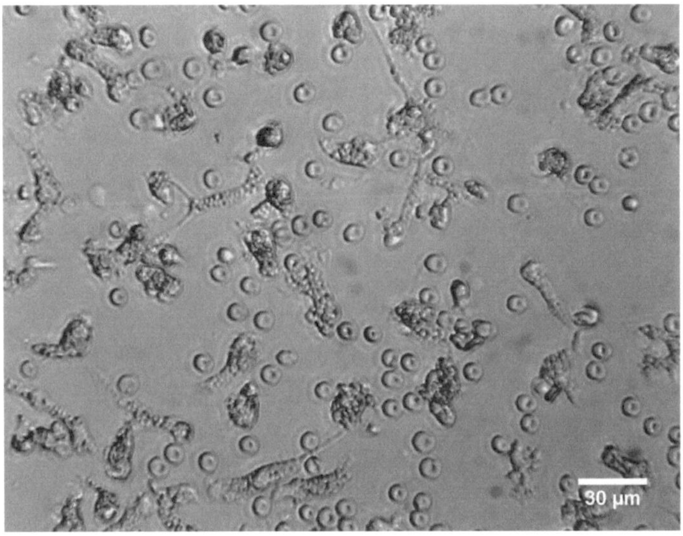

Fig. 11. Pilocytic astrocytoma cells in a day after passage

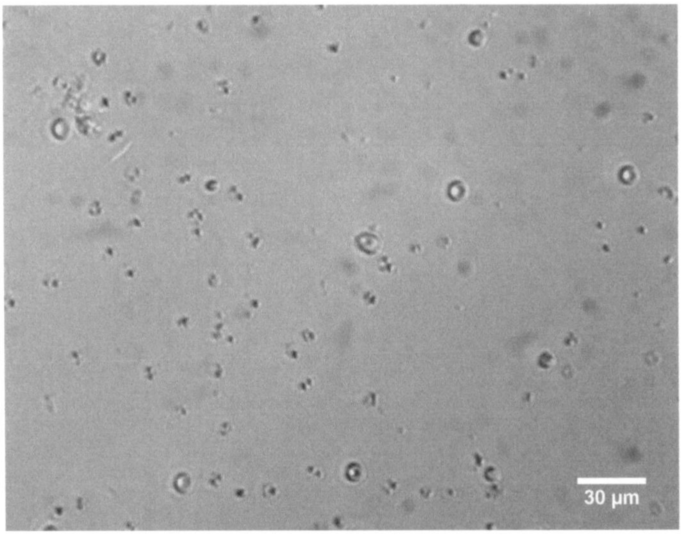

Fig. 12. Pilocytic astrocytoma cells in a day after application of Azide at a concentration of 1.0 mg / ml

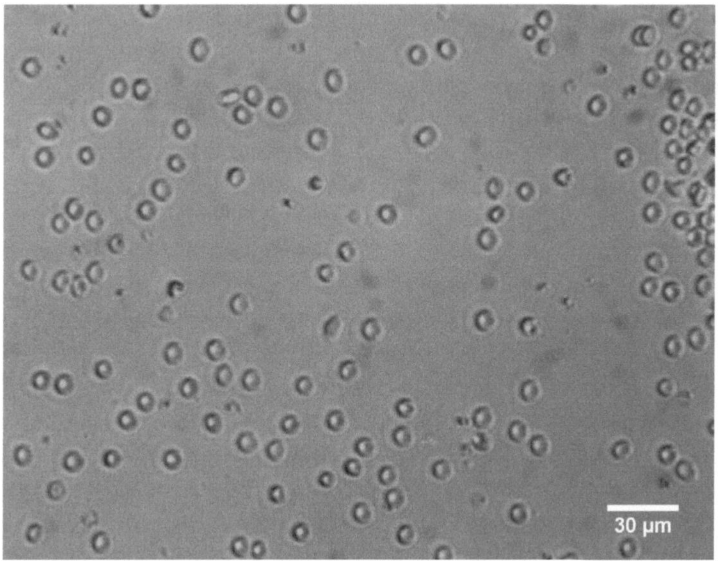

Fig. 13. Pilocytic astrocytoma cells in a day after application of Carbamide at a concentration of 1.0 mg / ml

4. Conclusion

The data obtained are the basis to discuss several aspects of increasing the chemotherapy effectiveness problem. Being general toxic poisons in the action by their nature, chemotherapy drugs come out as an essential attribute of anticancer therapy in accordance with the majority of the approved treatment protocols. There are no alternatives to their use considering the presence of appropriate evidence. In such a case, how can one reduce the general antineoplastic action of cytostatics and keep their strong anticancer effect? The anticancer effect is under discussion in respect of not only dividing tumor cells, but also stem tumor cells. The advantage of a mutual use of cytostatics and NGF compared with their individual use was confirmed in the work. It puts on the agenda the top-priority intensively developing problem, that is of improving the permeability of the blood-brain barrier at systemic application of chemotherapy and the search for "circuitous" ways to the desired delivery of biologically active compounds to tumor tissues (Alam et al., 2010; Chen et al., 2011; Gerstner & Fine, 2007). In order to implement the first plan several directions are supposed. One of them is to attract hyperosmotic solutions containing histamine, bradykinin, mannitol and so on, which will contribute to achieving the cytostatic targets in the brain at their systematic putting into operation (Kemper et al., 2004; Xie et al., 2005). But the transient opening by them of the entrance gate provides at the same time an opportunity of entering via them for the neurotoxic substance what is especially dangerous in case of a more complex operative procedure of an intracarotid infusion of chemotherapeutic agents. This may be accompanied by disorders of speech, movement, visual perception.

One more trend is based on creation of conjugates of an active commencement with proteins, which are able to recognize the integral components of cerebrovascular structures, such as antibodies to the receptor ferritin in relation to the NGF. This ensures its effectiveness in a rank of low concentrations. The simultaneous application of anticancer drugs with inhibitors of a large glycoprotein P, which prevents the movement of cytotoxic drugs through the blood-brain barrier (Gerstner & Fine, 2007; Kemper et al., 2004) is promising. Preclinical trials with Paclitaxel have confirmed the perspectives of such a method, making reasonable transition to clinical trials.

Attempts of a different kind are being made, namely the involvement of the bradykinin analog BMP-7, endowed with a more extended half-life period and with selectivity in respect to the receptor B2 in comparison with the being endogenously synthesized compound (Kemper et al., 2004; Ta et al., 2009; Xie et al., 2005). Being associated with them, BMP-7 leads to the opening of calcium channels in cells, an increase in their level of free cations. That leads to a reaction of endothelial cells and to weakening of intercellular contacts. The vascular permeability increases in addition. The recorded concentrations of growth factors were achieved in 30 minutes with the highest representation in the striatum, hippocampus, cerebral cortex and relatively low concentrations in the olfactory bulb, cerebellum and brainstem at joint custody of NGF and BMP-7 into stabilized liposomes, which are smaller than 100 nm. There was a good agreement between the permeability coefficient of the drug and its targeted action (Xie et al., 2005) at that. Under intracarotid administration of BMP-7 with Carboplatin in rat models of gliomas such a combination has significantly reduced the number of cytostatic normally used in humans. Phase II in clinical trials conducted on 87 patients with recurrence of malignant gliomas recorded a noticeable advantage of processing BMP-7 + Carboplatin before individually using only Carboplatin.

The advances in molecular biology and genetic engineering, which ensured the implementation of experimental and clinical use of low molecular weight peptides, proteins, oligonucleotides, monoclonal antibodies, etc. (Kruttgen et al., 2006; Xie et al., 2005) contributed to considerable progress in the development of a "roundabout" ways of delivery of drugs. In total they have created a fertile ground not only for in-depth understanding the basic mechanisms of carcinogenesis, but also simultaneously for widening the means of early diagnosis, the front of anticancer attack and optimization of medical schemes.

In a series of widely exploited methods there is a stereotactic implantation in the bed, formed after excision of tumor, indifferent biodegradable polymer substrates, impregnated in that or another way with an active principle. In this case, the cytostatic penetrates in measured doses into the surrounding tissue during a long period of time and destroy the remaining infected cells (Kemper et al., 2004; Ta et al., 2009). The concentration of drugs, developed in this case, can exceed observed ones with intravenous injection from 4 to 1200 times. In one of the clinical trial performed on 222 adult patients with recurrent gliomas mortality of persons who were within 6 months receiving such a method Cisplatin was 44% versus 67% among patients treated with placebo ($P < 0.02$).

The use of polymer capsules can also supply the brain with cells (transfected with viral vectors) which express a particular desired target gene which products act targeteous on the relevant parts of oncogenesis. The primary fibroblasts, astrocytes, ependimocytes, stem or progenitor cells serve as usual objects. For example, subclones Cyclin-Dependent Kinase 2 Interacting Protein (CINP) releasing *in vitro* NGF at 2 ng/ h/10^{-5} cells over 10 weeks was isolated from conventionally immortalized progenitor neuroblasts of the central nervous system of rat embryos with embedded DNA of growth factors. Being introduced into the brain such cells survived well, migrated at a distance of 15 mm from the implant site and integrated with the host tissue without any signs of growth or tumor formation.

Thus, we can conclude:

i. Sensitivity of glioma cells to chemotherapeutic agents, Nerve Growth Factor, and Dendrimers, Diamond like coated samples, heterocyclic compaunds *in vitro* depends on the origin, histological type tumors, the degree of malignancy, age and individual characteristics of patients;
ii. Combined application of Nerve Growth Factor and chemotherapy increases the percentage of dying in a culture of cellular elements;
iii. A complementary effect of Nerve Growth Factor appears to enhance cytotoxic effects of chemotherapy. This addictiveness reduces the effective dose of cytotoxic drugs in more than 10 times;
iv. The presence of growth factor and/or Dendrimers, heterocyclic compounds do reduce the toxic dose of the chemotherapeutic drugs simultaneously maintaining a high cytostatic effect;
v. Detection *in vitro* of high individual sensitivity of brain tumors to cytostatics confirms the hypothesis concerning polymorphism in mechanisms of carcinogenesis;
vi. It is appropriate to take into account the results of experiments in order to determine the sensitivity of tumor cells of primary culture to cytostatic drugs in the development of new specialized treatment protocols for brain tumors (mono- or polychemotherapy).

5. Acknowledgment

We express our deep appreciation to Professor Joseph Zalutsky for supporting this work, and Professor Eugene Cherstvoy for the attention and assistance in the histological studies.

6. References

Alam, M.I.; Beg, S.; Samad, A.; Baboota, S.; Kohli, K.; Ali, J.; Ahuja, A. & Akbar, M. (2010). Strategy for effective brain drug delivery. *European Journal of Pharmaceutical Sciences*, Vol.40, No.5, pp. 385-403.

Alomar, S.A. (2010). Clinical manifestation of central nervous system tumor. *Seminars in Diagnostic Pathology*, Vol.27, No.2, pp. 97-104.

Antonelli, A.; Lenzi, L.; Nakagawara, A.; Osaki, T.; Chiaretti, A. & Aloe, M. (2007). Tumor suppressor proteins are differentially affected in human ependymoblastoma and medulloblastoma cells exposed to nerve growth factor. *Cancer Investigation*, Vol.25, No.2, pp. 94-101.

Barnes, M.; Eberhart, C.G.; Collins, R. & Tihan, T. (2009). Expression of p75NTR in fetal brain and medulloblastomas: evidence of a precursor cell marker and its persistence. *Journal of Neurooncology*, Vol.92, No.2, pp. 193-201.

Beebe, J.S.; Jani, J.P.; Knauth, E.; Goodwin, P.; Higdon, C.; Rossi, A.M.; Emerson, E.; Finkelstein, M.; Floyd, E.; Harriman, S.; Atherton, J.; Hillerman, S.; Soderstrom, C.; Kou, K.; Gan,t T.; Noe, M.C.; Foster, B.; Rastinejad, F.; Marx, M.A.; Schaeffer, T.; Whalen, P.M. & Roberts,W.G. (2003). Pharmacological characterization of CP-547,632, a novel vascular endothelial growth factor receptor-2 tyrosine kinase inhibitor for cancer therapy. *Cancer Research*, Vol.63, No.21, pp. 7301-7309.

Bei, D.; Meng, J. & Youan, B.B. (2010). Engineering nanomedicines for improved melanoma therapy: progress and promises. *Nanomedicine* (Lond), Vol.5. No.9. pp. 1385-1399.

Blum, R. & Konnerth, A. (2005). Neurotrophin-mediated rapid signaling in the central nervous system: mechanisms and functions. *Physiology*, Vol.20, pp. 70-78.

Brossard, D.; El Kihel, L.; Clément, M.; Sebbahi, W.; Khalid, M.; Roussakis, C.; Rault, S. (2010). Synthesis of bile acid derivatives and in vitro cytotoxic activity with pro-apoptotic process on multiple myeloma (KMS-11), glioblastoma multiforme (GBM), and colonic carcinoma (HCT-116) human cell lines. *European Journal of Medicinal Chemistry*, Vol.45, No.7, pp. 2912-2918.

Charles, N.A.; Holland, E.C.; Gilbertson, R.; Glass, R.; Kettenmann, H. (2011). The brain tumor microenvironment. *Glia*. Vol.59, No.8, pp. 1169-1180.

Chekan, N.M.; Beleauski, N.M.; Akulich, V.V.; Pozdniak, L.V.; Sergeeva, E.K.; Chernov, A.N.; Kazbanov, V.V. & Kulchitsky, V.A. (2009). Biological activity of silver-doped DLC films, *Diamond & Related Materials*, Vol.18. pp. 1006-1009.

Chen, C.H.; Chang, Y.J.; Ku, M.S.; Chung, K.T., Yang, J.T. (2011). Enhancement of temozolomide-induced apoptosis by valproic acid in human glioma cell lines through redox regulation. *The Journal of Molecular Medicine*, Vol.89, No.3, pp. 303-315.

Collins, V.P. (2004). Brain tumors: classification and genes. *Journal of Neurology and Neurosurgical Psychiatry*, Vol.75, Supplement 2, pp. 2-11.

Cragnolini, A.B. & Friedman, W.J. (2008). The function of p75NTR in glia. *Trends Neuroscience*, Vol.31, No.2, pp. 93-104.

Davis, M.E.; Mulligan Stoiber, A.M. (2011). Glioblastoma multiforme: enhancing survival and quality of life.*Clinical Journal of Oncology Nursing*, Vol.15, No.3, pp. 291-297.

Dunkel, I.J.; Gardner, S.L.; Garvin, J.H. Jr.; Goldman, S.; Shi, W. & Finlay, J.L. (2010). High-dose carboplatin, thiotepa, and etoposide with autologous stem cell rescue for patients with previously irradiated recurrent medulloblastoma. *Neurooncology*, Vol.12, No.3, pp. 297-303.

Erdlenbruch, B.; Jendrossek, V.; Eibl, H.; Lakomek, M. (2000). Transient and controllable opening of the blood-brain barrier to cytostatic and antibiotic agents by alkylglycerols in rats. *Experimental Brain Research*, Vol.135, No.3, pp. 417-422.

Evangelopoulos, M.E.; Weis, J. & Kruttgen, A. (2004). Neurotrophin effects on neuroblastoma cells: correlation with Trk and p75NTR expression and influence of Trk receptor bodies. *Journal of Neurooncology*, Vol.66, No.1-2, pp. 101-110.

Frank, N.Y.; Schatton, T. & Frank, M.H. (2010). The therapeutic promise of the cancer stem cell concept, *Journal of Clinical Investigation*, Vol.120, No.1, pp. 41-50.

Gerstner, E.R. & Fine, R.L. (2007). Increased permeability of the blood-brain barrier to chemotherapy in metastatic brain tumors: establishing a treatment paradigm. *Journal of Clinical Oncology*, Vol.25, No.16, pp. 2306-2312.

Hirose, Y.; Yoshida, K. (2006). Chromosomal abnormalities subdivide neuroepithelial tumors into clinically relevant groups. *Keio Journal of Medicine*, Vol.55, No.2, pp. 52-58.

Kang, C.; Yuan, X.; Li, F.; Pu, P.; Yu, S.; Shen, C.; Zhang, Z.; Zhang, Y. (2010). Evaluation of folate-PAMAM for the delivery of antisense oligonucleotides to rat C6 glioma cells in vitro and in vivo. *The Journal of Biomedical Materials Research A*. Vol.93, No.2, pp. 585-594.

Kemper, E.M.; Boogerd, W.; Thuis, I.; Beijnen, J,H, & van Tellingen, O. (2004). Modulation of the blood-brain barrier in oncology: therapeutic opportunities for the treatment of brain tumours? *Cancer Treatment Reviews*, Vol.30, No.5, pp. 415-423.

Krűttgen, A.; Schneider, I. & Weis, J. (2006). The dark side of the NGF family: neurotrophins in neoplasias. *Brain Pathology*, Vol.16, No.4, pp. 304-310.

Liu, Y.; Li, C.; Lin, J. (2010). STAT3 as a Therapeutic Target for Glioblastoma. *Anticancer Agents in Medicinal Chemistry*, Vol.10, No.7, pp. 512-519.

Morgan, M.T.; Nakanishi, Y.; Kroll, D.J.; Griset, A.P.; Carnahan, M.A.; Wathier, M.; Oberlies, N.H.; Manikumar, G.; Wani, M.C.; Grinstaff, M.W. (2006). Dendrimer-encapsulated camptothecins: increased solubility, cellular uptake, and cellular retention affords enhanced anticancer activity in vitro. *Cancer Research*, Vol.66, No.24, pp. 11913-11921.

Myung, J.; Cho, B.K.; Kim, Y.S. & Park, S.H. (2010). Snail and Cox-2 expressions are associated with WHO tumor grade and survival rate of patients with gliomas, *Neuropathology*, Vol.30, No.3. pp. 224-231.

Nakagawara, A. (2001). Trk receptor tyrosine kinases: a bridge between cancer and neural development. *Cancer Letters*, Vol.169, No.2, pp. 107-114.

Nicholas, M.K.; Lukas, R.V.; Chmura, S.; Yamini, B.; Lesniak, M.; Pytel, P. (2011). Molecular heterogeneity in glioblastoma: therapeutic opportunities and challenges. *Seminars in Oncology*, Vol.38, No.2, pp. 243-253.

Poluha, W.; Poluha, D.K. & Ross, A.H. (1995). TrkA neurogenic receptor regulates differentiation of neuroblastoma cells. *Oncogene*, Vol.10, No.1, pp. 185-189.

Rosenfeld, A.; Kletzel, M.; Duerst, R.; Jacobsohn, D,; Haut, P.; Weinstein, J.; Rademaker, A.; Schaefer, C.; Evans, L.; Fouts, M. & Goldman S. (2010). A phase II prospective study of sequential myeloablative chemotherapy with hematopoietic stem cell rescue for the treatment of selected high risk and recurrent central nervous system tumors. *Journal of Neurooncology*, Vol.97, No.2, pp. 247-255.

Schatton, T.; Frank, M.H. (2009). Antitumor immunity and cancer stem cells, *Annals of the New York Academy of Sciences*, Vol.1176, pp. 154-169.

Schatton, T.; Frank, N.Y.; Frank, M.H. (2009). Identification and targeting of cancer stem cells, *Bioessays*, Vol.31, No.10, pp. 1038-1049.

Ta, H.T.; Dass, C.R.; Larson I.; Choong, P.F.; Dunstan, D.E. (2009). A chitosan hydrogel delivery system for osteosarcoma gene therapy with pigment epithelium-derived factor combined with chemotherapy. *Biomaterials*, Vol.30, No.21, pp. 4815-4823.

Van den Eynde, M.; Baurain, J.F.; Mazzeo, F.; Machiels, J.P. (2011). Epidermal growth factor receptor targeted therapies for solid tumors. *Acta Clinica Belgica*, Vol.66, No.1, pp. 10-17.

Vega, J.A.; Garcia-Suarez, O.; Hannestad, J. ; Pérez-Pérez, M.; Germanà, A. (2003).Neurotrophins and immune system. *Journal of Anatomy*, Vol.203, No.1, pp. 1-19.

Vinores, S.A.; Perez-Polo, J.R. (1983). Nerve growth factor and neural oncology. *Journal of Neuroscience Research*. Vol.9, No.1, pp. 81-100.

Waite, C.L.; Roth, C.M. (2009). PAMAM-RGD conjugates enhance siRNA delivery through a multicellular spheroid model of malignant glioma. *Bioconjugate chemistry*. Vol.20, No.10, pp. 1908-1916.

Xie, Y.; Ye, L.; Zhang, X.; Cui, W.; Lou, J.; Nagai, T.; Hou, X. (2005). Transport of nerve growth factor encapsulated into liposomes across the blood-brain barrier: In vitro and in vivo studies. *Journal of Control Release*, Vol.105, No.1-2, pp. 106-119.

Yaeger, M.J.; Koestner, A.; Marushige, K.; Marushide, J. (1992). The use of nerve growth factor as a reserve transforming agent for the treatment of neurogenic tumors: in vivo results. *Acta of Neuropathology*, Vol. 83, No 6, pp. 624-629.

Yamaguchi, Y.; Tabata, K.; Asami, S.; Miyake, M.; Suzuki, T. (2007). A novel cyclophane compound? CPPy, facilitates NGF-induced TrkA signal transduction and induces cell differentiation in neuroblastoma. *Biological Pharmaceutical Bulletin*, Vol.30, No.4, pp. 638-643.